RECENT TRANSLATIONAL RESEARCH IN HIV/AIDS

Edited by **Yi-Wei Tang**

Recent Translational Research in HIV/AIDS
Edited by Yi-Wei Tang

Published by InTech
Janeza Trdine 9, 51000 Rijeka, Croatia

Publishing Process Manager Silvia Vlase

Technical Editor Teodora Smiljanic

Cover Designer InTech Design Team

Additional hard copies can be obtained from orders@intechopen.com

Recent Translational Research in HIV/AIDS, Edited by Yi-Wei Tang
p. cm.
ISBN 978-953-307-719-2

For EU product safety concerns:
IN TECH d.o.o., Prolaz Marije Krucifikse Kozulić 3, 51000 Rijeka, Croatia,
info@intechopen.com or visit our website at intechopen.com.

Meet the editor

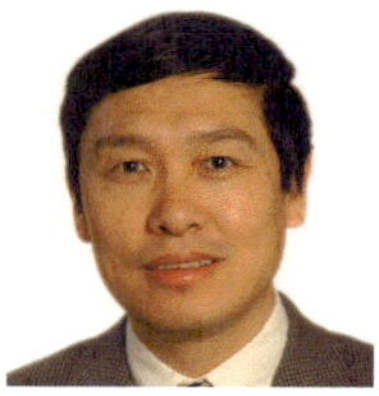

Dr. Yi-Wei Tang is currently the Chief of the Clinical Microbiology Service at the Memorial Sloan Kettering Cancer Center and a Professor of Laboratory Medicine at the Weill Cornell Medical College in New York City, USA. Dr. Tang ranks among the top scientists in the field of clinical microbiology, as evidenced by his election as an Editor for the Journal of Clinical Microbiology and a Fellow of the American Academy for Microbiology and of the Infectious Disease Society of America. During the past 20 years, Dr. Tang authored over 150 peer-reviewed articles and 38 book chapters, and has been recognized for his extraordinary expertise in the molecular microbiology diagnosis and monitoring. Dr. Tang has also served as an editor for the following books: "Molecular Microbiology: Diagnostic Principle and Practice", "Diagnostic Microbiology in Immunocompromised Host", and "Advanced Techniques in Diagnostic Microbiology".

Contents

Preface

A translational research serves a bench-to-bedside 'translation' of basic scientific research to practicable diagnostic procedure and therapies with meaningful improvements in physical, mental, or social health outcomes. To improve human health, scientific discoveries must be translated into practical applications. Such discoveries typically begin at "the bench" with basic research in which scientists study disease at a molecular or cellular level and then progress to the clinical level, or the patient's "bedside." Basic scientists provide clinicians with new tools for use in patients and for assessment of their impact, and clinical researchers make novel observations about the nature and progression of the disease that often stimulate basic investigations.

Translational research is a way of thinking about and conducting a much broader scientific research, which is practiced in the natural, biological, behavioural, and social sciences. HIV/AIDS is a perfect area to conduct translational researches. This InTech book, entitled "Recent Translational Research in HIV/AIDS", includes 27 chapters covering HIV/AIDS translational researches on pathogenesis, diagnosis, treatment and prevention, and also those beyond conventional fields. These chapters, which are divided into nine sections, provide excellent examples of translational research for HIV/AIDS. These are by no means inclusive, but they do offer a good foundation for the development of clinical patient care.

The first section on *Pathogenesis and epidemiology* comprises three chapters. Benjelloun and colleagues from the University of Saint-Etienne, France, provided an excellent review on HIV-1 glycoprotein immunogenicity. Williams and colleagues from the University of Oxford and other institutes in Oxford, UK, described characterisation, evaluation and clinical significance of latent HIV-1 reservoir and therapeutic strategies for HIV eradication. Kiptoo from Kenya Medical Research Institute overviewed changing trends of HIV subtypes and its implication on mother-to-child transmission.

In the *Pharmacology and host interaction* section (Chapters 4-5), Redzic and Misirlic Dencic from Kuwait University, Kuwait, and Belgrade University, Serbia, provided a comprehensive review on transport mechanisms of nucleosides and nucleoside analogues reverse transcriptase inhibitors in the brain. Eugenia Barros from CSIR

Biosciences, Pretoria, South Africa provided a comprehensive review on interaction of traditional remedies against HIV, nutrients and ARVs.

In the next section on *Opportunistic microbial infections* (Chapters 6-8), Rodriguez-Gomez and colleagues from two hospitals in Spain covered current status of syphilis in men infected with HIV-1. Cases are presented with a focus on diagnosis and treatment. Barth and colleagues from the University of Florida, USA, focused their chapter on rifamycin used in HIV-infected patients with tuberculosis. Interactions between rifamycin and antiretroviral drugs were illustrated in details. Menezes and colleagues from Oswaldo Cruz Foundation, Brazil explored reversal reaction as a manifestation of immune reconstitution inflammatory syndrome focusing on leprosy and other mycobacterial infections.

Diagnosis plays a bridge role in the translational researches. Chapters 9-11 are included in the section on *Laboratory diagnosis*. Jehuda-Cohen from Technion Israel Institute of Technology, Haifa, Israel, provided a comprehensive review on the HIV seronegative window period in relation to diagnostic challenges and solutions. My long-term collaborator Lu from Shanghai Public Health Clinical Center of Fudan University, China, used clinical case-based approach to summarize potential pitfalls of currently used HIV serology testing. Patient care providers should keep in mind that serology false negative results can happen in the clinical setting. Romero-Guadarrama from National Autonomous University of Mexico, Mexico provided unique comments on surgical pathology in HIV infection in the era of antiretroviral therapy.

Antiretroviral therapy (ART) is the center of the HIV-1 infection treatment thereby playing a critical role in the HIV translational researches. In Chapter 12, Martinez and Imbroda from Cuenca, Spain, provided a comprehensive review on simplification of ART in order to improve the quality of life, facilitate adherence and prevent or reverse some adverse effects. Zha and colleagues from Virginia Commonwealth University and VA Medical Center in Richmond, USA (Chapter 13), described the relationship between highly active antiretroviral therapy (HAART) and metabolic complications. Blas-Garcia and colleagues from the University of Valencia, Spain, provided future perspectives in NNRTI-based therapy in relation to their toxicity (Chapter 14). In Chapter 15, Akay et al from the University of Pennsylvania, Philadelphia, USA, provided a thorough review on ART and HIV-associated neurocognitive disorders.

Special clinical cares section includes Chapters 16-18. Dola et al from Tulane University, New Orleans, USA, described special considerations in the management of HIV infection in pregnancy. Reid and Novak from the University of Illinois in Chicago, USA, described treatment options and management in HIV-1 treatment-experienced patients. An InforMatrix interactive matrix model was described in details by Schreij and Janknegt from the Netherlands.

Chapters 19-22 form the *New therapy strategies* section. Batchu and colleagues from Wayne State University and VA Medical Center in Detroit, USA, introduced crippling of HIV at multiple stages with recombinant adeno-associated viral mediated RNA interference. Two chapters, contributed by Ledger et al from the University of New South Wales, Sydney, Australia, and by Egerer et al from Innsbruck Medical University, Innsbruck, Austria, summarized from different angels the current status and future directions of gene therapy for HIV-1 infections. Abad and colleagues from the University Complutense, Madrid, Spain explored new HIV-screening strategies for the discovery of novel HIV-inhibitors.

An effective HIV vaccine is badly needed to help halt the inexorable spread of HIV/AIDS. Translational-research programs need to be expanded to connect basic science with existing vaccine-development tools, including hypothesis-driven clinical trials to assess novel immunogen designs. There are only two chapters in the section on *Vaccine development*. In Chapter 23, De Almeida and colleagues from the University of Sao Paulo, Brazil, provided a comprehensive review on HIV vaccine covering major challenges, current status, future strategies and methods. In Chapter 24, Sommerfelt from Bionor Pharma ASA, Norway, introduced the potential contribution of therapeutic vaccination as a functional cure for HIV infection.

An important component of translational researches in HIV/AIDS is to study those *Beyond "conventional"* (Chapters 25-27). Jariwalla and colleagues from Dr. Rath Research Institute in Santa Clara, California, USA, described micronutrient synergy in the control of HIV infection and AIDS. As indicated by the authors, in the absence of an effective cure or vaccine and in the face of the toxicity and limited efficacy of ARVs, micronutrients provide a safe, effective and affordable way to halt progression towards and even reduce the symptoms of the AIDS disease and to improve the quality of life of AIDS patients. Kresina and colleagues from Health Resources and Services Administration in USA described substance abuse treatment utilizing medication assisted treatment as an HIV prevention strategy. Rodriguez and others from Health Institute Carlos III, Spain, described the pertinence of applying qualitative investigation strategies in the design and evaluation of HIV prevention policies.

I would like to share with our readers my appreciation for the InTech's tremendous efforts to collect and publish scientific books under Open Access model. I hope our readers will agree with me that this book consists of high quality chapters contributed by a group of authoritative authors. It is worth to point out that, thanks to the powerful, Internet-based, Open Access approach, readers around the world will be able to enjoy these wonderful color figures through the entire book, especially those in Chapters 6, 23 and 25.

The translational model forms the basis for progressing HIV/AIDS clinical research. When linked to the care of the patients, translational researches should result in a direct benefit for HIV/AIDS patients. At the time of the preface preparation, I am in a career transition and translocation myself from the Vanderbilt University Medical Center in Nashville to the Memorial Sloan Kettering Cancer Center in the New York City. I am looking forward to applying strategies and techniques described in this book to conduct translational researches in diagnostic microbiology field in immunocomprised hosts, including patients receiving chemotherapy and stem cell transplantation.

Yi-Wei Tang, MD, PhD, F(AAM), FIDSA
Chief of Clinical Microbiology Service
Memorial Sloan Kettering Cancer Center
Professor of Laboratory Medicine and Medicine
Weill Cornell Medical College
New York, NY,
USA

Part 1

Pathogenesis and Epidemiology

1

HIV-1 Glycoprotein Immunogenicity

Fahd Benjelloun, Christian Genin and Stephane Paul
University of Saint-Etienne (UPRES LYON)
Group of Mucosal Immunity and Pathogens GIMAP EA3064
France

1. Introduction

The Human Immunodeficiency Virus type 1 (HIV-1) is a C-type enveloped retrovirus (classification based on morphology of retroviruses electron microscopy) of the *Retroviridae* family. It's consisting in a genome of 2 positive stranded RNA molecules and a specific polymerase reverse transcriptase enzyme (RT). The viral RNA is reverse transcribed by RT into a double-stranded DNA molecule which is then integrated into the genome of infected cells (figure 1). The virus is wrapped by a bilayer membrane derived from the host cell. Homotrimers of the viral glycoprotein gp160 are inserted in the envelope (figure 1). Several cellular proteins are also incorporated into the viral membrane with relative abundance, including MHC class I and II molecules and intracellular adhesion molecule. Lentiviruses, to which HIV belongs, cause disease with a 'slow' evolution preceded by a period of clinical latency. Apart from humans, lentiviruses infect several other species of mammals such as

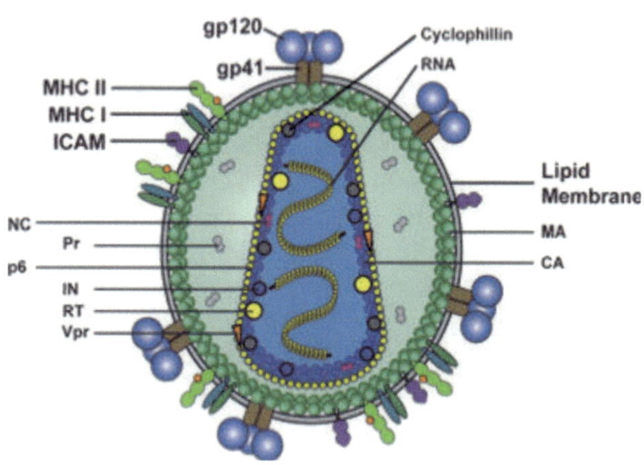

Fig. 1. Schematic representation of the HIV-1 particle. Two copies of the viral positive stranded RNA genome are packed in the capsid. Viral enzymes: reverse transcriptase (RT), integrase (IN), protease (Pr) and structural proteins; capsid (CA), nucleocapsid (NC), matrix (MA) and p6 are inside the particle together with the viral regulatory protein Vpr and the cellular protein cyclophilin (Phogat et al., 2007).

primates (Simian Immunodeficiency Virus, SIV), feline and ovine. Infection by HIV-1 causes a very rapid destruction of the majority of T cells memory $CD4^+/CCR5^+$ and especially those residing in the intestinal mucosa.
Although antiretroviral therapy for HIV infection prevents AIDS-related complications and prolongs life, it does not fully restore health. Long-term treated patients remain at higher than expected risk for a number of complications typically associated with aging, including cardiovascular disease, cancer, osteoporosis, and other end-organ diseases. The potential effect of HIV on health is perhaps most clearly exhibited by a number of immunologic abnormalities that persist despite effective suppression of HIV replication. These changes are consistent with some of the changes to the adaptive immune system that are seen in the very old ("immunosenescence") and that are likely related in part to persistent inflammation. HIV-associated inflammation and immunosenescence have been implicated as causally related to the premature onset of other end-organ diseases.
This review summarizes the importance to generate immune responses against HIV-1 glycoprotein in further vaccinal approaches and detail the complexity of the envelope structure and the relative high HIV-1 glycoprotein immunogenicity.

2. Molecular basis of HIV envelope glycoprotein

2.1 HIV-1 envelope glycoprotein

The gp120 (SU) and gp41 (TM) envelope glycoproteins are encoded by the HIV gene *env*. This gene codes for an Env precursor polyprotein (p90) which undergoes post-transcriptional modifications as glycosylations resulting in the gp160 precursor. It is interesting to note that the HIV cleavage sequence is highly conserved (Veronese et al., 1985) and is included in one of the most conserved domains within gp120 (C5). Gp160 is produced as an inactive precursor in the rough endoplasmic reticulum and subjected to extensive N-glycosylation resulting in high mannose chains linked to Asn residues at either Asn-X-Ser or Asn-X-Thr glycosylation sites. The gp160 are sorted through the constitutive secretory pathway of the infected cells (Moulard and Decroly, 2000). Once transported to the cellular plasma membrane, trimeric gp120–gp41 complexes are incorporated into budding virus for the release of new infectious particles. Before its anchoring on the surface, gp160 is cleaved by a host protease named furine in two sub-units associated by non-covalent interactions (gp120 on the surface and the transmembrane gp 41) (Hallenberger et al., 1992). Envelope glycoproteins form trimeric spicules of gp120-gp41 complexes on the surface of the virus conferring viral tropism (Chan and Kim, 1998). Env is also involved in the interaction, recognition and the fusion of the viral and cellular membranes leading to the introduction of the viral genome into the cytoplasm of the target cells. The Env spikes are thought to be trimeric and structure-based models have been proposed (figures 2&3). Cryoelectronic microscopy tomography shows heterotrimeric complexes (Roux and Taylor, 2007; Briggs et al., 2009). However, despite intensive efforts, the arrangement and orientation of the loop-deleted gp120 core atomic structures within a native Env spike and their association with the gp41 subunits have remained largely speculative.
The entry of virus into the target cell involves the fusion of cell membranes and the viral envelope. Whereas, the recognition of the target cell by the gp120 is not sufficient to directly cause membrane fusion and mediate the injection of viral genome. The adsorption of HIV-1 on cell surface is mediated by interactions between envelope glycoproteins and two types of surface molecules: attachment factors (or adhesion receptors) and coreceptors (figure2).

Coreceptors are actively involved in the penetration of the virus and are selective for the entry of the virion into the host cells depending on their tropism.

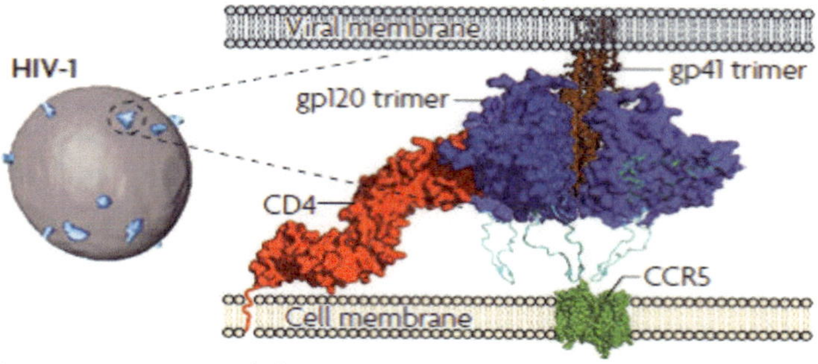

Fig. 2. Schematic representation of the interaction between envelope glycoprotein and viral receptors. On the left, a surface rendered cryo-electron microscopy tomographic image of HIV-1. Viral spikes are blue and the viral surface is grey. On the right is shown a structure-based model of the envelope glycoproteins of HIV. Trimeric HIV-1 gp120 proteins shown in cyan bind to the primary receptor, CD4. Following conformational changes, the gp120–CD4 complex binds the chemotaxis receptor adapted from (Karlsson Hedestam et al., 2008).

2.2 Gp120 envelope glycoprotein

Gp 120 glycoprotein represents the external part of the envelope glycoprotein of HIV with a molecular weight of 120 kDa. It contains 480aa with 9 disulfide bridges and 20 to 24 N-glycosylation sites. Gp120 is involved in the earlier steps of the infection of target cells. HIV-1-receptor binding is mediated by external Env gp120, which binds the CD4 primary on target cells. Then, a series of Env conformational changes occur that result in exposure of a transient binding site allowing the virus to interact with its co-receptor, usually the chemokine receptor CCR5 or CXCR4, to initiate another cycle of infection (figure 3A, B). HIV-1 gp120 consists of five conserved (C1-C5) and five extremely variable (V1-V5) domains. The conserved domains contribute to the core of gp120, while the variable domains (and numerous N-linked glycosylation sites) are located near the surface of the molecule. The gp120 is extensively glycosylated with N-linked glycan host derived carbohydrates. The role of these modification is to mask them and their micro-heterogeneities form a perfect immunological shield that allow a decrease of the immune response against viral particles (Pancera et al., 2010) The presence of glycosylation sites in the V3 region seems to affect the viral tropism. Removal of the glycosylation site at position 301 allows the chimeric virus to evolve to X4 phenotype (Pollakis et al., 2001). The removal of three amino acids on different glycosylation sites of gp120 from the laboratory strain X4R5 HIV89.6 tropism results in the loss of tropism for CCR5 (Yang et al., 2010). This phenomenon could be due to the unmasking of neighboring basic amino acids or the loss of negative charges located on the glycoprotein. Moreover, the number of glycosylations present on gp120 influences its secondary structure, which could alter the interactions between the V3 region and neighboring regions (figure 3F). The ability of some strains to be infectious and replicate even in the absence of V3 loop has been described (Cormier & Dragic, 2002)(Lin et al., 2007). The V3 region (35 amino acids) plays a significant role in the recognition and interaction with the cellular receptors of the target cell. This region also contains at its extremity a highly conserved sequence of amino acids (GPGRAF). This pattern is surrounded by variable amino acids which alter the viral tropism through interaction of gp120 with the cellular chemokine CCR5 and CXCR4. The V1-V5 regions form exposed loops anchored at their bases by disulfide bonds (Teixeira et al., 2011). Crystal structure of gp120 shows that this protein is folded as a connection of four β elements called "bridging sheet"with an inner and an outer domain (Kwong et al., 1998). The internal domain is a near point of contact with gp41 and the N and C-Term of gp120. In the native conformation, trimers are more stable due to the interaction with gp41 and V1-V2 loops. Oligomeric gp120 protein can adopt a conformation called 'closed' as in primary isolates resulting in masking the receptor binding site of CD4 in V1 and V2 regions while gp120 of TCLA viruses preferentially adopt an 'open' shape thereby reducing its affinity for this receptor. Finally the interaction with CD4 gives rise to an open structure enabling the link of viral and cellular membrane and an exposition of the V3 loop (Roux & Taylor, 2007).

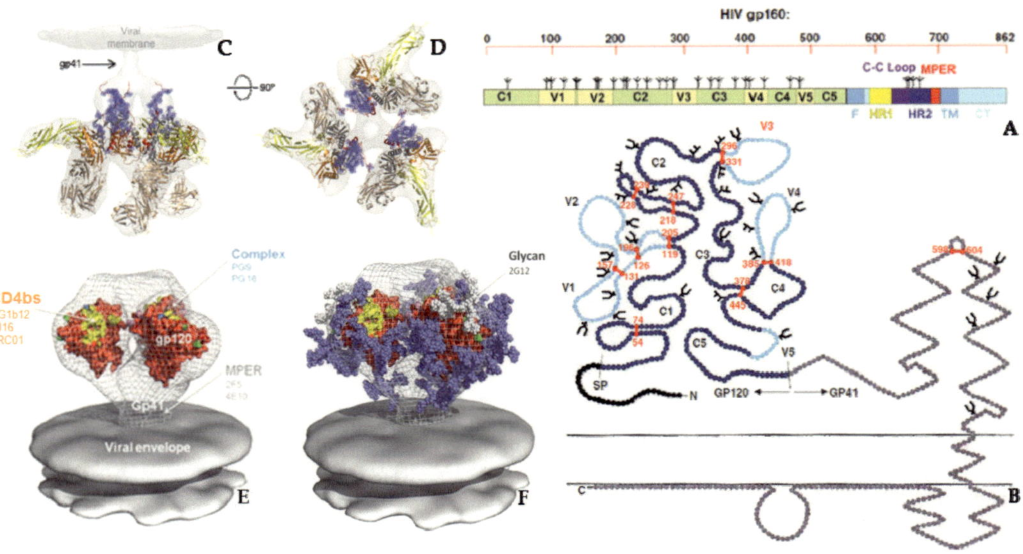

Fig. 3. Schematic representations of HIV-1 envelope glycoprotein A) Glycosylations sites present on gp160 glycoprotein B) Structure of the gp120-gp41 glycoprotein envelope of HIV (Pancera, 2005). C, D, E, F are obtained by cryo-electron tomography C) Structure of an HIV-1 gp120 core with intact gp41-interactive region D) 90° rotation of C placement of the gp120-CD4 complex in the electron density map (light gray), residues involved in gp41 interactions are colored with blue (Pancera et al., 2010) E) Schematic representation of HIV-1 native viral spike. The glycoprotein is shown as a transparent framework and represents three gp120 molecules non-covalently linked to three gp41. Epitopes of broadly neutralizing monoclonal antibodies on gp120 (red) or gp41 are labelled with arrows. The IgG1b12-binding surface is labelled yellow, and the bases of the variable regions (missing in this structure) are labelled blue, green, and pink. (F) The same model with the gp120 glycans shown in blue reveals the extensive glycosylation present as an antibody evasion mechanism on Env, and glycans implicated in BNMAb 2G12 binding are highlighted in white and labelled with an arrow. HIV-1, human immunodeficiency virus type-1; MPER membrane-proximal external region patterns obtained from the works of (Sattentau & McMichael, 2010).

CD4 receptor binding site

The main receptor of HIV is the CD4 membrane glycoprotein. Binding to CD4 initiates the process of infection. Different models forecast the exact configuration of some regions of the gp120 protein whereas they all show clearly the important structural differences in the organization of the trimer between the free and the associated form with CD4. The CD4 molecule binds with high affinity to gp120 protein (Klatzmann et al., 1984). The CD4 binding site is composed of relatively conserved regions located between the two domains of gp120, and the β inter-domains sheet. The contact areas are discontinuous in the native three-dimensional structure of protein. The CD4 binding domain is located in the D1 domain of the CDR2 loop (Complementarity Determining Region 2), on the opposite side of HLA type II binding domain (Fleury et al., 1991). In this area, two residues, Phe43 and Arg59, are particularly important in establishing interactions with gp120 residues of the CD4 binding site (including Glu^{370}, Trp^{427} and Asp^{368}) (Tachibana et al., 2000). The affinity of CD4 to the envelope glycoprotein of HIV is highly variable depending on its quaternary structure (monomeric or oligomeric) and tropism. In addition, gp120 is conformationally flexible, the site of initial CD4 attachment is conformationally inert (Zanetti et al., 2006; Zhu et al., 2006; Roux & Taylor, 2007).

Co-receptors of HIV

The two main HIV co-receptors are the chemokine receptors CXCR4 and CCR5 (figure7). CXCR4 and CCR5 are ubiquitously expressed in immune cells. CXCR4 and CCR5 belong to the superfamily of receptors linked to G proteins and are characterized by a structure comprising an extracellular N-Term segment, seven transmembrane domains in helices, three extracellular loops or ECL, three intracytoplasmic loops or ICL (intracellular loop) and an intracytoplasmic C-Term segment. The N-Term segment and extracellular loops are responsible for receptor affinity for its ligand (Allen et al., 2007).

The natural ligand for CXCR4 is the SDF-1 molecule (Stromal Derived Factor-1), a chemokine α of CXC type (presence of two cysteines separated by one amino acid). As a ligand, it induces internalization of CXCR4 by a process of vesicle clathrin-dependent endocytosis, resulting to its degradation. CCR5 is the receptor of three chemokine β of CC-type (with two adjacent cysteines), all produced by CD8 T cells: RANTES (Regulated upon Activation, Normal T-cell Expressed and secreted), MIP-1α and β (Macrophage Inflammatory Protein-1). RANTES induces CCR5 internalization and is recycled to the cell membrane without being degraded. According to the coreceptor involved in HIV entry into the target cell, the virus is classified depending on its tropism. Thus, viruses use the CCR5 receptor (expressed by monocytes, macrophages, activated T cells or memories and DC) are called 'CCR5-tropic' (or virus type 'R5') and those using the CXCR4 coreceptor (expressed by T cells, monocytes and DCs) are appointed, CXCR4-tropic '(or virus 'X4'). CXCR4 is the coreceptor identified as responsible for the entry of HIV in the lymphoid lineages adapted X4 viruses are also called 'T-tropic' or 'lymphocytotropic', whereas R5 viruses are called 'M-tropic' or 'monocytotropic'. Some isolates are capable of using both CXCR4 and CCR5 coreceptor and are referred as' X4R5' or ‘dual-tropic'. This classification has replaced an old classification based on the ability of the virus or not to induce syncytium formation (a reaction resulting in the cytopathic membrane fusion of several adjacent cells leading to the formation of a 'giant cell' multinucleate) at a T cell line (MT-2). It is now accepted that viruses using the CXCR4 coreceptor to enter target cells induce the formation of syncytia (SI virus like 'Syncytium Inducing virus') in contrast to viruses using exclusively CCR5 (NSI viruses for 'No Syncytium Inducing virus').

2.3 Alternative receptors

However, cells which not express the CD4 molecule on their surface can also be infected, at least *in vitro*. The CD4 is not the only molecule favoring infection by HIV-1.

2.3.1 Interaction with Galactosyl-ceramide (α-GalCer)

Surface molecules such as the α-GalCer glycolipid or lactosylceramide sulfate, present on different tissues (brain, intestine, epithelium and cervix) are capable of binding to gp160 protein V3 loop. These molecules can be considered as alternative receptors for HIV. The α-GalCer is a glycosphingolipid (GSL) most commonly involved in the interactions between cells lacking CD4 and HIV. It binds to the V3 region of gp120 (Harouse et al., 1995). These sequences form a conformational site exposed on the gp120 surface which interact with the galactose residue of GalCer. The affinity of gp120 to GalCer was higher than for other GSL (Long et al., 1994). Saturating the V3 area of gp120 with GalCer analogs can prevent the infection of $CD4^+$ T cells and $CD4^-$ by HIV (Fantini et al., 1997). GalCer is also capable of binding to gp41 domain located in a 35 amino acids region containing the ELDKWA epitope (Alfsen and Bomsel, 2002). This interaction takes place only after fixation on gp120 and GalCer stabilization. The α-GalCer/gp120 or gp41 interaction is also essential for viral particles transmission during endocytosis or transcytosis. The GSL are constituents of the lipid bilayer of the cell membrane and are associated with glycophospholipides (LPG) and cholesterol. This association form within the membrane microdomains distinct called "lipid rafts" (or 'rafts') (Simons and Ikonen, 1997). These lipid rafts traffic areas are preferred across the cell membrane for various pathogens or their toxins that use protein or lipid components of these micro-domains like receptors (Van der Goot & Harder, 2001). Lipid rafts are involved in the infectious cycle of HIV, particularly for the entry into target cells (Campbell et al., 2001). In the case of CD4-dependent infection and after fixation of the gp120 on CD4, an interaction between the central portion of the V3 region and the GSL would be essential to the establishment of the association between gp120 and coreceptors (Nehete et al., 2002). GSL present in lipid rafts can stabilize the attachment of the virus to the cell surface and to ensure migration of gp120-CD4 complex to a co-receptor. Rafts can move within the membrane and facilitate conformational change of gp120 leading to the insertion of the fusion peptide.

2.3.2 Interaction with C-type lectins

C-type lectins (CLR, C-type Lectin Receptor) are proteins that attach, with a calcium-dependent way, the carbohydrated residues through their CRD domain (Carbohydrate Recognition Domain). They are particularly expressed on dendritic cells where they play a key role in capturing pathogens by binding carbohydrates present on micro-organisms (Weis et al., 1998). There are two categories of CLR: CLR's type I which exposed their N-Term part outside the cell and the type II CLR with intracellular N-Term domain. The majority of CLR binds D-mannose, D-glucose or D-galactose and their derivatives. Four CLR type lectins have the ability to bind to gp120: MMR, MBL, DC-SIGN and Langerin.

Lectin MMR (Macrophage Mannose Receptor, or CD206) is highly expressed by dendritic cells generated *in vitro* from monocytes but not expressed by those of blood. Macrophages are capable of transferring HIV to cells expressing CD4 using this receptor (Nguyen and Hildreth, 2003).

MBL (Mannose Binding Lectin) is a CLR type I present in serum as a soluble form where it can bind to pathogens and initiate their attack by the complement system. It is capable of

binding to HIV through highly mannosylated oligosaccharides residues contains in the gp120 (Saifuddin et al., 2000).
The CLR type II DC-SIGN (Dendritic Cell-Specific ICAM-3 Grabbing Non-integrin, or CD209), is expressed as tetramers in lipid rafts of immature dendritic cells (Cambi et al., 2004). Its natural ligand is ICAM-3 (intercellular adhesion molecule-3 or CD50) also present on T cells which allow its interaction with dendritic cells (Geijtenbeek et al., 2000a; Geijtenbeek et al., 2000b). Like MBL, DC-SIGN binds mannose residues embedded into more internal patterns and more complex than MMR. DC-SIGN binds to Gp120 from many strains of HIV and SIV which harbor many oligosaccharides rich in mannose residues (Geijtenbeek et al., 2000b). Finally, Langerin (or CD207) is a CLR type receptor specifically expressed by Langerhans cells. Langerin is responsible for the formation of Birbeck granules (Valladeau et al., 2000) and contains a specific region which interacts with gp120 (Turville et al., 2002).

2.3.3 Interaction with the α4β7 integrin

It was recently demonstrated that gp120 activated form is also able to bind α4β7 integrin expressed on gut-homing T and B lymphocytes and CD4+ NK cells (figure4). A tri-peptide loop (Leu-Asp-Val) at the V2 loop, mimicking the binding motif of the natural ligands of α4β7, is involved in this interaction. This binding enables the formation of viral synapse through the activation of LFA-1 (Arthos et al., 2008). By this way, HIV-1 induces a massive depletion of gut CD4+ T cells which participate to the immune dysfunction in HIV patients.

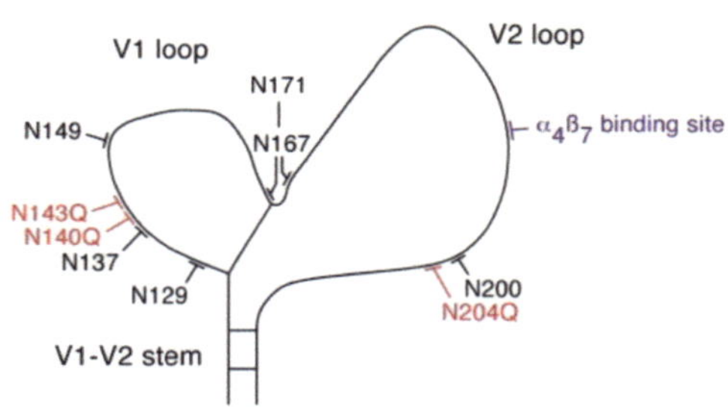

Fig. 4. Positions of all potential N-Glycosylation and α4β7 binding sites located in the V1/V2 loop gp120 (Nawaz et al., 2011).

2.4 Gp41 envelope glycoprotein

The binding of gp 120 to CD4 and coreceptors permits its conformational changes and triggers the establishment of the fusion complex compounds by trimers of gp41 (figure6). (Salzwedel et al., 1999, Munoz-Barroso et al., 1999, Dwyer et al., 2003). Gp41 is the transmembrane domain of the entire envelope glycoprotein which anchors the viral spikes in the bilayer lipid membrane of viral particles and plays an important role in membrane fusion and cell entry. Gp41 is composed by 345 amino acids (512 to 856 of HIV-1 HXB2 strain) with a molecular mass of about 41KDa. Gp41 presents an extracellular domain or ectodomain, a transmembrane domain or membrane spanning domain, and an intracytoplasmic domain (figure5). Gp41 sequences are clearly more conserved than gp120 and also contain only four N-glycosylation sites on its ectodomain. These glycosylation sites are highly conserved and appeared to contribute to optimal viral replication efficiency (Johnson et al., 2001).

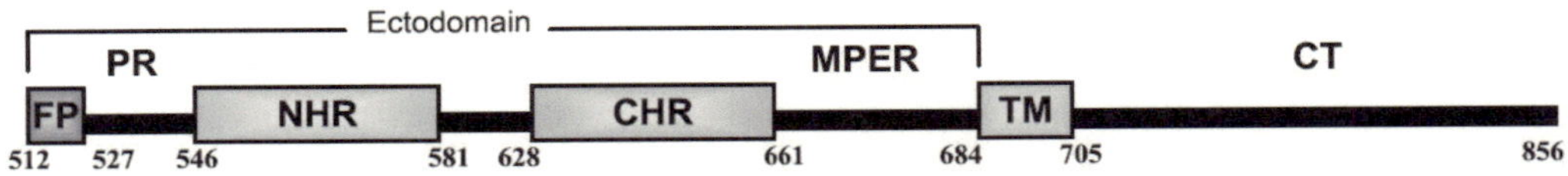

Fig. 5. Schematic representation of gp41 domains. Gp41 is divided in 3 regions. The ectodomain contains the fusion peptide (FP), a polar region (PR), N and C-terminal heptad repeat regions separated by an immunodominant region (NHR & CHR), a rich tryptophane highly conserved region (MPER), a transmembrane region (TM) and an intracytoplasmic tail (CT) (Montero et al., 2008).

Gp41 contains different domains involved in the fusion process of viral and host cell membrane. The N-Term hydrophobic region consist in the fusion peptide (512–527), a polar region (525-543) called the Fusion Peptide Proximal Region (FPPR) or Polar Region (PR), the N-Term heptad repeat (NHR or HR1) (546– 581) and C-Term heptad repeat (CHR or HR2). These regions are folded as α-helix and linked by a loop called immunodominant loop (598-604) containing a disulfide bridge. A highly conserved Tryptophan Rich Membrane Proximal Ectodomain/External Region (MPER) (660-683) is also present (Chan et al., 1997). Finally, the membrane spanning domain or transmembrane (MSD/TM) and the intracytoplasmic tail or C-tail are two other hydrophobic regions present at the C-Term portion of gp41 (figure5). A complete description of the whole molecule gp41 is not clearly defined. A crystallized intact trimer would be structurally definitive, but it's seems that large regions appear to be in constant motion as part of the conformational masking defence of potential epitopes from Abs. It is widely assumed that the failure of Env-based vaccine candidates to date relates, in part, to the difficulty in generating soluble versions of Env proteins that faithfully mimic key structural features of native *in situ* Env.

2.4.1 Fusion peptide (FP)

The FP corresponds to the first N-Term domain of the gp41 ectodomain (figure5). FP is highly conserved among HIV-1 clades and other viruses. For example, GFLG is a pattern found among fusion peptides of different retroviruses such as HIV-1, HIV-2, SIV and HBV (Durell et al., 1997). A mutation in the GFLG alters the fusogenicity of the FP (Pritsker et al., 1999). Other studies of HIV with truncated or mutated FP showed that it's crucial to the fusion process and viral entry into host cells (Qiang et al., 2009).

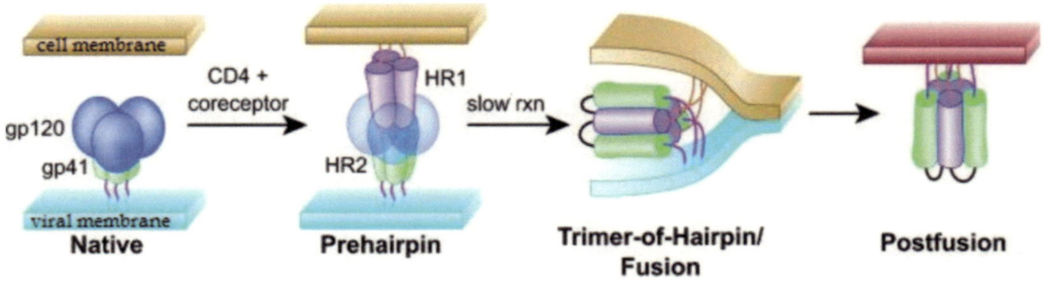

Fig. 6. Model of HIV entry pathway and gp41 conformational intermediates. Gp41 HR1 and HR2 regions are depicted in magenta and green, respectively (Miller et al., 2005).

FP is mostly hydrophobic (Del Angel et al., 2002). The substitution of glycine residues results in a fusogenicity decrease (Vanlandschoot et al., 1998). It has been suggested that the succession of FP glycines is involved in the oligomerization of fusion peptides, in the balance of amphipathicity necessary for membrane fusion and/or orientation of fusion peptides in the membrane (Delahunty et al., 1996). Recent studies showed that FP can also change its conformation according to the biochemical environment ((Buzon et al., 2005; Gordon et al., 2008). Solid-state nuclear magnetic resonance (MNR) spectroscopy (Zheng et al., 2006) confirmed that the FP oscillates from an α-helical state in low concentration of cholesterol to the β-strand form what reveals a high playing a crucial role during the viral fusion process. There are also controversies over the functional structure and the size of the FP it could have a different length and by the way a different sequence as 16 aa (Kamath and Wong, 2002), 23 aa (Delahunty et al., 1996; Gordon et al., 2002) or 33 aa (Pritsker et al., 1999) . To date the native structure in prefusogenic and fusogenic state remains unravelled.

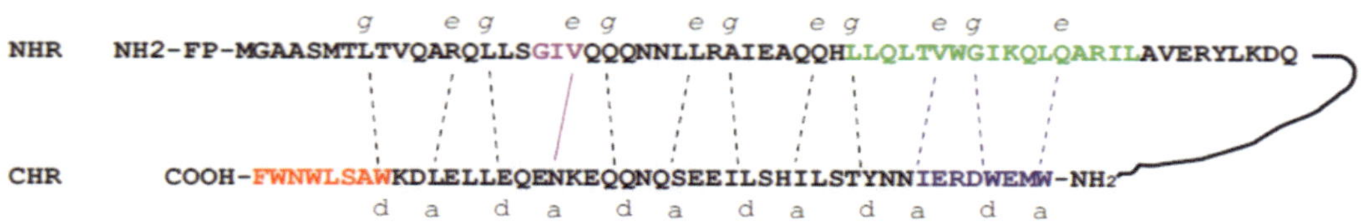

Fig. 7. Interaction between critical sequences in NHR and CHR regions of gp41 fusion intermediate. Dashed lines between the NHR and CHR domains indicate the interaction between the residues located at the e, g and a, d positions in the helical spiral of NHR and CHR domains, respectively. The critical sequences in NHR and CHR include: GIV (residues 547–549, *red*) is a determinant of resistance to T-20 in NHR region, LLQLTVWGIKQLQARIL (residues 565–581, *green*) is the cavity-forming sequence in NHR region, WMEWDREI (residues 628–635, *orange*) is the cavity binding sequence in CHR region; and WASLWNWF (residues 666–673, *pink*) is a partial tryptophan-rich sequence (Pan et al., 2010).

2.4.2 N-heptad repeat (NHR) / C-heptad repeat (CHR) regions

Adjacent to the FP is the first of two HR's (N and C-HR, respectively) that play critical roles in the fusion activity of gp41 (figures5, 6). HR motifs contain a characteristic repeating pattern of seven residues (abcdefg). Amino acid sequence of these segments is composed of seven AA which occupy seven positions on the fusogenic structure forming a pattern. This pattern repeats 7 times hence the name seven-repeat (heptad repeat). In the CHR, AA in position "a" and "d" are generally apolar or hydrophobic and are crucial for stabilizing trimers (figures7, 8). The "e" and "g" residues in NHR frequently interact with residues in the "a" and "d" positions. Characteristic packing of the hydrophobic side chains as the HR in a helical configuration stabilizes the coiled-coil structures N-HR (aa 541-581). Two binding sites have been characterized which bind the CHR region (aa 610-683) through the residues "g" and "e" or the endogenous homotrimeric NHR region through the residues "a" and "d" (Bewley et al., 2002).

A five-amino acid hydrophilic loop containing two cysteine residues with an intramolecular bisulfure bridge links the two HR regions together. These cysteines are highly conserved among retroviruses. It has been proposed that this loop creates a 'knob-like' protrusion in the TM subunit that permits packing in a cavity 'socket' in the surface subunit (figure6). This region is disordered in high-resolution studies of the gp41 ectodomain and has been reported to lead to aggregation of the protein (Caffrey et al., 2000). Structures of pre-fusion forms of gp41 are undetermined. Nevertheless the crystal structure of gp41 and X-ray and NMR structures determines its 6Helix Bundle and final states this studies revealed that three NHR are folded into a central triple-stranded coiled coil of α-helices, and three CHR are packed, anti-parallel, as α-helix into the three channels of the coiled-coil (figures6, 7, 8A) (Chan et al., 1997). The inner-helical NHR trimer in the 6HB structures has been used to model the receptor-activated state of gp41 and to design several mimetics of the NHR coiled-coil that can potently inhibit fusion like the T20 or N36 peptides. This 6HB is thermally stable and can confidently be considered a final structure. The formation of 6HBs was originally accepted as being the process that brings the viral and the cellular membranes together and allows the aggregation of several activated Env complexes to form a pore, leading to the entry of the nucleocapsid into the cell (Markosyan et al., 2009).

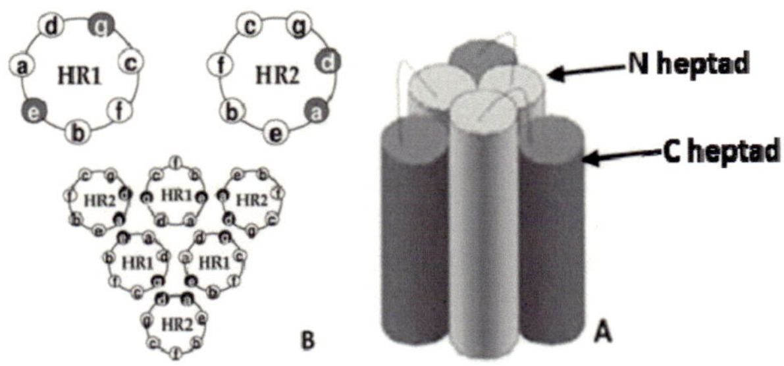

Fig. 8. Schematic representations of the six-helix bundle (6HB) in gp41 at the fusogenic state. A) Description of the six helix bundle: describes the N-(bright) and C-(dusky) heptad repeats that fold in an anti-parallel shape (hairpin). Three monomers of NHR form a α-helix trimer in the central triple-stranded coiled coil and the C-HR region comes to bind the grooves of this structure to form the final state of 6HB. The link between the two heptad repeat regions is involved in the aggregation of this complex. (Weiss, 2003) B) Overview of depiction of a 6 helix bundle. Three NHR from each gp41 monomer form grooves and to complete the bundle three HR2 dock in them (Markosyan et al., 2009).

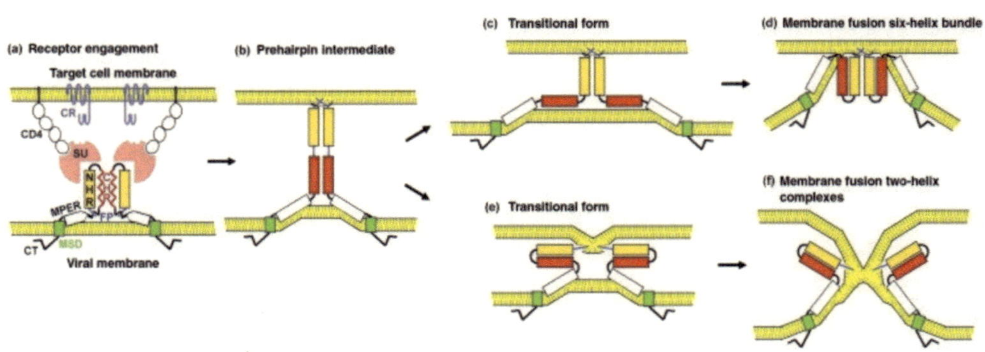

Fig. 9. Schematic speculative representation of topological questions related to single-spike-mediated fusion mechanisms. a,b) gp120 interacts with CD4 then with a co-receptor CR. The binding of the fusion peptide segment allows a changing of conformation and the HR regions form pre-hairpin shapes. c, d) Model where conformational changes undergo easily but require membrane breaks to form the 6HB. E, f), Second model where the membranes remain intact during the folding of gp41. CHR and NHR helix bind together and form the fusion pore. NHR, gold; CHR, red (Roux & Taylor, 2007).

2.4.3 The Membrane Proximal Ectodomain/external Region (MPER)

The MPER segment or Membrane-Proximal External Region is bordered by HR2 region and TM segment of gp41 (figures5, 9). This region is rich in tryptophan residues and interacts with cholesterol in the lipid bilayer cell membrane playing an important role in the viral fusion process and infectivity of HIV-1 (Salzwedel et al., 1999). MPER seems to be involved in the early steps of viral fusion and syncytium formation (Munoz-Barroso et al., 1999).

Mutations in MPER induce a decrease of the virus ability to cause syncytium formation in infected cells due to the inability to form the fusion complex (Zwick et al., 2001; Veiga and Castanho, 2007). MPER is highly conserved and represents a major target for therapeutic approaches. MPER sequence (^{663}ELDKWASLWNWFNITNWLWYIK^{683}) is the same in most HIV-1 strains and includes epitopes of 3 well described human broadly neutralizing monoclonal Abs as (ELDKWA) for the 2F5 and WF(N/D)IT for 4E10 and Z13 (figure12)(Ofek et al., 2004; Zwick and Burton, 2007). MPER has also been described as α-helix or as an extenteded β-turn. Recent studies have revealed that MPER adopts a helical form that is kinked and somewhat L-shaped and the segment that contains the epitope of 4E10 is embedded within the bilayer lipid membrane (Sun et al., 2008; Franquelim et al., 2011). The structure of the MPER in the context of lipids is well known, but the question of its native structure(s) on the cell surface in the context of gp41 remains open.

2.4.4 Transmembrane (TM) or Membrane spanning domain (MSD)

The TM region or MSD contains 25aa (aa681–705) is surrounded at its N-Term side by MPER and by the cytoplasmic domain at its C-Term tail (figures5, 9). This region is encrusted in the viral bilayer lipid membrane and anchors the gp41 into the membrane. This highly conserved region is composed mostly of neutral and hydrophobic AA (figure10). Two models have been proposed to explain the conformation assumed by MSD: a stable sloping α-helical conformation and a metastable kinked curved conformation and the MSD seem to switches from one to another while conformational changes of the gp41 (Gangupomu and Abrams, 2010).

Fig. 10. AA sequence of HIV-1 membrane spanning domains: The consensus sequence of the HIV-1 MSD was generated by the alignment of the Env MSD sequences of all M and N groups HIV-1 isolates from the Los Alamos HIV database. The graphic shows the percentage of conserved residues among isolates from (Shang et al., 2008).

The MSD contains two common features of lentiviral MSD, a basic charged residue Arg^{694} buried in bilayer lipid membrane (Shang et al., 2008) and a very conserved motif ^{688}GXXXG ^{694}. The loss of this feature doesn't affect the formation of glycoprotein Env trimers during the transport from the endoplasmic reticulum to the Golgi apparatus. However, it alters the membrane fusion and viral infectivity such as the loss of Lys^{681}, Arg ^{694} or Arg^{705} (Shang et al., 2008). The MSD or TM plays a very important role in viral fusion (figure9) (Miyauchi et al., 2010). Truncation studies on HIV-1 Env revealed that only 17 amino acid residues (Lys^{681}-Ala^{697}) are needed for a stable anchoring of the gp41 in the membrane and mediating cell to cell fusion (Yue et al., 2009). Small deletions (three amino acid residues) in the region between Arg^{694} and Arg^{705} showed normal cell to cell fusion, while larger deletions were more deleterious, suggesting that, the length of this region is more important than its AA sequence (Owens et al., 1994). Substitution of all leucine residues or two other highly conserved residues, Phe^{683} with Val^{687} AA residues in the helical core of MSD is critical for the fusogenicity of Env complexes and infectivity (Shang et al., 2008).

2.4.5 The C-Term tail / intra cytoplasmic tail (CT/ICS)

Lentiviruses, including HIV-1, have TM envelope (Env) glycoproteins with cytoplasmic tails (CT) that are quite long compared with those of other retroviruses. The gp41 CT is remarkably long and follows the MSD. CT is a hydrophobic region of 150 AA inserted into the plasma membrane (figure9A, 11) (Viard et al., 2008). The CT contains three regions called lentiviral lytic peptide and form amphipathic helices. The LLP1 and LLP2 regions have high hydrophobic properties. It have been admitted that the CT is entirely contained inside the cell or virion (Gallaher, 1987). Whereas it have been revealed that there are Abs directed to an epitope in the CT and some of them present neutralization properties on HIV virions (Cleveland et al., 2003; Mclnerney et al., 1999; McLain et al., 2001; Reading et al., 2003). Then, since antibodies do not traverse the membrane and infectious virus are by definition intact, this suggests that part of the tail is exposed on the virion surface allowing antibody binding and neutralization, thus contrasting with the traditional intracytoplasmic location of the entire C-Term sequence of gp41 (Hollier & Dimmock, 2005). Studies have attempted to address this divergence between the old model of an exclusively intracytoplasmic tail and an alternative model with external segments of the CT, as the Kennedy peptide (aa731-752) (Kennedy et al., 1986) containing three patterns a conserved one ^{741}EEEGGE^{746} and two others ^{747}QDRDRS^{752} or ^{731}PRGPDRPGRI^{740}. At the early steps of the viral entry, CT is implicated in the regulating of the kinetics of fusion and in the ability of Env to promote syncytia (Edwards et al., 2002; Wyss et al., 2005). Mutational studies have revealed that long CT interacts with domains of HIV matrix like the p55 Gag protein during the budding and this interaction is required for the envelope incorporation into the virion (Dubay et al., 1992; Yu et al., 1993).

3. Envelope glycoprotein immunogenicity

HIV -1 patients generate strong Ab responses to the viral envelope glycoprotein. However, these antibodies are generally strain-specific or non-neutralizing what disable the immune system to install a protective or a preventive immune response (Kwong et al., 2002; Wei et al., 2003). Most of the monoclonal antibodies raised against the env glycoprotein seems to be shaped by 1F7 (IgM) idiotypic dominance (Zhou et al., 2010). Evidence suggests that anti-HIV broadly neutralizing Abs requires high levels of somatic hypermutation and polyreactivity. However it is unclear if Abs without 1F7 idiotype also requires these characteristics to neutralize a broad spectrum of viral variants. It is also unknown whether BnAbs not expressing the 1F7 idiotype are any easier, or even possible, to induce by vaccination than idiotypic BnAbs, if the 1F7 idotype is suppressed (Parsons,M.S. et al., 2011). Genetic sequence variability created by its error prone reverse transcriptase and by host immune pressure lead to the evolution of the HIV-1 into multiple subtypes or clades with circulating recombinant forms. A fundamental barrier to HIV-1 vaccine development lies with the unique properties of the virus to predominantly enter through mucosal surfaces, to target preferentially human CD4+ T cells, and to establish quickly a persistent reservoir of latently infected cells. Properties of transmitted (founder) viruses from mucosal transmission indicate that in 70–80% of cases, a single virus or virus-infected cell establishes productive clinical infection (Fischer et al., 2010). Such viruses typically exhibit C-C chemokine receptor type 5 (CCR5)-dependence. Mask functional envelope trimers needed to trigger efficient antibody response, and undergo rapid mutation as productive infection ensues (Goonetilleke et al., 2009; Keele et al., 2008). These viral properties narrow innate and adaptive immune pathways that can efficiently defend against HIV-1 entry and productive infection. Because of this global diversity (up to 35% in envelope gp120), it may impossible to design a single vaccine candidate that can induce potent effector immunity to multiple key antigenic determinants among worldwide circulating infecting HIV-1 strains. Although innate immune mechanisms contribute to HIV-1 control (Alter et al., 2007; Alter & Moody, 2010), it remains unclear whether recapitulating these responses with a vaccine will enhance protection against HIV-1 acquisition.

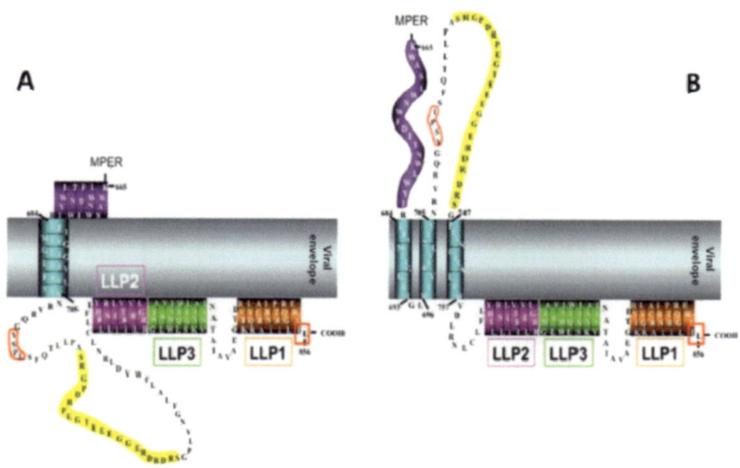

Fig. 11. Schematic models of the HIV-1 CT. A) A total intracytoplasmic localization of the CT with one membrane-spanning α-helix sequence (Traditional model). B) Alternative model with 3 MSD β-sheets and an extracellular segment that bears the Kennedy peptide Adapted from (Steckbeck et al., 2010).

3.1 Gp120 immunogenicity

During HIV-1 infection, gp120-specific Abs are generated and some of them are directed to conserved sites on Env crucial to host receptor recognition or viral fusion (table 2) Conventional insight suggests that constant rather than variable regions of Env should be targeted by the immune system to elicit broad responses against diverse HIV strains. However, these regions were classified on single criteria as the sequence and for only a few virus strains (Zolla-Pazner and Cardozo, 2010). Whereas immunological and 3-D structural studies of Env have shown that these regions were flexible and variable to interact with other surface molecules thus explaining how Abs specific for some variable regions have neutralizing activity against diverse viruses. Although, gp120-specific Abs typically recognize type-specific neutralizing epitopes located on variable loops (Davis et al., 2009) or recognize dominant non-neutralizing conserved epitopes in gp120 (Palker et al., 1987) or gp41 (Gnann et al., 1987). Inducing neutralizing antibodies that target these epitopes using rationally designed immunogens has, so far, been unsuccessful (Selvarajah et al., 2005; Selvarajah et al., 2008; Wu et al., 2010).

This provides a rational basis for understanding the immunological cross-reactivity of many monoclonal Abs targeting the second (V2) and third (V3) variable loops of gp120, and the quaternary neutralization epitopes (QNEs) formed by V2 and V3. The glycan-rich outer face of gp120 is also the target of 2G12 broadly neutralizing mAb (Calarese et al., 2003; Huskens et al., 2007; Scanlan et al., 2002; Trkola et al., 1995). The V3 and the "bridging sheet" contain the binding site for co-receptor (CCR5 or CXCR4), but Abs against these targets are typically weakly neutralizing due to limited epitope exposure on native Env, and steric and kinetic restrictions post-CD4 engagement (Binley et al., 2004; Hartley et al., 2005; Reeves et al., 2005)

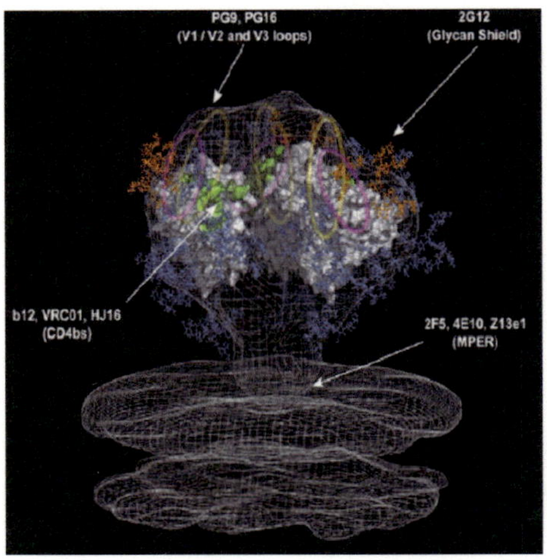

Fig. 12. Epitope modeling of HIV-1 trimer-specific neutralizing antibodies. The above model is adapted from a recent cryoelectron tomographic structure of the HIV-1 trimer (Liu et al., 2008; Schief et al., 2009). The crystal structure of the b12-bound monomeric gp120 core has been fitted into the density map (Zhou et al., 2007). The V1/V2 and V3 loops, which are not resolved in the structure, are represented as yellow and magenta ovals, respectively. The red structure located above the trimer is representative of a human IgG1 molecule. The approximate locations of the epitopes targeted by the existing NAbs are indicated with arrows. Carbohydrate chains are shown in blue, and the oligomannose cluster targeted by mAb 2G12 is shown in orange (Walker and Burton, 2010)

3.1.1 Receptor-binding sites

Binding of gp120 to CD4 results in gp120 conformational changes that expose the binding site for a secondary co-receptor, which is either of the chemokine receptors CCR5 or CXCR4 (Sterjovski et al., 2011). Crystallographic and biochemical studies of gp120 have provided valuable insights into mechanisms involved in CD4-binding and CD4-induced conformational changes that result in formation and exposure of the co-receptor binding site (Huang et al., 2005; Myszka et al., 2000). The unbound gp120 core consists of a highly conserved inner domain, which faces the trimer axis, and a heavily glycosylated, outer domain, which is mostly exposed on the surface of the trimmer (Kwong et al., 1998; Teixeira et al., 2011; Zolla-Pazner and Cardozo, 2010). CD4 binding site represents the encounter of three separate regions *via* their surface-exposed residues. These regions are distributed over 6 segments of gp120. These regions include the α-helices of the inner domain, the CD4-binding loop of outer domain, and the β20–β21 ribbon, that incorporate the gp120 bridging sheet, which is a structural element of gp120 formed after CD4 binding that is involved in co-receptor binding. Otherwise, thermodynamic and structural analysis of the interaction between gp120–CD4 showed evidence of a structured CD4-binding pocket on the unloaded gp120, and that CD4 binding site elements that influence gp120–CD4 affinity are formed from conformational alterations that occur after gp120 has encountered CD4 (Kwong et al., 1998; Myszka et al., 2000). All these structures occur in the very early steps of the recognition (tropism) and anchorage process and provoke broad immune response. However, Abs remains interesting due to their large capacity to neutralize HIV-1 (table 1). The antibody IgG1b12 recognizes an epitope that overlaps the binding site of gp120 to the CD4 receptor. Several antibodies specific of the CD4 binding site have been described by several teams as the 15th, F105, F91, 1125H, 21H, 654-30D and Fab b6. All these antibodies show responsiveness to monomeric gp120 from different isolates of HIV-1 while this response disappears with trimeric gp120 which is present on the viral envelope spikes. Only the b12 antibody binds these two forms, and neutralizes many strains of HIV-1 (Zwick et al., 2003). Recently, the VRC01 Ab has been identified by screening of sera from infected individuals. It could be detected with high proportion and titers in patients. VRC01 Ab has been mapped to the CD4 binding site of gp120 (Wu et al., 2010; Zhou et al., 2010). In these studies it was observed that among 190 circulating HIV-1 isolates tested for sensitivity to VRC01, 173 were neutralized and only 17 were resistant. A structural analysis of these 17 resistant isolates by threading their sequences onto the gp120 structure showed important variations in the V5 region. However, the low VRC01 resistance frequency suggests that VRC01 use a recognition mechanism that allows binding despite V5 variation. Study of VRC01 interaction with V5 shows that VRC01 recognition of V5 is different than CD4. The V5 loop fits into the gap between heavy and light chains. Interaction with the more conserved residues at the loop base is sufficient for the VRC01 activity independently of variation in the top of the V5 loop.

Neutralizing Abs directed against CD4 binding site have been recently compared (Pietzsch et al., 2010). Around 30% of high titers of broadly HIV-neutralizing Abs expressed by memory B cells in HIV+ patients recognize one or more "core" epitopes that were not defined. Some of them recognize the ^{474}DMR^{476} motif on the gp120 which is conserved in different strains and its mutation alters the viral fusion process. For example, HJ6 exhibit a breadth neutralizing activity comparable to, and could be considered as complementary to b12. HJ16 also showed selective neutralization (Corti et al., 2010).

3.1.2 CD4-induced region

The receptor-binding structures of gp120 are conserved among diverse viral isolates and represent functionally constrained regions that might serve as targets of broadly neutralizing antibodies. However, structural evidence suggests that, within functional spike, the CD4-binding site (CD4bs) is a recessed pocket and the co-receptor-binding site (CD4-induced region) is either not formed or not exposed until gp120 engages CD4 on target cells (Kwong et al., 1998). Numerous Abs were described for their binding to the CD4-induced site and the most interesting by their breadth neutralizing capacities are the 17b, X5, m18, and m14 which all contains long H3s playing a major role in their mechanism of binding (table 1). The H3s region of X5, m6 and m9 appear to be very flexible and highly potent to neutralize the virus (Wen et al., 2010; Zhu et al., 2006)

3.1.3 V1/V2 regions

The V1/V2 loops are less investigated even if several studies have shown that the V1/V2 domain of the HIV-1 gp120 envelope protein is involved in viral tropism during infection. V1V2 region interfere by masking conserved neutralizing epitopes, in the conformational changes occurring after co-receptor binding.
As V1/V2 domain is highly glycosylated, numerous studies have determined the influence of carbohydrates on neutralizing antibodies production. As an example, mucosal secretory IgA from parotid saliva and also seric IgG from seropositives present differences in their neutralization properties in fuction of the clade and glycosylation state. (Granados-Gonzalez et al., 2009)

Epitope	Monoclonal antibody	Epitope on	Region(s) recognized	Epitope type
CD4-binding site	IgG1b12 HJ16 VRC01 VRC03	Gp120	C2, C3, C4, V5 and C5	Discontinuous
CD4-induced region	17b X5	Gp120	Binding Sheet	Discontinuous
Complex carbohydrate	2G12	Gp120	Carbohydrate moieties in C2, C3 and V4	Discontinuous
V3	447/52-D 2219 3074 HGN194	Gp120	V3 loop	Linear (conformational)
Quaternary neutralizing epitope	2909 PG9 PG16	Gp120 Trimer	V2-V3	Quaternary
Membrane-proximal external region	2F5 4E10 Z13	Gp41	Protein and lipid	Linear (conformational)

Table 1. Main HIV-1 Env-specific neutralizing human monoclonal Abs.

3.1.4 V3 region

The b12 (CD4bs) and 2G12 (glycan) epitopes are presently the most attractive targets for vaccine design owing to their highly conserved nature. Although other sites seems present an interest in the immune response to gp120 as epitopes in the V3 region. This region is recognized by an antibody called 447- 52D (table 1) (Dhillon et al., 2008). Its core epitope is the Gly-Pro-Gly-Arg (GPGR) motif which is located at the center of the V3 region. This recognition is altered with the substitution of AA at the N-Term segment of the V3 region (Rosen et al., 2005). This Ab neutralize both X4 and R5 primary isolates, making it one of the most effective anti-V3 Ab. X-ray crystal structure of 447- 52D in complex with a V3 peptide indicates how this antibody may have the capacity to neutralize more clade B viruses than other anti-V3. Since the binding interaction between the antibody and the peptide is mediated by main chain contacts, which enlarges the ability of the antibody to recognize a variety of V3 sequences (Stanfield et al., 2004). The only side-chain interactions are with the Pro and Arg-residues in the GPGR sequence; the side chains from both residues form extensive interactions with residues in the Ab combining site. The side chain of the Arg residue in the GPGR sequence is oriented in the opposite direction in the 447-52D complex relative to its orientation in the other complexes with anti-V3 antibodies and V3 (Binley et al., 2004; Rosen et al., 2005). However, exposure of the V3 region during infection seems to occur exclusively in the context of gp120 oligomer on the virus and may be influenced by the presence of glycan moieties. Given these caveats, the V3 region may be a target that only yields antibodies with restricted neutralizing ability. It is worth noting here that a 447-52D equivalent has not been identified so far for non-clade B viruses. A novel human monoclonal Ab HGN194 was isolated from memory B cells of a long-term non-progressor infected with a HIV-1 clade AG circulating recombinant form (CRF). This Ab recognizes a conformational epitope in the V3 and neutralizes all tier 1 viruses which are relatively neutralization-sensitive but only 11% of the tier 2 viruses tested. Tier 2 strains are more difficult to neutralize and reflect the majority of primary HIV-1 isolates. (Watkins et al., 2011) After massive immunization in Rhesus monkeys with the IgG1HGN194, the authors describe the absence of virus reservoirs after HGN194 was cleared. HGN194 seems to be an interesting cross-clade Nabs.

3.1.5 Impact of glycosylations

HIV uses glycans to occlude Ab epitopes on gp120. Around 50% of the molecule is covered with carbohydrates that render the underlying protein surface masked from the immune system and inaccessible (figure12). The virus can also shift the locations of its glycans *in vivo* (Nawaz et al., 2011). These observations gave a non static model called evolving glycan-shield model by which, through the continuous repositioning of its N-glycosylations positons, HIV is able to escape from a specific neutralizing Ab response. Thus, the developed resistance is not a comprehensive one but, instead, a specific adaptation to the particular Ab response in each infected individual (Wei et al., 2003). In addition to being involved in blocking neutralizing Ab responses, glycan repositioning also may compensate for conformational changes in the envelope glycoprotein caused by localized AA changes directly related to virus escape from neutralizing antibody. The works of Trkola led to the characterization of the human monoclonal Ab 2G12 directed against the envelope glycoprotein gp120 of HIV-1. This antibody recognizes clustered $\alpha 1 \rightarrow 2$-linked mannose residues on the distal ends of oligomannose sugars located on the carbohydrate-covered silent face of the gp120 outer domain. It confers neutralizing activity *in vitro* on T cells infected with HIV-1 primary isolates from clade A or B. This study has demonstrated the ability of 2G12 to induce an immune response as "antibody-dependent cellular cytotoxicity ADCC" directed against infected cells or by activation of the complement system (Trkola et al., 1996). The epitope of 2G12 is described as a dependent structure of N-glycans in the C2, C3, V3, V4 and C4 regions of gp120. Other studies have described that the epitope recognized by monoclonal antibody 2G12 contains mannose type glycans at multiple sites of N-glycosylation (Calarese et al., 2003; Scanlan et al., 2002). This is not aware that the glycosylated epitopes contain microheterogenities at various carbohydrates which can lead to an escape from immune response. Only deletion of N392 glycosylation site is sufficient for decrease drastically 2G12 activies, which may explain the emergence of new strains viral resistance (Huskens et al., 2007; Scanlan et al., 2002).

3.1.6 Quaternary neutralizing epitope

Quaternary epitopes are formed by interactions between proteins during multimerization. It is as a result of such reorganization that many proteins (such as enzymes and the trimeric gp120 spike of HIV-1) carry out their physiological function. An Ab that reacts with a true quaternary epitope will not interact with the individual monomeric subunits. Monoclonal antibodies mAb2909 and PG16 (figure 13), react with the trimeric form of gp120 on the surface of HIV-1 virions or *env*-transfected cells but not with monomeric gp120 (Gorny et al., 2005; Walker et al., 2009). However, some Abs that react with quaternary epitopes binds preferentialy the trimers rather than monomeric subunits. This seems to be true for the monoclonal antibody PG9. Trimerization can result in changes in quaternary structure within individual subunits or through reorientation of the subunits against each other, so regions contributing to the quaternary epitope can be inter-molecular (*trans*) or intra-molecular (*cis*). Recently, a human mAb (mAb 2909) (figure 13) has been described to bind to a quaternary structure only on virion but not to soluble monomeric gp120 (Changela et al., 2011; Gorny et al., 2005). It has been discovered by immortalization of PBMC from HIV 1 patients asymptomatic and drug-naïve (Gorny et al., 1991). It demonstrates a high neutralizing activity for primary isolate such as SF162 (picomolar concentrations) and specificity for a complex epitope consisting of V2, V3, and the CD4 binding site that is present exclusively on the surfaces of intact virions but not on soluble viral proteins (Gorny et al., 2005). The neutralizing activity of MAb 2909 against pseudovirus SF162 is 750- to 100,000-fold more potent than those of other well-characterized. The occurrence of mAb 2909 suggests the possible existence of additional Abs that are oligomer-specific. Such Abs, in contrast to mAb2909, may possess broader neutralizing activity.

Moreover, two potent broadly neutralizing monoclonal antibodies, PG9 and PG16, have been discovered recently both targeting highly conformational, discontinuous epitopes involving the V2 and V3 loops (Walker et al., 2009). These antibodies have been characterized after a large screening of 1800 sera from HIV- and HIV+ donors from all over the world (Thailand, Australia, and United Kingdom etc). Only donors that exhibit broad and potent neuralizing serum activity were selected. Analysis of the antibody variable genes revealed two pairs of somatic variants, each one contained long, heavy-chain complementaritydetermining region 3 (CDRH3) loops (PG9 and PG16). Long CDRH3 loops have been previously associated with polyreactivity. PG9 and PG16 are somatically related and appear to be derived from the same recombination of heavy and light chains. The both Abs recognize a site on gp120 composed of elements from the V2 and V3 variable regions. Despite the vaunted diversity of the HIV-1 gp120 envelope and the even higher sequence variability in the V2 and V3 regions (Walker et al., 2009), neutralization assays indicate that the recognized epitope is conserved in 70 to 80% of circulating viral isolates. Neutralization by PG9 correlates strongly with that of PG16, indicating that these Abs recognize a common HIV-1 epitope. This suggests that a common surface of the paratope on PG9 and PG16 might be involved in recognition of HIV-1. Substantial differences in sequence are found between PG9 and PG16 (Doria-Rose et al., 2010; Pancera et al., 2010).

3.2 Gp41 immunogenicity

Gp41 is largely occluded by quaternary interactions within native Env (Sougrat et al., 2007; Zanetti et al., 2006; Zhu et al., 2006). During the fusion process, different gp41 regions are exposed and elicit while the changing of conformation due to the intercation with gp120 antibodies. Some of them are very essential and present interesting capacities to block the infection and neutralizing the virus. The neutralizing Abs 2F5, Z13e1 and 4E10 directed against the membrane-proximal external region (MPER) in the C-Term portion of the gp41 ectodomain can bind Env and block a late stage of fusion (table 1) (Nelson et al., 2007;

Stiegler et al., 2001; Dimitrov et al., 2007; Zwick et al., 2005). Despite great efforts, high neutralizing Abs titers against any of the conserved sites on Env have not yet been elicited (Kim et al., 2007; Phogat and Wyatt, 2007).

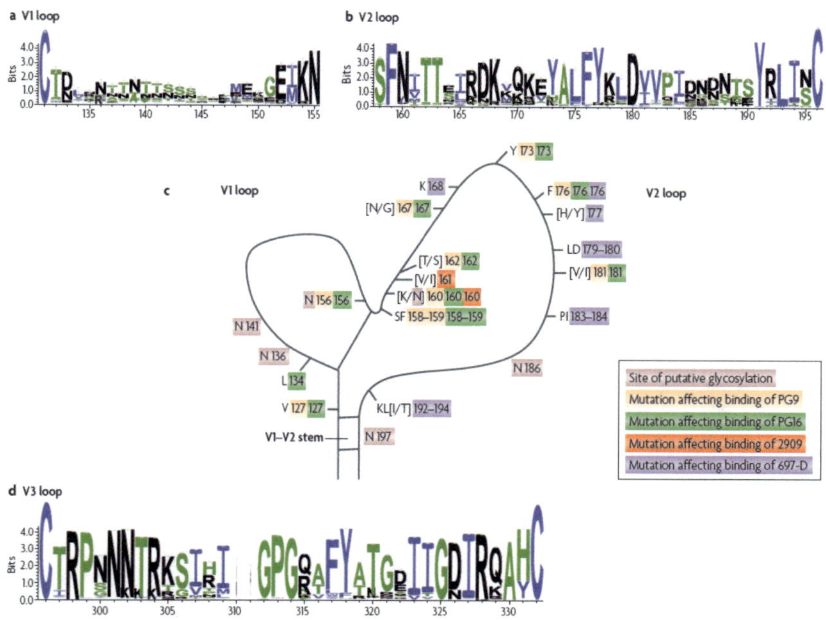

Fig. 13. Conserved and variable residues in the V1, V2 and V3 loops of gp120. A, b, d) Sequence logo describs the AA conservation pattern across a multiple alignment of many V1, V2 and V3 loops. The height of the letter indicates the degree of conservation of the most common amino acid at that position. Data obtained from the Los Alamos National Laboratory, New Mexico, USA. AA are colored according to their chemical properties. C) AA positions and sites of glycosylation that are implicated in binding of the V2-specific monoclonal Ab 697-D and the Quaternay Neutralizing epitopes-specific monoclonal Abs PG9, PG16 and 2909 are mapped onto a schematic illustration. Square brackets indicate more than one commonly occurring AA at a single position. The individual sites associated with binding of each single Ab are distributed throughout the V1–V2 primary sequence linearly but, in 3D space, must group into one or a few overlapping epitopes (adapted from (Zolla-Pazner and Cardozo, 2010)

3.2.1 Polar region (PR)

Only one study described PR-specific Abs in HIV-1+ patients. However, these Abs remains poorly neutralizing (Buchacher et al., 1994).

3.2.2 N-Heptad Repeat region

Cross-reactive antibodies to the NHR have been detected in HIV-1-positive sera, indicating its immunogenic characteristics (Poumbourios et al., 1992). Moreover, the D5 NAb was generated from a native single-chain variable fragment library. D5 has been shown to bind to the NHR trimer and, like the T-20 peptide, inhibits the assembly of the fusion intermediate *in vitro* (Miller et al., 2005). Those studies indicate the potential of the inner NHR trimer as a target for vaccine design. D5 was derived from B cells of HIV-naive subjects and has not been subject to extensive somatic hypermutation, with only seven non-complementarity-determining regions (CDR) amino acid changes from germline sequences (four changes in VH and three in VL). Unlike b12, 2F5, and 4E10, D5 does not have an atypically long heavy chain CDR3 region. Unlike 2G12, D5 does not require a "domain-swapped" structure for neutralization. Unlike X5, D5 retains antiviral activity against primary HIV isolates when converted to an IgG1 format. Finally, and most importantly, D5 was elected by binding to IZN36 and 5H which are synthetic antigens with well defined structures mimicing the 6 helix bundle structure. In addition, new NAbs with limited potency against the NHR trimer of HIV-1 have been isolated by screening phage-display library (Nelson et al., 2008). Ag-binding and monoclonal Ab-competition experiments using 8K8, DN9 and D5 strongly suggest that the epitopes of 8K8 and DN9 are more closely related to each other than to that of D5. Although, D5 has a preference to bind NHR mimetics in the absence of CHR peptide thus indicating a significant cross-reactivity of D5 with immobilized 6-Helix (Luftig et al., 2006; Miller et al., 2005),. Similarly, C34 HR2 peptide competes efficiently with 8K8 and DN9 binding to immobilized NHR mimetics (e.g. 5-Helix and IZN36), but not with D5. Another antibody, Fab 3764, has been shown to bind to the NHR region with the same efficiency on free (N35CCG-N13) or interacting with CHR peptide in the form of a 6-Helix Bundle (Gustchina et al., 2007; Gustchina et al., 2010). Further more absence of detectable cardiolipin reactivity with 8K8 178 170–183 suggests that autoreactivity, at least to cardiolipin cannot explain the weak titers of 8K8-like Abs in the rabbits (Haynes et al., 2005; Scherer et al., 2007). Three-dimensional structural informations of the mAb-mimetic complexes may be used to better predict the accessibility to the NHR on fusogenic gp41 for prospective next-generation Abs. Recently, the HK20 gp41-specific antibody was obtained from immortalized memory B cells of an HIV-1 infected individual (Corti et al., 2010). This Ab targets the conserved hydrophobic pocket in HR1. Crystal structure of HR1-specific human mAb HK20 in complex with 5-Helix shows that HK20 binds to the same region recognized by D5 but differs significantly in the contact sites and shows a role for somatic mutations in affinity maturation (Luftig et al., 2006). These aspects influence both potency and breadth of neutralization, which are higher for HK20 compared to D5 and depend on somatically mutated residues. In addition, we show that in case of HK20 the scFv is at least 15-fold more potent in neutralization than IgG, consistent with a limited accessibility to the target site. The gp41 footprints of HK20 and D5 and the global structural principles employed by both antibodies are similar.

3.2.3 Immunodominant loop

This region located between the two heptad repeat region N-HR and C-HR was identified during serum-mapping studies (reviewed in Girard et al., 2006; Montero et al., 2008). Even if the response to this region is very frequent most of the Abs elicited do not present neutralization capacities but instead shown enhancement of infection (Robinson et al., 1990). Only one MAb (clone3) neutralize T-cell laboratory adapted viruses from clade B and three primary isolates from group O (Ferrantelli et al., 2004).

3.2.4 C-Heptad repeat region (C-HR)

Considering that MPER is not included in C-HR, no CHR-specific Ab has been described. The poor immunogenicity of this region may be attributed to its lack of exposure on the surface of the native virus and is exposed only if gp120/CD4 interaction occurred. This region is probably masked by gp120 (Nyambi et al., 2000; Pietzsch et al., 2010).

3.2.5 Fusogenic 6 helix-bundle form

The gp41 TM subunit, which anchors the spikes in the viral envelope, maintains their trimeric organization, and plays a major role in fusion of the virus and host cell membrane through its hydrophobic N-Term fusion peptide and a fusion active hairpin structure involving the HR that can fold into a six-helix coiled-coil bundle. This pattern plays an important role in both the early and late stages of the membrane fusion (Chan and Kim, 1998; Johnson et al., 2001; Liu et al., 2005; Lu et al., 1995; Munoz-Barroso et al., 1998). This process can also participate in the formation of the fusion pore through direct protein-membrane interactions (Munoz-Barroso et al., 1998; Shnaper et al., 2004). Different studies have shown the immunogenicity of the fusogenic complex and describe Abs direct against this structure (Gustchina et al., 2010; Opalka et al., 2004; Vincent et al., 2008). Authors were confronted to the difficulty of the construction of a native form of the fusogenic complex with 6 helix-bundle and used a five helix-bundle (Gustchina et al., 2010) or synthetic peptide that mimic the N-HR like (peptide N36) or mimic C-HR (peptides C34 or T20). Abs directed against the complex do not always recognize the HR1 or HR2 individually. The Abs have shown low neutralizing activity excepted in one study with Nabs against primary isolates (Vincent et al., 2008), and the work of Gustchina *et al.*, with a monoclonal antibody Fab 3674 that neutralize diverse laboratory-adapted B strains of HIV-1 and primary isolates of subtypes A, B, and C (Gustchina et al., 2007). When gp41 switches from the native conformation to the fusion structure, there are probably several intermediate structures, which can be a target for Abs. Several studies indicate that the prehairpin intermediate state is accessible to Abs and that the access is not restricted (Louis et al., 2003). Therefore, the gp41 6-HB core may serve as an attractive target for development of anti-HIVmolecules.

3.2.6 MPER (membrane-proximal external region)

The Membrane Proximal Ectodomain Region contains the epitopes of three broadly neutralizing Abs, 2F5, 4E10, and Z13 (Buchacher et al., 1994; Zwick et al., 2001) (figure 15). MPER is not highly immunogenic like the N-HR, ID loop or the gp120. Specific anti-MPER Abs present in natural infection are not as broadly neutralizing as 2F5, 4E10 (Braibant et al., 2006; Muhlbacher et al., 1999). Both 2F5 and 4E10 neutralize a broad range of both laboratory adapted and primate isolates of HIV-1 (Mascola et al., 2000; Stiegler et al., 2001). 2F5 is the most potent NAb, whereas 4E10 neutralizes a broader range of HIV-1 isolates, as shown by pseudovirus studies using an extensive panel of Envs derived from primary isolates (Binley et al., 2004). The 2F5 Ab could also be detected at low level in the sera of HIV long term progressors (Braibant et al., 2006). The frequency of seroreactivity to MPER is about 56% in 50 HIV-1-positive subjects. Most of the Abs are specific for the C-Term region of the ELDKWA sequence just preceding the 2F5 epitope. In addition, more than 30% of sera were reactive to the ELDKWA 2F5 epitope. Furthermore, serum reactivity against an MPER peptide (aa 642 to 673) in patients could be correlated to the recognition of infected T cells and to CD4 cell counts (Muhlbacher et al., 1999). There is a possibility that NAbs against MPER are present in low titers or with low affinities in serum that they are not sufficiently neutralizing to inhibit HIV-1 infection and are therefore undetectable in neutralization assays. However, recent studies using chimeric pseudoviruses with epitopes in a context more closely related to the MPER structure (figure 15B) suggest that MPER-specific NABs are relatively rare or absent during natural infection. Moreover, the fact that new NAbs are mapping to a different region in MPER than 2F5 and 4E10 provides hopes by suggesting that vaccine-induced neutralizing antibodies are achievable (Haynes and Montefiori, 2006;

Li et al., 2006). To date, the lack of broadly neutralizing activity shown by MPER binding sera could be due to low titers or absence of NAbs. This issue of quantity *versus* quality has not been fully resolved but has significant implications for vaccine design.

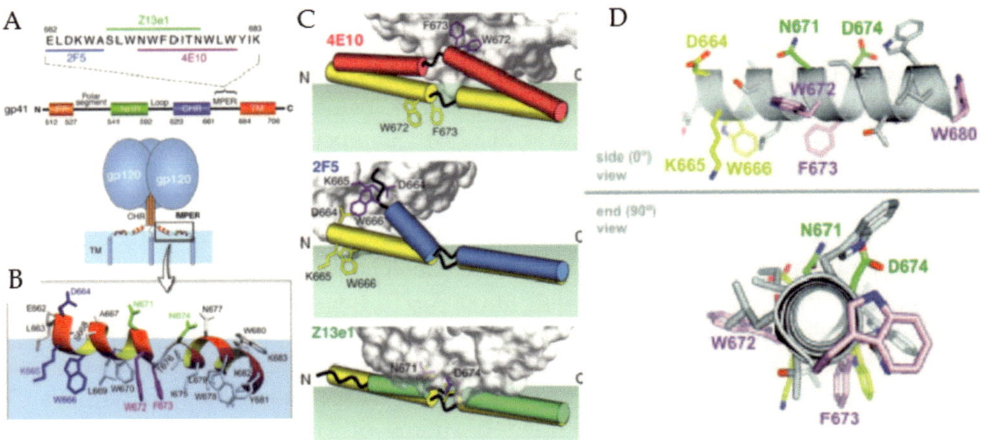

Fig. 15. Different representations of MPER interaction with 2F5 4E10 and Z13 Abs A) Schematic diagram of HIV-1 gp41. FP, fusion peptide region; NHR and CHR, N- and C-terminal-helices of heptad repeat, respectively; and TM, transmembrane domain. The minimal peptide epitopes are indicated for 2F5 (blue), Z13e1 (green), and 4E10 (magenta). B) A simple model of env including MPER and TM based on 3D structural features of HIV-1/SIV-1 trimeric env and the NMR structure of the HxB2 MPER in a virion mimic surface (blue plane). N674 rather than D674 is shown. C) Artistic rendering of MPER orientation changes induced by 4E10, 2F5, and Z13e1. Unbound MPER peptides (yellow tubes) are immersed in the lipid bilayers (light green panel). Red, blue, and green tubes represent the membrane orientation of schematic MPER segments in complex with 4E10, 2F5, and Z13e1 (gray surface area). Several key binding residues positions are indicated before (yellow) and after (purple) antibody binding (Song et al., 2009). D) Hypothetical model of the MPER (DKWASLWNWFDITNWLW) and the 2F5, Z13e and 4E10 cores epitope with the core residues colored in yellow, green and violet, respectively described by (Nelson et al., 2007).

As said before 2F5 Ab has broad neutralizing activity. In animal models it could interrupt the mucosal transmission and confers protection against SHIV infection (Mascola et al., 2000). The 2F5 antibody was isolated from human immortalized B cells. It recognizes an epitope lying between glutamic acid 662 and alanine 667 (ELDKWA). Studies have shown, for expression library and protection against proteases, that this epitope is wider (EQELLELDKWASLWN). By addition of a leucine at each side (LELDKWASL), the affinity for its epitope is increased by more than 2000 times (Ofek et al., 2004; Parker et al., 2001; Tian et al., 2002). In models that study the involvement of the viral membrane using POPC (1-oleyl-2-palmolityl-sn-glycero-3-phosphocholine) and POPC/cholesterol in the recognition and binding to its epitope, it has been shown that 2F5 does not interact with the membrane before fixation (Veiga and Castanho, 2006). In the absence of an hydrophobic environment, 2F5 and 4E10 are unable to bind to MPER (Ofek et al., 2004). This study demonstrate that the recognition of 2F5 and 4E10 epitopes depend on their integrity and conformational context. Recently, it was shown that the binding of 2F5 causes peptide docking on the membrane and increase the ability of the Mab to be intrusive (Franquelim et al., 2011). The 2F5 induces a confined local disorder in the membrane which can promote the exposure and interaction with gp41. However, the role of the presence of lipids in recognition of epitopes during the membrane fusion has not yet been clearly elucidated. The 2F5 epitope contains a β-turn conformation and antigen which is presented in a similar context may better mimic the epitope and consequently improve the binding of this Ab (Tian et al., 2002). Several difficulties rise to make a stable immunogen, flexible and mimicking faithfully the MPER in a native conformation sported during the steps of rapprochement and viral fusion process. Moreover, the polyspecificity of 2F5 and 4E10 and autoreactivity by binding to cardiolipin could explain the low activity of these antibodies *in vivo* as the immune system deplete all B cells which produce auto-reactive Abs (Haynes et al., 2005).

Another promising MPER-specific Ab (4E10) was isolated from B cells of HIV patients. It binds a deeper epitope in the MPER and presents neutralizing abilities. The 4E10 is highly protective against infection with primary isolates and laboratory strains of HIV-1. The 4E10 binds to a highly conserved linear epitope on MPER ^{671}NWF (D/N) IT^{676} (Zwick et al., 2001). Crystallographic structures of the epitope have been characterized and form a large helical shape with all the important AA on the same side of the helix (Hager-Braun and Tomer, 2005)(figure 15D). The antigen reacts only with residues of the base and the center of the loop of CDR H3. However much of this loop is not involved in its binding to the antigen. The top of the loop of CDR H3 of 4E10 and this residue is removed from the apolar binding site epitope which suggest a possible interaction with the membrane of the virus. Structural models predict that the formation of the epitope of 2F5 and 4E10 would be highly dependent on the presence of a membrane. The affinity of 4E10 increases in the presence of lipids (Lorizate et al., 2006). The W^{672}, F^{673}, T^{676} residues seems to be crucial for 4E10 binding since their substitution by alanine residues reduce drastically the affinity (Brunel et al., 2006). The sequence ^{671}NWFDITNWLWYIK^{683} is optimal for 4E10 recognition. In resistant strains, the pattern NWF(N/D)IT indicate that the 4E10 epitope is more complex and would be even discontinuous (Hager-Braun and Tomer, 2005). Mass spectrometry studies reveal that 4E10 binds to the N-Term of gp120 and gp41 on the native conformation (Stiegler et al., 2001). It has been suggested that the pattern NWF (N/D)IT forms a cryptic epitope accessible only during the intermediate stages of the merger. It seems that 4E10 has higher affinity to the membrane than 2F5 and that unlike 2F5, 4E10 promotes peptide extraction from the bilayer lipid membrane (Franquelim et al., 2011). The 4E10 Ab has also a polyspecificity for autoantigens as histone or DNA in systemic lupus erythematosus. Several *in vivo* pharmacokinetic studies and phase I/II clinical trials phases I and II with combination of 4E10, 2F5 and 2G12 showed that these three Abs are able to maintain undetectable viral load in patients where the infection has been suppressed by antiviral therapy (Joos et al., 2006). These studies also showed that 4E10 administration is not highly immunogenic with rare IgM against 4E10 but no IgG. Clearance and half-life of 4E10 are identical to those of other classical therapeutic Abs.

One other described MPER-specific Ab is the Z13 Fab. This Ab derived from an expression library recognizes an epitope located on the C-Term of 2F5 epitope and which overlaps 4E10 epitope. The epitope of Z13 is centered around the sequence ^{671}NWFDIT^{676} but this would be dependent on the conformation of this motif and changes such as N-glycosylation of asparagine (D) ^{674} or exposure to a native protein (Zwick et al., 2001).This Ab is able to neutralize weakly several clades such as B, C and D.

3.2.7 The C-Term tail

The external tail loop within the CT of the gp41 TM subunit of the HIV-1 envelope protein comprises approximately 40 AA, and within are 18 AA (^{734}PDRPEGIEEEGGERDRDR ^{751}) including three interesting regions. The antigenicity of this segment of the CT is very complex, and changes according to the biological context of gp41 (Reading et al., 2003). The Kennedy sequence, ^{731}PRGPDRPEGIEEEGGERDRDRS^{752}, is exposed on the outer surface (Kennedy et al., 1986). It was observed that 3 epitopes ^{734}PDRPEG^{739}, ^{740}IEEE^{743}, ^{746}ERDRD^{750} are mostly recognized in the Kennedy sequences (Chen et al., 2001; McLain et al., 2001). Kennedy-specific NAbs could be elicited in different conditions of exposure.

The ^{746}ERDRD^{750} epitope is exposed constitutively and does not require contact with cell receptors or an elevated temperature (Cleveland et al., 2003). ^{734}PDRPEG^{739} is recognised by the non-neutralizing Ab C8, ^{740}IEEE^{743} by the non-neutralizing Ab 1575 (Abacioglu et al., 1994), ^{746}ERDRD^{750} by the non-neutralising Abs 1577 and 1583 (Vella et al., 1993), and the neutralizing EPES (epitope purified and ERDRD specific) and SAR1 antibodies. EPES and SAR1 Abs were both obtained by immunisation of mice with cowpea mosaic virus (CPMV) chimeras expressing short, ERDRD-containing gp41 sequences. EPES is the only Kennedy-specific polyclonal IgG described to have a strong neutralizing activity against primary isolates. It was also shown that some of the IgA from infected patients parotid saliva or sera are able to recognize the linear peptides ^{731}PEGIEEEGGERDRDTSGRLV^{750} or ^{741} RDRDTSGRLVHGFLAIIWVD^{762} (Vincent et al., 2004). IEEE epitope is antigenically dominant , and competes with the binding of ERDRD-specific antibodies. This situation in humans is not known. It is interesting that MAb 1575 appears to have no biological activity other than suppression of the antibody response to ERDRD. Furthermore, the sequence ERDRD is involved in at least three epitopes. These epitopes may be occulted or exposed as a result of conformational changes occurring in another part of gp41, or may be hidden by the associated gp120 and exposed when that gp120 is shed. In addition epitopes may be modulated by conformational changes that affect the ERDRD sequence directly. (Hollier & Dimmock, 2005).

4. Conclusions

The development of an HIV vaccine has proven to be a formidable scientific challenge given the extreme genetic variability of the virus, lack of good animal models, lack of knowledge of all mechanisms involved in immunity or limitations of the technology. However, passive administration of rare human anti-Env monoclonal broadly neutralizing antibodies with titers that can be achieved by immunization can protect against SHIV challenge in rhesus macaques (Hessell et al., 2007; Hessell et al., 2009a; Mascola and Montefiori, 2010; Montefiori and Mascola, 2009). Thus, a major goal of HIV-1 vaccine development is to design highly immunogenic Env antigens capable of inducing Abs that can broadly neutralize HIV-1 (Mascola and Montefiori, 2010; Stamatatos et al., 2009).

According to the clinicaltrials.gov database, more than 543 clinical trials were performed in the field of HIV vaccines. During these last ten years, only one vaccine candidate seems to give objective protection. This prophylactic vaccine from Sanofi Pasteur is composed by an heterologous prime-boost vaccine with a priming with VaxGen gp120 B/E (AIDSVAX B/E) protein and a boost with live recombinant ALVAC-HIV (vCP1521). This trial (RV144) has involved 16,403 individuals and was conducted in Thailand and completed in October 2009,. Vaccination appeared to reduce about 31.2% the rate of acquisition of HIV-1 infection but had no significant effect on viral loads or on CD4+ T cell counts. This "weak" efficacy is the first indication that effective vaccination against HIV-1 could be reach and give rease for hopes in the developpement of anti-HIV vaccines. The immunological correlates in this trial indicate that induction of Nabs is important for vaccine efficacy but not sufficient. Induction of polyspecific virus-specific CD8+ T cell responses is also an important actor of vaccine efficacy. So the scope of action that remains for an effective vaccination is restricted to early stages of infection before the virus infects lymphoid organs and mucosal tissue. In addition, HIV has developed during its evolution, an immune system circumvent strategies that really works. The data from human clinical trials demonstrate that the first generation of soluble protein and vectored Env immunogens was safe and immunogenic. However, generated Abs are only effective on highly sensitive strains of HIV-1. One of the major goal in the development of an effective vaccine remain to develop a mimetic immunogen similar to viral proteins as the most accurate meaning can replicate all possible conformations in steps of infection Indeed, conserved Env epitopes targeted by NAbs are poorly immunogenic because they either are masked by glycan similar to host carbohydrates (Binley et al., 2010; Wei et al., 2003), appear transiently (Frey et al., 2008), are sterically hindered (Schief et al., 2009), or must overcome entropy for Ab binding. Another important point is that conserved epitopes (more in the gp41) present homologies with self-proteins which could trigger tolerance mechanisms (Haynes et al., 2005; Verkoczy et al., 2010). Finally, even when Abs can neutralize the infecting strains, their effect is transient due to escape mutations (Richman et al., 2003; Wei et al., 2003). Thus, immunization of non-human primates and humans with HIV-1 Env monomers or trimers has failed to induce broadly NAbs. Induced Abs are mainly effective on easily neutralized strains also called Tier 1 strains but have weak neutralization abilities for Tier 2 and Tier 3 strains (Gilbert et al., 2010; Mascola and Montefiori, 2010). The explanation for the poor cross-reactivity of vaccine-elicited Nabs appears to be related to the restricted repertoire of induced Abs and to the complexity of the native viral spike structure. NAbs against HIV-1 play an important role in preventing viral infections. Less clear is their role in the containment of viral replication in infected individuals.

However, evidence is accumulating that NAbs may help the cellular arm of the immune response to prevent or delay the progression to AIDS. Detection of NAbs depends on the *in vitro* neutralization assays used, and standardization of the assays is essential in order to be able to compare the magnitude and quality of a NAb response in sera or other fluids from HIV-infected patients, uninfected HIV-1 exposed persons, or vaccinated animals/persons. Viral mechanisms to prevent neutralization include high variability and extensive glycosylation of the Envelope proteins, Envelope trimerization and shedding as well as late exposure of functionally important entry domains by conformational changes induced upon CD4 binding. These are also the difficulties encountered in the design of immunogens able to induce neutralizing antibodies upon vaccination.

5. Acknowledgements

We would like to thank the Cluster 10 of Infectiology of the region Rhône-Alpes and Sidaction to fund our works.

6. References

Abacioglu, Y.H., Fouts, T.R., Laman, J.D., Claassen, E., Pincus, S.H., Moore, J.P., Roby, C.A., Kamin-Lewis, R., and Lewis, G.K. (1994). Epitope mapping and topology of baculovirus-expressed HIV-1 gp160 determined with a panel of murine monoclonal antibodies. AIDS Res. Hum. Retroviruses *10*, 371-381.

Alfsen, A., and Bomsel, M. (2002). HIV-1 gp41 envelope residues 650-685 exposed on native virus act as a lectin to bind epithelial cell galactosyl ceramide. J. Biol. Chem. *277*, 25649-25659.

Allen, S.J., Crown, S.E., and Handel, T.M. (2007). Chemokine: receptor structure, interactions, and antagonism. Annu. Rev. Immunol. *25*, 787-820.

Alter, G., Martin, M.P., Teigen, N., Carr, W.H., Suscovich, T.J., Schneidewind, A., Streeck, H., Waring, M., Meier, A., Brander, C., *et al.* (2007). Differential natural killer cell-mediated inhibition of HIV-1 replication based on distinct KIR/HLA subtypes. J. Exp. Med. *204*, 3027-3036.

Alter, G., and Moody, M.A. (2010). The humoral response to HIV-1: new insights, renewed focus. J. Infect. Dis. *202 Suppl 2*, S315-22.

Arthos, J., Cicala, C., Martinelli, E., Macleod, K., Van Ryk, D., Wei, D., Xiao, Z., Veenstra, T.D., Conrad, T.P., Lempicki, R.A., *et al.* (2008). HIV-1 envelope protein binds to and signals through integrin alpha4beta7, the gut mucosal homing receptor for peripheral T cells. Nat. Immunol. *9*, 301-309.

Bewley, C.A., Louis, J.M., Ghirlando, R., and Clore, G.M. (2002). Design of a novel peptide inhibitor of HIV fusion that disrupts the internal trimeric coiled-coil of gp41. J. Biol. Chem. *277*, 14238-14245.

Binley, J.M., Ban, Y.E., Crooks, E.T., Eggink, D., Osawa, K., Schief, W.R., and Sanders, R.W. (2010). Role of complex carbohydrates in HIV-1 infection and resistance to antibody neutralization. J. Virol. *84*, 5637-5655.

Binley, J.M., Wrin, T., Korber, B., Zwick, M.B., Wang, M., Chappey, C., Stiegler, G., Kunert, R., Zolla-Pazner, S., Katinger, H., Petropoulos, C.J., and Burton, D.R. (2004). Comprehensive cross-clade neutralization analysis of a panel of anti-HIV-1 monoclonal antibodies. J. Virol. *78*, 13232-13252.

Braibant, M., Brunet, S., Costagliola, D., Rouzioux, C., Agut, H., Katinger, H., Autran, B., and Barin, F. (2006). Antibodies to conserved epitopes of the HIV-1 envelope in sera from long-term non-progressors: prevalence and association with neutralizing activity. AIDS *20*, 1923-1930.

Briggs, J.A., Riches, J.D., Glass, B., Bartonova, V., Zanetti, G., and Krausslich, H.G. (2009). Structure and assembly of immature HIV. Proc. Natl. Acad. Sci. U. S. A. *106*, 11090-11095.

Brunel, F.M., Zwick, M.B., Cardoso, R.M., Nelson, J.D., Wilson, I.A., Burton, D.R., and Dawson, P.E. (2006). Structure-function analysis of the epitope for 4E10, a broadly neutralizing HIV-1 antibody. J. Virol. *80*, 1680-1687.

Buchacher, A., Predl, R., Strutzenberger, K., Steinfellner, W., Trkola, A., Purtscher, M., Gruber, G., Tauer, C., Steindl, F., and Jungbauer, A. (1994). Generation of human monoclonal antibodies against HIV-1 proteins; electrofusion and Epstein-Barr virus transformation for peripheral blood lymphocyte immortalization. AIDS Res. Hum. Retroviruses *10*, 359-369.

Buzon, V., Padros, E., and Cladera, J. (2005). Interaction of fusion peptides from HIV gp41 with membranes: a time-resolved membrane binding, lipid mixing, and structural study. Biochemistry *44,* 13354-13364.

Caffrey, M., Braddock, D.T., Louis, J.M., Abu-Asab, M.A., Kingma, D., Liotta, L., Tsokos, M., Tresser, N., Pannell, L.K., Watts, N., *et al.* (2000). Biophysical characterization of gp41 aggregates suggests a model for the molecular mechanism of HIV-associated neurological damage and dementia. J. Biol. Chem. *275,* 19877-19882.

Calarese, D.A., Scanlan, C.N., Zwick, M.B., Deechongkit, S., Mimura, Y., Kunert, R., Zhu, P., Wormald, M.R., Stanfield, R.L., Roux, K.H., *et al.* (2003). Antibody domain exchange is an immunological solution to carbohydrate cluster recognition. Science *300,* 2065-2071.

Cambi, A., de Lange, F., van Maarseveen, N.M., Nijhuis, M., Joosten, B., van Dijk, E.M., de Bakker, B.I., Fransen, J.A., Bovee-Geurts, P.H., van Leeuwen, F.N., Van Hulst, N.F., and Figdor, C.G. (2004). Microdomains of the C-type lectin DC-SIGN are portals for virus entry into dendritic cells. J. Cell Biol. *164,* 145-155.

Campbell, S.M., Crowe, S.M., and Mak, J. (2001). Lipid rafts and HIV-1: from viral entry to assembly of progeny virions. J. Clin. Virol. *22,* 217-227.

Chan, D.C., Fass, D., Berger, J.M., and Kim, P.S. (1997). Core structure of gp41 from the HIV envelope glycoprotein. Cell 89, 263-273

Chan, D.C., and Kim, P.S. (1998). HIV entry and its inhibition. Cell *93,* 681-684.

Changela, A., Wu, X., Yang, Y., Zhang, B., Zhu, J., Nardone, G.A., O'Dell, S., Pancera, M., Gorny, M.K., Phogat, S., *et al.* (2011). Crystal structure of human antibody 2909 reveals conserved features of quaternary structure-specific antibodies that potently neutralize HIV-1. J. Virol. *85,* 2524-2535.

Chen, S.S., Lee, S.F., and Wang, C.T. (2001). Cellular membrane-binding ability of the C-terminal cytoplasmic domain of HIV-1 envelope transmembrane protein gp41. J. Virol. *75,* 9925-9938.

Cleveland, S.M., McLain, L., Cheung, L., Jones, T.D., Hollier, M., and Dimmock, N.J. (2003). A region of the C-terminal tail of the gp41 envelope glycoprotein of HIV-1 contains a neutralizing epitope: evidence for its exposure on the surface of the virion. J. Gen. Virol. *84,* 591-602.

Cormier, E.G., and Dragic, T. (2002). The crown and stem of the V3 loop play distinct roles in HIV-1 envelope glycoprotein interactions with the CCR5 coreceptor. J. Virol. *76,* 8953-8957.

Corti, D., Langedijk, J.P., Hinz, A., Seaman, M.S., Vanzetta, F., Fernandez-Rodriguez, B.M., Silacci, C., Pinna, D., Jarrossay, D., Balla-Jhagjhoorsingh, S., *et al.* (2010). Analysis of memory B cell responses and isolation of novel monoclonal antibodies with neutralizing breadth from HIV-1-infected individuals. PLoS One *5,* e8805.

Davis, K.L., Gray, E.S., Moore, P.L., Decker, J.M., Salomon, A., Montefiori, D.C., Graham, B.S., Keefer, M.C., Pinter, A., Morris, L., Hahn, B.H., and Shaw, G.M. (2009). High titer HIV-1 V3-specific antibodies with broad reactivity but low neutralizing potency in acute infection and following vaccination. Virology *387,* 414-426.

Del Angel, V.D., Dupuis, F., Mornon, J.P., and Callebaut, I. (2002). Viral fusion peptides and identification of membrane-interacting segments. Biochem. Biophys. Res. Commun. *293,* 1153-1160.

Delahunty, M.D., Rhee, I., Freed, E.O., and Bonifacino, J.S. (1996). Mutational analysis of the fusion peptide of the HIV-1: identification of critical glycine residues. Virology *218,* 94-102.

Dhillon, A.K., Stanfield, R.L., Gorny, M.K., Williams, C., Zolla-Pazner, S., and Wilson, I.A. (2008). Structure determination of an anti-HIV-1 Fab 447-52D-peptide complex from an epitaxially twinned data set. Acta Crystallogr. D Biol. Crystallogr. *D64,* 792-802.

Dimitrov, A.S., Jacobs, A., Finnegan, C.M., Stiegler, G., Katinger, H., and Blumenthal, R. (2007). Exposure of the membrane-proximal external region of HIV-1 gp41 in the course of HIV-1 envelope glycoprotein-mediated fusion. Biochemistry *46,* 1398-1401.

Doria-Rose, N.A., Klein, R.M., Daniels, M.G., O'Dell, S., Nason, M., Lapedes, A., Bhattacharya, T., Migueles, S.A., Wyatt, R.T., Korber, B.T., Mascola, J.R., and Connors, M. (2010). Breadth of human immunodeficiency virus-specific neutralizing activity in sera: clustering analysis and association with clinical variables. J. Virol. *84,* 1631-1636.

Dubay, J.W., Roberts, S.J., Brody, B., and Hunter, E. (1992). Mutations in the leucine zipper of the HIV-1 transmembrane glycoprotein affect fusion and infectivity. J. Virol. *66,* 4748-4756.

Durell, S.R., Martin, I., Ruysschaert, J.M., Shai, Y., and Blumenthal, R. (1997). What studies of fusion peptides tell us about viral envelope glycoprotein-mediated membrane fusion (review). Mol. Membr. Biol. *14,* 97-112.

Dwyer, J.J., Hasan, A., Wilson, K.L., White, J.M., Matthews, T.J., and Delmedico, M.K. (2003). The hydrophobic pocket contributes to the structural stability of the N-terminal coiled coil of HIV gp41 but is not required for six-helix bundle formation. Biochemistry *42,* 4945-4953.

Edwards, T.G., Wyss, S., Reeves, J.D., Zolla-Pazner, S., Hoxie, J.A., Doms, R.W., and Baribaud, F. (2002). Truncation of the cytoplasmic domain induces exposure of conserved regions in the ectodomain of HIV-1 envelope protein. J. Virol. *76,* 2683-2691.

Fantini, J., Hammache, D., Delezay, O., Yahi, N., Andre-Barres, C., Rico-Lattes, I., and Lattes, A. (1997). Synthetic soluble analogs of galactosylceramide (GalCer) bind to the V3 domain of HIV-1 gp120 and inhibit HIV-1-induced fusion and entry. J. Biol. Chem. *272,* 7245-7252.

Ferrantelli, F., Kitabwalla, M., Rasmussen, R.A., Cao, C., Chou, T.C., Katinger, H., Stiegler, G., Cavacini, L.A., Bai, Y., Cotropia, J., Ugen, K.E., and Ruprecht, R.M. (2004). Potent cross-group neutralization of primary HIV-1isolates with monoclonal antibodies--implications for acquired immunodeficiency syndrome vaccine. J. Infect. Dis. *189,* 71-74.

Fischer, W., Ganusov, V.V., Giorgi, E.E., Hraber, P.T., Keele, B.F., Leitner, T., Han, C.S., Gleasner, C.D., Green, L., Lo, C.C., *et al.* (2010). Transmission of single HIV-1 genomes and dynamics of early immune escape revealed by ultra-deep sequencing. PLoS One *5,* e12303.

Fleury, S., Lamarre, D., Meloche, S., Ryu, S.E., Cantin, C., Hendrickson, W.A., and Sekaly, R.P. (1991). Mutational analysis of the interaction between CD4 and class II MHC: class II antigens contact CD4 on a surface opposite the gp120-binding site. Cell *66,* 1037-1049.

Franquelim, H.G., Chiantia, S., Veiga, A.S., Santos, N.C., Schwille, P., and Castanho, M.A. (2011). Anti-HIV-1 antibodies 2F5 and 4E10 interact differently with lipids to bind their epitopes. AIDS *25,* 419-428.

Frey, G., Peng, H., Rits-Volloch, S., Morelli, M., Cheng, Y., and Chen, B. (2008). A fusion-intermediate state of HIV-1 gp41 targeted by broadly neutralizing antibodies. Proc. Natl. Acad. Sci. U. S. A. *105,* 3739-3744.

Gallaher, W.R. (1987). Detection of a fusion peptide sequence in the transmembrane protein of human immunodeficiency virus. Cell *50,* 327-328.

Gangupomu, V.K., and Abrams, C.F. (2010). All-atom models of the membrane-spanning domain of HIV-1 gp41 from metadynamics. Biophys. J. *99,* 3438-3444.

Geijtenbeek, T.B., Kwon, D.S., Torensma, R., van Vliet, S.J., van Duijnhoven, G.C., Middel, J., Cornelissen, I.L., Nottet, H.S., KewalRamani, V.N., Littman, D.R., Figdor, C.G., and van Kooyk, Y. (2000a). DC-SIGN, a dendritic cell-specific HIV-1-binding protein that enhances trans-infection of T cells. Cell *100,* 587-597.

Geijtenbeek, T.B., Torensma, R., van Vliet, S.J., van Duijnhoven, G.C., Adema, G.J., van Kooyk, Y., and Figdor, C.G. (2000b). Identification of DC-SIGN, a novel dendritic cell-specific ICAM-3 receptor that supports primary immune responses. Cell *100,* 575-585.

Gilbert, P., Wang, M., Wrin, T., Petropoulos, C., Gurwith, M., Sinangil, F., D'Souza, P., Rodriguez-Chavez, I.R., DeCamp, A., Giganti, M., *et al.* (2010). Magnitude and breadth of a nonprotective neutralizing antibody response in an efficacy trial of a candidate HIV-1 gp120 vaccine. J. Infect. Dis. *202,* 595-605.

Girard, M.P., Osmanov, S.K., and Kieny, M.P. (2006). A review of vaccine research and development: the HIV. Vaccine *24,* 4062-4081.

Gnann, J.W.,Jr, Nelson, J.A., and Oldstone, M.B. (1987). Fine mapping of an immunodominant domain in the transmembrane glycoprotein of human immunodeficiency virus. J. Virol. *61,* 2639-2641.

Goonetilleke, N., Liu, M.K., Salazar-Gonzalez, J.F., Ferrari, G., Giorgi, E., Ganusov, V.V., Keele, B.F., Learn, G.H., Turnbull, E.L., Salazar, M.G., *et al.* (2009). The first T cell response to transmitted/founder virus contributes to the control of acute viremia in HIV-1 infection. J. Exp. Med. *206,* 1253-1272.

Gordon, L.M., Mobley, P.W., Pilpa, R., Sherman, M.A., and Waring, A.J. (2002). Conformational mapping of the N-terminal peptide of HIV-1 gp41 in membrane environments using (13)C-enhanced Fourier transform infrared spectroscopy. Biochim. Biophys. Acta *1559,* 96-120.

Gordon, L.M., Nisthal, A., Lee, A.B., Eskandari, S., Ruchala, P., Jung, C.L., Waring, A.J., and Mobley, P.W. (2008). Structural and functional properties of peptides based on the

N-terminus of HIV-1 gp41 and the C-terminus of the amyloid-beta protein. Biochim. Biophys. Acta *1778,* 2127-2137.

Gorny, M.K., Stamatatos, L., Volsky, B., Revesz, K., Williams, C., Wang, X.H., Cohen, S., Staudinger, R., and Zolla-Pazner, S. (2005). Identification of a new quaternary neutralizing epitope on HIV-1 virus particles. J. Virol. *79,* 5232-5237.

Gorny, M.K., Xu, J.Y., Gianakakos, V., Karwowska, S., Williams, C., Sheppard, H.W., Hanson, C.V., and Zolla-Pazner, S. (1991). Production of site-selected neutralizing human monoclonal antibodies against the third variable domain of the HIV-1 envelope glycoprotein. Proc. Natl. Acad. Sci. U. S. A. *88,* 3238-3242.

Granados-Gonzalez, V., Piedrahita, L.D., Martinez, M., Genin, C., Riffard, S., and Urcuqui-Inchima, S. (2009). Role of the HIV-1 gp120 V1/V2 domains in the induction of neutralizing antibodies]. Enferm. Infecc. Microbiol. Clin. *27,* 523-530.

Gustchina, E., Li, M., Louis, J.M., Anderson, D.E., Lloyd, J., Frisch, C., Bewley, C.A., Gustchina, A., Wlodawer, A., and Clore, G.M. (2010). Structural basis of HIV-1 neutralization by affinity matured Fabs directed against the internal trimeric coiled-coil of gp41. PLoS Pathog. *6,* e1001182.

Gustchina, E., Louis, J.M., Lam, S.N., Bewley, C.A., and Clore, G.M. (2007). A monoclonal Fab derived from a human nonimmune phage library reveals a new epitope on gp41 and neutralizes diverse HIV-1 strains. J. Virol. *81,* 12946-12953.

Hager-Braun, C., and Tomer, K.B. (2005). Determination of protein-derived epitopes by mass spectrometry. Expert Rev. Proteomics *2,* 745-756.

Hallenberger, S., Bosch, V., Angliker, H., Shaw, E., Klenk, H.D., and Garten, W. (1992). Inhibition of furin-mediated cleavage activation of HIV-1 glycoprotein gp160. Nature *360,* 358-361.

Harouse, J.M., Collman, R.G., and Gonzalez-Scarano, F. (1995). HIV-1 infection of SK-N-MC cells: domains of gp120 involved in entry into a CD4-negative, galactosyl ceramide/3' sulfo-galactosyl ceramide-positive cell line. J. Virol. *69,* 7383-7390.

Hartley, O., Klasse, P.J., Sattentau, Q.J., and Moore, J.P. (2005). V3: HIV's switch-hitter. AIDS Res. Hum. Retroviruses *21,* 171-189.

Haynes, B.F., Fleming, J., St Clair, E.W., Katinger, H., Stiegler, G., Kunert, R., Robinson, J., Scearce, R.M., Plonk, K., Staats, H.F., *et al.* (2005). Cardiolipin polyspecific autoreactivity in two broadly neutralizing HIV-1 antibodies. Science *308,* 1906-1908.

Haynes, B.F., and Montefiori, D.C. (2006). Aiming to induce broadly reactive neutralizing antibody responses with HIV-1 vaccine candidates. Expert Rev. Vaccines *5,* 579-595.

Haynes, B.F., Moody, M.A., Verkoczy, L., Kelsoe, G., and Alam, S.M. (2005). Antibody polyspecificity and neutralization of HIV-1: a hypothesis. Hum. Antibodies *14,* 59-67.

Hessell, A.J., Hangartner, L., Hunter, M., Havenith, C.E., Beurskens, F.J., Bakker, J.M., Lanigan, C.M., Landucci, G., Forthal, D.N., Parren, P.W., Marx, P.A., and Burton, D.R. (2007). Fc receptor but not complement binding is important in antibody protection against HIV. Nature *449,* 101-104.

Hessell, A.J., Poignard, P., Hunter, M., Hangartner, L., Tehrani, D.M., Bleeker, W.K., Parren, P.W., Marx, P.A., and Burton, D.R. (2009a). Effective, low-titer antibody protection against low-dose repeated mucosal SHIV challenge in macaques. Nat. Med. *15,* 951-954.

Hessell, A.J., Rakasz, E.G., Poignard, P., Hangartner, L., Landucci, G., Forthal, D.N., Koff, W.C., Watkins, D.I., and Burton, D.R. (2009b). Broadly neutralizing human anti-HIV antibody 2G12 is effective in protection against mucosal SHIV challenge even at low serum neutralizing titers. PLoS Pathog. *5,* e1000433.

Hollier, M.J., and Dimmock, N.J. (2005). The C-terminal tail of the gp41 transmembrane envelope glycoprotein of HIV-1 clades A, B, C, and D may exist in two conformations: an analysis of sequence, structure, and function. Virology *337,* 284-296.

Huang, C.C., Tang, M., Zhang, M.Y., Majeed, S., Montabana, E., Stanfield, R.L., Dimitrov, D.S., Korber, B., Sodroski, J., Wilson, I.A., Wyatt, R., and Kwong, P.D. (2005). Structure of a V3-containing HIV-1 gp120 core. Science *310,* 1025-1028.

Huskens, D., Van Laethem, K., Vermeire, K., Balzarini, J., and Schols, D. (2007). Resistance of HIV-1 to the broadly HIV-1-neutralizing, anti-carbohydrate antibody 2G12. Virology *360,* 294-304.

Johnson, W.E., Sauvron, J.M., and Desrosiers, R.C. (2001). Conserved, N-linked carbohydrates of HIV-1 gp41 are largely dispensable for viral replication. J. Virol. *75,* 11426-11436.

Joos, B., Trkola, A., Kuster, H., Aceto, L., Fischer, M., Stiegler, G., Armbruster, C., Vcelar, B., Katinger, H., and Gunthard, H.F. (2006). Long-term multiple-dose pharmacokinetics of human monoclonal antibodies (MAbs) against HIV-1 envelope gp120 (MAb 2G12) and gp41 (MAbs 4E10 and 2F5). Antimicrob. Agents Chemother. *50,* 1773-1779.

Kamath, S., and Wong, T.C. (2002). Membrane structure of the HIVgp41 fusion domain by molecular dynamics simulation. Biophys. J. *83,* 135-143.

Karlsson Hedestam, G.B., Fouchier, R.A., Phogat, S., Burton, D.R., Sodroski, J., and Wyatt, R.T. (2008). The challenges of eliciting neutralizing antibodies to HIV-1 and to influenza virus. Nat. Rev. Microbiol. *6,* 143-155.

Keele, B.F., Giorgi, E.E., Salazar-Gonzalez, J.F., Decker, J.M., Pham, K.T., Salazar, M.G., Sun, C., Grayson, T., Wang, S., Li, H., *et al.* (2008). Identification and characterization of transmitted and early founder virus envelopes in primary HIV-1 infection. Proc. Natl. Acad. Sci. U. S. A. *105,* 7552-7557.

Kennedy, R.C., Henkel, R.D., Pauletti, D., Allan, J.S., Lee, T.H., Essex, M., and Dreesman, G.R. (1986). Antiserum to a synthetic peptide recognizes the HTLV-III envelope glycoprotein. Science *231,* 1556-1559.

Kim, M., Qiao, Z., Yu, J., Montefiori, D., and Reinherz, E.L. (2007). Immunogenicity of recombinant HIV-1-like particles expressing gp41 derivatives in a pre-fusion state. Vaccine *25,* 5102-5114.

Klatzmann, D., Champagne, E., Chamaret, S., Gruest, J., Guetard, D., Hercend, T., Gluckman, J.C., and Montagnier, L. (1984). T-lymphocyte T4 molecule behaves as the receptor for human retrovirus LAV. Nature *312,* 767-768.

Kwong, P.D., Doyle, M.L., Casper, D.J., Cicala, C., Leavitt, S.A., Majeed, S., Steenbeke, T.D., Venturi, M., Chaiken, I., Fung, M., *et al.* (2002). HIV-1 evades antibody-mediated neutralization through conformational masking of receptor-binding sites. Nature *420,* 678-682.

Kwong, P.D., Wyatt, R., Robinson, J., Sweet, R.W., Sodroski, J., and Hendrickson, W.A. (1998). Structure of an HIV gp120 envelope glycoprotein in complex with the CD4 receptor and a neutralizing human antibody. Nature *393,* 648-659.

Li, B., Decker, J.M., Johnson, R.W., Bibollet-Ruche, F., Wei, X., Mulenga, J., Allen, S., Hunter, E., Hahn, B.H., Shaw, G.M., Blackwell, J.L., and Derdeyn, C.A. (2006). Evidence for potent autologous neutralizing antibody titers and compact envelopes in early infection with subtype C HIV-1. J. Virol. *80,* 5211-5218.

Lin, G., Bertolotti-Ciarlet, A., Haggarty, B., Romano, J., Nolan, K.M., Leslie, G.J., Jordan, A.P., Huang, C.C., Kwong, P.D., Doms, R.W., and Hoxie, J.A. (2007). Replication-competent variants of HIV-2 lacking the V3 loop exhibit resistance to chemokine receptor antagonists. J. Virol. *81,* 9956-9966.

Liu, S., Lu, H., Niu, J., Xu, Y., Wu, S., and Jiang, S. (2005). Different from the HIV fusion inhibitor C34, the anti-HIV drug Fuzeon (T-20) inhibits HIV-1 entry by targeting multiple sites in gp41 and gp120. J. Biol. Chem. *280,* 11259-11273.

Long, D., Berson, J.F., Cook, D.G., and Doms, R.W. (1994). Characterization of HIV-1 gp120 binding to liposomes containing galactosylceramide. J. Virol. *68,* 5890-5898.

Lorizate, M., Cruz, A., Huarte, N., Kunert, R., Perez-Gil, J., and Nieva, J.L. (2006). Recognition and blocking of HIV-1 gp41 pre-transmembrane sequence by monoclonal 4E10 antibody in a Raft-like membrane environment. J. Biol. Chem. *281,* 39598-39606.

Louis, J.M., Nesheiwat, I., Chang, L., Clore, G.M., and Bewley, C.A. (2003). Covalent trimers of the internal N-terminal trimeric coiled-coil of gp41 and antibodies directed against them are potent inhibitors of HIV envelope-mediated cell fusion. J. Biol. Chem. *278,* 20278-20285.

Lu, M., Blacklow, S.C., and Kim, P.S. (1995). A trimeric structural domain of the HIV-1 transmembrane glycoprotein. Nat. Struct. Biol. *2,* 1075-1082.

Luftig, M.A., Mattu, M., Di Giovine, P., Geleziunas, R., Hrin, R., Barbato, G., Bianchi, E., Miller, M.D., Pessi, A., and Carfi, A. (2006). Structural basis for HIV-1 neutralization by a gp41 fusion intermediate-directed antibody. Nat. Struct. Mol. Biol. *13,* 740-747.

Markosyan, R.M., Leung, M.Y., and Cohen, F.S. (2009). The six-helix bundle of HIVEnv controls pore formation and enlargement and is initiated at residues proximal to the hairpin turn. J. Virol. *83,* 10048-10057.

Mascola, J.R. (2002). Passive transfer studies to elucidate the role of antibody-mediated protection against HIV-1. Vaccine *20,* 1922-1925.

Mascola, J.R., Frankel, S.S., and Broliden, K. (2000). HIV-1 entry at the mucosal surface: role of antibodies in protection. AIDS *14 Suppl 3,* S167-74.

Mascola, J.R., and Montefiori, D.C. (2010). The role of antibodies in HIV vaccines. Annu. Rev. Immunol. *28,* 413-444.

McInerney, T.L., Brennan, F.R., Jones, T.D., and Dimmock, N.J. (1999). Analysis of the ability of five adjuvants to enhance immune responses to a chimeric plant virus displaying an HIV-1 peptide. Vaccine *17,* 1359-1368.

McLain, L., Brown, J.L., Cheung, L., Reading, S.A., Parry, C., Jones, T.D., Cleveland, S.M., and Dimmock, N.J. (2001). Different effects of a single amino acid substitution on three adjacent epitopes in the gp41 C-terminal tail of a neutralizing antibody escape mutant of HIV-1. Arch. Virol. *146,* 157-166.

Miller, M.D., Geleziunas, R., Bianchi, E., Lennard, S., Hrin, R., Zhang, H., Lu, M., An, Z., Ingallinella, P., Finotto, M., *et al.* (2005). A human monoclonal antibody neutralizes diverse HIV-1 isolates by binding a critical gp41 epitope. Proc. Natl. Acad. Sci. U. S. A. *102,* 14759-14764.

Miyauchi, K., Curran, A.R., Long, Y., Kondo, N., Iwamoto, A., Engelman, D.M., and Matsuda, Z. (2010). The membrane-spanning domain of gp41 plays a critical role in intracellular trafficking of the HIV envelope protein. Retrovirology *7,* 95.

Montefiori, D.C., and Mascola, J.R. (2009). Neutralizing antibodies against HIV-1: can we elicit them with vaccinesand how much do we need? Curr. Opin. HIV. AIDS. *4,* 347-351.

Montero, M., van Houten, N.E., Wang, X., and Scott, J.K. (2008). The membrane-proximal external region of the HIV-1 envelope: dominant site of antibody neutralization and target for vaccine design. Microbiol. Mol. Biol. Rev. *72,* 54-84, table of contents.

Moulard, M., and Decroly, E. (2000). Maturation of HIV envelope glycoprotein precursors by cellular endoproteases. Biochim. Biophys. Acta *1469,* 121-132.

Muhlbacher, M., Spruth, M., Siegel, F., Zangerle, R., and Dierich, M.P. (1999). Longitudinal study of antibody reactivity against HIV-1 envelope and a peptide representing a conserved site on Gp41 in HIV-1-infected patients. Immunobiology *200,* 295-305.

Munoz-Barroso, I., Durell, S., Sakaguchi, K., Appella, E., and Blumenthal, R. (1998). Dilation of the HIV-1 envelope glycoprotein fusion pore revealed by the inhibitory action of a synthetic peptide from gp41. J. Cell Biol. *140,* 315-323.

Munoz-Barroso, I., Salzwedel, K., Hunter, E., and Blumenthal, R. (1999). Role of the membrane-proximal domain in the initial stages of HIV-1 envelope glycoprotein-mediated membrane fusion. J. Virol. *73,* 6089-6092.

Myszka, D.G., Sweet, R.W., Hensley, P., Brigham-Burke, M., Kwong, P.D., Hendrickson, W.A., Wyatt, R., Sodroski, J., and Doyle, M.L. (2000). Energetics of the HIV gp120-CD4 binding reaction. Proc. Natl. Acad. Sci. U. S. A. *97,* 9026-9031.

Nawaz, F., Cicala, C., Van Ryk, D., Block, K.E., Jelicic, K., McNally, J.P., Ogundare, O., Pascuccio, M., Patel, N., Wei, D., Fauci, A.S., and Arthos, J. (2011). The Genotype of Early-Transmitting HIV gp120s Promotes alpha(4)beta(7) -Reactivity, Revealing alpha(4)beta(7)/CD4 T cells As Key Targets in Mucosal Transmission. PLoS Pathog. *7,* e1001301.

Nehete, P.N., Vela, E.M., Hossain, M.M., Sarkar, A.K., Yahi, N., Fantini, J., and Sastry, K.J. (2002). A post-CD4-binding step involving interaction of the V3 region of viral gp120 with host cell surface glycosphingolipids is common to entry and infection by diverse HIV-1 strains. Antiviral Res. *56,* 233-251.

Nelson, J.D., Brunel, F.M., Jensen, R., Crooks, E.T., Cardoso, R.M., Wang, M., Hessell, A., Wilson, I.A., Binley, J.M., Dawson, P.E., Burton, D.R., and Zwick, M.B. (2007). An affinity-enhanced neutralizing antibody against the membrane-proximal external region of HIV-1 gp41 recognizes an epitope between those of 2F5 and 4E10. J. Virol. *81,* 4033-4043.

Nelson, J.D., Kinkead, H., Brunel, F.M., Leaman, D., Jensen, R., Louis, J.M., Maruyama, T., Bewley, C.A., Bowdish, K., Clore, G.M., *et al.* (2008). Antibody elicited against the gp41 N-heptad repeat (NHR) coiled-coil can neutralize HIV-1 with modest potency but non-neutralizing antibodies also bind to NHR mimetics. Virology *377,* 170-183.

Nguyen, D.G., and Hildreth, J.E. (2003). Involvement of macrophage mannose receptor in the binding and transmission of HIV by macrophages. Eur. J. Immunol. *33,* 483-493.

Nyambi, P.N., Mbah, H.A., Burda, S., Williams, C., Gorny, M.K., Nadas, A., and Zolla-Pazner, S. (2000). Conserved and exposed epitopes on intact, native, primary HIV-1 virions of group M. J. Virol. *74,* 7096-7107.

Ofek, G., Tang, M., Sambor, A., Katinger, H., Mascola, J.R., Wyatt, R., and Kwong, P.D. (2004). Structure and mechanistic analysis of the anti-HIV-1 antibody 2F5 in complex with its gp41 epitope. J. Virol. *78,* 10724-10737.

Opalka, D., Pessi, A., Bianchi, E., Ciliberto, G., Schleif, W., McElhaugh, M., Danzeisen, R., Geleziunas, R., Miller, M., Eckert, D.M., *et al.* (2004). Analysis of the HIV-1 gp41 specific immune response using a multiplexed antibody detection assay. J. Immunol. Methods *287,* 49-65.

Owens, R.J., Burke, C., and Rose, J.K. (1994). Mutations in the membrane-spanning domain of the HIV envelope glycoprotein that affect fusion activity. J. Virol. *68,* 570-574.

Palker, T.J., Matthews, T.J., Clark, M.E., Cianciolo, G.J., Randall, R.R., Langlois, A.J., White, G.C., Safai, B., Snyderman, R., and Bolognesi, D.P. (1987). A conserved region at the COOH terminus of HIVgp120 envelope protein contains an immunodominant epitope. Proc. Natl. Acad. Sci. U. S. A. *84,* 2479-2483.

Pan, C., Liu, S., and Jiang, S. (2010). HIV-1 gp41 fusion intermediate: a target for HIV therapeutics. J. Formos. Med. Assoc. *109,* 94-105.

Pancera, M. (2005).Structure, fonction et antigénicité des glycoprotéines d'enveloppe du virus de l'immunodéficience humaine de type 1 (VIH1). Virologie *9,* 457-472.

Pancera, M., Majeed, S., Ban, Y.E., Chen, L., Huang, C.C., Kong, L., Kwon, Y.D., Stuckey, J., Zhou, T., Robinson, J.E., *et al.* (2010). Structure of HIV-1 gp120 with gp41-interactive region reveals layered envelope architecture and basis of conformational mobility. Proc. Natl. Acad. Sci. U. S. A. *107,* 1166-1171.

Parker, C.E., Deterding, L.J., Hager-Braun, C., Binley, J.M., Schulke, N., Katinger, H., Moore, J.P., and Tomer, K.B. (2001). Fine definition of the epitope on the gp41 glycoprotein of HIV-1 for the neutralizing monoclonal antibody 2F5. J. Virol. *75,* 10906-10911.

Parsons, M.S., Rouleau, D., Routy, J.P., LeBlanc, R., Grant, M.D., and Bernard, N.F. (2011). Selection of human anti-HIV broadly neutralizing antibodies occurs within the context of frozen 1F7-idiotypic repertoire. AIDS *25,* 1249-1264

Phogat, S., and Wyatt, R. (2007). Rational modifications of HIV-1 envelope glycoproteins for immunogen design. Curr. Pharm. Des. *13,* 213-227.

Phogat, S., Wyatt, R.T., and Karlsson Hedestam, G.B. (2007). Inhibition of HIV-1 entry by antibodies: potential viral and cellular targets. J. Intern. Med. *262,* 26-43.

Pietzsch, J., Scheid, J.F., Mouquet, H., Klein, F., Seaman, M.S., Jankovic, M., Corti, D., Lanzavecchia, A., and Nussenzweig, M.C. (2010). Human anti-HIV-neutralizing antibodies frequently target a conserved epitope essential for viral fitness. J. Exp. Med. *207,* 1995-2002.

Pollakis, G., Kang, S., Kliphuis, A., Chalaby, M.I., Goudsmit, J., and Paxton, W.A. (2001). N-linked glycosylation of the HIV type-1 gp120 envelope glycoprotein as a major determinant of CCR5 and CXCR4 coreceptor utilization. J. Biol. Chem. *276,* 13433-13441.

Poumbourios, P., McPhee, D.A., and Kemp, B.E. (1992). Antibody epitopes sensitive to the state of HIV-1 gp41 oligomerization map to a putative alpha-helical region. AIDS Res. Hum. Retroviruses *8,* 2055-2062.

Pritsker, M., Rucker, J., Hoffman, T.L., Doms, R.W., and Shai, Y. (1999). Effect of nonpolar substitutions of the conserved Phe11 in the fusion peptide of HIV-1 gp41 on its function, structure, and organization in membranes. Biochemistry *38,* 11359-11371.

Qiang, W., Sun, Y., and Weliky, D.P. (2009). A strong correlation between fusogenicity and membrane insertion depth of the HIV fusion peptide. Proc. Natl. Acad. Sci. U. S. A. *106,* 15314-15319.

Reading, S.A., Heap, C.J., and Dimmock, N.J. (2003). A novel monoclonal antibody specific to the C-terminal tail of the gp41 envelope transmembrane protein of HIV-1 that preferentially neutralizes virus after it has attached to the target cell and inhibits the production of infectious progeny. Virology *315,* 362-372.

Reeves, J.D., Lee, F.H., Miamidian, J.L., Jabara, C.B., Juntilla, M.M., and Doms, R.W. (2005). Enfuvirtide resistance mutations: impact on HIVenvelope function, entry inhibitor sensitivity, and virus neutralization. J. Virol. *79,* 4991-4999.

Richman, D.D., Wrin, T., Little, S.J., and Petropoulos, C.J. (2003). Rapid evolution of the neutralizing Ab response to HIV type 1 infection. Proc. Natl. Acad. Sci. U. S. A. *100,* 4144-4149.

Robinson, W.E.,Jr, Kawamura, T., Gorny, M.K., Lake, D., Xu, J.Y., Matsumoto, Y., Sugano, T., Masuho, Y., Mitchell, W.M., and Hersh, E. (1990). Human monoclonal antibodies to the HIV-1 (HIV-1) transmembrane glycoprotein gp41 enhance HIV-1 infection in vitro. Proc. Natl. Acad. Sci. U. S. A. *87,* 3185-3189.

Rosen, O., Chill, J., Sharon, M., Kessler, N., Mester, B., Zolla-Pazner, S., and Anglister, J. (2005). Induced fit in HIV-neutralizing antibody complexes: evidence for alternative conformations of the gp120 V3 loop and the molecular basis for broad neutralization. Biochemistry *44,* 7250-7258.

Roux, K.H., and Taylor, K.A. (2007). AIDS virus envelope spike structure. Curr. Opin. Struct. Biol. *17,* 244-252.

Saifuddin, M., Hart, M.L., Gewurz, H., Zhang, Y., and Spear, G.T. (2000). Interaction of mannose-binding lectin with primary isolates of HIV-1. J. Gen. Virol. *81,* 949-955.

Salzwedel, K., West, J.T., and Hunter, E. (1999). A conserved tryptophan-rich motif in the membrane-proximal region of the HIV-1 gp41 ectodomain is important for Env-mediated fusion and virus infectivity. J. Virol. *73,* 2469-2480.

Sattentau, Q.J., and McMichael, A.J. (2010). New templates for HIV-1 antibody-based vaccine design. F1000 Biol. Rep. *2,* 60.

Scanlan, C.N., Pantophlet, R., Wormald, M.R., Ollmann Saphire, E., Stanfield, R., Wilson, I.A., Katinger, H., Dwek, R.A., Rudd, P.M., and Burton, D.R. (2002). The broadly neutralizing anti-HIV-1 Ab 2G12 recognizes a cluster of alpha1-->2 mannose residues on the outer face of gp120. J. Virol. *76,* 7306-7321.

Scherer, E.M., Zwick, M.B., Teyton, L., and Burton, D.R. (2007). Difficulties in eliciting broadly neutralizing anti-HIV antibodies are not explained by cardiolipin autoreactivity. AIDS *21,* 2131-2139.

Schief, W.R., Ban, Y.E., and Stamatatos, L. (2009). Challenges for structure-based HIV vaccine design. Curr. Opin. HIV. AIDS. *4,* 431-440.

Selvarajah, S., Puffer, B., Pantophlet, R., Law, M., Doms, R.W., and Burton, D.R. (2005). Comparing antigenicity and immunogenicity of engineered gp120. J. Virol. *79,* 12148-12163.

Selvarajah, S., Puffer, B.A., Lee, F.H., Zhu, P., Li, Y., Wyatt, R., Roux, K.H., Doms, R.W., and Burton, D.R. (2008). Focused dampening of Ab response to the immunodominant variable loops by engineered soluble gp140. AIDS Res. Hum. Retroviruses *24,* 301-314.

Shang, L., Yue, L., and Hunter, E. (2008). Role of the membrane-spanning domain of HIV-1 envelope glycoprotein in cell-cell fusion and virus infection. J. Virol. *82,* 5417-5428.

Shnaper, S., Sackett, K., Gallo, S.A., Blumenthal, R., and Shai, Y. (2004). The C- and the N-terminal regions of glycoprotein 41 ectodomain fuse membranes enriched and not enriched with cholesterol, respectively. J. Biol. Chem. *279,* 18526-18534.

Simons, K., and Ikonen, E. (1997). Functional rafts in cell membranes. Nature *387,* 569-572.

Song, L., Sun, Z.Y., Coleman, K.E., Zwick, M.B., Gach, J.S., Wang, J.H., Reinherz, E.L., Wagner, G., and Kim, M. (2009). Broadly neutralizing anti-HIV-1 antibodies disrupt a hinge-related function of gp41 at the membrane interface. Proc. Natl. Acad. Sci. U. S. A. *106,* 9057-9062.

Sougrat, R., Bartesaghi, A., Lifson, J.D., Bennett, A.E., Bess, J.W., Zabransky, D.J., and Subramaniam, S. (2007). Electron tomography of the contact between T cells and SIV/HIV-1: implications for viral entry. PLoS Pathog. *3,* e63.

Stamatatos, L., Morris, L., Burton, D.R., and Mascola, J.R. (2009). Neutralizing antibodies generated during natural HIV-1 infection: good news for an HIV-1 vaccine? Nat. Med. *15,* 866-870.

Stanfield, R.L., Gorny, M.K., Williams, C., Zolla-Pazner, S., and Wilson, I.A. (2004). Structural rationale for the broad neutralization of HIV-1 by human monoclonal Ab 447-52D. Structure *12,* 193-204.

Steckbeck, J.D., Sun, C., Sturgeon, T.J., and Montelaro, R.C. (2010). Topology of the C-terminal tail of HIV-1 gp41: differential exposure of the Kennedy epitope on cell and viral membranes. PLoS One *5,* e15261.

Sterjovski, J., Churchill, M.J., Roche, M., Ellett, A., Farrugia, W., Wesselingh, S.L., Cunningham, A.L., Ramsland, P.A., and Gorry, P.R. (2011). CD4-binding site alterations in CCR5-using HIV-1 envelopes influencing gp120-CD4 interactions and fusogenicity. Virology *410,* 418-428.

Stiegler, G., Kunert, R., Purtscher, M., Wolbank, S., Voglauer, R., Steindl, F., and Katinger, H. (2001). A potent cross-clade neutralizing human monoclonal Ab against a novel epitope on gp41 of HIV-1. AIDS Res. Hum. Retroviruses *17,* 1757-1765.

Sun, Z.Y., Oh, K.J., Kim, M., Yu, J., Brusic, V., Song, L., Qiao, Z., Wang, J.H., Wagner, G., and Reinherz, E.L. (2008). HIV-1 broadly neutralizing Ab extracts its epitope from a kinked gp41 ectodomain region on the viral membrane. Immunity *28,* 52-63.

Tachibana, M., Siddiqi, M.A., Ikegami, Y., Eshima, K., Shirota-Someya, Y., Tahara-Hanaoka, S., Koito, A., Iizuka, M., and Shinohara, N. (2000). Coreceptor function of mutant human CD4 molecules without affinity to gp120 of human immunodeficiency virus. J. Biol. Chem. *275,* 20288-20294.

Teixeira, C., Gomes, J.R., Gomes, P., and Maurel, F. (2011). Viral surface glycoproteins, gp120 and gp41, as potential drug targets against HIV-1: Brief overview one quarter of a century past the approval of zidovudine, the first anti-retroviral drug. Eur. J. Med. Chem. *46,* 979-992.

Tian, Y., Ramesh, C.V., Ma, X., Naqvi, S., Patel, T., Cenizal, T., Tiscione, M., Diaz, K., Crea, T., Arnold, E., Arnold, G.F., and Taylor, J.W. (2002). Structure-affinity relationships in the gp41 ELDKWA epitope for the HIV-1 neutralizing monoclonal Ab 2F5: effects of side-chain and backbone modifications and conformational constraints. J. Pept. Res. *59,* 264-276.

Trkola, A., Pomales, A.B., Yuan, H., Korber, B., Maddon, P.J., Allaway, G.P., Katinger, H., Barbas, C.F.,3rd, Burton, D.R., and Ho, D.D. (1995). Cross-clade neutralization of primary isolates of HIV-1 by human monoclonal antibodies and tetrameric CD4-IgG. J. Virol. *69,* 6609-6617.

Trkola, A., Purtscher, M., Muster, T., Ballaun, C., Buchacher, A., Sullivan, N., Srinivasan, K., Sodroski, J., Moore, J.P., and Katinger, H. (1996). Human monoclonal Ab 2G12 defines a distinctive neutralization epitope on the gp120 glycoprotein of HIV-1. J. Virol. *70,* 1100-1108.

Turville, S.G., Cameron, P.U., Handley, A., Lin, G., Pohlmann, S., Doms, R.W., and Cunningham, A.L. (2002). Diversity of receptors binding HIV on dendritic cell subsets. Nat. Immunol. *3,* 975-983.

Valladeau, J., Ravel, O., Dezutter-Dambuyant, C., Moore, K., Kleijmeer, M., Liu, Y., Duvert-Frances, V., Vincent, C., Schmitt, D., Davoust, J., *et al.* (2000). Langerin, a novel C-type lectin specific to Langerhans cells, is an endocytic receptor that induces the formation of Birbeck granules. Immunity *12,* 71-81.

van der Goot, F.G., and Harder, T. (2001). Raft membrane domains: from a liquid-ordered membrane phase to a site of pathogen attack. Semin. Immunol. *13,* 89-97.

Vanlandschoot, P., Beirnaert, E., Barrere, B., Calder, L., Millar, B., Wharton, S., Jou, W.M., and Fiers, W. (1998). An Ab which binds to the membrane-proximal end of influenza virus haemagglutinin (H3 subtype) inhibits the low-pH-induced conformational change and cell-cell fusion but does not neutralize virus. J. Gen. Virol. *79,* 1781-1791.

Veiga, A.S., and Castanho, M.A. (2007). The influence of cholesterol on the interaction of HIV gp41 membrane proximal region-derived peptides with lipid bilayers. FEBS J. *274,* 5096-5104.

Veiga, A.S., and Castanho, M.A. (2006). The membranes' role in the HIV-1 neutralizing monoclonal Ab 2F5 mode of action needs re-evaluation. Antiviral Res. *71,* 69-72.

Vella, C., Ferguson, M., Dunn, G., Meloen, R., Langedijk, H., Evans, D., and Minor, P.D. (1993). Characterization and primary structure of a HIV-1 (HIV-1) neutralization domain as presented by a poliovirus type 1/HIV-1 chimera. J. Gen. Virol. *74 (Pt 12),* 2603-2607.

Verkoczy, L., Diaz, M., Holl, T.M., Ouyang, Y.B., Bouton-Verville, H., Alam, S.M., Liao, H.X., Kelsoe, G., and Haynes, B.F. (2010). Autoreactivity in an HIV-1 broadly reactive neutralizing Ab variable region heavy chain induces immunologic tolerance. Proc. Natl. Acad. Sci. U. S. A. *107,* 181-186.

Veronese, F.D., DeVico, A.L., Copeland, T.D., Oroszlan, S., Gallo, R.C., and Sarngadharan, M.G. (1985). Characterization of gp41 as the transmembrane protein coded by the HTLV-III/LAV envelope gene. Science *229,* 1402-1405.

Viard, M., Ablan, S.D., Zhou, M., Veenstra, T.D., Freed, E.O., Raviv, Y., and Blumenthal, R. (2008). Photoinduced reactivity of the HIV-1 envelope glycoprotein with a membrane-embedded probe reveals insertion of portions of the HIV-1 Gp41 cytoplasmic tail into the viral membrane. Biochemistry *47,* 1977-1983.

Vincent, N., Kone, A., Chanut, B., Lucht, F., Genin, C., and Malvoisin, E. (2008). Antibodies purified from sera of HIV-1-infected patients by affinity on the heptad repeat region 1/heptad repeat region 2 complex of gp41 neutralize HIV-1 primary isolates. AIDS *22,* 2075-2085.

Vincent, N., Malvoisin, E., Pozzetto, B., Lucht, F., and Genin, C. (2004). Detection of IgA inhibiting the interaction between gp120 and soluble CD4 receptor in serum and saliva of HIV-1-infected patients. AIDS *18,* 37-43.

von Andrian, U.H., and Mackay, C.R. (2000). T-cell function and migration. Two sides of the same coin. N. Engl. J. Med. *343,* 1020-1034.

Walker, L.M., and Burton, D.R. (2010). Rational Ab-based HIV-1 vaccine design: current approaches and future directions. Curr. Opin. Immunol. *22,* 358-366.

Walker, L.M., Phogat, S.K., Chan-Hui, P.Y., Wagner, D., Phung, P., Goss, J.L., Wrin, T., Simek, M.D., Fling, S., Mitcham, J.L., *et al.* (2009). Broad and potent neutralizing Abs from an African donor reveal a new HIV-1 vaccine target. Science *326,* 285-289.

Watkins, J.D., Siddappa, N.B., Lakhashe, S.K., Humbert, M., Sholukh, A., Hemashettar, G., Wong, Y.L., Yoon, J.K., Wang, W., Novembre, F.J., *et al.* (2011). An Anti-HIV-1 V3 Loop Ab Fully Protects Cross-Clade and Elicits T-Cell Immunity in Macaques Mucosally Challenged with an R5 Clade C SHIV. PLoS One *6,* e18207.

Wei, X., Decker, J.M., Wang, S., Hui, H., Kappes, J.C., Wu, X., Salazar-Gonzalez, J.F., Salazar, M.G., Kilby, J.M., Saag, M.S., *et al.* (2003). Antibody neutralization and escape by HIV-1. Nature *422,* 307-312.

Weis, W.I., Taylor, M.E., and Drickamer, K. (1998). The C-type lectin superfamily in the immune system. Immunol. Rev. *163,* 19-34.

Weiss, R.A. (2003). HIV and AIDS: looking ahead. Nat. Med. *9*, 887-891.

Wen, M., Arora, R., Wang, H., Liu, L., Kimata, J.T., and Zhou, P. (2010). GPI-anchored single chain Fv--an effective way to capture transiently-exposed neutralization epitopes on HIV-1 envelope spike. Retrovirology *7*, 79.

Wu, X., Yang, Z.Y., Li, Y., Hogerkorp, C.M., Schief, W.R., Seaman, M.S., Zhou, T., Schmidt, S.D., Wu, L., Xu, L., *et al.* (2010). Rational design of envelope identifies broadly neutralizing human monoclonal antibodies to HIV-1. Science *329*, 856-861.

Wyss, S., Dimitrov, A.S., Baribaud, F., Edwards, T.G., Blumenthal, R., and Hoxie, J.A. (2005). Regulation of HIV-1 envelope glycoprotein fusion by a membrane-interactive domain in the gp41 cytoplasmic tail. J. Virol. *79*, 12231-12241.

Yang, P., Ai, L.S., Huang, S.C., Li, H.F., Chan, W.E., Chang, C.W., Ko, C.Y., and Chen, S.S. (2010). The cytoplasmic domain of HIV-1 transmembrane protein gp41 harbors lipid raft association determinants. J. Virol. *84*, 59-75.

Yu, X., Yuan, X., McLane, M.F., Lee, T.H., and Essex, M. (1993). Mutations in the cytoplasmic domain of HIV-1 transmembrane protein impair the incorporation of Env proteins into mature virions. J. Virol. *67*, 213-221.

Yue, L., Shang, L., and Hunter, E. (2009). Truncation of the membrane-spanning domain of HIV-1 envelope glycoprotein defines elements required for fusion, incorporation, and infectivity. J. Virol. *83*, 11588-11598.

Zanetti, G., Briggs, J.A., Grunewald, K., Sattentau, Q.J., and Fuller, S.D. (2006). Cryo-electron tomographic structure of an immunodeficiency virus envelope complex in situ. PLoS Pathog. *2*, e83.

Zheng, Z., Yang, R., Bodner, M.L., and Weliky, D.P. (2006). Conformational flexibility and strand arrangements of the membrane-associated HIV fusion peptide trimer probed by solid-state NMR spectroscopy. Biochemistry *45*, 12960-12975.

Zhou, T., Georgiev, I., Wu, X., Yang, Z.Y., Dai, K., Finzi, A., Kwon, Y.D., Scheid, J.F., Shi, W., Xu, L., *et al.* (2010). Structural basis for broad and potent neutralization of HIV-1 by antibody VRC01. Science *329*, 811-817.

Zhou, T., Xu, L., Dey, B., Hessell, A.J., Van Ryk, D., Xiang, S.H., Yang, X., Zhang, M.Y., Zwick, M.B., Arthos, J., *et al.* (2007). Structural definition of a conserved neutralization epitope on HIV-1 gp120. Nature *445*, 732-737.

Zhu, P., Liu, J., Bess, J.,Jr, Chertova, E., Lifson, J.D., Grise, H., Ofek, G.A., Taylor, K.A., and Roux, K.H. (2006). Distribution and three-dimensional structure of AIDS virus envelope spikes. Nature *441*, 847-852.

Zolla-Pazner, S., and Cardozo, T. (2010). Structure-function relationships of HIV-1 envelope sequence-variable regions refocus vaccine design. Nat. Rev. Immunol. *10*, 527-535.

Zwick, M.B., and Burton, D.R. (2007). HIV-1 neutralization: mechanisms and relevance to vaccine design. Curr. HIV. Res. *5*, 608-624.

Zwick, M.B., Jensen, R., Church, S., Wang, M., Stiegler, G., Kunert, R., Katinger, H., and Burton, D.R. (2005). Anti-HIV-1 (HIV-1) antibodies 2F5 and 4E10 require surprisingly few crucial residues in the membrane-proximal external region of glycoprotein gp41 to neutralize HIV-1. J. Virol. *79*, 1252-1261.

Zwick, M.B., Labrijn, A.F., Wang, M., Spenlehauer, C., Saphire, E.O., Binley, J.M., Moore, J.P., Stiegler, G., Katinger, H., Burton, D.R., and Parren, P.W. (2001). Broadly neutralizing antibodies targeted to the membrane-proximal external region of HIV-1 glycoprotein gp41. J. Virol. *75*, 10892-10905.

Zwick, M.B., Parren, P.W., Saphire, E.O., Church, S., Wang, M., Scott, J.K., Dawson, P.E., Wilson, I.A., and Burton, D.R. (2003). Molecular features of the broadly neutralizing immunoglobulin G1 b12 required for recognition of HIV-1 gp120. J. Virol. *77*, 5863-5876.

2

Characterisation, Evaluation and Clinical Significance of Latent HIV-1 Reservoirs and Therapeutic Strategies for HIV Eradication

James Williams[1], Sarah Fidler[2] and John Frater[1,3]
[1]*Peter Medawar Building for Pathogen Research, Nuffield Department of Medicine, University of Oxford, Oxford*
[2]*Division of Medicine, Wright Fleming Institute, Imperial College, St. Mary's Hospital, Norfolk Place, Paddington, London, United Kingdom*
[3]*Oxford NIHR Comprehensive Biomedical Research Centre, Oxford United Kingdom*

1. Introduction

HIV induces persistent infection and, despite improvements in mortality and morbidity conferred by Highly Active Antiretroviral Therapy (HAART), there is currently no cure [1]. The immune system controls HIV only partially, and plasma HIV and proviral DNA can be detected from acute primary infection to end-stage AIDS [2]. More than 99% of HIV replication has been demonstrated in activated and infected CD4+ T-cells [3]. These are the very cells that are instrumental in the clearance of virus through the host's adaptive immune response. Gradually, throughout the course of infection, repeated rounds of CD4+ T cell infection lead to an overall and marked decrease in the total number of CD4+ T cells [4] and this has been linked to the clinical manifestations of HIV disease [5]. HIV-1 replicates rapidly in infected patients, with a virion half-life of less than 6 hours in plasma [6], and a half-life of 1-2 days in proliferating infected cells [7] [8] [9], corresponding to the short-lived population that produces most of the HIV-1

The major problem with eradication of HIV lies with the existence of a pool of latently infected cells. Retroviral latency occurs when a provirus infects and integrates into the genomic DNA of its target cell, but is transcriptionally silent [10]. These cells are able to persistently produce infectious HIV virions when activated, even from patients on highly active antiretroviral therapy (HAART), and are a potential source of rebounded virus after HAART treatment is interrupted [3]. There are myriad cells and tissue types in which HIV can integrate, and it is at these sites that the long-term preservation of replication-competent HIV can occur [11].

Infectious virus within HIV reservoirs has a longer half life than the virus in cells where there is active viral replication [12]. The half life of the viral reservoir has been estimated at 43.9 months during three years of HAART, [13] and 44.2 months whilst on seven years of HAART [14]. Thus, it had been estimated to take possibly as long as 60 years to eradicate the virus using HAART alone [13]. In other studies , the reservoir half life in patients with optimal suppression of viral replication was estimated to be as little as 6 months [15] [16].

HAART usually consists of a combination of at least three antiretroviral drugs, typically two nucleoside analogue reverse transcription inhibitors and a third drug, either a protease or non nucleoside reverse transcriptase inhibitor [17-18]. There are currently 22 licensed antiretroviral drugs [19] which fall into the following categories; Nucleoside reverse transcription inhibitors (NRTI), non-nucleoside reverse transcriptase inhibitors (NNRTI), protease, integrase, entry and maturation inhibitors. Antiretroviral drug therapy (ART) has led to a significant decline in morbidity and mortality in HIV-1 infected individuals in the developed world [20], with mortality in 1255 studied patients falling from 29.4 per 100 person-years in the first quarter of 1996 to 8.8 per 100 person years in the second quarter of 1997 [21]. In this study, Mycobacterium avium complex disease, and cytomegalovirus retinitis incidence declined from 21.9 per 100 person-years in 1994 to 3.7 per 100 person-years in mid-1997. The actual HAART regime was shown not to impact on residual viremia [22]

There is contradictory evidence supporting the use of HAART in early, or 'primary', HIV infection. In one study when HAART was initiated in patients during primary HIV infection, the formation of a latently infected CD4+ T-cell reservoir was not inhibited, despite the control of plasma HIV viremia levels [23]. However, in another study, 5/32 patients who received very early and prolonged (77 month) HAART exhibited sustained immuno-virological control of HIV, after treatment interruption. This subset of patients did not exhibit the genetic characteristics of elite controllers, so were termed 'post treatment controllers', a distinct population. The viral reservoir amongst the 'post treatment controllers' was very low and stable, suggesting that early therapy could cause a reduction in the viral reservoir [24], perhaps to a point where the immune system can control HIV infection without HAART. The rapid initiation of antiretroviral drugs after initial HIV infection was therefore hypothesised to prevent damage of the immune system and minimise the size of the latent reservoir [25].

However, despite HAART regimes having reduced the frequency of HIV-infected cells to fewer than 1 cell per 10^6 resting CD4+ T-cells [13-14, 26], when HAART is interrupted, in most cases, rapid viral rebound from the latent HIV reservoir still occurs [27]. The life expectancy of patients on HAART is still less than that for uninfected people [28]. There is also morbidity in patients on HAART that is not explained by drug toxicities, mostly due to cardiovascular and metabolic complications [29-30], as well as renal and hepatic toxicities, osteoporosis, dementia and ageing [31]. Also, the logistics of providing HAART to developing regions are currently extremely challenging [32]. Collectively, these data show that HAART mediated eradication of HIV is unlikely and that there is a real need for new therapies if the goal of HIV eradication is ever to be achieved.

2. HIV-I latency

Despite the wealth of experimental evidence to suggest that productive HIV-1 infection occurs in activated CD4+ T-cells [33], there are many points at which integration of HIV into the genome, and thus latency can be blocked. The presence of small nucleotide pools [34] coupled with an inability to import the pre-integration complex into the nucleus [35] results in inefficient reverse transcription of the HIV genome and a latent viral phenotype [36-37]. However, this pre-integration latency is a labile form of latency and rapidly decays on HAART, and is unlikely to contribute to residual or rebound virus [36, 38-39].

In post integration latency, HIV-1 must infect an activated CD4+ T-cell, so that efficient reverse transcription and nuclear import can occur, leading to the integration of HIV-DNA into the host genome. However, for a latent phenotype to emerge, the infected cell must then return to a quiescent (G0) or resting state. Generally, HIV-infected activated CD4+ T cells die due to the cytopathic effect of virus, or from host-mediated immune killing, however, some infected activated CD4+ T-cells may survive just long enough to revert to the resting state [40]. The fact that resting CD4+ T-cells were shown to contain integrated HIV provirus [41] supports this theory. Subtle differences in HIV integration sites between activated and resting CD4+ T-cells were discovered through 454-pyrosequencing, with insertion into actively transcribing gene sites most favoured, although in resting CD4+ T-cells, integrated DNA was more commonly found in regions suboptimal for the expression of proviral genes [42].

3. Characterisation and evaluation of HIV-1 reservoirs

When HAART is initiated, four plasma virus decay phases have been described. Firstly, there is an initial rapid decline in plasma virus, with a half-life of around 2 days [6, 8, 43-44]. Treatment with ABT-538, an HIV-1 protease inhibitor, caused an exponential decrease in plasma HIV-1, with an estimated half life of 2.1 +/- 0.4 days, and a substantial increase in CD4 lymphocyte counts [7]. This initial decline is thought to be due to the elimination of short-lived HIV-infected cells of the lymphocyte lineage, including activated CD4+ lymphocytes, due to the cytopathic effect of HIV, or through immune-mediated destruction [1]. A biphasic decay in plasma viremia was seen in 7 acute seroconverters who received HAART shortly after initial symptoms. The first phase was thought to reflect the loss of virus from productively infected cells and the second phase, loss of virus from latently infected cells [45]. However, many studies have shown that the HIV viral reservoir need not be restricted to that of the lymphocyte lineage and virus has been discovered in a vast array of different cell types, discussed later. The source of the virus contributing to the third and fourth phases is less clear, but may include macrophages, tissue sanctuary sites and sporadic activation of latently infected memory lymphocytes.

3.1 The resting CD4+ T-cell reservoir

A major HIV reservoir is thought to be latently infected resting memory CD4+ T-cells [26, 46]. Persistently infected resting CD4+ T-cells have been isolated from peripheral blood samples of HIV-infected patients whose HAART regimes resulted in very low plasma viremia levels [47]. Another study showed that the activation of CD4+ T-cells with anti-CD3 and anti-CD28 antibodies and depletion of CD8+ T-cells from six patients who maintained undetectable viral levels under HAART for 2 years, could release PBMC-derived replication-competent virus [48]. In a study of 22 successfully HAART treated patients, replication-competent virus was isolated from infected CD4+ T-cells, although the frequency of these latently infected cells was low - around 0.2 to 16.4 per 10^6 cells. While patients were on therapy, this reservoir of latently infected CD4+ T-cells was shown not to decline with time [46]. In another study, the CD4+ T-cells isolated from all 13 HAART-receiving patients with undetectable plasma viremia carried integrated proviral HIV-DNA, and on cellular activation, were shown to release viable virus [26]. This latent viral reservoir in memory T-cells was shown to be established very early in HIV infection [23] and the activation of these resting T cells by proinflammatory cytokines induced in vitro release of infectious HIV [49].

Replication-competent latent provirus has been mostly recovered from patients on suppressive HAART in resting (CD45RO) CD4+ T-cells, although low levels of virus have been discovered in resting naïve (CD45RA) CD4+ T-cells [10]. Since the infection of naïve T-cells is a rare event, most resting CD4+ T-cells will have been infected with HIV when they were in a prior activated state, suggesting that these infected activated CD4+ T-cells can revert back to a naïve state, conducive for HIV latency [50]. Thymocytes, a haematopoietic progenitor cell type found in the thymus of adults and children naturally develop into naïve T-cells in the T-lymphocyte developmental pathway, so the presence of proviral DNA in naïve T-cells could be explained by latently infected thymocytes developing into naïve T-cells, which still contain the latently infected proviral DNA [51].

A recent study has identified subsets of CD4+ T-cells as distinct reservoir locations. Central memory (TCM) and Transitional memory T cells (TTM) were found to constitute major HIV reservoirs. In patients who had started HAART early, the viral reservoir was located in the long-lived TCM cells. Cytotoxic T cell killing, apoptosis and cytopathic viral effects were hypothesised to reduce this reservoir, as TCM cells may be able to mount an antigen-induced response. However, in patients who started therapy late, the reservoir was mostly present in TTM cells, attributable to greater CD4+ T-cell proliferation. TTM cells have been shown to proliferate at low levels, through IL-7-induced mitosis and thus may be able to act as a continuously replenishing reservoir [52].

3.2 Macrophages, monocytes and partially activated T-cells

The second phase of decline in plasma virus levels on HAART [6] has an estimated half life in the range of 1-4 weeks, and is thought to represent virus present in infected macrophages and monocytes, which are known to be more resistant to the cytopathic effects of HIV infection [53-54] and which, once terminally differentiated, have a turnover rate of approximately two weeks [55]. Replication competent HIV has been isolated from peripheral blood monocytes of HAART-treated patients [53] and infected monocytes have been isolated from patients on effective HAART [56]. There is evidence for HIV replication in vivo in CD14+ monocytes [57], infectious HIV has been shown to assemble in late endosomes in primary macrophages [58], and virions persisting in monocyte-derived macrophages have been shown to retain infectivity for weeks [59], thus suggesting possible new mechanisms for HIV persistence. However, the theory that macrophages, monocytes or partially activated CD4+ T-cells could represent a separate source of virus is disputed, since in two studies using Raltegravir, an integrase inhibitor, no second phase decay kinetics on treatment were observed [60-61]. It is also possible that this second decay phase in plasma viremia levels could also reflect the destruction of other viral reservoirs, for example the release of virus after activation of partially activated T-lymphocytes [40].

By extrapolating the first and second phase decay kinetics, it was initially suggested that HAART alone may be able to eradicate virus from infected individuals, since virus levels could fall to below detectable levels after 2 months of therapy [44]. However, this prediction was based on the assumption that HAART completely inhibits all viral replication and that no viral reservoirs with a half life longer than a few days exist in infected patients [62]. Despite the initial thought that HIV could be eradicated with HAART [6], this has shown to be false extremely unlikely, since other reservoirs with longer half-lives have been detected.

3.3 Follicular dendritic cells

Follicular Dendritic cells (FDC) have been suggested to contribute to the second and third phase decay in plasma viremia, since infectious virus [63] binds through the viral envelope proteins to DC-SIGN receptors, expressed on the FDC cell surface [64]. This more prolonged third decay phase has been estimated to have a half-life of around six months [43, 65], although a half-life of 30 months during HAART was estimated in another study [66], and mathematical modelling studies have shown HIV:FDC interactions to persist for years, despite effective HAART [67]. Through phylogenetic analysis of the HIV that interacts with FDCs isolated from 2 out of 4 patients, the virus present was similar to the virus isolated 22 months earlier, which suggests long-term FDC sequestration of replication-competent HIV [68]. However, other studies have shown DC-SIGN being unable to protect against virion degradation, since loss of HIV infectivity was reported over a course of hours [69].

3.4 Other HIV reservoirs

3.4.1 Gut - Associated Lymphoid Tissue (GALT)

There is evidence for the presence of HIV-1 DNA and RNA in the duodenum, ileum, colon and rectum, from gut biopsy studies. The concentration of HIV-1 DNA increases from duodenum to rectum [70] and there is evidence for ongoing residual HIV replication in the ileum [71]. Mucosal lymphoid tissues may be an important reservoir outside of the peripheral blood for residual HIV viremia whilst patients are on HAART, since the GALT contains the highest level of activated CD4+ T-cells, which can support HIV replication [72]. In SIV infection, the gastrointestinal (GI) tract was shown to be a major site of CD4+ T-cell depletion and viral replication [73], and viral replication was found to be disproportionally higher in the GALT than in the blood [74]. Rapid accumulation and early establishment of HIV-1 in the lymphatic system has also been observed after HIV infection [75].

3.4.2 CD34+ multipotent hematopoietic progenitor cells

CD34+ multipotent haematopoietic progenitor cells have shown to be permissive to HIV infection, but it is not know whether a latent phenotype can emerge or whether this potential reservoir can contribute to persistent viremia seen in patients on HAART [76]. Since HIV-infected monocytes were discovered in HAART treated patients, and since their short halflife in the blood, this could also be evidence that monocyte precursor cells were infected [56].

3.4.3 Mast cells

Mast cells from human tissue have been shown to be an inducible reservoir of persistent HIV infection [77].

3.4.4 Urogenital tract

Through the longitudinal analysis of gp120 in five acute HIV seroconverters, it was discovered that the HIV populations present in genital secretions were different to that extracted from blood plasma. This indicated that the male urogenital tract could act as a separate reservoir to resting CD4+ T-cells [78]. HIV has also been found in seminal fluid, T cells and macrophages isolated from the seminal fluids of patients of HAART [79-80].

3.4.5 Central Nervous system (CNS)

Different HIV sub-populations have been isolated from the CNS and peripheral blood. CNS HIV was less able to infect T-cell lines, modulate CD4 antigen expression in infected cells and neutralise serum, as well as having reduced cytopathogenicity, whereas blood-isolated HIV replicated better in T-cell and glioma cell lines [81]. HIV has been shown to persist in nervous tissue, such as microglia, astrocytes and in cells contained within the cerebrospinal fluids [82-84].

3.4.6 Kidney

A possible HIV reservoir exists in tubular epithelial kidney cells [85], as viral replication, through hybridisation studies, has been detected in patients on suppressive HAART [86-87]. In the study by Marras et al, kidney cells were shown to be permissive for viral replication and represented a phylogenetically distinct HIV reservoir.

3.5 Residual viremia

After around 12 to 16 weeks of HAART, the levels of HIV RNA fall below the limit of detection of many clinical assays (less than 20-50 RNA copies/ml) [88]. Following this, slow viral decay, with a half life of between 39 and infinite weeks, reflects the release and clearance of HIV contained within the latently infected lymphocyte reservoir - the third and fourth decay phases of plasma HIV decline [89-90]. However, through the use of low copy viral load assays [91], most (80%) patients on HAART treatment have detectable persistent viraemia [92-93]. Palmer et al demonstrated this viraemia to persist at an average level of 0.781 copies/ml in 15 patients on HAART treatment using a low copy viral load assay, despite having clinically undetectable viral RNA levels using standard clinical assays. Viremia was shown to persist at low levels for at least 7 years in patients on suppressive HAART [94].

The single copy assay was used to analyze longitudinally sampled plasma HIV RNA levels in 40 patients enrolled in the Abbott M97-720 trial [91] and 77% of patient samples were found to have detectable low level viremia. In another study using the single copy analysis, 80% of patients on suppressive HAART had >1 viral RNA copy (with a median of 3.1 copies) per ml of plasma with no decrease in plasma viremia up to 60-110 weeks after starting therapy [22]. Kinetic examinations of viral decay revealed a two-stage decline in plasma RNA levels from HAART treated patients, sampled at 60 and 384-week intervals. This suggested that two cell compartments could potentially give rise to the low level decline of HIV persistent viremia. The first compartment represents a productively infected cell type from which virus is produced and released from cells, but is not able to re-infect naïve cells due to the inhibitory nature of HAART. This causes a decline in virus production over time. The second compartment reflects a reservoir of latently infected cells where the production of virus remains stable for at least seven years [94].

A novel ultrasensitive isothermal transcription-mediated amplification (TMA) assay was used to identify HIV-1 RNA levels in patient plasma samples over 12 years. Virus and antibody levels whilst on HAART was shown to decrease during the first 12 months, then remained stable with a seemingly infinite half-life in a steady-state 'set point' during HAART combination therapy [95].

It is not known whether the residual viremia that is seen in plasma samples of long-term HAART-treated patients reflects replication-competent virions. However, a study using recombinant viral clones isolated from a single patient show that viable virus can be isolated from the plasma of patients on HAART [96].

3.5.1 Source of residual viremia

The cellular and anatomical source of this residual virus also remains unknown. A phylogenetic analysis comparing residual plasma virus and CD4+ T-cell associated virus revealed two genetically distinct viral populations, in four out of five patients [96]. It was also shown that viral plasma sequences during HAART treatment and scheduled treatment interruption (STI) studies were both produced from a compartment, different to that of the circulating CD4+ T-cells, suggesting residual plasma virus production from a cellular source, yet to be identified, and that may contribute to the rapid viral rebound seen in patients undergoing STI studies [96]. Residual viremia was demonstrated to be genetically distinct from proviral DNA isolated from monocytes, unfractioned PBMCs and resting and activated CD4+ T-cells, where the viruses belonged to the same population, also suggesting that residual viremia is produced from a cellular source that is not the CD4+ T-cell compartment [97].

On analysis of HIV *Pol* gene sequences from plasma virus and resting CD4+ T-cell proviral DNA from HAART-treated patients, the plasma viremia in most patients was not related to, and was rarely found in resting CD4+ T-cells, but instead was dominated by a 'small number of invariant clones' [98]. Since the 'predominant plasma sequences' did not evolve whilst patients remained on HAART treatment, the persistent residual viremia was concluded to just arise from the prolonged production of a small number of viral clones in a compartment different to that of the resting CD4+ T-cell. Shen and Siliciano hypothesised that rare HIV infection of and integration into the DNA of a cell type with proliferative capacities, for example stem cells or macrophage/monocyte lineage progenitor cells, could give rise to these predominant plasma clones. The infected cell can then proliferate, copying the viral genome without error induction and thus give rise to myriad differentiated progeny cells, all that are latently infected and all that can potentially contribute to residual viremia [19].

3.5.2 Sporadic release of latent virus from reservoirs

There is much debate as to whether the persistent, residual viremia observed in patients under HAART is produced from new cycles of viral replication or from sporadic release of latent virus [19]. Drug regime and treatment intensification had no effect on reducing this residual viraemia in one study [99], and this may be because HAART only blocks new rounds of HIV infection but does not prevent sporadic HIV release from the latently infected cell reservoirs. Variation in residual viremia levels between patients correlates with the pre-HAART treatment viral loads, suggesting HIV is spontaneously and sporadically released from the latent reservoirs [94]. Also, it was suggested that HAART drugs may suppress HIV viremia to a baseline level, proportional to the initial extent of the pre-therapy latent reservoir, because of similar observed levels of residual viremia in patients with varying expected levels of anti-HIV activity [91].

The low level-viremia seen in HAART-treated adults and children was shown to be related to pre-HAART virus, with no evidence of drug-resistant mutation selection. Since there was no virus evolution, it has been suggested that no residual virus replication was occurring [100]. A novel RT-PCR method for genotyping the HIV-1 *protease* gene at low viral loads (5 copies/ml) revealed that children who began successful inhibitory HAART soon after birth, also did not exhibit drug-resistance mutations to the protease inhibitor nelfinavir and the virus resembled that found in resting CD4+ T-cells [101]. A longitudinal study has again shown lack of evolution in residual viraemia through analysis of drug resistance mutations in *reverse transcriptase* and *protease* sequences from eight patients who maintained undetectable viraemia for 15 months [102]. Also, no viral evolution was observed between *polymerase* gene sequences in patients on HAART, isolated from longitudinally sampled plasma and CD4+ T-cells [98].

A number of people receiving HAART experience viral 'blips' or increases in plasma viral load to detectable levels. These viral blips have been postulated to be because of emerging drug resistant viruses [103], [104]. However, it was discovered that these viral blips do not contain new drug resistant mutations, which supports the spontaneous viral release model [105] and most 'blips' are within expected statistical fluctuations [19].

3.5.3 On-going replication?

Despite evidence of no viral evolution whilst on HAART, some studies that assess other parameters of viral replication suggest that there may be on-going replication. For example, inflammatory markers (hsCRP, Il-6, d-dimer and Cystatin-C) are elevated in treated HIV patients, compared to untreated, suggesting low grade immune activation, despite therapy [106].

Evidence of continued viral replication was gleaned in a study whereby the PBMCs of 138 patients on suppressive HAART who have undetectable plasma HIV levels, were examined for intracellular HIV-RNA. In all 138 patients, intracellular HIV-RNA was detected, which in the absence of plasma HIV-RNA represents newly synthesised RNA, and provides evidence for new rounds of viral replication while on HAART therapy [107]. New rounds of HIV replication were discovered in the lymph nodes and PBMCs of 10 patients on up to 52 weeks of HAART, even after 1 year, and where there was incomplete inhibition of viral replication, resistance mutations emerged [108]. In two patients, sequence evolution was demonstrated in PBMCs, and in one patient, there was evidence of persistent replication but no viral drug resistance in the lymph nodes [15]. In another study comparing the HIV-1 C2-V3 envelope regions, between baseline and residual virus in six patients after two years of HAART, viral evolution was observed in half of the patients and correlated with incomplete viral suppression indicated by the speed of initial virus decline and intermittent rebound events, whilst on HAART [109]. Also, there was persistent HIV transcription in PBMCs from patients on HAART, based on DNA and mRNA analysis on longitudinal samples from 5 men [110].

Ongoing HIV replication was discovered through four viral genetic analyses in a subset of children, over 5.1 years of HAART [111]. The presence of unintegrated proviral DNA seen in one study [26] could be evidence of ongoing viral replication in patients on HAART. Also, 2-LTR circles were seen in the CD4+ T-cells of patients receiving HAART. This viral DNA is formed through the self-ligation and circularisation of proviral HIV DNA by host cell ligase enzymes. Since 2-LTR circles are thought to have a short half life, this could be evidence of ongoing viral replication [112], however, the half-life of LTR circles has been shown to be considerably longer than previously thought and may not always be indicative of recent infection [113-114].

Low levels of viral replication were shown to persist in patients receiving HAART, which could replenish the viral reservoir, thus increasing its half-life [16]. In a cohort of patients, aviremic under HAART treatment for up to 9.1 years, higher levels of HIV proviral DNA were discovered in their activated CD4+ T-cells compared to resting CD4+ T-cells. There was phylogenetic evidence for cross infection between resting and activated cells, which suggests there is an ongoing reactivation of latently infected CD4+ T-cells, potentially causing further infection of virus into activated CD4+ T-cells. It was suggested that these events may contribute to the replenishment of the CD4+ T-cell reservoir, and may 'reset' the half-life of the latently infected resting CD4+ T-cells [115]. In the GALT of HAART treated patients, who were aviremic for up to 9.9 years, incomplete recoveries of CD4+ T-cells were demonstrated. Interestingly, higher frequencies of HIV infection were demonstrated in the gut, compared to in PBMCs and cross infection between the GALT and PBMCs was observed, suggesting a novel role for the GALT in maintenance of the viral reservoirs [74].

It has been demonstrated through mathematical modelling that the unique sequences of HIV predominant plasma clones, which are not found in the reservoir could act as labels for the kinetics of cell entry into the viral reservoir [98]. It was calculated that 0-70 cells are able to enter the reservoir per day in HAART treated patients, which is considerably lower than the total viral reservoir. It was concluded that viral replication cannot replenish the reservoir and therefore cannot contribute to the stability of the reservoir [116]. The influx of cells was shown to represent less than 0.0001% of the total viral reservoir [47], which suggests that the reservoir cannot be replenished by replicating virus [19].

3.6 HAART intensification studies

Poor HAART drug potency or pharmacodynamics could lead to suboptimal drug penetration into 'sanctuary sites' and could be responsible for the viral replication observed in the above studies [117]. Tissues bordering blood-tissue barriers, secondary to cell tight junctions were theorised to be unpermissive to drug penetration [10], and thus act as drug sanctuary sites for continued viral replication. Tissues such as the central nervous system, retina [118] and testes [119] could represent such sites. The latter study discovered replication competent HIV in the seminal cells of some men on HAART and it was found that penetration of the HIV protease inhibitor into the male genital tract was poor [120]. However, in another study, the HIV-RNA levels in semen [121] and in the cervico-vaginal fluids [122] of HIV-infected patients were shown to fall to below detectable levels on HAART. However, studies have shown a decrease in tissue and CSF viremia induced by HAART, in parallel with that seen in plasma, suggesting that antiretroviral drugs do penetrate these sanctuary sites, but possibly at suboptimal concentrations [43]. However, drug penetration to sites such as the gut, CNS and brain have yet to be fully elucidated. It could be that residual viremia is expressed sporadically from the latent reservoirs and also replicates, possibly in drug sanctuary sites and in other viral reservoirs, suggesting the possibility that both sporadic release of virus from latent reservoirs and de novo infection and viral replication might be occurring together [123].

HAART intensification regimes were devised to see if a greater effect on inhibition of viral production could be demonstrated. However, the intensification of antiretroviral drugs therapy in nine HIV-1 infected individuals on successful ART therapy showed no change in persistent virus levels as measured by the single copy assay [99].

Raltegravir is a potent HIV integrase inhibitor, and since integrated proviral DNA is present in infected T-cells, the inclusion of Raltegravir into HAART regimens was hypothesised to impact on latency [61, 124]. However, short-course (28 day) Raltegravir intensification studies on 10 subjects already receiving HAART, with long term suppression, was shown not to reduce their persistent viremia, compared to pre-intensification levels [125]. A recent randomised controlled and double-blinded clinical trial investigating the effect of 12 weeks of Raltegravir intensification on low-level residual viremia in HIV-infected patients did not demonstrate a reduction in plasma HIV-1 levels [126]. On another Raltegravir intensification regime, a transient, but specific increase in episomal cDNA was seen in 30% of the HAART suppressed subjects tested, especially in those that received a protease inhibitor intensification regime. In subjects with high levels of episomal cDNA, the immune activation was higher than baseline levels, and normalised after drug intensification. This may be evidence that viral replication continues, although changes in plasma viremia were not observed [127].

The HIV-RNA levels in plasma, PBMC, duodenal, ileal, colonic and rectal biopsies from seven patients on intensified raltegravir-containing HAART regimes, revealed evidence for residual HIV replication in the ileum, where a decrease in unspliced HIV levels and increase in CD4+ T-cells was discovered, although it is unknown whether this local virus contributes to plasma viremia [71]. Although subsets of patients have ongoing viral replication during therapy, this does not seem to impact on viral plasma RNA levels [127] and it is thus apparent that eradication of HIV through intensification regimes with existing antiretroviral drugs is unlikely [128].

3.7 Viral rebound and its origin

When HAART is discontinued, most patients, even those who suppress viral load to below detectable levels, will experience rapid viral rebound (mean time 9-17 days) [27] [129] and high plasma HIV levels. However, if HAART treatment is initiated early, some patients are able to suppress virus rebound for extended periods of time after scheduled treatment interruptions (STI), although this is rare [24]. In another recent study, eight patients out of 45 had undetectable plasma viraemia and in these, those that started HAART early had a significantly lower amount of latently infected cells. Also, one patient who had undetectable plasma and tissue HIV levels the virus rebounded 50 days after STI, suggesting early HAART treatment may help reduce the latent reservoir in a select few [130]. As well as in patients, this has also been observed in acutely SIV-infected macaques, where early treatment correlated with a more active SIV-specific immune response on commencement of STIs [131]. The rebounding virus could potentially be an early viral clone, whose virus-specific T cell was killed during the acute phase of HIV infection [132], an escape mutant that is unrecognised by pre-existing antibodies or cytotoxic CD8+ T cells (CTLs) [133] or from HIV-specific B and T cells, 'exhausted' from chronic antigen exposure [1].

In a study by Zhang et al, the rebounding virus, after HAART discontinuation in five aviremic patients was identical to that found in the latent viral reservoir. However, in three patients who showed some residual viral replication, the rebounded virus was genetically distinct to that found in the latent reservoir, but related to viral variants isolated in the lymphoid tissues [134]. No genetic variation was seen in HIV Env C2-V3-C2 regions during HAART suppression, when the viral diversity between pre-treatment and scheduled two-week structured treatment interruptions was examined longitudinally in 20 chronically HIV-infected patients [135]. The rebounding virus was shown to be homogenous, suggesting a clonal origin post-reactivation. Also, expansion of distinct clonal HIV lineages during STIs was seen, suggesting stochastic reactivation of different clones from latently infected cells. Diversity increased slowly after treatment was stopped, although 2.5 years elapsed before the viral diversity reached the same levels as found in pre-treatment samples [135]. However, in order to study rebounded virus, there are ethical issues.

Other studies show that any rebound virus observed after STIs does not originate from PBMC or the lymph system, although this may be due to sampling error. Chun et al showed, using tracking and heteroduplex mobility assays that latent HIV present in resting CD4+ T-cells was genetically distinct to the rebounding virus seen in the majority of patients with discontinued HAART treatment and it was suggested that other persistent HIV reservoirs could be responsible for viral rebound after HAART cessation [136]. In another study, envelope gene sequence homology was identified in 12 patients, who received regular cycling scheduled HAART interruptions, at various time points. HIV populations in three quarters of patients diverged between STI cycles, hinting that multiple compartments could contribute to rebounding virus diversity [137]. Through the phylogenetic analysis of HIV polymerase during STI studies, it was discovered that rebounding HIV variants were not related directly to their temporal ancestor, but formed a separate population cluster, which indicates re-emergence of a latent viral population [138]. Also, the genetic diversity, as discovered by tracking and heteroduplex assays, of HIV in lymph node B and CD4+ T-cells were similar, but more distantly related to peripheral blood-derived B and CD4+ T cells in chronically infected patients, suggesting B and T cell 'cross-talk' in lymph nodes [139].

A recent longitudinal study has revealed the gut mucosal viral reservoir not to represent the major viral sequences obtained in plasma, post STI, although it was shown to be an early and stable reservoir in the three patients studied pre and post HAART interruption. Rebound viremia varients also did not replenish the GALT HIV-reservoir. Also, inflammatory responses and a severe loss in gut mucosal CD4+ T-cells were observed on STI induction at the gut mucosa [140].

In six patients whose HIV viremia was controlled for at least 20 months, the episomal and proviral HIV-DNA pre-STI were analysed phylogenetically and compared to rebound virus sequences isolated during a STI study [141]. It appeared, in this study, that the rebounded sequences clustered with envelope regions of pre-rebound episomal DNA, and since episomes are evidence of recent HIV-infection, they may represent a reservoir that contributes to viral rebound after the cessation of HAART and that can lead to treatment failure [141]. This supports the idea that low level viral replication on HAART contributes to viral rebound, as in another study the rebounded sequences of HIV quasispecies closely resembled the sequences observed in replicating virus, before STI [142].

In a further study, HAART-treated patients with undetectable viremia were treated with Didanosine and Hydroxyurea, followed by low dose OKT-3 and IL-2 therapy for 2 weeks, after which treatment was discontinued. 6 months after viral rebound, a shift towards dual tropism in semen cell-associated, but not plasma HIV-1 proviral DNA was detected through the appearance of an X4 provirus. Also, the virus responsible for plasma rebound was not represented in the semen microenvironment, suggesting that there is viral compartmentalization after an intensification and stimulatory HIV-1 eradication protocol [80] [143].

4. Approaches to HIV eradication

Approaches to HIV eradication have focused on the induction of T-cell activation, induction of viral expression with and without activation of the host cell, and a selection of other novel therapeutic strategies [3]. It should be noted that HIV has been 'eradicated' in one HIV-infected patient who was also diagnosed with acute myeloid leukemia resulting in a CCR5 delta32 stem cell transplant. CCR5 is a key co-receptor that HIV uses for cellular entry, and homozygosity for a 32bp deletion in the CCR5 gene results in resistance to HIV-1 infection. This patient remains free from viral rebound 20 months after the stem cell transplant and in the absence of HAART [144].

4.1 Induction of T-cell activation

The theory behind this therapeutic strategy is that activation of resting CD4+ T-cells could induce HIV LTR transcription and hence viral expression, thus clearing virus from latently infected cells [3]. Immune activation therapy, involving agents such as IL-2 and OKT3 (an anti T-cell receptor antibody) could activate T-cell receptors (TCRs) and through multiple signalling pathways could induce histone acetylation of the integrated HIV-DNA site, thus stimulating viral transcription and viral eradication from the latently infected cell. IL-2 therapy was shown to temporarily induce HIV transcription in 4/10 patients and CD4+ T-cell expansion to levels 50% higher than at baseline [145] and 94.8% higher than baseline after 6 months on high level IL-2 doses [146]. Through CD4+ T-cell labelling, naïve and TCM cells were preferentially expanded and had a more prolonged survival time [147]. IL-2 treatment also induced prolonged CD4+ T-cell survival, in combination with the antiretroviral drugs, Zidovudine and Didanosine, and viremia remained undetectable [148]. The amount of latently infected cells in patients receiving IL-2 therapy in combination with HAART drug regimens was shown to decrease, relative to patients receiving HAART alone [149]. However, in patients who received HAART and IL-2 within 6 months of primary HIV infection, no decrease in the amount of latently infected cells was seen compared to HAART-only treated patients [150]. In other studies, early HAART treatment was able to restore CD4+ T-cells to near normal levels, although virus rebounded rapidly after the treatment was interrupted [151-152]. Also, IL-2 therapy in two HIV-infected patients was shown to induce a population of T-cells that expressed the transcription factor, FOXP3 [153], and it has shown elsewhere that FOXP3 can repress HIV expression [154].

In studies attempting viral 'purging' where HIV infected patients were treated with IL-2, HAART and OKT-3 to deplete T cells, cytokine storms were induced and severe toxicities resulted [155], with the added issue that CD4+ cell levels were shown to never fully recover in a separate study after OKT3 treatment [156]. If OKT-3 is used at lower concentrations, it was discovered that rebounded virus genotypes were vastly different to those isolated before treatment, indicating the drug regime had altered the viral pool but not eradicated the virus [151]. In another study, commencement of Didanosine and Hydroxyurea treatment on HAART-treated patients who maintained viral RNA levels below 50 copies/ml for a month, followed by low dose OKT-3 therapy with IL-2 did not stop rebound viremia after STIs [143]. Intensification studies with hydroxyurea, didanosine and low-dose OKT3 also did not to fully ablate HIV-1 reservoirs in vivo [151].

4.2 Induction of viral expression

During HIV infection, plasma levels of IL-7, a cytokine necessary for T cell homeostasis, increase as CD4+ T-cell counts fall [157], and once CD4+ T-cell levels start to increase on HAART, levels of IL-7 have been shown to decline [158]. IL-7 was shown using the SCID-hu mouse model to stimulate the expression of latent HIV from primary human T cells and thymocytes, with little effect on the cell phenotype, highlighting IL-7 as a possible therapeutic agent [159]. Studies have shown that IL-7 can induce latent virus expression ex vivo from CD4+ T-cells from patients who are receiving HAART, although to differing extents. For example, there was no statistically significant difference in viral re-expression between Il-7 and mitogen-treated latently infected CD4 cells, although IL-7 itself could induce viral recovery [160]. It was also found that IL-7 could induce the expression of unique viral isolates through activation of the JAK/STAT pathway, and could thus be of clinical significance [161]. However, IL-7 has also been shown to promote proliferation of latently HIV-infected cells, thus causing doubt as to whether it is clinically useful [52].

HIV proviral expression from HAART-treated patient cell lines and primary cells can also be induced without cellular proliferation through PKC and NF-kB signalling, mediated by prostratin, a phorbol ester isolated from the Samoan medicinal plant 'Homolanthus nutans' [162-163]. The usefulness of prostratin as a drug was restricted because of its limited supply, however synthesis of prostratin has recently been developed synthetically [164]. In cell lines, prostratin can stimulate HIV transcription through NF-kB activation, mediated by PKC [165]. Prostratin has also been shown in other studies to reactivate latent HIV from primary blood lymphocytes and lymphoid tissue and inhibit infection of HIV by down-regulating the expression of the co-receptors CXCR4 and CD4, thus increasing the chance of HIV purging without the risk of new rounds of HIV infection [166-167]. Prostratin, alone, has been shown to reactivate latent HIV from thymocytes and primary human peripheral blood lymphocytes in the SCID-hu (Thy/Liv) model, in the absence of cellular proliferation [168]. Recently, the PKC activator, bryostatin-1, which has well documented pharmacokinetic and toxicity profiles, has been shown to reactivate HIV-1 from Jurkat-LAT-GFP cells through a PKC mediated mechanism and to synergise with other HDAC inhibitors such as VPA. Byrostatin-1 downregulates CD4 and CXCR4 and was thus able to prevent de novo HIV infection [192].

Hexamethylene bisacetamide (HMBA) can also induce the expression of the HIV-LTR, through the modulation of PKC, in rat and human fibroblasts [169] by modulating the PI3-K signalling cascade [170]. It downregulates CD4 expression, thus preventing new rounds of de novo infection and propagation in PBMC cell cultures [171] and is well tolerated in phase II clinical trials, despite being tested as a potential anti-cancer drug [172]. Unlike Prostratin which operates via Tat, an HIV protein that enhances the RNAP II elongation step of the viral DNA template, HMBA activates proviral transcription in the absence of Tat [173], and high-level viral reactivation is Tat dependant [174]. High levels of Tat can out-compete HEXIM and recruit pTEFb to the HIV promoter [175]. HMBA can induce liberation of pTEFb from the inhibitor HEXIM in the absence of Tat, so pTEFb can bind to the HIV LTR and induce processive viral transcription from abortive transcription [176].

4.3 Induction of viral expression without host cell activation

The problem with inducing cellular activation as well as viral reactivation from latency is the increase in *de novo* activated CD4+ T-cells - the targets for HIV infection [3]. This global T-cell activation could result in an increase the number of cells susceptible to HIV infection at a level that HAART may not be able to contain [149], thereby enhancing rather than reducing the reservoir. Approaches, therefore, need to be developed which result in viral transcription without widespread T cell activation.

Pyrrole imidazole polyamides are small molecule drugs that can recognise specific HIV sequences [177] and targeting of these small molecules to sequences in the HIV promoter has been shown to block histone deacetylase (HDAC) recruitment, resulting in increased HIV-LTR expression [178]. Viable virus was recovered from pyrrole imidazole polyamide-treated cell cultures of resting CD4+ T-cells, that were originally isolated from aviremic patients on HAART [179].

HDAC inhibitors have also been shown to release integrated HIV from latency in the HIV reservoir [180]. TNF-a was found to cause a disruption in chromatin packaging of the HIV-1 promoter region, specifically at nucleosome-1 (nuc-1), suggesting that chromatin plays an important role in the repression of HIV transcription and thus, induction of latency [181]. Trichostatin A, a HDAC inhibitor, was shown to induce acetylation of histone proteins, also at nuc-1, independent of NF-kB and caused transcriptional activation of the HIV-1 promoter in a dose dependant manner [182]. Also, TSA was shown to synergise with TNF-a to cause NF-kB mediated re-expression of the HIV-LTR [183].

Valproic acid (VPA), also an HDAC inhibitor, has been shown to increase HIV gene expression and virus production in cultured latently infected cells [184-185]. VPA was shown in another study to induce the expression of HIV from resting CD4+ T-cells, isolated from patients receiving HAART treatment without fully activating the cells or enhancing new rounds of HIV infection [186]. An accelerated and significant decline in the number of replication competent virions in resting CD4+ T-cells was observed in three out of four patients who received a combination of intensified HAART (enfurvitide) and an HDAC inhibitor (VPA) [187]. However, VPA itself, without ART intensification, was found not to be sufficient for a reduction in HIV infection of CD4+ T-cells from the majority (7/11) HAART treated patients, although in the absence of low level viremia, there was an associated reduction in T-cell infection [188]. The infection rates of resting CD4+ T-cells from patients on standard HAART and from patients receiving HAART in combination with VPA, prescribed for neurological or mood disorders, were not sufficiently different [189] and in a study of seven patients who had 5.1 months of drug treatment, no change in CD4+ T-cell levels were observed. On comparison of total cellular HIV DNA and HIV RNA isolated from resting CD4+ T-cells from 10 patients on HAART alone and 10 patients receiving ART in combination with VPA for seizure treatment, no difference in levels of total and integrated HIV DNA or HIV RNA was observed [190]. HAART treatment intensification with VPA in chronic HIV disease also did not significantly reduce levels of resting T-cell infection or impact plasma viral load [191].

Suberoylanilide hydroxamic acid (SAHA), also known as Vorinostat, is a selective class I HDAC inhibitor and has been shown to induce HIV outgrowth from infected J89 Jurkat T cell lines. SAHA also induced HIV production from cells from ART-treated chronically HIV-infected patients, including from memory T-cells and PBMCs [193-194]. Preclinical and clinical trials have shown that the drug is well tolerated and shows little major toxicity at effective concentrations [195].

Oxamflatin, belongs to a novel hydroxamate class of HDAC inhibitor drugs, and has FDA approval in the treatment of solid tumours and haematological malignancies. In the latently infected ACH2 and Jurkat cell lines, it has a EC50 of 3.5uM/L [196] and can induce HIV-1 transcription through the modulation of histone H3 and H4 acetylation in latently infected cells [197]. Another novel HDAC NCH-51 was shown to activate latent HIV-1 gene expression with minimal cytotoxicity, through SP1 sites [198].

The 5'LTR of HIV is CpG hypermethylated. The DNA methylation inhibitor 5-aza-2'-deoxycytidine (aza-CdR) when combined with HDACs, PKC agonists or TNF-a may cause HIV reactivation, especially in combination with SAHA [199]. Aza-CdR was shown to reactivate HIV-1 from latency through inhibition of MBD2 and HDAC2 recruitment to methylated CpG islands. The drug could also potently synergise with the NF-kB activators, prostratin or TNF-a [200].

Screening studies have been performed to isolate potent small molecule drugs that can reactivate HIV from primary human CD4+ T-cells, transfected with BCL2 to increase cell survival. It was discovered in this study that 5HN (5-hydroxynaphthalene-1,4-dione), a natural quinone found in the bark and roots of the black walnut tree, could reactivate latent HIV-1 in a similar manner to anti-CD3 and anti-CD28 antibody combinations, without inducing global T-cell activation [201].

4.4 Combination therapy

Ex vivo studies have shown that a combination of prostratin with VPA or SAHA was more efficient at reactivating latently infected CD8+ T-cell-depleted PBMCs from HAART-treated patients, who had plasma RNA levels below 50 copies/ml [202]. In one study, a synergistic relationship in reactivating latent HIV from PBMCs between SAHA and prostratin was observed, and it was discovered that this combination of drugs could target a wide range of latently integrated sites, irrespective of some viral variants and subtypes [203]. Also, the novel hydroxamate class HDAC inhibitor Oxamflatin has demonstrated synergistic effects with TNF-a, prostratin and aza-cdr [197].

4.5 Novel, and new therapies used for eradication studies

The immunotoxin 3B3(Fv)-PE38, a recombinant derivative of Pseudomonas aeruginosa exotoxin A and gp120 targeting moieties can selectively kill HIV-1 infected cells *in vitro,* and potently inhibits the spread of viral infection in primary human macrophages, with little or no toxicity in non-human primates [204]. If CD4+ memory T cells are destroyed, then the reservoir of latent HIV would be removed. This theory led to the development of the anti-CD45RO ricin immunotoxin. An *ex vivo* study with latently infected CD4+ T-cells from patients with undetectable plasma viral loads showed a specific CD4+ memory cell decrease with little decrease in CD8+ memory T cells. However this therapy would not be able to discriminate between infected and uninfected memory T-cells and would severely compromise broader immunological memory [205].

The P-glycoprotein, expressed in cell membranes, can pump antiretroviral drugs, such as HIV protease inhibitors, out of the cell, reducing drug concentrations to sub-therapeutic levels [206]. A possible solution to this could be biodegradable Tat peptide-conjugated nanoparticles. These can be loaded with anti-HIV drugs and can enhance drug transport across the blood brain barrier, resulting in increased bioavailability of drugs to the CNS, a known reservoir for HIV [207]. Nanoparticles with special optical properties called quantum rods (QRs), conjugated to the antiretroviral drug Saquinavir and the Transferrin receptor (to mediate its transport across the blood-brain barrier), decreased HIV p24 production by 63% and the HIV-1 LTR gene expression by 93% in infected monocytes [208].

Various anticancer drugs such as 5-azacytidine (5-AZC), 5-fluorouracil, (5-FU), methotrexate, cytoine arabinoside and vinblastine, as well as phorbol myristate acetate (PMA) and phytohemagglutinin (PHA) could induce the expression of HIV-1 from a latently infected ACH2 cell line [209]. Based on previous observations, where IVIG treatment for patients with Guillain Barre syndrome led to an increase in plasma HIV RNA levels in patients who were HIV positive, IVIG therapy has recently been shown to reduce the latent viral reservoir levels in half of the HAART-treated patients studied [210].

5. Concluding remarks

Despite the success of HAART in controlling HIV viraemia, it is clear that current drug strategies will not eradicate HIV from an infected individual and thus cure the disease. In fact, more people contract HIV daily, than initiate HAART [211]. The main barrier to viral eradication lies with the persistent and sporadic release of virus from long term viral reservoirs, such as the latently infected resting CD4+ T-cell population, or from residual virus replication in drug sanctuary sites due to poor HAART penetration, pharmacokinetics and bioavailability [3]. A sustained background low level viraemia (median of 3.34 copies / ml) with an 'infinite half life' in patients on HAART was reported in a 7 year study [94] and was confirmed in a similar 11 year study [95]. It is not known whether these virions represent a replication competent form of virus, however viable virus has been isolated from the plasma of a single HAART treated patient using recombinant clones [96], which may suggest that residual viraemia does contribute to rebounded viremia once therapy is stopped. The source of residual and rebounded virus is not presently known.

The theory that the source of residual viremia seen in patients on HAART represents spontaneous release of virus from the latent cell reservoirs is more likely than there being residual viral replication since drug intensification studies have not shown a reduction in plasma viral load [191], and no evidence for viral evolution has been gleaned in phylogenetic analyses of residual viremia [97-98, 135]. It may be that the amount of intensification needed to completely inhibit viral replication at such low levels has been underestimated. The argument for on-going viral replication on HAART is supported by studies showing transient increases in 2-LTR circles following treatment intensification with Raltegravir [127], and that the episomal sequences may reflect a separate reservoir [141]. It may be more likely that residual viraemia arises from a combination of both processes [123].

Therapies to target the latent viral reservoir have focused around the forced re-expression of virus from latently infected cells, using global T-cell activators such as IL-2, or by using compounds such as IL-7, prostratin or HBMA, that can also induce T cell activation [3]. However the main issue surrounding these drugs is that they also potentially create more potential target cells for HIV infection [3, 149]. Current research is focussed around FDA approved HDAC inhibitors like Valproic Acid and SAHA and their role in forcing viral expression through epigenetic mechanisms at the chromatin level. However VPA has enjoyed limited success in all but one clinical trial [187, 189-191], and the need for the development of more potent HDACs remains a high priority. It is likely that a cocktail of potent anti-latency compounds will be needed in concert with intensified HAART regimes to eradicate HIV. However at the moment, with current knowledge, the eradication of HIV from infected patients remains a formidable challenge.

6. References

[1] Trono, D., et al., HIV persistence and the prospect of long-term drug-free remissions for HIV-infected individuals. Science, 2010. 329(5988): p. 174-80.

[2] Piatak, M., Jr., et al., High levels of HIV-1 in plasma during all stages of infection determined by competitive PCR. Science, 1993. 259(5102): p. 1749-54.

[3] Bowman, M.C., N.M. Archin, and D.M. Margolis, Pharmaceutical approaches to eradication of persistent HIV infection. Expert Rev Mol Med, 2009. 11: p. e6.

[4] Stebbing, J., B. Gazzard, and D.C. Douek, Where does HIV live? N Engl J Med, 2004. 350(18): p. 1872-80.
[5] Douek, D.C., L.J. Picker, and R.A. Koup, T cell dynamics in HIV-1 infection. Annu Rev Immunol, 2003. 21: p. 265-304.
[6] Perelson, A.S., et al., Decay characteristics of HIV-1-infected compartments during combination therapy. Nature, 1997. 387(6629): p. 188-91.
[7] Ho, D.D., et al., Rapid turnover of plasma virions and CD4 lymphocytes in HIV-1 infection. Nature, 1995. 373(6510): p. 123-6.
[8] Wei, X., et al., Viral dynamics in human immunodeficiency virus type 1 infection. Nature, 1995. 373(6510): p. 117-22.
[9] Zhang, Z., et al., Sexual transmission and propagation of SIV and HIV in resting and activated CD4+ T cells. Science, 1999. 286(5443): p. 1353-7.
[10] Pomerantz, R.J., Reservoirs, sanctuaries, and residual disease: the hiding spots of HIV-1. HIV Clin Trials, 2003. 4(2): p. 137-43.
[11] Nickle, D.C., et al., Importance and detection of virus reservoirs and compartments of HIV infection. Curr Opin Microbiol, 2003. 6(4): p. 410-6.
[12] Blankson, J.N., D. Persaud, and R.F. Siliciano, The challenge of viral reservoirs in HIV-1 infection. Annu Rev Med, 2002. 53: p. 557-93.
[13] Finzi, D., et al., Latent infection of CD4+ T cells provides a mechanism for lifelong persistence of HIV-1, even in patients on effective combination therapy. Nat Med, 1999. 5(5): p. 512-7.
[14] Siliciano, J.D., et al., Long-term follow-up studies confirm the stability of the latent reservoir for HIV-1 in resting CD4+ T cells. Nat Med, 2003. 9(6): p. 727-8.
[15] Zhang, L., et al., Quantifying residual HIV-1 replication in patients receiving combination antiretroviral therapy. N Engl J Med, 1999. 340(21): p. 1605-13.
[16] Ramratnam, B., et al., The decay of the latent reservoir of replication-competent HIV-1 is inversely correlated with the extent of residual viral replication during prolonged anti-retroviral therapy. Nat Med, 2000. 6(1): p. 82-5.
[17] Bartlett, J.G., New guidelines for the use of antiretroviral agents in HIV-infected adults and adolescents. Hopkins HIV Rep, 2001. 13(2): p. 1, 15.
[18] Hammer, S.M., et al., Treatment for adult HIV infection: 2006 recommendations of the International AIDS Society--USA panel. Top HIV Med, 2006. 14(3): p. 827-43.
[19] Shen, L. and R.F. Siliciano, Viral reservoirs, residual viremia, and the potential of highly active antiretroviral therapy to eradicate HIV infection. J Allergy Clin Immunol, 2008. 122(1): p. 22-8.
[20] Gulick, R.M., et al., Treatment with indinavir, zidovudine, and lamivudine in adults with human immunodeficiency virus infection and prior antiretroviral therapy. N Engl J Med, 1997. 337(11): p. 734-9.
[21] Palella, F.J., Jr., et al., Declining morbidity and mortality among patients with advanced human immunodeficiency virus infection. HIV Outpatient Study Investigators. N Engl J Med, 1998. 338(13): p. 853-60.
[22] Maldarelli, F., et al., ART suppresses plasma HIV-1 RNA to a stable set point predicted by pretherapy viremia. PLoS Pathog, 2007. 3(4): p. e46.
[23] Chun, T.W., et al., Early establishment of a pool of latently infected, resting CD4(+) T cells during primary HIV-1 infection. Proc Natl Acad Sci U S A, 1998. 95(15): p. 8869-73.

[24] Hocqueloux, L., et al., Long-term immunovirologic control following antiretroviral therapy interruption in patients treated at the time of primary HIV-1 infection. AIDS, 2010. 24(10): p. 1598-601.
[25] Haase, A.T., Targeting early infection to prevent HIV-1 mucosal transmission. Nature, 2010. 464(7286): p. 217-23.
[26] Chun, T.W., et al., Presence of an inducible HIV-1 latent reservoir during highly active antiretroviral therapy. Proc Natl Acad Sci U S A, 1997. 94(24): p. 13193-7.
[27] Harrigan, P.R., M. Whaley, and J.S. Montaner, Rate of HIV-1 RNA rebound upon stopping antiretroviral therapy. AIDS, 1999. 13(8): p. F59-62.
[28] Lohse, N., et al., Survival of persons with and without HIV infection in Denmark, 1995-2005. Ann Intern Med, 2007. 146(2): p. 87-95.
[29] Fantoni, M., C. Del Borgo, and C. Autore, Evaluation and management of metabolic and coagulative disorders in HIV-infected patients receiving highly active antiretroviral therapy. AIDS, 2003. 17 Suppl 1: p. S162-9.
[30] Barbaro, G., Metabolic and cardiovascular complications of highly active antiretroviral therapy for HIV infection. Curr HIV Res, 2006. 4(1): p. 79-85.
[31] Volberding, P.A. and S.G. Deeks, Antiretroviral therapy and management of HIV infection. Lancet, 2010. 376(9734): p. 49-62.
[32] Hecht, R., et al., Critical choices in financing the response to the global HIV/AIDS pandemic. Health Aff (Millwood), 2009. 28(6): p. 1591-605.
[33] McDougal, J.S., et al., Cellular tropism of the human retrovirus HTLV-III/LAV. I. Role of T cell activation and expression of the T4 antigen. J Immunol, 1985. 135(5): p. 3151-62.
[34] Korin, Y.D. and J.A. Zack, Nonproductive human immunodeficiency virus type 1 infection in nucleoside-treated G0 lymphocytes. J Virol, 1999. 73(8): p. 6526-32.
[35] Bukrinsky, M.I., et al., Active nuclear import of human immunodeficiency virus type 1 preintegration complexes. Proc Natl Acad Sci U S A, 1992. 89(14): p. 6580-4.
[36] Zack, J.A., et al., HIV-1 entry into quiescent primary lymphocytes: molecular analysis reveals a labile, latent viral structure. Cell, 1990. 61(2): p. 213-22.
[37] Zack, J.A., et al., Incompletely reverse-transcribed human immunodeficiency virus type 1 genomes in quiescent cells can function as intermediates in the retroviral life cycle. J Virol, 1992. 66(3): p. 1717-25.
[38] Pierson, T.C., et al., Molecular characterization of preintegration latency in human immunodeficiency virus type 1 infection. J Virol, 2002. 76(17): p. 8518-31.
[39] Lassen, K., et al., The multifactorial nature of HIV-1 latency. Trends Mol Med, 2004. 10(11): p. 525-31.
[40] Marcello, A., Latency: the hidden HIV-1 challenge. Retrovirology, 2006. 3: p. 7.
[41] Chun, T.W., et al., In vivo fate of HIV-1-infected T cells: quantitative analysis of the transition to stable latency. Nat Med, 1995. 1(12): p. 1284-90.
[42] Brady, T., et al., HIV integration site distributions in resting and activated CD4+ T cells infected in culture. AIDS, 2009. 23(12): p. 1461-71.
[43] Cavert, W., et al., Kinetics of response in lymphoid tissues to antiretroviral therapy of HIV-1 infection. Science, 1997. 276(5314): p. 960-4.
[44] Perelson, A.S., et al., HIV-1 dynamics in vivo: virion clearance rate, infected cell life-span, and viral generation time. Science, 1996. 271(5255): p. 1582-6.

[45] Blankson, J.N., et al., Biphasic decay of latently infected CD4+ T cells in acute human immunodeficiency virus type 1 infection. J Infect Dis, 2000. 182(6): p. 1636-42.
[46] Finzi, D., et al., Identification of a reservoir for HIV-1 in patients on highly active antiretroviral therapy. Science, 1997. 278(5341): p. 1295-300.
[47] Chun, T.W., et al., Quantification of latent tissue reservoirs and total body viral load in HIV-1 infection. Nature, 1997. 387(6629): p. 183-8.
[48] Wong, J.K., et al., Recovery of replication-competent HIV despite prolonged suppression of plasma viremia. Science, 1997. 278(5341): p. 1291-5.
[49] Chun, T.W., et al., Induction of HIV-1 replication in latently infected CD4+ T cells using a combination of cytokines. J Exp Med, 1998. 188(1): p. 83-91.
[50] Pierson, T., et al., Characterization of chemokine receptor utilization of viruses in the latent reservoir for human immunodeficiency virus type 1. J Virol, 2000. 74(17): p. 7824-33.
[51] Brooks, D.G., et al., Generation of HIV latency during thymopoiesis. Nat Med, 2001. 7(4): p. 459-64.
[52] Chomont, N., et al., HIV reservoir size and persistence are driven by T cell survival and homeostatic proliferation. Nat Med, 2009. 15(8): p. 893-900.
[53] Sonza, S., et al., Monocytes harbour replication-competent, non-latent HIV-1 in patients on highly active antiretroviral therapy. AIDS, 2001. 15(1): p. 17-22.
[54] Gartner, S., et al., The role of mononuclear phagocytes in HTLV-III/LAV infection. Science, 1986. 233(4760): p. 215-9.
[55] Ho, D.D., T.R. Rota, and M.S. Hirsch, Infection of monocyte/macrophages by human T lymphotropic virus type III. J Clin Invest, 1986. 77(5): p. 1712-5.
[56] Mavigner, M., et al., HIV-1 residual viremia correlates with persistent T-cell activation in poor immunological responders to combination antiretroviral therapy. PLoS One, 2009. 4(10): p. e7658.
[57] Zhu, T., HIV-1 in peripheral blood monocytes: an underrated viral source. J Antimicrob Chemother, 2002. 50(3): p. 309-11.
[58] Pelchen-Matthews, A., B. Kramer, and M. Marsh, Infectious HIV-1 assembles in late endosomes in primary macrophages. J Cell Biol, 2003. 162(3): p. 443-55.
[59] Sharova, N., et al., Macrophages archive HIV-1 virions for dissemination in trans. EMBO J, 2005. 24(13): p. 2481-9.
[60] Markowitz, M., et al., Rapid and durable antiretroviral effect of the HIV-1 Integrase inhibitor raltegravir as part of combination therapy in treatment-naive patients with HIV-1 infection: results of a 48-week controlled study. J Acquir Immune Defic Syndr, 2007. 46(2): p. 125-33.
[61] Murray, J.M., et al., Antiretroviral therapy with the integrase inhibitor raltegravir alters decay kinetics of HIV, significantly reducing the second phase. AIDS, 2007. 21(17): p. 2315-21.
[62] Chun, T.W. and A.S. Fauci, Latent reservoirs of HIV: obstacles to the eradication of virus. Proc Natl Acad Sci U S A, 1999. 96(20): p. 10958-61.
[63] Heath, S.L., et al., Follicular dendritic cells and human immunodeficiency virus infectivity. Nature, 1995. 377(6551): p. 740-4.
[64] Geijtenbeek, T.B., et al., Identification of DC-SIGN, a novel dendritic cell-specific ICAM-3 receptor that supports primary immune responses. Cell, 2000. 100(5): p. 575-85.

[65] Hlavacek, W.S., et al., Influence of follicular dendritic cells on decay of HIV during antiretroviral therapy. Proc Natl Acad Sci U S A, 2000. 97(20): p. 10966-71.

[66] Hlavacek, W.S., C. Wofsy, and A.S. Perelson, Dissociation of HIV-1 from follicular dendritic cells during HAART: mathematical analysis. Proc Natl Acad Sci U S A, 1999. 96(26): p. 14681-6.

[67] Hlavacek, W.S., et al., Retention of antigen on follicular dendritic cells and B lymphocytes through complement-mediated multivalent ligand-receptor interactions: theory and application to HIV treatment. Math Biosci, 2002. 176(2): p. 185-202.

[68] Keele, B.F., et al., Characterization of the follicular dendritic cell reservoir of human immunodeficiency virus type 1. J Virol, 2008. 82(11): p. 5548-61.

[69] Moris, A., et al., DC-SIGN promotes exogenous MHC-I-restricted HIV-1 antigen presentation. Blood, 2004. 103(7): p. 2648-54.

[70] Yukl, S.A., et al., Differences in HIV burden and immune activation within the gut of HIV-positive patients receiving suppressive antiretroviral therapy. J Infect Dis, 2010. 202(10): p. 1553-61.

[71] Yukl, S.A., et al., Effect of raltegravir-containing intensification on HIV burden and T-cell activation in multiple gut sites of HIV-positive adults on suppressive antiretroviral therapy. AIDS, 2010. 24(16): p. 2451-60.

[72] Mowat, A.M. and J.L. Viney, The anatomical basis of intestinal immunity. Immunol Rev, 1997. 156: p. 145-66.

[73] Veazey, R.S., et al., Gastrointestinal tract as a major site of CD4+ T cell depletion and viral replication in SIV infection. Science, 1998. 280(5362): p. 427-31.

[74] Chun, T.W., et al., Persistence of HIV in gut-associated lymphoid tissue despite long-term antiretroviral therapy. J Infect Dis, 2008. 197(5): p. 714-20.

[75] Schacker, T., et al., Rapid accumulation of human immunodeficiency virus (HIV) in lymphatic tissue reservoirs during acute and early HIV infection: implications for timing of antiretroviral therapy. J Infect Dis, 2000. 181(1): p. 354-7.

[76] Carter, C.C., et al., HIV-1 infects multipotent progenitor cells causing cell death and establishing latent cellular reservoirs. Nat Med, 2010. 16(4): p. 446-51.

[77] Sundstrom, J.B., et al., Human tissue mast cells are an inducible reservoir of persistent HIV infection. Blood, 2007. 109(12): p. 5293-300.

[78] Zhu, T., et al., Genetic characterization of human immunodeficiency virus type 1 in blood and genital secretions: evidence for viral compartmentalization and selection during sexual transmission. J Virol, 1996. 70(5): p. 3098-107.

[79] Craigo, J.K., et al., Persistent HIV type 1 infection in semen and blood compartments in patients after long-term potent antiretroviral therapy. AIDS Res Hum Retroviruses, 2004. 20(11): p. 1196-209.

[80] Nunnari, G., et al., Residual HIV-1 disease in seminal cells of HIV-1-infected men on suppressive HAART: latency without on-going cellular infections. AIDS, 2002. 16(1): p. 39-45.

[81] Cheng-Mayer, C., et al., Isolates of human immunodeficiency virus type 1 from the brain may constitute a special group of the AIDS virus. Proc Natl Acad Sci U S A, 1989. 86(21): p. 8575-9.

[82] Kramer-Hammerle, S., et al., Cells of the central nervous system as targets and reservoirs of the human immunodeficiency virus. Virus Res, 2005. 111(2): p. 194-213.

[83] Lambotte, O., et al., Persistence of replication-competent HIV in the central nervous system despite long-term effective highly active antiretroviral therapy. AIDS, 2005. 19(2): p. 217-8.

[84] Bell, J.E., An update on the neuropathology of HIV in the HAART era. Histopathology, 2004. 45(6): p. 549-59.

[85] Bruggeman, L.A., et al., Renal epithelium is a previously unrecognized site of HIV-1 infection. J Am Soc Nephrol, 2000. 11(11): p. 2079-87.

[86] Marras, D., et al., Replication and compartmentalization of HIV-1 in kidney epithelium of patients with HIV-associated nephropathy. Nat Med, 2002. 8(5): p. 522-6.

[87] Winston, J.A., et al., Nephropathy and establishment of a renal reservoir of HIV type 1 during primary infection. N Engl J Med, 2001. 344(26): p. 1979-84.

[88] Finzi, D. and R.F. Siliciano, Viral dynamics in HIV-1 infection. Cell, 1998. 93(5): p. 665-71.

[89] Muller, V., J.F. Vigueras-Gomez, and S. Bonhoeffer, Decelerating decay of latently infected cells during prolonged therapy for human immunodeficiency virus type 1 infection. J Virol, 2002. 76(17): p. 8963-5.

[90] Strain, M.C., et al., Heterogeneous clearance rates of long-lived lymphocytes infected with HIV: intrinsic stability predicts lifelong persistence. Proc Natl Acad Sci U S A, 2003. 100(8): p. 4819-24.

[91] Palmer, S., et al., New real-time reverse transcriptase-initiated PCR assay with single-copy sensitivity for human immunodeficiency virus type 1 RNA in plasma. J Clin Microbiol, 2003. 41(10): p. 4531-6.

[92] Dornadula, G., et al., Residual HIV-1 RNA in blood plasma of patients taking suppressive highly active antiretroviral therapy. JAMA, 1999. 282(17): p. 1627-32.

[93] Di Mascio, M., et al., In a subset of subjects on highly active antiretroviral therapy, human immunodeficiency virus type 1 RNA in plasma decays from 50 to <5 copies per milliliter, with a half-life of 6 months. J Virol, 2003. 77(3): p. 2271-5.

[94] Palmer, S., et al., Low-level viremia persists for at least 7 years in patients on suppressive antiretroviral therapy. Proc Natl Acad Sci U S A, 2008. 105(10): p. 3879-84.

[95] Hatano, H., et al., Evidence of persistent low-level viremia in long-term HAART-suppressed, HIV-infected individuals. AIDS, 2010. 24(16): p. 2535-9.

[96] Sahu, G.K., et al., Low-level plasma HIVs in patients on prolonged suppressive highly active antiretroviral therapy are produced mostly by cells other than CD4 T-cells. J Med Virol, 2009. 81(1): p. 9-15.

[97] Brennan, T.P., et al., Analysis of human immunodeficiency virus type 1 viremia and provirus in resting CD4+ T cells reveals a novel source of residual viremia in patients on antiretroviral therapy. J Virol, 2009. 83(17): p. 8470-81.

[98] Bailey, J.R., et al., Residual human immunodeficiency virus type 1 viremia in some patients on antiretroviral therapy is dominated by a small number of invariant clones rarely found in circulating CD4+ T cells. J Virol, 2006. 80(13): p. 6441-57.

[99] Dinoso, J.B., et al., Treatment intensification does not reduce residual HIV-1 viremia in patients on highly active antiretroviral therapy. Proc Natl Acad Sci U S A, 2009. 106(23): p. 9403-8.

[100] Hermankova, M., et al., HIV-1 drug resistance profiles in children and adults with viral load of <50 copies/ml receiving combination therapy. JAMA, 2001. 286(2): p. 196-207.

[101] Persaud, D., et al., Continued production of drug-sensitive human immunodeficiency virus type 1 in children on combination antiretroviral therapy who have undetectable viral loads. J Virol, 2004. 78(2): p. 968-79.

[102] Kieffer, T.L., et al., Genotypic analysis of HIV-1 drug resistance at the limit of detection: virus production without evolution in treated adults with undetectable HIV loads. J Infect Dis, 2004. 189(8): p. 1452-65.

[103] Cohen Stuart, J.W., et al., Transient relapses ("blips") of plasma HIV RNA levels during HAART are associated with drug resistance. J Acquir Immune Defic Syndr, 2001. 28(2): p. 105-13.

[104] Havlir, D.V., et al., Prevalence and predictive value of intermittent viremia with combination hiv therapy. JAMA, 2001. 286(2): p. 171-9.

[105] Nettles, R.E., et al., Intermittent HIV-1 viremia (Blips) and drug resistance in patients receiving HAART. JAMA, 2005. 293(7): p. 817-29.

[106] Neuhaus, J., et al., Markers of inflammation, coagulation, and renal function are elevated in adults with HIV infection. J Infect Dis, 2010. 201(12): p. 1788-95.

[107] Natarajan, V., et al., HIV-1 replication in patients with undetectable plasma virus receiving HAART. Highly active antiretroviral therapy. Lancet, 1999. 353(9147): p. 119-20.

[108] Wong, J.K., et al., Reduction of HIV-1 in blood and lymph nodes following potent antiretroviral therapy and the virologic correlates of treatment failure. Proc Natl Acad Sci U S A, 1997. 94(23): p. 12574-9.

[109] Gunthard, H.F., et al., Evolution of envelope sequences of human immunodeficiency virus type 1 in cellular reservoirs in the setting of potent antiviral therapy. J Virol, 1999. 73(11): p. 9404-12.

[110] Furtado, M.R., et al., Persistence of HIV-1 transcription in peripheral-blood mononuclear cells in patients receiving potent antiretroviral therapy. N Engl J Med, 1999. 340(21): p. 1614-22.

[111] Frenkel, L.M., et al., Multiple viral genetic analyses detect low-level human immunodeficiency virus type 1 replication during effective highly active antiretroviral therapy. J Virol, 2003. 77(10): p. 5721-30.

[112] Sharkey, M.E., et al., Persistence of episomal HIV-1 infection intermediates in patients on highly active anti-retroviral therapy. Nat Med, 2000. 6(1): p. 76-81.

[113] Butler, S.L., E.P. Johnson, and F.D. Bushman, Human immunodeficiency virus cDNA metabolism: notable stability of two-long terminal repeat circles. J Virol, 2002. 76(8): p. 3739-47.

[114] Pierson, T.C., et al., Intrinsic stability of episomal circles formed during human immunodeficiency virus type 1 replication. J Virol, 2002. 76(8): p. 4138-44.

[115] Chun, T.W., et al., HIV-infected individuals receiving effective antiviral therapy for extended periods of time continually replenish their viral reservoir. J Clin Invest, 2005. 115(11): p. 3250-5.

[116] Sedaghat, A.R., et al., Limits on replenishment of the resting CD4+ T cell reservoir for HIV in patients on HAART. PLoS Pathog, 2007. 3(8): p. e122.
[117] Pierson, T., J. McArthur, and R.F. Siliciano, Reservoirs for HIV-1: mechanisms for viral persistence in the presence of antiviral immune responses and antiretroviral therapy. Annu Rev Immunol, 2000. 18: p. 665-708.
[118] Pomerantz, R.J., et al., Infection of the retina by human immunodeficiency virus type I. N Engl J Med, 1987. 317(26): p. 1643-7.
[119] Zhang, H., et al., Human immunodeficiency virus type 1 in the semen of men receiving highly active antiretroviral therapy. N Engl J Med, 1998. 339(25): p. 1803-9.
[120] Taylor, S., et al., Poor penetration of the male genital tract by HIV-1 protease inhibitors. AIDS, 1999. 13(7): p. 859-60.
[121] Barroso, P.F., et al., Effect of antiretroviral therapy on HIV shedding in semen. Ann Intern Med, 2000. 133(4): p. 280-4.
[122] Cu-Uvin, S., et al., Effect of highly active antiretroviral therapy on cervicovaginal HIV-1 RNA. AIDS, 2000. 14(4): p. 415-21.
[123] Tobin, N.H., et al., Evidence that low-level viremias during effective highly active antiretroviral therapy result from two processes: expression of archival virus and replication of virus. J Virol, 2005. 79(15): p. 9625-34.
[124] Stevenson, M., HIV-1 pathogenesis. Nat Med, 2003. 9(7): p. 853-60.
[125] McMahon, D., et al., Short-course raltegravir intensification does not reduce persistent low-level viremia in patients with HIV-1 suppression during receipt of combination antiretroviral therapy. Clin Infect Dis, 2010. 50(6): p. 912-9.
[126] Gandhi, R.T., et al., The effect of raltegravir intensification on low-level residual viremia in HIV-infected patients on antiretroviral therapy: a randomized controlled trial. PLoS Med, 2010. 7(8).
[127] Buzon, M.J., et al., HIV-1 replication and immune dynamics are affected by raltegravir intensification of HAART-suppressed subjects. Nat Med, 2010. 16(4): p. 460-5.
[128] Josefsson, L., V. Dahl, and S. Palmer, Can HIV infection be eradicated through use of potent antiviral agents? Curr Opin Infect Dis, 2010. 23(6): p. 628-32.
[129] Davey, R.T., Jr., et al., HIV-1 and T cell dynamics after interruption of highly active antiretroviral therapy (HAART) in patients with a history of sustained viral suppression. Proc Natl Acad Sci U S A, 1999. 96(26): p. 15109-14.
[130] Chun, T.W., et al., Rebound of plasma viremia following cessation of antiretroviral therapy despite profoundly low levels of HIV reservoir: implications for eradication. AIDS, 2010. 24(18): p. 2803-8.
[131] Lori, F., et al., Control of SIV rebound through structured treatment interruptions during early infection. Science, 2000. 290(5496): p. 1591-3.
[132] Douek, D.C., et al., HIV preferentially infects HIV-specific CD4+ T cells. Nature, 2002. 417(6884): p. 95-8.
[133] Kawashima, Y., et al., Adaptation of HIV-1 to human leukocyte antigen class I. Nature, 2009. 458(7238): p. 641-5.
[134] Zhang, L., et al., Genetic characterization of rebounding HIV-1 after cessation of highly active antiretroviral therapy. J Clin Invest, 2000. 106(7): p. 839-45.
[135] Joos, B., et al., HIV rebounds from latently infected cells, rather than from continuing low-level replication. Proc Natl Acad Sci U S A, 2008. 105(43): p. 16725-30.

[136] Chun, T.W., et al., Relationship between pre-existing viral reservoirs and the re-emergence of plasma viremia after discontinuation of highly active anti-retroviral therapy. Nat Med, 2000. 6(7): p. 757-61.
[137] Dybul, M., et al., Genetic characterization of rebounding human immunodeficiency virus type 1 in plasma during multiple interruptions of highly active antiretroviral therapy. J Virol, 2003. 77(5): p. 3229-37.
[138] Kijak, G.H., et al., Origin of human immunodeficiency virus type 1 quasispecies emerging after antiretroviral treatment interruption in patients with therapeutic failure. J Virol, 2002. 76(14): p. 7000-9.
[139] Malaspina, A., et al., Human immunodeficiency virus type 1 bound to B cells: relationship to virus replicating in CD4+ T cells and circulating in plasma. J Virol, 2002. 76(17): p. 8855-63.
[140] Lerner, P., et al., Gut mucosal viral reservoir in HIV infected patients is not the major source of rebound plasma viremia following HAART interruption. J Virol, 2011.
[141] Sharkey, M., et al., Episomal Viral cDNAs Identify a Reservoir That Fuels Viral Rebound after Treatment Interruption and That Contributes to Treatment Failure. PLoS Pathog, 2011. 7(2): p. e1001303.
[142] Imamichi, H., et al., Human immunodeficiency virus type 1 quasi species that rebound after discontinuation of highly active antiretroviral therapy are similar to the viral quasi species present before initiation of therapy. J Infect Dis, 2001. 183(1): p. 36-50.
[143] Geeraert, L., G. Kraus, and R.J. Pomerantz, Hide-and-seek: the challenge of viral persistence in HIV-1 infection. Annu Rev Med, 2008. 59: p. 487-501.
[144] Hutter, G., et al., Long-term control of HIV by CCR5 Delta32/Delta32 stem-cell transplantation. N Engl J Med, 2009. 360(7): p. 692-8.
[145] Kovacs, J.A., et al., Increases in CD4 T lymphocytes with intermittent courses of interleukin-2 in patients with human immunodeficiency virus infection. A preliminary study. N Engl J Med, 1995. 332(9): p. 567-75.
[146] Davey, R.T., Jr., et al., A randomized trial of high- versus low-dose subcutaneous interleukin-2 outpatient therapy for early human immunodeficiency virus type 1 infection. J Infect Dis, 1999. 179(4): p. 849-58.
[147] Kovacs, J.A., et al., Induction of prolonged survival of CD4+ T lymphocytes by intermittent IL-2 therapy in HIV-infected patients. J Clin Invest, 2005. 115(8): p. 2139-48.
[148] Simonelli, C., et al., Interleukin-2 in combination with zidovudine and didanosine is able to maintain high levels of CD4 cells and undetectable HIV viraemia. AIDS, 1998. 12(1): p. 112-3.
[149] Chun, T.W., et al., Effect of interleukin-2 on the pool of latently infected, resting CD4+ T cells in HIV-1-infected patients receiving highly active anti-retroviral therapy. Nat Med, 1999. 5(6): p. 651-5.
[150] Dybul, M., et al., Pilot study of the effects of intermittent interleukin-2 on human immunodeficiency virus (HIV)-specific immune responses in patients treated during recently acquired HIV infection. J Infect Dis, 2002. 185(1): p. 61-8.
[151] Kulkosky, J., et al., Intensification and stimulation therapy for human immunodeficiency virus type 1 reservoirs in infected persons receiving virally suppressive highly active antiretroviral therapy. J Infect Dis, 2002. 186(10): p. 1403-11.

[152] Stellbrink, H.J., et al., Effects of interleukin-2 plus highly active antiretroviral therapy on HIV-1 replication and proviral DNA (COSMIC trial). AIDS, 2002. 16(11): p. 1479-87.
[153] Sereti, I., et al., In vivo expansion of CD4CD45RO-CD25 T cells expressing foxP3 in IL-2-treated HIV-infected patients. J Clin Invest, 2005. 115(7): p. 1839-47.
[154] Grant, C., et al., Foxp3 represses retroviral transcription by targeting both NF-kappaB and CREB pathways. PLoS Pathog, 2006. 2(4): p. e33.
[155] Prins, J.M., et al., Immuno-activation with anti-CD3 and recombinant human IL-2 in HIV-1-infected patients on potent antiretroviral therapy. AIDS, 1999. 13(17): p. 2405-10.
[156] van Praag, R.M., et al., OKT3 and IL-2 treatment for purging of the latent HIV-1 reservoir in vivo results in selective long-lasting CD4+ T cell depletion. J Clin Immunol, 2001. 21(3): p. 218-26.
[157] Napolitano, L.A., et al., Increased production of IL-7 accompanies HIV-1-mediated T-cell depletion: implications for T-cell homeostasis. Nat Med, 2001. 7(1): p. 73-9.
[158] Llano, A., et al., Interleukin-7 in plasma correlates with CD4 T-cell depletion and may be associated with emergence of syncytium-inducing variants in human immunodeficiency virus type 1-positive individuals. J Virol, 2001. 75(21): p. 10319-25.
[159] Scripture-Adams, D.D., et al., Interleukin-7 induces expression of latent human immunodeficiency virus type 1 with minimal effects on T-cell phenotype. J Virol, 2002. 76(24): p. 13077-82.
[160] Lehrman, G., et al., Interleukin-7 induces HIV type 1 outgrowth from peripheral resting CD4+ T cells. J Acquir Immune Defic Syndr, 2004. 36(5): p. 1103-4.
[161] Wang, F.X., et al., IL-7 is a potent and proviral strain-specific inducer of latent HIV-1 cellular reservoirs of infected individuals on virally suppressive HAART. J Clin Invest, 2005. 115(1): p. 128-37.
[162] Kulkosky, J., et al., Prostratin: activation of latent HIV-1 expression suggests a potential inductive adjuvant therapy for HAART. Blood, 2001. 98(10): p. 3006-15.
[163] Kulkosky, J., et al., Expression of latent HAART-persistent HIV type 1 induced by novel cellular activating agents. AIDS Res Hum Retroviruses, 2004. 20(5): p. 497-505.
[164] Wender, P.A., J.M. Kee, and J.M. Warrington, Practical synthesis of prostratin, DPP, and their analogs, adjuvant leads against latent HIV. Science, 2008. 320(5876): p. 649-52.
[165] Williams, S.A., et al., Prostratin antagonizes HIV latency by activating NF-kappaB. J Biol Chem, 2004. 279(40): p. 42008-17.
[166] Biancotto, A., et al., Dual role of prostratin in inhibition of infection and reactivation of human immunodeficiency virus from latency in primary blood lymphocytes and lymphoid tissue. J Virol, 2004. 78(19): p. 10507-15.
[167] Gulakowski, R.J., et al., Antireplicative and anticytopathic activities of prostratin, a non-tumor-promoting phorbol ester, against human immunodeficiency virus (HIV). Antiviral Res, 1997. 33(2): p. 87-97.
[168] Korin, Y.D., et al., Effects of prostratin on T-cell activation and human immunodeficiency virus latency. J Virol, 2002. 76(16): p. 8118-23.

[169] Zoumpourlis, V. and D.A. Spandidos, Hexamethylene bisacetamide stimulates the expression of human immunodeficiency virus long terminal repeat sequences in rat and human fibroblasts. Anticancer Drugs, 1992. 3(2): p. 163-7.

[170] Contreras, X., et al., HMBA releases P-TEFb from HEXIM1 and 7SK snRNA via PI3K/Akt and activates HIV transcription. PLoS Pathog, 2007. 3(10): p. 1459-69.

[171] Klichko, V., et al., Hexamethylbisacetamide remodels the human immunodeficiency virus type 1 (HIV-1) promoter and induces Tat-independent HIV-1 expression but blunts cell activation. J Virol, 2006. 80(9): p. 4570-9.

[172] Andreeff, M., et al., Hexamethylene bisacetamide in myelodysplastic syndrome and acute myelogenous leukemia: a phase II clinical trial with a differentiation-inducing agent. Blood, 1992. 80(10): p. 2604-9.

[173] Sung, T.L. and A.P. Rice, Effects of prostratin on Cyclin T1/P-TEFb function and the gene expression profile in primary resting CD4+ T cells. Retrovirology, 2006. 3: p. 66.

[174] Pearson, R., et al., Epigenetic silencing of human immunodeficiency virus (HIV) transcription by formation of restrictive chromatin structures at the viral long terminal repeat drives the progressive entry of HIV into latency. J Virol, 2008. 82(24): p. 12291-303.

[175] He, N., A.C. Pezda, and Q. Zhou, Modulation of a P-TEFb functional equilibrium for the global control of cell growth and differentiation. Mol Cell Biol, 2006. 26(19): p. 7068-76.

[176] Choudhary, S.K., N.M. Archin, and D.M. Margolis, Hexamethylbisacetamide and disruption of human immunodeficiency virus type 1 latency in CD4(+) T cells. J Infect Dis, 2008. 197(8): p. 1162-70.

[177] Cho, J., M.E. Parks, and P.B. Dervan, Cyclic polyamides for recognition in the minor groove of DNA. Proc Natl Acad Sci U S A, 1995. 92(22): p. 10389-92.

[178] Coull, J.J., et al., Targeted derepression of the human immunodeficiency virus type 1 long terminal repeat by pyrrole-imidazole polyamides. J Virol, 2002. 76(23): p. 12349-54.

[179] Ylisastigui, L., et al., Polyamides reveal a role for repression in latency within resting T cells of HIV-infected donors. J Infect Dis, 2004. 190(8): p. 1429-37.

[180] Archin, N.M. and D.M. Margolis, Attacking latent HIV provirus: from mechanism to therapeutic strategies. Curr Opin HIV AIDS, 2006. 1(2): p. 134-40.

[181] Verdin, E., P. Paras, Jr., and C. Van Lint, Chromatin disruption in the promoter of human immunodeficiency virus type 1 during transcriptional activation. EMBO J, 1993. 12(8): p. 3249-59.

[182] Van Lint, C., et al., Transcriptional activation and chromatin remodeling of the HIV-1 promoter in response to histone acetylation. EMBO J, 1996. 15(5): p. 1112-20.

[183] Quivy, V., et al., Synergistic activation of human immunodeficiency virus type 1 promoter activity by NF-kappaB and inhibitors of deacetylases: potential perspectives for the development of therapeutic strategies. J Virol, 2002. 76(21): p. 11091-103.

[184] Moog, C., et al., Sodium valproate, an anticonvulsant drug, stimulates human immunodeficiency virus type 1 replication independently of glutathione levels. J Gen Virol, 1996. 77 (Pt 9): p. 1993-9.

[185] Witvrouw, M., et al., Cell type-dependent effect of sodium valproate on human immunodeficiency virus type 1 replication in vitro. AIDS Res Hum Retroviruses, 1997. 13(2): p. 187-92.

[186] Ylisastigui, L., et al., Coaxing HIV-1 from resting CD4 T cells: histone deacetylase inhibition allows latent viral expression. AIDS, 2004. 18(8): p. 1101-8.

[187] Lehrman, G., et al., Depletion of latent HIV-1 infection in vivo: a proof-of-concept study. Lancet, 2005. 366(9485): p. 549-55.

[188] Archin, N.M., et al., Valproic acid without intensified antiviral therapy has limited impact on persistent HIV infection of resting CD4+ T cells. AIDS, 2008. 22(10): p. 1131-5.

[189] Siliciano, J.D., et al., Stability of the latent reservoir for HIV-1 in patients receiving valproic acid. J Infect Dis, 2007. 195(6): p. 833-6.

[190] Sagot-Lerolle, N., et al., Prolonged valproic acid treatment does not reduce the size of latent HIV reservoir. AIDS, 2008. 22(10): p. 1125-9.

[191] Archin, N.M., et al., Antiretroviral intensification and valproic acid lack sustained effect on residual HIV-1 viremia or resting CD4+ cell infection. PLoS One, 2010. 5(2): p. e9390.

[192] Perez, M., et al., Bryostatin-1 Synergizes with Histone Deacetylase Inhibitors to Reactivate HIV-1 from Latency. Curr HIV Res, 2010. 8(6): p. 418-29.

[193] Archin, N.M., et al., Expression of latent HIV induced by the potent HDAC inhibitor suberoylanilide hydroxamic acid. AIDS Res Hum Retroviruses, 2009. 25(2): p. 207-12.

[194] Contreras, X., et al., Suberoylanilide hydroxamic acid reactivates HIV from latently infected cells. J Biol Chem, 2009. 284(11): p. 6782-9.

[195] Marks, P.A. and R. Breslow, Dimethyl sulfoxide to vorinostat: development of this histone deacetylase inhibitor as an anticancer drug. Nat Biotechnol, 2007. 25(1): p. 84-90.

[196] Shehu-Xhilaga, M., et al., The novel histone deacetylase inhibitors metacept-1 and metacept-3 potently increase HIV-1 transcription in latently infected cells. AIDS, 2009. 23(15): p. 2047-50.

[197] Yin, H., et al., Histonedeacetylase inhibitor Oxamflatin increase HIV-1 transcription by inducing histone modification in latently infected cells. Mol Biol Rep, 2010.

[198] Victoriano, A.F., et al., Novel histone deacetylase inhibitor NCH-51 activates latent HIV-1 gene expression. FEBS Lett, 2011.

[199] Blazkova, J., et al., CpG methylation controls reactivation of HIV from latency. PLoS Pathog, 2009. 5(8): p. e1000554.

[200] Kauder, S.E., et al., Epigenetic regulation of HIV-1 latency by cytosine methylation. PLoS Pathog, 2009. 5(6): p. e1000495.

[201] Yang, H.C., et al., Small-molecule screening using a human primary cell model of HIV latency identifies compounds that reverse latency without cellular activation. J Clin Invest, 2009. 119(11): p. 3473-86.

[202] Reuse, S., et al., Synergistic activation of HIV-1 expression by deacetylase inhibitors and prostratin: implications for treatment of latent infection. PLoS One, 2009. 4(6): p. e6093.

[203] Burnett, J.C., et al., Combinatorial latency reactivation for HIV-1 subtypes and variants. J Virol, 2010. 84(12): p. 5958-74.

[204] Kennedy, P.E., et al., Anti-HIV-1 immunotoxin 3B3(Fv)-PE38: enhanced potency against clinical isolates in human PBMCs and macrophages, and negligible hepatotoxicity in macaques. J Leukoc Biol, 2006. 80(5): p. 1175-82.
[205] Saavedra-Lozano, J., et al., An anti-CD45RO immunotoxin kills HIV-latently infected cells from individuals on HAART with little effect on CD8 memory. Proc Natl Acad Sci U S A, 2004. 101(8): p. 2494-9.
[206] Huisman, M.T., J.W. Smit, and A.H. Schinkel, Significance of P-glycoprotein for the pharmacology and clinical use of HIV protease inhibitors. AIDS, 2000. 14(3): p. 237-42.
[207] Rao, K.S., et al., TAT-conjugated nanoparticles for the CNS delivery of anti-HIV drugs. Biomaterials, 2008. 29(33): p. 4429-38.
[208] Mahajan, S.D., et al., Enhancing the delivery of anti retroviral drug "Saquinavir" across the blood brain barrier using nanoparticles. Curr HIV Res, 2010. 8(5): p. 396-404.
[209] O'Brien, M.C., et al., HIV-1 expression induced by anti-cancer agents in latently HIV-1-infected ACH2 cells. Biochem Biophys Res Commun, 1995. 207(3): p. 903-9.
[210] Lindkvist, A., et al., Reduction of the HIV-1 reservoir in resting CD4+ T-lymphocytes by high dosage intravenous immunoglobulin treatment: a proof-of-concept study. AIDS Res Ther, 2009. 6: p. 15.
[211] Margolis, D.M., Eradication Therapies for HIV Infection: Time to Begin Again. AIDS Res Hum Retroviruses, 2011. 27(4): p. 347-53.

3

The Changing Trends of HIV Subtypes and Its Implication on Mother-to-Child Transmission

Michael Kiptoo
Kenya Medical Research Institute
Kenya

1. Introduction

The first cases of Acquired Immune Deficiency Syndrome (AIDS) were described in the United States in 1981[1]. In Kenya, the first case was recognized in 1984[2] and since that time, Human Immunodeficiency Virus (HIV)/AIDS still remains a huge barrier to social and economic development. It is estimated that 33.4 million people worldwide were living with HIV by December 2008. During 2008 more than two and a half million adults and children became infected with HIV. Sub-Saharan Africa remains the epicenter[3]. Recent data show HIV prevalence in Kenya of 7.4%, resulting in 1.4 million Kenyans living with HIV. An estimated 190,000 HIV-infected Kenyans receive Antiretroviral therapy (ART), representing 44% of those in need of treatment[4]. Access to ART in Kenya has significantly increased since the start of the World Health Organization (WHO) 3 by 5 initiative. The Kenya AIDS indicator survey of 2007 showed that of the estimated 392,000 Kenyan adults in need of ART, 138,000 (35%) had received the treatment by September 2007[4].

Human immunodeficiency virus is a highly variable virus due to rapid mutation. This results in many different strains of HIV, even within the body of a single infected person. There are two types of HIV: HIV-1 and HIV-2. Both types are transmitted by sexual contact, through blood, and from mother to child, and they cause clinically indistinguishable AIDS. However, HIV-2 is less easily transmitted, and the period between initial infection and illness is longer in the case of HIV-2. Worldwide, the predominant virus is HIV-1. The relatively uncommon HIV-2 type is concentrated in West Africa and is rarely found elsewhere[5].

The strains of HIV-1 are classified into three groups: the "major" group M, the "outlier" group O and the "new" group N. These three groups represent three separate introductions of SIV into humans. Members of HIV-1 group O have been recovered from individuals living in Cameroon, Gabon, and Equatorial Guinea with the genomes sharing less than 50% identity with group M viruses[6]. The group N HIV-1 strains have been identified in infected Cameroonians[7]. In 2009, a newly-analyzed HIV sequence was reported to have greater similarity to a Simian Immunodeficiency Virus (SIV) recently discovered in wild gorillas (SIVgor) than to SIVs from chimpanzees (SIVcpz). The virus had been isolated from a Cameroonian woman residing in France who was diagnosed with HIV-1 infection in 2004. The scientists reporting this sequence placed it in a proposed Group P "pending the identification of further human cases[8].

More than 90% of HIV-1 infections belong to HIV-1 group M. Within group M there are nine genetically distinct subtypes (or clades) of HIV-1. These are subtypes A, B, C, D, F, G, H, J and K[9]. The HIV-1 population present within an individual can vary from 6% to 10% in nucleotide sequences. Human immunodeficiency virus type 1 isolates within a clade may exhibit nucleotide distances of 15% in *gag* and up to 30% in gp 120 coding sequences. One obvious consequence of the genetic diversity of HIV-1 is the potential impact on the efficacy of a future vaccine. Less obvious and largely controversial is the impact of genetic diversity on disease progression, vertical transmission, response to antiretroviral therapy and drug-resistance pathways.

2. Viral variation

High rates of genetic variation are a hallmark of retroviruses[10]. The molecular basis for variation is the error-prone nature of the reverse transcriptase enzyme and the absence of any exonucleolytic proof-reading mechanisms to correct the errors. The ability of HIV to generate extremely large numbers of diverse variants is an advantage to the virus in its continuous effort to adapt to local environments or respond to selection pressures. Viral variation in HIV is as a result of mutation and recombination. Due to the lack of proof-reading ability of the HIV-1 reverse transcriptase enzyme, several mutations are generated. These point mutations are base-pair substitutions, and base-pair insertions or deletions. Recombination occurs frequently during reverse transcription, a consequence of having two RNA genomes packaged per virion[11].

A significant fraction of the HIV-1 group M global diversity includes interclade viral recombinants (Figure 1). These HIV-1 recombinants are found in geographic areas such as Africa, South America and Southeast Asia where multiple subtypes co-exist and account for 10% of circulating HIV-1 strains. The HIV-1 recombinants are known as "circulating recombinant forms" or CRFs. Most HIV-1 recombinants have arisen from Africa and a majority contains segments originally derived from clade A viruses[12].

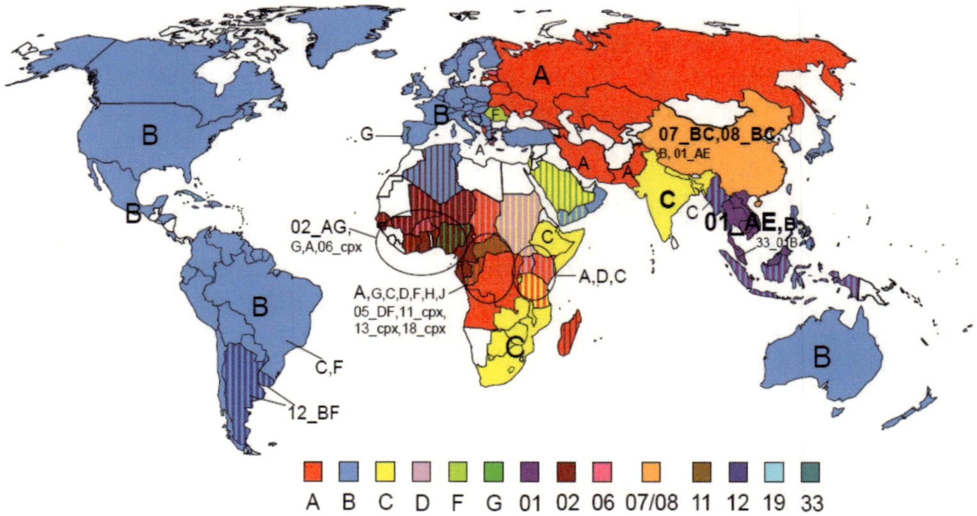

Fig. 1. Geographical distribution of HIV-1 subtypes (Adapted from WHO-UNAIDS HIV Vaccine Initiative)

In Thailand, for example, the predominant circulating strain consists of a clade A *gag* plus *pol* gene segment and a clade E *env* gene (CRF01_AE) [13]. Within subtypes A and F, there are separate sub-clusters that are related closely to each other than to other subtypes. They are designated A1, A2 and F1, F2 respectively. Within subtypes B, C and G there are geographically localized sub-clusters that share a common ancestry as suggested in phylogenetic trees: subtype B from Thailand, subtype C from India and Ethiopia, and subtype G from Spain and Portugal. The classification of HIV strains into subtypes, sub-subtypes and CRFs is a complex issue and the definitions are subject to change as new discoveries are made. These subtypes are generally confined to specific geographical regions with some of these subtypes having been characterized in Kenya.

3. HIV-1 diversity in Kenya

Kenya has about 2.2 million people living with HIV/AIDS. In 2003, the first national HIV prevalence survey was carried out, which estimated that 7% of adults aged 15-49 years in Kenya were infected[14]. Several studies on the HIV molecular epidemiology in Kenya has been done mostly based on partial sequencing of the *env*, *gag* or *pol* regions.

In a study carried out between 1990 and 1992, 22 HIV-1-seropositive pregnant women and 1 HIV-1-infected baby attending the Pumwani Maternity Hospital of Nairobi were studied as part of a cohort study of maternal risk factors in mother-to-child transmission. A 250-base pair (bp) fragment of the *env* gene encoding C2V3 was amplified mostly from Deoxyribonucleic Acid (DNA) isolated from primary peripheral blood mononuclear cells and subsequently sequenced. The results revealed that 19 were classified in subtype A versus 3 in subtype D, together with a much larger variation between subtype A strains as compared to subtype D strains, which suggested an earlier introduction of a subtype A strain, multiple introductions of subtype A strains, and/or faster diversification of subtype A strains as compared to subtype D strains [15].

Another study carried out in 1996 revealed that 71% of the viruses were clade A and 29% were clade D. The most divergent clade A isolate identified in the study grouped closely with two other taxa previously reported as having no distinct clade affiliation[16]. These findings signaled the emergence of an outlier group of clade A variants or a new subtype of HIV-1. The first two virtually full-length genome sequences from HIV-1 subtype G were isolated in Sweden and Finland but originated in Congo and Kenya [17].

In another study, HIV-1 subtype was determined among 320 women from Nairobi by a combination of heteroduplex mobility assays and sequence analyses of envelope genes, using geographically diverse subtype reference sequences as well as envelope sequences of known subtype from Kenya. The distribution of subtypes in this population was as follows: subtype A, 225 (70.3%); subtype D, 65 (20.5%); subtype C, 22 (6.9%); and subtype G, 1 (0.3%). Intersubtype recombinant envelope genes were detected in 2.2% of the sequences analyzed[18]. This study also addressed whether infection with a particular subtype is associated with differences in disease stage. It was found out that the plasma viral RNA levels were highest in women infected with subtype C virus, and women infected with subtype C virus had significantly lower CD4 lymphocyte levels than women infected with the other subtypes.

To further define the genetic diversity of HIV-1 in Kenya, purified peripheral blood mononuclear cell DNA from 41 HIV-1 positive blood donations collected from six hospitals across southern Kenya was used to amplify near full-length genomes by nested PCR.

Among 41 near full-length genomes, 25 were non-recombinant (61%) and 16 were recombinant (39%). Of the 25 pure subtypes, 23 were subtype A, one was subtype C and one was subtype D. Most recombinants consisted of subtype A and either subtype C or subtype D; a few contained A2, a recently identified sub-subtype. Two A2/D recombinants had identical breakpoints and may represent a circulating recombinant form. A third A2/D recombinant had the same structure as a previously described Korean isolate, and these may constitute a second A2-containing circulating recombinant form[19]. The latter has been designated as CRF16.

Our group further analyzed samples from pregnant women in rural western Kenya based on the envelope region (C2V3) and we identified for the first time the presence of CRF10 which had been identified previously in Tanzania. The following were the other subtypes: 20 subtype Al, 2 subtype D, 1 subtype C, 1 subtype G, 2A/D, 2A/C, and 2 were unclassified[20]. In order to investigate the *in vivo* evolution of recombinant HIV, we followed up on a mother who was initially co-infected with subtypes A and D in Kenya. Blood samples were obtained in 1996 and 2002, and HIV *pol* and *env* genes were amplified by PCR, cloned, sequenced, and phylogenetically analyzed. In this study, the clones (1996) generated from the *pol* and *env* genes clustered either with subtypes A and D reference strains. However, two clones from the *pol* gene were found to be independent recombinants between subtypes A and D by RIP analysis, suggesting active generation of recombinant forms. As for the 2002 sample, all the clones from the *pol* gene clustered only with the subtype A reference strain, while all the *env* clones clustered only with subtype D, denoting a dominance of an A/D recombinant form[21].

A detailed molecular epidemiological investigation on HIV-1-infected women attending an antenatal clinic in Kisumu, based on gag-p24 region from 460 specimens revealed that 310 (67.4%) were A, 94 (20.4%) were D, 28 (6.1%) were C, 9 (2.0%) were A2, 8 (1.7%) were G, and 11 (2.4%) were unclassifiable. Analysis of the env -gp41 region revealed that 326 (70.9%) were A, 85 (18.5%) D, 26 (5.7%) C, 9 (2.0%) each of A2 and G, 4(0.9%) unclassifiable, and 1 (0.2%) CRF02_AG. Parallel analyses of the gag-p24 and env-gp41 regions indicated that 344 (74.8%) were concordant subtypes, while the remaining 116 (25.2%) were discordant subtypes. The most common discordant subtypes were D/A (40, 8.7%), A/D (27, 5.9%), C/A (11, 2.4%), and A/C (8, 1.7%) [22].

In 2003/4, we carried out a study in northern Kenya, especially areas bordering Ethiopia, Sudan and Somalia to determine the circulating HIV-1 subtypes. This study revealed that 50% were subtype A, 39% subtype C and 11% subtype D based on the analysis of partial *env* (C2V3) sequences[23]. This showed that subtype A and C are the dominant strains in circulation unlike the other regions with subtype A being dominant and followed by subtype D. We carried out a study in 2005 to establish HIV-1 subtype diversity among patients with sexually transmitted infections in Nairobi. In this study, 140 samples were collected and partial *pol* gene sequencing done. From the analysis it was established that subtype A1 was the major subtype (64%) followed by D (17%), C (9%), G (1%), and recombinants AD (4%), AC (3%), CRF02_AG (1%), and CRF16_A2D (1%) [24].

From April 2005 to July 2006 we carried a study in North Rift to determine the subtypes circulating based on the *pol* region (RT). This was part of a study to explore the status of nevirapine resistant HIV genotypes in rural hospitals in North Rift Valley Province of Kenya. Of the total of 39 HIV infected mother and child samples successfully amplified and sequenced , 28 were subtype A1 (72 %), 5 subtype D (13%), 3 subtype C (8%), 1 subtype A2 (3%) and one subtype G (3%).Our analysis shows that like other parts of the country the predominant circulating subtype in North Rift was A1[25]. This clearly shows that the HIV epidemic in Kenya is a dynamic one and is continually evolving. This observation is applicable to other countries where different subtypes are circulating.

4. Antiretroviral therapy

The development of antiretroviral therapy has been one of the most dramatic progressions in the history of medicine. The early years, 1987-90, brought great hope and the first modest advances using monotherapy[26]. The use of combination therapies became widely used in 1996. Within only three years, from 1994-1997, the proportion of untreated patients in Europe decreased from 37% to 9%, whilst the proportion of highly active antiretroviral therapy (HAART) patients rose from 2% to 64%. Almost all compounds used as part of HAART are either nucleoside reverse transcriptase inhibitors (NRTIs), non-nucleoside reverse transcriptase inhibitors (NNRTIs), or protease inhibitors (PIs). These three classes of drugs target intracellular steps in the viral life cycle mediated by two viral enzymes, reverse transcriptase (RT) and HIV protease. The fusion inhibitors have been introduced recently and block the viral entry[27,28].

4.1 Reverse transcriptase inhibitors

The reverse transcriptase inhibitors (RTI) are divided into nucleoside/nucleotide reverse transcriptase inhibitors (NRTI/NtRTI) and non-nucleoside reverse transcriptase inhibitors (NNRTI). The NRTI mimic the naturally occurring building blocks of DNA. After conversion to their triphosphate form, they compete with natural deoxynucleoside for binding to reverse transcriptase (RT), the necessary enzyme for HIV multiplication within the human cell. The NRTI also compete with deoxynucleoside triphosphates for incorporation into newly synthesized viral DNA chains, resulting in chain termination[29].

Seven compounds of the NRTI class have been approved by the US Food and Drug Administration (FDA): zidovudine (ZDV/AZT), stavudine (d4T), didanosine (ddI), zalcitabine (ddc), lamivudine (3TC), abacavir (ABC) and emtricitabine (FTC). The NRTI are divided into thymidines such as zidovudine (ZDV) and stavudine (d4T) which act preferentially on activated CD4 cells and non-thymidines such as didanosine (ddI), zalcitabine (ddc) and lamivudine (3TC) which act on resting and activated CD4 cells[29]. There is also a new class of anti-HIV drugs called nucleotide reverse transcriptase inhibitors which includes tenofovir. The concentration of NRTIs in cerebrospinal fluid (CSF) varies, but, thus far, zidovudine is the only drug with proven efficacy against the neurological complications of HIV[30].

The NNRTI target the reverse transcriptase enzyme. The NNRTI bind directly and non-competitively to the enzyme at a position in close proximity to the substrate-binding site for nucleosides. The resulting complex blocks the catalyst-activated binding site of the reverse transcriptase, which can thus bind fewer nucleosides, and polymerization is slowed down significantly. These include efavirenz (EFZ), nevirapine (NVP) and delaviridine (DLV).

4.2 Protease inhibitors

The HIV protease cleaves the viral *gag-pol* polyprotein into its functional subunits. Inhibition of the protease, preventing proteolytic splicing and maturation, leads to the release of virus particles, which are non-infectious. Knowledge of the protease substrate and protease inhibitor structures has led to successful development of protease inhibitors[31]. The protease inhibitors (PI) work against HIV in the late stage of viral replication to prevent infectious virus production from infected cells. They block the protease enzyme, which is necessary for the production of mature virions[32]. Seven compounds of the PI class have been approved by the US Food and Drug Administration (FDA): saquinavir (SQV), indinavir (IDV), ritonavir (RTV), nelfinavir (NFV), amprenavir (AMP), lopinavirritonavir (LPV), and atazanavir (ATV).

4.3 Fusion inhibitors

The fusion inhibitors block the attachment of the viral envelope to the cell membrane and the first to be approved was enfuvirtide (Fuzeon) by the US Food and Drug Administration (FDA) [33]. The availability of these drugs has changed the treatment of HIV-1 infected patients. Escalating drug resistance in treatment-experienced HIV-1-infected patients has made management increasingly difficult. In clinical trials, tripanavir/enfuvirtide based salvage regimens have produced potent and durable responses[34]. Multiple observations in a variety of settings have demonstrated a decrease in mortality due to HIV related illnesses, and the incidence of HIV-1 related opportunistic infections has decreased[35].
However, the efficacy of these antiretroviral treatments is impaired by poor compliance with treatment regimens, sub-optimal antiviral potency and drug concentrations, and selection of drug-resistant HIV quasi species[36, 37].

5. Mechanisms of HIV drug resistance

Human immunodeficiency virus replication is a highly dynamic process whereby large numbers of virions are created and destroyed by the immune system each day[38]. Mutations in the HIV genome are primarily generated during the initial steps of HIV replication cycle. The genomic ribonucleic acid (RNA) carried by HIV is copied into DNA early in the replication cycle. The RT makes spontaneous errors when copying the RNA, placing the incorrect nucleotide in the growing DNA strand about once in every 10,000 to 30,000 nucleotides[39].
These nucleotide errors may cause changes in the amino-acid coding of the HIV proteins made from the HIV DNA, potentially altering the structure and/ or function of these proteins and affecting the replication competence of the viral strain. Since mutations in the proteins cause changes in drug susceptibility, the nomenclature for drug resistance mutations refers to the changes in the amino acid sequence of the proteins. Viral mutations are described in the format M184V, where the initial letter represents the wild-type amino-acid of the particular protein, the number represents the mutated codon, or position of the protein and the end letter represents the mutant amino acid that is present[40].
In uncontrolled HIV infection, the high HIV replication rate generates a large pool of genetically but distinct HIV strains called quasispecies, each with potential to develop into the dominant strain. A strain possessing a mutation that provides a growth advantage in a particular environment such as in the presence of antiretroviral drugs out competes the other quasispecies and become the dominant viral strain in the population[41].

6. Mother-To-Child Transmission of HIV (MTCT)

6.1 Pathogenesis of MTCT

Human Immunodeficiency Virus can be transmitted from a HIV-infected mother to the infant during pregnancy (*in utero*), during delivery (*intra partum*) or via breastfeeding (*post partum*). The precise mechanisms responsible for *in utero* and *intra partum* MTCT remain uncertain. The placenta is an effective barrier to infection, but conditions that compromise the placental unit such as vasoactive drug use or chorio-amnionitis, may allow mixture of maternal and foetal blood[42].

Virus in vaginal secretions, mother's blood and breast milk may penetrate the infant's mucosal tissues either during or after delivery. After penetrating the mucosal tissues, langerhans cells and key immune cells such as dendritic cells, macrophages and lymphocytes (CD4 T cells) take up the virus. These cells transport the virus to the lymph nodes where it replicates. In 5-7 days post exposure, HIV appears in the blood within infected CD4 T cells or as free virions[43].

6.2 Risk factors for MTCT

In non-breastfed populations, 25-30% of infected infants have detectable provirus in their peripheral blood lymphocytes at birth, suggesting *in utero* infection[44]. The detection of HIV RNA or provirus after a week or two suggests *intra partum* transmision of HIV-1. In breastfed populations, approximately 15% of infections are thought to occur *in utero*, 65-70% during delivery, and 15-20% during *post partum* through breastfeeding[45].

Maternal plasma HIV-1 viral load is one of the strongest predictors of MTCT[46]. Mother-to-child transmission of HIV can occur at any maternal viral load, but the risk of transmission increases with increasing maternal plasma HIV-1 load. Mothers with a high viral load during pregnancy are more likely to transmit virus to their infants during the *in utero* or *intra partum* periods, particularly if they seroconvert while pregnant[47]. Prolonged labour accounts for MTCT during delivery. An increased risk of MTCT has been observed in first-born twins[48]. In addition, cervico-vaginal ulcers or high maternal cervical or vaginal HIV-1 proviral copy numbers have been significantly associated with MTCT, independent of maternal plasma HIV-1 load[49].

Available data suggests that most breast milk transmission occurs within the first months of life. Longer durations of breastfeeding are associated with increased risk of HIV-1 transmission to infants[50]. The maternal factors associated with breastfeeding transmission include younger age and higher parity, maternal HIV disease stage and breast health. Advanced disease stage is a risk factor associated with postnatal transmission of HIV-1. This is associated with low blood CD4+ cell counts and higher maternal peripheral blood or milk viral load[51, 52].

Several studies have established the association between transmission of HIV-1 through breastfeeding with maternal breast abnormalities such as breast abscesses, mastitis and nipple lesions. In Kenya, for example, mastitis and breast abscesses were associated with late postnatal transmission of HIV-1[53]. In Malawi, women with increased milk sodium concentrations consistent with subclinical mastitis had higher milk viral load[47]. In another study in Kenya, maternal nipple lesions and mastitis were associated with increased risk of postnatal transmission. Oral candidiasis in infants before 6 months of age was associated with postnatal transmission[54]. A study in the Ivory Coast suggested maternal breast abscesses, cracked nipples and oral candidiasis in infants as risk factors for late postnatal transmission of HIV-1 through breastfeeding[55].

7. Strategies for reduction of MTCT

7.1 Behavioural Intervention

Counselling and testing in the antenatal clinic offers an opportune time to discuss prevention of primary HIV infection. For women who are found to be HIV-negative, safe sexual behaviour should be reinforced.

7.2 Nutritional intervention

Low Vitamin A levels have been associated with higher rates of MTCT and with higher levels of virus in breast milk[56]. Among HIV-infected pregnant women, low selenium status increases risk of MTCT and poor pregnancy outcomes[57]. Therefore, HIV positive pregnant women should maintain adequate nutritional status.

7.3 Obstetric intervention

Studies have shown that vaginal cleansing with antiseptic is associated with reduced MTCT and improved perinatal outcome[58]. The other obstetric intervention is elective caesarean section (CS). Prospective cohort studies have shown that the rate of perinatal transmission among women undergoing elective CS delivery was significantly lower than among women undergoing non-elective CS or vaginal delivery[59].

7.4 Antiretroviral prophylaxis

The use of antiretroviral prophylactic therapies to reduce MTCT came into effect following studies by Paediatrics AIDS Clinical Trial Group 076[60]. In this trial, zidovudine (ZDV) was given to mothers beginning at 14-34 weeks of pregnancy, intravenously during labour and for 6 weeks to infants. This resulted in 68% reduction in MTCT. Owing to the high cost and complexity of the regimen, recommendations were made for shorter and simplified forms to be tried in developing countries. A trial in Thailand showed a 50% reduction in mother-to-child transmission of HIV in non-breastfeeding women who took an exclusive oral ZDV regimen twice a day beginning at 36 weeks gestation and every 3 hours during labour[61].
An identical regimen on breastfeeding populations in two areas of West Africa showed high efficacy rates by 3-6 months[62, 63]. In the perinatal transmission trial (PETRA®) carried out in Eastern and Southern African countries, a combination of zidovudine and lamivudine had efficacies beyond 65% at 18 months[64]. In Kenya, a study was carried out to determine the feasibility of using short-course zidovudine to prevent MTCT in a breastfeeding population in a rural area. The mothers were given a daily dose of 400 mg of ZDV starting at 36 weeks of gestation and another 300 mg every three hours *intra partum*. No ZDV was administered to infants after delivery. Even though not all the mothers took ZDV, the HIV vertical transmission rate was reduced by 65.6% [65]. In the ultra-short nevirapine (NVP) HIVNET 012® trial in Uganda, one dose given to the mother during labour combined with one dose given to the neonate within 72 hours of birth reduced 3-month transmission by 47% [66]. These studies have formed the basis of recommendations on the use of short course antiretroviral therapies for prevention of mother-to-child transmission of HIV in developing countries[45, 67].

8. Drug resistance, viral subtypes and implications on MTCT

Drug resistance is one of the greatest threats to successful long-term antiretroviral therapy (ART). Combination ART delays the onset of drug resistance, but drug resistance can still develop and lead to a reduction in drug efficacy. Once resistance has developed to a drug or drug class, resistant viruses are archived in lymphoid tissue, and responses to the drug or drug class are compromised indefinitely[68]. Because cross-resistance may also limit the efficacy of unused ART agents, many persons infected with HIV can exhaust effective ART treatment options quickly if careful selection and monitoring of initial ART are not undertaken.
Many studies have shown the existence of polymorphisms among non-B strains, especially naturally occurring minor mutations in the protease gene, as well as atypical substitutions in

protease (PR) and reverse transcriptase (RT) at positions associated with resistance[69]. Accessory (or minor) mutations may not result in a significant decrease in susceptibility[70], but may be associated with an increase in viral fitness (replication capacity) and/or increase in resistance level associated with major mutations, and thus long-term failure of therapy. It is not clear whether differences exist among the various forms of HIV-1 (groups, subtypes, and CRFs) in terms of transmissibility, pathogenicity, and responses to antiretroviral therapy, but some *in vitro* and *in vivo* observations suggest that certain variants may respond differently to certain antiretroviral drugs[71].

There is a solid body of evidence to indicate that drug resistance pathways vary between different subtypes. One classic example is that of the development of NFV resistance in subtypes B and G. Patients with subtype B tend to preferentially develop the D30N mutation, whereas those with other subtypes including G tend to preferentially develop L90M. Even in cases where the first mutation is L90M in both B and G subtypes, subsequent mutations differ significantly. In subtype B, L63P is the second mutation and occurs in almost 100% of cases, suggesting that the progression of resistance is dependent on the emergence of this mutation, followed by the selection of V77I and other mutations. In subtype G, L89I follows the emergence of L90M, and is present in almost 100% of cases suggesting a role in subtype G similar to that of L63P in subtype B. The third mutation can be either A71V or I54V[72, 73].

The HIV-1 group O and HIV-2 strains are naturally resistant to non-nucleoside reverse transcriptase inhibitors (NNRTIs). Human immunodeficiency virus type 2 variants carry the major NNRTI resistance mutations, Y181I, Y188L, and G190A, in addition to the minor mutations, K101A, V106I, and V179I. Human immunodeficiency virus type 2 isolates show 1000–10,000-fold resistance to first and second-generation NNRTIs. These observations clearly shows that the use of NNRT's to reduce the transmission rates of mother-to-child will not work among women infected with HIV-2. Subtype O viruses show resistance to NNRTIs through two distinct mutational profiles involving the NNRTI secondary mutations, A98G, K103R, and I79E, in the presence or absence of Y181C. Subtype O viruses without Y181C show greater than 100-fold and greater than 500-fold resistance to nevirapine and efavirenz, respectively[74].

Clinical trials demonstrate a disparity in the frequency of primary nevirapine resistance, involving K103N or Y181C in 65–69, 36, 19 and 21% in women with subtype C, D, A and CRF02_AG infections, respectively[75,76,77,78]. Subtype C viruses have a signature valine codon polymorphism absent in other non-B subtypes. This subtype C polymorphism facilitates the acquisition of V106M upon selective drug pressure with efavirenz but not nevirapine. The V106M confers cross-resistance to NNRTIs[79].

A rapid selection of K65R is observed in subtype C strains compared with the slow evolution of K65R in subtype B[80]. Subtype G strains are less susceptible *in vitro* to protease inhibitors (PIs), the rate of occurrence of nevirapine resistance-associated mutations after a single dose is significantly higher in women with HIV-1 subtype C than in women with subtype A or D[81, 82].

Nevirapine prophylaxis used in the HIVNET 012 [66] has been reported to result in selection of single point mutations strongly associated with high resistance to non-nucleoside reverse transcriptase inhibitors that were detectable in 19% of the mothers and 46% of the infants[83]. By contrast with HIVNET 012®, where *intra partum* and neonatal exposure to nevirapine or zidovudine was limited, the PETRA® interventions led to ongoing maternal exposure to zidovudine plus lamivudine from 36 weeks gestation. It has been postulated that induction of significant single mutation (M184V) lamivudine resistance will occur[84].

Viral genetic diversity seems to have an important role on MTCT and in timing of transmission. In a study by Kwiek and colleagues, among HIV-1 subtype C infected mothers, they observed different diversity patterns during intrauterine and intrapartum transmissions. Intrauterine infected-infants tended to be infected by one single variant that was more detected in the mother's plasma, whereas intrapartum infected-infants showed multiple variants of detected and undetected variants of the mother's quasispecies. Regardless of the time of transmission, nearly 50% of the quasispecies included the transmission of variants that were not detected in the mother's blood plasma, suggesting a genetic bottleneck and arguing against a stochastic model of vertical transmission[85].
A number of studies have been carried out to determine the role of HIV-1 subtypes on MTCT. A study carried out in Kenya among 414 women, MTCT rates were higher among women with subtype D compared with subtype A in either the gp41[86]. Such differences may be caused by altered cellular tropism for placental cell types. However, a study carried out in Uganda found no significant difference in the rate of MTCT in women with subtype A versus D[87]. Several HIV-1 structural, regulatory and accessory genes are highly conserved following MTCT. In addition, HIV-1 sequences from non-transmitting mothers are less heterogeneous compared with transmitting mothers, suggesting that a higher level of viral heterogeneity influences MTCT.
The mechanism through which MTCT occurs seems not to be fully clear, and should be a focus point for researches to understand the biology of viral transmission and also attempt to eliminate one of transmission routes. Further studies are needed regarding the mechanisms that determine the moment of transmission, and the influence of the viral subtype, the influence of host immunity, recombination and drug resistance on MTCT may provide insight into new prevention strategies and the development of an effective vaccine[88]. Early and universal access to ARV during pregnancy is the most important measure to achieve a decrease in vertical transmission in areas where clade distribution differs[89].

9. References

[1] Centres for Disease Control (1981). *Pneumocystis pneumonia*--Los Angeles. *Morbidity and Mortality Weekly Report*; 30: 250-252.
[2] Obel A., Shariff S.M., Gitonga E., Shah M. and Gitau W. (1984). Acquired immune deficiency syndrome in an African. *East African Medical Journal*; 61: 724-730.
[3] UNAIDS/WHO AIDS epidemic update December 2008. *www.unaids.org*.
[4] *Kenya AIDS Indicator Survey 2007* Nairobi Kenya: National AIDS and STI Control Programme, *Ministry of Health Kenya (NASCOP)*; 2008.
[5] Peeters M., Piot P. and van der Groen G (1991). Variability among HIV and SIV strains of African origin. *AIDS*; 5 (Suppl.1): S29-S36.
[6] Subbarao S. and Schochetman G. (1996). Genetic variability of HIV-1. *AIDS*; 10 (Suppl. A): S13-S23.
[7] Simon F., Mauclere P., Roques P., Loussert-Ajaka I., Muller-Trutwin M.C., Saragosti S., Georges-Courbot M.C., Barre-Sinoussi F. and Brun-Vezinet F.(1998). Identification of a new Human Immunodeficiency Virus type 1 distinct from group M and group O. *Nature Medicine*; 4 (9): 1032-1037.
[8] Plantier J.C., Leoz M., Dickerson J.E., De Oliveira F., Cordonnier F., Lemée V., Damond F., Robertson D.L. and Simon F. (2009). "A new human immunodeficiency virus derived from gorillas". *Nature Medicine*; 15 (8): 871-2.

[9] Tatt I.D., Barlow K.L., Nicoll A. and Chewley J.P. (2001). The public health significance of HIV-1 subtypes. *AIDS*; 15(Suppl.5): S59-S71.
[10] Coffin J.M. (1986). Genetic variation in AIDS viruses. *Cell*; 46 (1): 1-4.
[11] Mild M., Esbjornsson J., Fenyo E., and Medstrand P. (2007). Frequent intarpatient recombination between human Immunodeficiency virus type 1 R5 and X4 envelopes: implications for coreceptor switch. *Journal of Virology*; 81: 3369-3376.
[12] Gao F., Robertson D.L., Carruthers C.D., Morrison S.G., Jian B., Chen Y., Barre-Sinoussi F., Girard M., Srinivasan A., Abimiku A.G., Shaw G.M., Sharp P.M. and Hahn B.H. (1998). A comprehensive panel of near-full-length clones and reference sequences for non-subtype B isolates of Human Immunodeficiency Virus type 1. *Journal of Virology*; 72(7): 5680-5698.
[13] Carr J.K., Salminen M.O., Koch C., Gotte D., Artenstein A.W., Hegerich P.A., St Louis D., Burke D.S. and McCutchan F.E. (1996). Full-length sequence and mosaic structure of a Human Immunodeficiency Virus type 1 isolate from Thailand. *Journal of Virology*; 70 (9): 5935-5943.
[14] Central Bureau of Statistics (2003). Kenya demographic and health survey 2003. Calverton, Maryland, USA: CBS, MOH, ORC MARCO.
[15] Janssens W., Heyndrickx L., Fransen K., Temmerman M., Leonaers A., Ivens T., Motte J., Piot P. and Van der Groen G. (1994). Genetic variability of HIV type 1 in Kenya. *AIDS Research and Human Retroviruses*; 10 (11):1577-9.
[16] Poss M., Gosink J., Thomas E., Kreiss J.K., Ndinya-Achola J., Mandaliya K., Bwayo J. and Overbaugh J. (1997). Phylogenetic evaluation of Kenyan HIV type 1 isolates. *AIDS Research and Human Retroviruses*; 13(6):493-9.
[17] Carr J.K., Salminen M.O., Albert J., Sanders-Buell E., Gotte D., Birx D.L. and McCutchan F. E. (1998). Full genome sequences of human immunodeficiency virus type 1 subtypes G and A/G intersubtype recombinants. *Journal of Virology*; 247(1):22-31.
[18] Neilson J.R., John G.C., Carr J.K., Lewis P., Kreiss J.K., Jackson S., Nduati R.W., Mbori-Ngacha D., Panteleeff D.D., Bodrug S., Giachetti C., Bott M.A., Richardson B.A., Bwayo J., Ndinya-Achola J. and Overbaugh J. (1999). Subtypes of human immunodeficiency virus type 1 and disease stage among women in Nairobi, Kenya. *Journal of Virology*; 73(5):4393-4403.
[19] Dowling W.E., Kim B., Mason C.J., Wasunna K.M., Alam U., Elson L., Birx D.L., Robb M.L., McCutchan F.E. and Carr J.K. (2002). Forty-one near full-length HIV-1 sequences from Kenya reveal an epidemic of subtype A and A-containing recombinants. *AIDS*; 16(13):1809-1820.
[20] Songok E.M., Lihana R.W., Kiptoo M.K., Genga I.O., Kibaya R., Odhiambo F., Kobayashi K., Ago Y., Ndembi N., Okoth F., Fujiyama Y., Imanishi J. and Ichimura H. (2003). Identification of env CRF-10 among HIV variants circulating in rural western Kenya. *AIDS Research and Human Retroviruses*; 19(2):161-1655.
[21] Songok E.M., Lwembe R.M., Kibaya R., Kobayashi K., Ndembi N., Kita K., Vulule J., Oishi I, Okoth F, Kageyama S. and Ichimura H. (2004). Active generation and selection for HIV intersubtype A/D recombinant forms in a co-infected patient in Kenya. *AIDS Research and Human Retroviruses*; 20(2):255-258.
[22] Yang C., Li M., Shi Y.P., Winter J., van Eijk A.M., Ayisi J., Hu D.J., Steketee R., Nahlen B.L. and Lal R.B. (2004). Genetic diversity and high proportion of intersubtype recombinants among HIV type 1-infected pregnant women in Kisumu, western Kenya. *AIDS Research and Human Retroviruses*; 20(5):565-574.
[23] Khamadi S.A., Ochieng W., Lihana R.W., Kinyua J., Muriuki J., Mwangi J., Lwembe R, Kiptoo M., Osman S., Lagat N., Pelle R., Muigai A., Carter J.Y., Oishi I., Ichimura H.,

Mwaniki D.L., Okoth F.A., Mpoke S. and Songok E.M. (2005). HIV type 1 subtypes in circulation in northern Kenya. *AIDS Research and Human Retroviruses*; 21(9): 810-4.

[24] Lihana R.W., Khamadi S.A., Kiptoo M.K., Kinyua J.G., Lagat N., Magoma G.N., Mwau M.M., Makokha E.P., Onyango V., Osman S., Okoth F.A. and Songok E.M. (2006). HIV type 1 subtypes among STI patients in Nairobi: a genotypic study based on partial pol gene sequencing. *AIDS Research and Human Retroviruses*; 22(11):1172-7.

[25] Kiptoo M.K., Ichimura H., Raphael L., Ng'ang'a Z, Mueke J., Kinyua J., Lagat N.,Okoth F. and Songok E.M. (2008). Prevalence of Nevirapine-Associated Resistance Mutations after Single Dose Prophylactic Treatment among Antenatal Clinic Attendees in North Rift Kenya. *AIDS Research and Human Retroviruses;* 24(12):1555-1559.

[26] Volberding P.A., Lagakos S.W., Koch M.A., Pettinelli C., Myers M.W., Booth D.K., Balfour H.H. Jr, Reichma R.C., Bartleth J.A. and Hirsch M.S. (1990). Zidovudine in asymptomatic HIV infection. A controlled trial in persons with fewer than 500 CD4-positive cells per cubic millimeter. *New England Journal of Medicine*; 322(14): 941-949.

[27] Rusconi S., Scozzafava A., Mastrolorenzo A. and Supuran C.T. (2007). An update in the development of HIV entry inhibitors. *Current Topics in Medicinal Chemistry*; 7(13): 1273-1289.

[28] Barbaro G., Scozzafava A., Mastrolorenzo A. and Supuran C.T. (2005). Highly active antiretroviral therapy: current state of the art, new agents and their pharmacological interactions useful for improving therapeutic outcome. *Current Pharmaceutical Design*; 11(14): 1805-1843.

[29] Richman D.D. (2001). HIV chemotherapy. *Nature*; 410(6831): 995-1001.

[30] Bean P. (2005). New Drug Targets for HIV. *Clinical Infectious Diseases*; 41: S96–S100.

[31] Eron J.J. Jr. (2000). HIV-1 protease inhibitors. *Clinical Infectious Diseases*; 30 (Suppl. 2): S160-S170.

[32] Venaud S., Yahi N., Fehrentz J.L., Guettari N., Nisato D., Hirsch I. and Chermann J.C. (1992). Inhibition of HIV by anti-HIV protease synthetic peptide blocks an early step of viral replication. *Research in Virology*; 143(5): 311-319.

[33] Burton A. (2003). Enfuvirtide approved for defusing HIV. *Lancet Infectious Diseases*; 3 (5): 260.

[34] Gupta R.K., Loveday C., Kalindi U., Lechelt M., Skinner C. and Orkin C. (2007). Tipranavir/T20-based salvage regimens highly effective and durable against HIV-1 with evidence for genotypic predictability of response in clinal practice. *International Journal of STD & AIDS*; 18(9): 630-632.

[35] Hogg R.S., Heath K.V., Yip B., Craib K.J., O'Shaughnessy M.V., Schechter M.T. and Montaner J.S. (1998). Improved survival among HIV-infected individuals following initiation of antiretroviral therapy. *Journal of the American Medical Association*; 279(6): 450-454.

[36] Murphy D.A., Greenwell L. and Hoffman D. (2002). Factors associated with antiretroviral adherence among HIV-infected women with children. *Journal of Women & Health*; 36(1): 97-111.

[37] Miller V. and Larder B.A. (2001). Mutational patterns in the HIV genome and cross-resistance following nucleoside and nucleotide analogue drug exposure. *Antiviral Therapy*; 6 (Suppl.3): 25-44.

[38] Perelson A.S., Neumann A.U., Markowitz M., Leonard J.M. and Ho D.D. (1996). HIV-1 dynamics in vivo: virion clearance rate, infected cell life span, and viral generation time. *Science*; 271(5255): 1582-1586.

[39] Mansky L.M. and Temin H.M. (1995). Lower in vivo mutation rate of Human Immunodeficiency Virus type 1 than that predicted from the fidelity of purified reverse transcriptase. *Journal of Virology*; 69(8): 5087-5094.

[40] Naeger L.K., Margot N.A. and Miller M.D. (2001). Increased susceptibility of HIV-1 reverse transcriptase mutants containing M184V and zidovudine-associated mutations: analysis of enzyme processivity, chain-terminator removal and viral replication. *Antiviral Therapy*; 6 (2): 115-126.

[41] Coffin J.M. (1995). HIV population dynamics *in vivo*: Implications for genetic variation, pathogenesis, and therapy. *Science*; 367: 483-489.

[42] Van Dyke R., Korber B., Popek E., Macken C., Widmayer S.M., Bardeguez A., Hansan I.C., Wiznia A., Luzuriaga K., Visearello R.R. and Wolinsky S. (1999). The Arie Project: A prospective cohort study of maternal-child transmission of Human Immunodeficiency Virus type 1 in the era of maternal antiretroviral therapy. *Journal of Infectious Diseases*; 179(2): 319-328.

[43] Lewis P., Nduati R., Kreiss J.K., John G.C., Richardson B.A., Mbori-Ngacha D., Ndinya-Achola J. and Overbaugh J. (1998). Cell free HIV-1 in breast milk. *Journal of Infectious Diseases*; 177(1): 34-39.

[44] Luzuriaga K. and Sullivian J. (1996). DNA polymerase chain reaction for the diagnosis of vertical HIV infection. *Journal of the American Medical Association*; 275: 1360-1361.

[45] De Cock K.M., Fowler M.G., Mercier E., de Vincenzi I., Saba J., Hoff E., Alnwick D.J., Rogers M. and Shaffer N. (2000). Prevention of mother-to- child transmission of HIV in resource poor countries: translating research into policy and practice. *Journal of the American Medical Association*; 283: 1175-1182.

[46] Garcia P., Kalish L., Pitt J., Minkoff H., Quinin T.C., Burchett S.K., Kornegay J., Jackson B., Moye J., Hanson C., Zorilla C. and Lewis J.F. (1999). Maternal levels of plasma Human Immunodeficiency Virus type 1 RNA and the risk of perinatal transmission. *New England Journal of Medicine*; 341(6): 394-402.

[47] Sperling R.S., Shapiro D.E., Coombs R.W., Todd J.A., Herman S.A., McSherry G.D., O'Sullivan M.J., Van Dyke R.B., Jimenez E., Rouzioux C., Flynn P.M. and Sullivan J.L. (1996). Maternal viral load, zidovudine treatment and risk of transmission of HIV from mother to child. *New England Journal of Medicine*; 335: 1621-1629.

[48] Goedert J., Duliege A.M. and Amos C. (1991). High risk HIV-1 infection for first-born twins. *Lancet*; 338(8781): 1471-1475.

[49] John G.C., Nduati R., Mbori-Ngacha D., Richardson B.A., Panteleff D., Mwatha A., Overbaugh J., Bwayo J., Ndinya-Achola J.O. and Kreiss J.K. (2001). Correlates of mother-to-child Human Immunodeficiency Virus type 1 (HIV-1) transmission: association with maternal plasma HIV-1 RNA load, genital HIV-1 DNA shedding, and breast infections. *Journal of Infectious Diseases*; 183 (2): 206-212.

[50] Miotti P.G., Taha T.E., Kumwenda N.I., Broadhead R., Mtimavalye L.A., Van der Hoeven L., Chiphangwi J.D., Liomba G. and Biggar R.J. (1999). HIV transmission through breastfeeding: a study in Malawi. *Journal of the American Medical Association*; 282(8): 744-749.

[51] Semba R.D., Kumwenda N., Hoover D.R., Taha T.E., Quinn T.C., Mtimavalye L., Biggar R.J., Broadhead R., Miotti P.G., Sokoll L.J., Hoeven L. and Chiphangwi J.D. (1999). Human Immunodeficiency Virus load in breast milk, mastitis, and mother-to-child transmission of Human Immunodeficiency Virus type 1. *Journal of Infectious Diseases*; 180(1): 93-98.

[52] Richardson B.A., John-Stewart G.C., Hughes J.P., Nduati R., Mbori-Ngacha D., Overbaugh J. and Kreiss J.K. (2003). Breast-milk infectivity in Human Immunodeficiency Virus type 1. *Journal of Infectious Diseases*; 187(5): 736-740.

[53] John G.C., Richardson B.A., Nduati R.W., Mbori-Ngacha D. and Kreiss J.K. (2001). Timing of breast milk HIV-1 transmission: a meta-analysis. *East African Medical Journal*; 78 (2): 75-79.

[54] Embree J.E., Njenga S., Datta P., Nagelkerke N.J., Ndinya-Achola J.O., Mohammed Z., Ramdahin S., Bwayo J.J. and Plummer F.A. (2000). Risk factors for postnatal mother-to-child transmission of HIV-1. *AIDS*; 14(16): 2535-2541.

[55] Ekpini E.R., Wiktor S.Z., Satten G.A., Adjorlolo-Johnson G.T., Sibailly T.S., Ou C.Y., Karon J.M., Brattegaard K., Whitaker J.P., Gnaore E., De Cock K.M. and Greenberg A.E. (1997). Late postnatal mother-to-child transmission of HIV-1 in Abidjan, Cote d'Ivoire. *Lancet*; 349(9058): 1054-1059.

[56] Mills E. J., Wu P., Seely D. and Guyatt G.H. (2005). Vitamin supplementation for prevention of mother-to-child transmission of HIV and pre-term delivery: a systematic review of randomized trial including more than 2800 women. *AIDS Research and Therapy*; 2(1):4.

[57] Kupta R., Garland M., Msamanga G., Spiegelman D., Hunter D. and Fawzi W. (2005). Selenium status, pregnancy outcomes and mother-to-child transmission of HIV-1. *Journal of Acquired Immune Deficiency Sydrome*; 39 (2): 203-210.

[58] Taha T.E., Biggar R.J., Broadhead R.L., Mtimavalye L.A., Justesen A.B., Liomba G.N., Chiphangwi J.D. and Miotti P.G. (1997). Effect of cleansing the birth canal with antiseptic solution on maternal and newborn morbidity and mortality in Malawi: clinical trial. *British Medical Journal*; 315(7102): 216-219.

[59] The International Perinatal HIV Group (1999). The mode of delivery and risk of vertical transmission of Human Immunodeficiency Virus type 1 a meta-analysis of 15 prospective cohort studies. *New England Journal of Medicine*; 340(13): 977-987.

[60] Connor E.M., Sperling R.S., Gelbert R., Kiseleu P., O'Sullian M.J., Van Dyke R., Bey M., Shearer W., Jacobson R.L., Jimenez E., Basin B., Delfraissy J.F., Culnane M., Coombs R., Elkins M., Moye J., Stratton P. and Basley J. (1994). Reduction of maternal-infant transmission of Human Immunodeficiency Virus type 1 with zidovudine treatment. Pediatric AIDS Clinical Trials Protocol 076 study group. *New England Journal of Medicine*; 331: 1173-1180.

[61] Wiktor S.Z., Ekpini E., Karon J.M., Nkengasong J., Maurice C., Severin S.T., Roels T.H., Kouassi M.K., Lackritz E.M., Coulibaly I.M. and Greenberg A.E. (1999). Short course oral zidovudine for prevention of mother-to-child transmission of HIV-1 in Abidjan, Cote d'Ivoire: a randomised trial. *Lancet*; 353(9155): 781-785.

[62] Dabis F., Msellati P., Meda N., Welffens-Ekra C., You B., Manigart O., Leroy V., Simonon A., Cartoux M., Combe P., Ouangre A., Ramon R., Ky-Zebro O., Montcho C., Salamon R., Rouzioux C., Van de Perre P. and Mandelbrot L. (1999). Six-month efficacy, tolerance and acceptability of a short regimen of oral Zidovudine to reduce vertical transmission of HIV in breastfed children in Cote d'Ivoire and Burkina Faso: a double-blind placebo-controlled multicentre trial. *Lancet*; 353: 786-792.

[63] Leroy V., Karon J.M., Alioum A., Ekpini ER., Meda N., Greenberg A.E., Msellati P., Hudgens M., Dabis F. and Wiktor S.Z. (2002) . 24-month efficacy of a maternal short course zidovudine regimen to prevent mother-to-child transmission of HIV-1 in West Africa. *AIDS*; 16(4): 631-641.

[64] PETRA® (2002). Efficacy of three short-course regimens of Zidovudine and lamivudine in preventing early and late transmission of HIV-1 from mother-to-child in

Tanzania, South Africa and Uganda (Petra study): a randomised, double-blind placebo-controlled trial. *Lancet*; 359(9313): 1178-1186.

[65] Songok E.M., Fujiyama Y., Adungo N., Vulule J., Kiptoo M., Kobayashi N., Mpoke S., Genga I., Tukei P.M. and Ichimura H. (2003). The use of short course Zidovudine to prevent mother-to-child transmission of Human Immunodeficiency Virus in rural Kenya. *American Journal of Tropical Medicine and Hygiene*; 69 (1): 8-13.

[66] Guay L.A., Musoke P., Fleming T., Bagenda D., Allen M., Nakabiito C., Sherman J., Bakaki P., Ducar C., Deseyve M., Emel L., Mirochnick M., Fowler M.G., Mofenson L., Miotti P., Dransfield K., Bray D., Mmiro F. and Jackson B. (1999). Intrapartum and neonatal single dose nevirapine compared with zidovudine for prevention of mother-to-child transmission of HIV-1 in Kampala, Uganda: HIVNET 012 randomized trial. *Lancet*; 354(9181): 795-802.

[67] Fowler M.G. (2000). Prevention of perinatal infection. What do we know? Where should future research go? *Annals of the New York Academy of Sciences*; 918: 45-52.

[68] Fortin J.F., Cantin R., Lamontagne G. and Tremblay M. (1997). Host-derived ICAM-1 glycoproteins incorporated on Human Immunodeficiency Virus type 1 are biologically active and enhance viral infectivity. *Journal of Virology*; 71(5): 4847-4851.

[69] Kantor R. and Katzenstein D. (2003). Polymorphism in HIV-1 non-subtype B protease and reverse transcriptase and its potential impact on drug susceptibility and drug resistance evolution. *AIDS Reviews*; 5(1): 25-30.

[70] Adje-Toure C., Bile C.E., Borget M.Y., Hertog K., Maurice C., Nolan M.L. and Nkengasong J.N. (2003). Polymorphism in protease and reverse transcriptase and phenotypic drug resistance of HIV-1 recombinant CRF02_AG isolates from patients with no prior use of antiretroviral drugs in Abidjan, Cote d'Ivoire. *Journal of Acquired Immune Deficiency Syndrome*; 34(1): 111-113.

[71] Jülg B. and Goebel F.D. (2005). HIV genetic diversity: any implications for drug resistance? *Infection*; 33(4):299-301.

[72] Abecasis A.B., Deforche K. and Bacheler L.T. (2005). Lack of reduced susceptibility to PIs in wild-type non-B subtypes and detection of hypersusceptibility to nelfinavir in HIV-1 patients infected with CRFO2_AG. *Third European HIV Drug Resistance Workshop*, Athens, Abstr. 28.

[73] Kinomoto M., Appiah-Opong R. and Brandful J.A. (2005).HIV-1 Proteases from drug-naive West African patients are differentially less susceptible to protease inhibitors. *Clinical Infectious Diseases*; 41: 243–251.

[74] Brenner B. (2007). Resistance and viral subtypes: how important are the differences and why do they occur? *Current Opinion HIV/AIDS*; 2: 94–102.

[75] Eshleman S.H., Hoover D.R., Chen S., Hudelson S.E., Guay L.A., Mwatha A., Fiscus S.A., Mmiro F., Musoke P., Jackson J.B., Kumwenda N., and Taha T. (2005a). Nevirapine (NVP) resistance in women with HIV-1 subtype C, compared with subtypes A and D, after the administration of single-dose NVP. *Journal of Infectious Diseases*; 192(1): 30-36.

[76] Flys T., Nissley D.V., Claasen C.W., Jones D., Shi C., Guay L.A., Musoke P., Mmiro F., Strathern J.N., Jackson J.B., Eshleman J.R. and Eshleman S.H. (2005). Sensitive drug-resistance assays reveal long-term persistence of HIV-1 variants with the K103N nevirapine (NVP) resistance mutation in some women and infants after the administration of single-dose NVP: HIVNET 012. *Journal of Infectious Diseases*; 192: 24–29.

[77] Loubser S., Balfe P., Sherman G., Hammer S., Kuhn L. and Morris L. (2006). Decay of K103N mutants in cellular DNA and plasma RNA after single-dose nevirapine to reduce mother-to-child HIV transmission. *AIDS*; 20(7): 995-1002.

[78] Chaix M.L., Ekouevi D.K., Rouet F., Tonwe-Gold B., Viho I., Bequet L., Peytavin G., Toure H., Menan H., Leroy V., Dabis F. and Rouzioux C.(2006). Low risk of nevirapine resistance mutations in the prevention of mother-to-child transmission of HIV-1: ANRS Study, Abidjan, Cote d'Ivoire. *Journal of Infectious Diseases;* 193(4): 482–487.

[79] Brenner B., Turner D., Oliveira M, Moisi D., Detorio M., Carobene M., Marlink R.G., Schapiro J., Roger M. and Wainberg M.A.(2003). A V106M mutation in HIV-1 clade C viruses exposed to efavirenz confers cross-resistance to nonnucleoside reverse transcriptase inhibitors. *AIDS;* 17(1): F1–F5.

[80] Brenner B., Oliveira M., Doualla-Bell F., Moisi D.D., Ntemgwa M., Frankel F., Essex M. and Wainberg M.A. (2006). HIV-1 subtype C viruses rapidly develop K65R resistance to tenofovir in cell culture. *AIDS;* 20 (9): F9–F13.

[81] Descamps D., Collin G., Letourneur F., Apetrei C., Damond F., Loussert-Ajaka I., Simon F., Saragosti S. and Brun-Vezinet F. (1997). Susceptibility of Human Immunodeficiency Virus type 1 group O isolates to antiretroviral agents. *Journal of Virology* 71(11): 8893–8898.

[82] Eshleman S.H., Hoover D.R., Chen S., Hudelson S.E., Guay L.A., Mwatha A., Fiscus S.A., Mmiro F., Musoke P., Jackson J.B., Kumwenda N., and Taha T. (2005). Nevirapine (NVP) resistance in women with HIV-1 subtype C, compared with subtypes A and D, after the administration of single-dose NVP. *Journal of Infectious Diseases;* 192(1): 30-36.

[83] Jackson J.B., Becker-Pergola G., Guay L.A., Musoke P., Mracna M., Fowler M.G., Mofenson L.M., Mirochnick M., Mmiro F. and Eshleman S.H. (2000). Identification of the K103N resistance mutation in Ugandan women receiving nevirapine to prevent HIV-1 vertical transmission. *AIDS;* 14(11): F111-F115.

[84] Beckerman K.P. (2002). Mothers, orphans and prevention of pediatric AIDS. *Lancet* 359: 1168-1169.

[85] Kwiek J.J., Russell E.S., Dang K.K., Burch C.L., Mwapasa V., Meshnick S.R. and Swanstrom R. (2008). The molecular epidemiology of HIV-1 envelope diversity during HIV-1 subtype C vertical transmission in Malawian mother-infant pair. *AIDS;* 22:863-871.

[86] Yang C., Li M., Newman R.D., Shi Y.P., van Eijk A.M., Otieno J., Misore A.O., Steketee R.W. Nahlen B.L. and Lal R.B. (2003). Genetic diversity of HIV-1 in western Kenya: subtype-specific differences in mother-to-child transmission. *AIDS;* 17(11):1667-1674.

[87] Eshleman S.H., Guay L.A., Mwatha A., Brown E., Musoke P., Mmiro F. and Jackson J.B. (2005). Comparison of mother-to-child transmission rates in Ugandan women with subtype A versus D HIV-1 who received single-dose nevirapine prophylaxis: HIV Network for Prevention Trials 012. *Journal of Acquired Immune Deficiency Syndrome;* 39(5): 593-597.

[88] Bulterys P.L., Dalai S.C. and Katzenstein D.A. (2010). Viral sequence analysis from HIV-infected mothers and infants: molecular evolution, diversity, and risk factors for mother-to-child transmission. *Clinical Perinatology;* 37 (4): 739-750.

[89] Renaud Becquet, Didier K. Ekouevi, Elise Arrive, Jeffrey S. A. Stringer, Nicolas Meda, Marie-Laure Chaix, Jean-Marc Treluyer,Vale´ riane Leroy, Christine Rouzioux, Ste´phane Blanche, and Francois Dabis (2009). Universal Antiretroviral Therapy for Pregnant and Breast-Feeding HIV-1–Infected Women:Towards the Elimination of Mother-to-Child Transmission of HIV-1 in Resource-Limited Settings. *Clinical Infectious Diseases;* 49: 1936-1945.

Part 2

Pharmacology and Host Interaction

4

Transport Mechanisms of Nucleosides and Nucleoside Analogues Reverse Transcriptase Inhibitors in the Brain

Zoran B. Redzic[1] and Sonja Misirlic Dencic[2]
[1]*Department of Physiology, Faculty of Medicine, Kuwait University*
[2]*Department of Biochemistry, School of Medicine, Belgrade University*
[1]*Kuwait*
[2]*Serbia*

1. Introduction

Because of their hydrophilic natures, movements of nucleosides and many of their analogues across cellular membranes are mediated by nucleoside transporter (NT) proteins. Thus, NT proteins play an important role in physiological actions of nucleosides and in alterations of their function under various pathophysiological conditions. Also, these proteins are important for the therapeutic actions of some of synthetic nucleosides that have pharmacological actions and are thus used as drugs, including nucleoside analogues reverse transcriptase inhibitors (King et al., 2006, Zhang et al., 2007).

Before the "molecular biology" era, it was possible to explore nucleoside transport processes mainly by functional transport studies, which measured transcellular flux or cellular uptake of radiolabelled nucleosides. These early studies have identified two distinct transport processes in mammalian cells: the equilibrative bidirectional transport with lower affinity for naturally occurring nucleosides and the concentrative, unidirectional secondary active transport (Na^+/nucleoside cotransport) which revealed higher affinity for nucleosides (Hyde et al., 2004, Baldwin et al., 2004). Also, based on inhibition of these processes by synthetic analogues and based on substrate specificity and kinetics, it was recognized that both groups were heterogeneous: equilibrative nucleoside transport processes were further categorized as either nitrobenzylthioinosine (NBMPR)-sensitive (*es*) or NBMPR-insensitive (*ei*), while concentrative transport processes were categorized as either *cit* (concentrative, NBMPR insensitive, thymidine important substrate), *cif* (concentrative, NBMPR insensitive, formycin B important substrate) or *cib* (concentrative, NBMPR insensitive, broadly selective for purine and pyrimidine nucleosides) (Cass et al., 1998). Transport studies have also revealed that all these transport processes are not ubiquitously distributed in all mammalian cells; while equlibrative transport processes were more or less ubiquitous, concentrative transport processes were mainly found in epithelia, endothelial layers and in the liver (for an early review of nucleoside transport processes see Young and Jarvis 1983).

Development of molecular biology techniques has allowed identification of the proteins responsible for nucleoside transport processes (King et al., 2006). Purification and N-terminal sequencing of the *es* transporter from human erythrocytes enabled cloning a human placental

cDNA encoding the corresponding transporter in 1996 (Griffiths et al., 1997a). cDNA clones encoding one of the *ei*-type transporter were subsequently isolated (Griffiths et al., 1997b, Crawford et al., 1998), while the remaining two *ei*-type transporters were identified and isolated as a result of the completion of the human genome project (Hyde et al., 2001). The isoforms corresponding to pyrimidine-, purine- and broadly selective concentrative nucleoside transport have been cloned and their structure was defined (Che et al., 1995, Ritzel et al., 1997, Wang et al., 1997, Gerstin et al., 2000, Patel et al., 2000, Ritzel et al., 2001).
All these proteins are members of two structurally unrelated protein families that are named (according to processes that they mediate) as equilibrative nucleoside transporter family (ENT) and concentrative nucleoside transporter family (CNT). These two familes are members of a superfamily of solute carriers (SLC), which includes facilitated transporters, ion-coupled transporters and exchangers that do not require ATP; ENT-family and CNT-family are in humans known as SLC29 and SLC28, respectively.

2. Molecular biology of nucleoside transporters

So far, seven nucleoside transporter proteins were identified and described in mammals; four of them belong to the ENT family and are categorized as ENT1-4, while three of them belong to the CNT family and are categorized as CNT1-3.

2.1 Equilibrative nucleoside transporter family

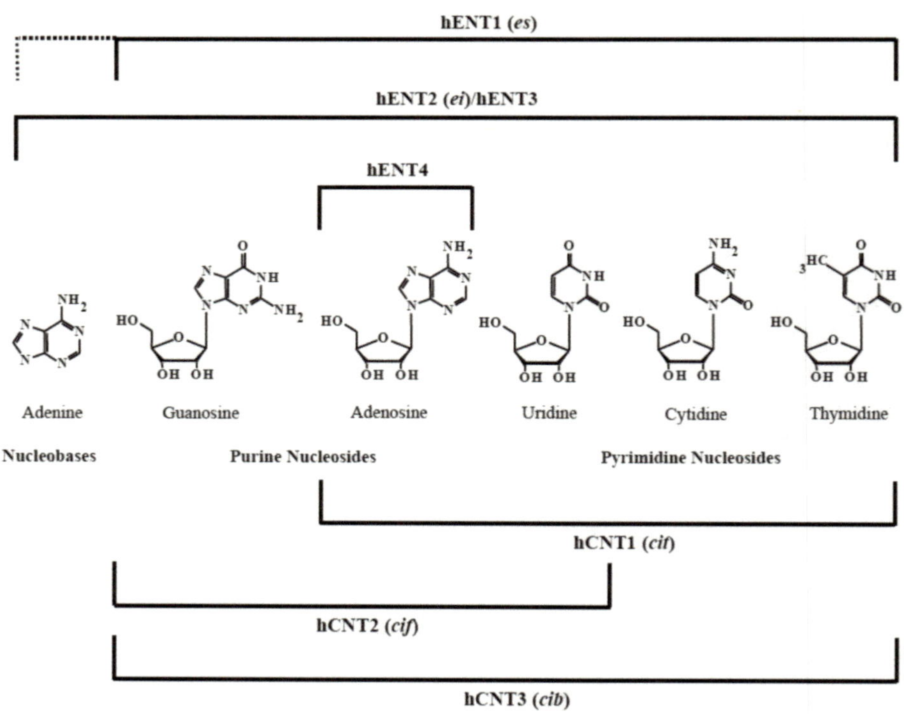

Fig. 1. Structures of naturally occurring nucleosides and nucleobases and their transport by human NT families. Reproduced with permission from Parkinson et al. (2011b).

Equilibrative nucleoside transporters are present in many cell types and they transport a broad range of purine and pyrimidine nucleosides (Griffits et al., 1997a, Griffits et al., 1997b); hENT2 also transports nucleobases (Figure 1) (Yao et al., 2002). hENT3 functions predominantly in intracellular membranes (Baldwin et al., 2005), while hENT4 is also known as plasma monoamino transporter and transport monoamines in the brain and heart, while it transports adenosine only at low pH (Barnes et al., 2006, Zhou et al., 2007).

2.1.1 Inhibition by synthetic analogues of nucleosides

As it was mentioned above, early transport studies have recognized that nucleoside analogue NBMPR, when present in nanomolar concentrations, inhibited partially equilibrative transport. It is known today that this molecule is highly specific inhibitor of nucleoside transport *via* ENT1 protein, which mediates *es*-type transport activity. Because hENT1 is inhibited by nanomolar NBMPR, whereas hENT2, hENT3 and hENT4 are either unaffected by NBMPR or inhibited by micromolar concentrations, this synthetic analogue was extensively used for studies of ENT1 protein.
Both ENT1 and ENT2 are also inhibited by drugs such as dipyridamole and dilazep, which are also used as coronary vasodilators because by blocking equilibrative uptake of adenosine they increase extracellular concentration of this nucleoside, thereby producing vasodilation; dilazep, dipirydamole and NBMPR bind either to or adjacent to the outward-facing region of the permeant-binding site (Baldwin et al., 2004). NBMPR and dipyridamole inhibit hENT1 with Ki values of <5 and 20 nM, respectively, and hENT2 with Ki values of >1 and 150 μM, respectively (Griffits et al., 1997a, Visser et al., 2002).
NBMPR is a membrane permeable nucleoside analogue; thus, if $[^3H]$NBMPR is used in a study, it will label all extracellular and intracellular binding sites, which makes relative quantification of extra- or intracellular binding sites impossible. To overcome this problem, a membrane-impermeant ENT1 ligand 5'-S-{2-(1-[(fluorescein-5-yl)thioureido]-hexanamido)ethyl}-6-N-(4-nitrobenzyl)-5'-thioadenosine (FTH-SAENTA) was developed (Visser et al., 2007). This ligand was used for competitive binding studies with a logic behind its application that in the absence of FTH-SAENTA, $[^3H]$NBMPR will bind for all binding sites (intracellularly and extracellularly), while in the presence of FTH-SAENTA, only intracellular binding sites will be labeled. This approach enabled differentiation of intra- and extracellular $[^3H]$NBMPR binding sites and revealed that the intracellular distribution of hENT1 varies largely in different cell types (Paproski et al., 2008), and was mainly confined to nuclear membranes (Mani et al., 1998) and mitochondria (Lee et al., 2006). hENT1 also undergoes intensive trafficking and recycling (see below) which could be another explanation for relatively high proportion of $[^3H]$NBMPR binding sites present intracellualrly.

2.2 Molecular properties, expression and mechanism of transport of ENTs

Four ENT proteins have been encoded in the human , rat and mouse genomes and the abbreviations used for those proteins are hENTs, rENTs and mENTs, respectively (Griffits et al., 1997a, Griffits et al., 1997b, Baldwin et al., 2005, Barnes et al., 2006). They have been also produced as recombinant proteins in African clawed frog (*Xenopus laevis)* oocytes, that allowed detailed kinetic studies of transport processes; data obtained mainly by this technique, which describe kinetics of transport of naturally occurring nucleosides and nucleobases towards hENTs are presented in Table 1, while kinetic of transport of synthetic analogues that are used as reverse transcriptase inhibitors drugs by hENTs are presented in Table 2.

Molecule	Nucleoside transporter that mediate transport	Available Km values (mM) (transporter is indicated in brackets)	Source
Nucleosides			
Adenosine	hENT1-4 & hCNT1-3	0.8 (hENT4), 0.008 (hCNT2), 0.015 (hCNT3)	Griffits et al., 1997a; 1997b; Baldwin et al., 2005; Barnes et al., 2006; Ritzel et al., 1997; 2001; Smith et al., 2004
Guanosine	hENT1-3, hCNT2, hCNT3	0.04 (hCNT3)	Griffits et al., 1997a; 1997b; Baldwin et al., 2005; Ritzel et al., 1997; 2001
Inosine	hENT1-3, hCNT1, hCNT3	0.005 (hCNT1), 0.05 (hCNT3)	Griffits et al., 1997a; 1997b; Baldwin et al., 2005; Ritzel et al., 1997; 2001
Uridine	hENT1-3, hCNT1-3	0.24 (hENT1), 0.2 (hENT2), 2.0 (hENT3), 0.03 (hCNT1), 0.04 (hCNT2), 0.015 (hCNT3)*	Griffits et al., 1997a; 1997b; Baldwin et al., 2005; Ritzel et al., 1997; 200; Slugoski et al., 2007, 2008;
Cytidine	hENT1-3, hCNT1, hCNT3	0.02 (hCNT1), 0.015 (hCNT3)	Griffits et al., 1997a; 1997b; Baldwin et al., 2005; Ritzel et al., 1997; 200; Slugoski et al., 2007, 2008;
Thymidine	hENT1-3, hCNT1, hCNT3	0.03 (hCNT1), 0.02 (hCNT3)	Griffits et al., 1997a; 1997b; Baldwin et al., 2005; Ritzel et al., 1997; 200; Slugoski et al., 2007, 2008;
Nucleobases			
Hypoxanthine	hENT2	0.7	Yao et al., 2002
Adenine	hENT3, hENT3	1.1 (hENT2)	Yao et al., 2002; Baldwin et al., 2005,
Thymine	hENT2	1.7	Yao et al., 2002
Uracil	hENT2	2.6	Yao et al., 2002

Table 1. Selectivity of human nucleoside transporters (expressed in Xenopus oocytes) for naturally occurring nucleosides and nucleobases. Affinity of ligands for transporters is also presented as Michaelis constant Km. * This value is for Na+ containing medium; in H+ containing medium Km is 0.06.

As mentioned above, the main location of ENT1 and ENT2 is the plasma membrane. However, immuno-staining and [^{3}H]NBMPR binding studies have often revealed a diffuse staining of cells. In example, when mouse CP was stained with these antibodies, obtained images revealed diffuse staining of CP epithelial cells in the case of mENT1 and disuse staining with a weak membrane staining of mENT2 (Parkinson et al., 2011). Such findings reflect, at least partially, abundant recycling and intracellular trafficking of those proteins. Studies that assessed NBMPR-binding in chromaffin cells suggested that NBMPR-binding disappears from the plasma membrane in about 5 hours, suggesting that ENT1 was internalized, with about 50% of this protein is recycled to the plasma membrane and the remaining protein probably degraded (Torres et al., 1992). A recent study has provided an important insight into the life cycle of human equilibrative nucleoside transporters (Nivillac et al., 2011). In this study, green fluorescence protein-tagged or FLAG- tagged hENT1 was transiently transfected into mammalian cells and the sequence of events regulating the hENT1 life cycle was studied; protein translocation to the plasma membrane was examined using fixed and live cell confocal microscopy (Nivillac et al., 2011). This study revealed that that the entire life cycle of the tagged-hENT1 protein was approximately 14 hours following translation, folding and ER export (Nivillac et al., 2011). After exiting the ER, hENT1 was translocated to the Golgi and glycosylated. Glycosylation probably plays a significant role in trafficking and function for a number of transporters including ENTs (Cai et al., 2005, Hendriks et al., 2004, Tanaka et al., 2004). hENT1 was then trafficked to the plasma membrane in association with the microtubule network in a variety of vesicles; in the plasma membrane hENT1 was co-localized with actin, which suggested that this transporter was anchored in the membrane by the actin cytoskeleton (Nivillac et al., 2011). This finding was consistent with previous observations for some other transporters, such as mouse GABA transporter 1 (Moss et al., 2009). After about an hour at the plasma membrane hENT1 internalized and interestingly only a proportion of the transporter population was recycled, which could indicate an efficient mechanism for fine-tuning, similar to what was described for the organic anion exchanger OAT1 (Zhang et al., 2008). Finally, internalized protein is degraded via the lysosomal pathway and observations suggest the complete life cycle of tagged hENT1 within these cells is approximately 14 hours.

In addition to studies on ENT 1 trafficking, efforts were also made to understand the mechanisms by which expression of ENT1 is modulated. A study investigated whether stress-activated kinases regulate ENT1 expression and function, using a mouse myeloid leukemic cell line as a model. It was revealed that Jun N-terminal kinase activation resulted in rapid loss of mENT1 function, mRNA expression and promoter activity; c-Jun decreased mENT1 promoter activity, which suggested a specific role for this transcription factor in mENT1 regulation. Overall, this study concluded that activation of JNK-cJun pathway negatively regulates mENT1(Leisewitz et al., 2011).

Current knowledge suggest that ENT3 is present in most tissues, including brain (Lu et al., 2004). It was found to co-localize with lysosomal markers and showed broad selectivity and low affinity towards the naturally occurring nucleosides and was unaffected by micromolar NBMPR, dipyridamole or dilazep (Baldwin et al., 2005). It was also indicated that hENT3 was found in mitochondrial membrane in several human cell lines (Govindarajan et al., 2009). Human and mouse ENT3 have a long hydrophilic N-terminus that contains a conserved characteristic of endosomal and /or lysosomal targeting sequences (Baldwin et al., 2005). Thus, when expressed in *Xenopus* oocytes, hENT3 and mENT3 did not have functional role in transport across the plasma membrane unless the N-terminus was modified (Baldwin et al., 2005). This transporter is activated at low pH (proton-dependent activation), which may be an important feature for its localization in acidic environment, like lysosomes and mitochondria. A physiological function of this transporter could be to transport nucleosides and nucleobases that are produced by nucleic acid breakdown in lysosomes and to provide material for mitochondrial DNA synthesis. A recent study revealed that hENT3 mRNA was the most abundant when compared to other hNTs mRNAs in human choroid plexus (Redzic et al., 2010).

Immunocytochemistry and immunonlotting have detected presence of ENT4 in human and mouse brain and in human, mouse and rat heart (Barnes et al., 2006). hENT4 revealed selectivity for adenosine, while mENT4 also shows affinity to transport adenine; affinity for substrates appears to be low and proton-dependent (Barnes et al., 2006). hENT4 is unaffected by as much as 1 μM NBMPR and only partially inhibited by micromolar dipyridamole. This transporter is also known as plasma membrane monoamine transporter (PMAT); experimental data also suggest that transport of substrates by h/mENT4 is inhibited by organic cation transporter inhibitor 1,1'-diethyl-2,2'-cyanine (decynium-22) and dopamine transporter inhibitor (Barnes et al., 2006). Structure analysis suggested that human and mouse ENT4 are closely related to ENT3 in a fruit fly (*Drosophila melanogaster*), rather than to human and mouse ENT1, a data that could suggest early divergence from other mammalian ENTs during the evolution (Barnes et al., 2006).

2.3 Molecular properties of transport by concentrative nucleoside transporters

CNT1 and CNT2 proteins are found primarily in epithelial tissues of small and large intestine, kidney, liver, heart (CNT2), pancreas (CNT2), skeletal muscle (CNT2), brain endothelial cells (CNT2) and choroid plexus (CNT2) (Gray et al., 2004, Redzic et al, 2005). CNT3 protein is found the pancreas, trachea, bone marrow, mammary gland and choroid plexus (Gray et al, 2004, Redzic et al., 2005, Redzic et al., 2010). Structure of human, rat and mouse CNTs is largely identical, with hCNT1 and rCNT1 being 83% identical at protein level, hCNT2 and rCNT2 being 81% identical and hCNT3 and mCNT3 being 78% identical (Gray et al., 2004). CNT1 is pyrimidine selective, but also transports adenosine with high-affinity and low capacity (Ritzel et al., 2001); CNT2 transport purine nucleosides and pyrimidine uridine (Wang et al., 1997, Ritzel et al., 1998), while CNT3 is broadly selective and transports both purine and pyrimidine nucleosides (Ritzel et al., 1997).

Membrane transport of nucleosides by CNTs takes place in symport with Na^+ and/or H^+. Thus, this process is electrogenic, since an uncharged particle (i.e. nucleoside) is transported together with an ion. If these transporters are produced as functional recombinant proteins in a heterologous expression system (i.e. *Xenopus* oocytes), molecular properties of nucleoside transport could be studied by steady-state electrophysiology techniques, using the two microelectrode voltage-clamp (Smith et al., 2005).

Using this approach, it has been shown that hCNT1 and hCNT2 are coupling nucleoside translocation to cotransport of Na^+ (i.e. they are Na+-specific) (Smith et al., 2004), while hCNT3 couples nucleoside translocation to cotransport of Na^+ and H^+ (Smith et al., 2005). For hCNT1 and hCNT2 the coupling ratio is 1:1, while for hCNT3 the Na^+:nucleoside coupling ration is 2:1, while the H^+:nucleoside coupling ratio is 1:1 (Smith et al., 2007).

Pre-steady-state currents measurements in hCNT-producing *Xenopus* oocytes revealed the transporter valence to be -1 and -2 for hCNT1 and hCNT3, respectively; it was estimated that 10^{10} to 10^{11} hCNT2 and hCNT3 transporters were present per oocyte (Smith et al., 2004, 2005). The sequence of events during CNTs-mediated transport has been elucidated partially. First Na^+ and/or H^+ bind to hCNT1 or hCNT3 and this event increases the affinity of these proteins for nucleoside substrates; in the case of hCNT3, after nucleoside binding it binds second Na^+ (Smith et al., 2004, 2005). Thus, the Na^+ coupling ratio for hCNT3 (2:1) if compared to the Na^+ coupling ratio for hCNT1 (1:1) suggests that the former one is more capable to transport nucleosides against their concentration gradient. Interestingly, H^+ binding for hCNT3 changes its conformation (when compared hCNT3 with Na^+ ion bound), so Na^+-coupled hCNT3 transports purine and pyrimidine nucleosides and also nucleoside analogue reverse transport inhibitor zidovudine, while H^+-coupled hCNT3 is selective for pyrimidines and does not transport zidovudine (Smith et al, 2005).

3. Distribution of nucleoside transporters in the brain

Expression of nucleoside transporters in the brain was mainly explored by techniques *in situ* (i.e. ligand binding and immunostaining of brain slices or various brain regions), immunoblotting and by *in vitro* techniques (i.e. cell cultures). Surprisingly, those approaches often produced conflicting results. In example, an *in situ* study that used polyclonal antibodies against rENT1 and rENT2 revealed that those transporters were present in all neurons explored, while only some astrocytes showed rENT1 staining, while rENT2 staining on astrocytes was observed only sporadically (Alanko et al., 2006) Contrary to this finding, a study that used immunoblotting on rat astrocytes in primary culture has clearly revealed that both rENT1 and rENT2 were present (Redzic et al., 2010b). Those discrepancies could be partially explained by dedifferentiation of cells in culture.

3.1 Equilibrative nucleoside transporter 1

ENT1 was by far the most well studied nucleoside transporter in the brain. This was largely because a specific ligand NBMPR that binds to this protein with high affinity was available (see above). Thus, most of our current knowledge was gained on studies that used brain sections that were incubated with [^{3}H]NBMPR, with unlabelled NMBPR being used to define non-specific binding and with autoradiography film being used to visualize the distribution of specific binding sites. These studies have revealed localized distribution of binding sites for this radioligand, indicating uneven distribution of ENT1 in rodent brain, which was unexpected because a general view was that ENT1 is an ubiquitous nucleoside transporter. High [^{3}H]NBMPR binding was detected in thalamus and superior colliculus, while low binding was detected in hippocampus, cerebral cortex and cerebellum; other regions show no ligand binding (Geiger et al., 1984, Parkinson et al., 1996, Bailey et al., 2002). Contrary to this, immunocytochemistry studies has revealed more even distribution of this transporter throughout the brain, with a strong signal being detected in cerebral cortex, hippocampus, striatum and cerebellum (Alanko et al., 2006).

In situ hybridization studies that detected distribution of mRNA encoding ENT1 have revealed its wide distribution in the brain with a strong signal being detected from hippocampus, cerebellum, cerebral cortex and striatum (Anderson et al., 1999). This technique has also detected ENT1 mRNA in astrocytes, and choroid plexus epithelial cells.

Distribution of hENT1 in human brain has also been investigated and these studies have revealed that hENT1 mRNA was very abundant in caudate nucleus, amygdale, hippocampus and thalamus, while it was scarce in *substantia nigra*; like in the rodent brain, there was no correlation between those findings and hENT1 protein distribution, which was greatest in several areas of cerebral cortex, much lower in thalamus and basal ganglia, and scarce in hippocampus and cerebellum (Jennings et al, 2001). However, in the human brain, a positive correlation was shown between hENT1 distribution and adenosine A1 receptors distribution (Jennings et al, 2001), which was opposite to findings in the rodent brain, where a correlation between rENT1 and A1 receptors distribution was either poor (Geiger et al., 1984, Bailey et al., 2002) or negative (Parkinson et al., 1996).

3.2 Equilibrative nucleoside transporter 2

Since there is no high-affinity ligand for ENT2 available so far, studies that explored distribution of ENT2 in the brain employed a strategy in which brain slices were probed with radiolabelled dipyridamole, a ligand that binds more or less equally to ENT1 and ENT2 and with radiolabelled dipyridamole in the presence of unlabelled NBMPR, which in nanomolar concentration binds to ENT1 (and thus block dipyridamole binding for this transporter). Under those circumstances, the detected radiligand binding that was not blocked by the presence of nanomolar NBMPR but was blocked by micromolar NBMPR could be largely attributed to ENT2. A problem with this strategy is that dipyridamole is very lipophilic and thus binds unspecifically, which limits usefulness of data drawn from these studies. Data available so far suggest that for guinea pig CNS membranes 40-50% of [^{3}H]dipyridamole binding could be attributed to ENT2 (Jones and Hammond, 1992).

Some studies have measured uptake of [^{3}H] adenosine in the presence of nanomolar NBMPR and in the presence of dipyridamole. The logic behind these studies was that adenosine cellular uptake *via* rENT1 would be inhibited by the presence of nanomolar NBMPR, while adenosine upake *via* both transporters would be inhibited in the presence of dipyridamole, so a difference between uptake rates under those two conditions could be credited to uptake via rENT2. Using this strategy it was revealed that [^{3}H] adenosine uptake by primary cultures of rat cerebral neurons and astrocytes was inhibited by >20 and >30% by the presence of nanomolar NBMPR, respectively, while dipyridamole inhibited more than 80% of uptake, which indicated that rENT2 was functionally more abundant than rENT1 in these cells (Parkinson et al., 2005).

Immunocytochemistry revealed that rENT2 had a widespread distribution of in rat brain and that this distribution largely overlapped with distribution of rENT1 (Alanko et al., 2006). Distribution of rENT2 mRNA in rat brain was widespread and more abundant than distribution of rENT1 and mRNA was localized in cerebral cortex, striatum, thalamus, hippocampus and cerebellum, choroid plexus and blood vessels (Anderson et al., 1999). Primary cultures of rat neurons and astrocytes also had more abundant mRNA for rENT2 than for rENT1, as revealed by quantitative RT-PCR (Parkinson et al., 2006).

3.3 Other equilibrative nucleoside transporters

It was revealed that rat and mouse brain express mRNA for ENT3 [Baldwin et al., 2005, Parkison et al., 2006). Human choroid plexus expressed abundantly hENT3 mRNA (Redzic et al., 2010a). However, so far there are no data demonstrating functional role of this transporter in the brain. Human, mouse and rat brain also express ENT4 mRNA that was widespread in neurons [Barnes et al., 2006, Parkinson et al., 2006, Vialou et al., 2007). Immunocytochemistry did not reveal presence of this transporter in astrocytes (Dahlin et al., 2007).

3.4 Concentrative nucleoside transporter 1

Amount of CNT1 mRNA in the brain was less abundant than in epithelia (Lu et al., 2004). In the brain, CNT1 mRNA was detected by in cerebral cortex, hypothalamus, hippocampus, cerebellum and choroid plexus (Lu et al., 2004). Rat astrocytes in primary culture express rCNT1 transcript, as revealed by RT-PCR, but the abundance was very low; however, rCNT1 protein was detected in these cells by immunoblotting (Redzic et al. 2010b).

3.5 Concentrative nucleoside transporter 2

The relative abundance of CNT2 mRNA in the rodent brain was low when compared to epithelial, barrier-forming layers, like intestine (Lu et al., 2004). RT-PCR revealed that distribution of rENT2 mRNA was widespread and uniform in all rat brain regions examined (Anderson et al., 1996). In situ hybridization revealed that neurons in the hippocampus, basal ganglia, cerebral cortex, hypothalamus and cerebellum had intense signal (Guillen-Gomez et al., 2004). Interestingly, in situ studies showed that CNT2 mRNA was not present in astrocytes (Guillen-Gomez et al., 2004), but it was present in primary cultures of mouse and rat astrocytes and functional activity of this transporter in those cells was revealed (Nagai et al., 2005, Peng et al., 2005, Redzic et al., 2010b). However, rCNT2 protein was absent from rat astrocytes in primary culture (Redzic et al., 2010b).

3.6 Concentrative nucleoside transporter 3

Rat and mouse brain revealed low abundance of CNT3 mRNA (Lu et al., 2004). mRNA was not detectable in primary cultures of rat neurons and astrocytes (Nagai et al., 2005, Redzic et al., 2010b), but surprisingly rCNT3 protein was detected in cultured rat astrocytes (Redzic et al., 2010b). Human brain contained hCNT3 transcripts, but with low abundance (Ritzel et al., 2001).

3.7 Expression of nucleoside transporters in the brain of ENT1-knockout mice

Genetic variation of equilibrative nucleoside transporters are very rare, which indicated that function of those proteins could be essential for the survival; thus, efforts were made to produce ENT1-knockout mouse, in order to analyze effects of mENT1 absence on homeostasis and on expression of other nucleoside transporters (for the procedure Choi et al., 2004). Surprisingly, it was found that mice lacking mENT1 have similar pattern of distribution of other nucleoside transporters as wild-type mice. A study that examined if the ENT1-null mouse heart was cardioprotected in response to ischemia showed that ENT1-null mouse hearts showed significantly less myocardial infarction (after 30-min coronary occlusion) compared with wild-type littermates (Rose et al., 2010). Wild-type adult mouse cardiomyocytes express predominantly ENT1 and this transporter was primarily responsible for purine nucleoside uptake; thus, ENT1-null cardiomyocytes exhibit severely impaired nucleoside transport that could cause a higher increase in extracellular adenosine following ischemia than in wild-type mouse (Rose et al., 2010). However, adenosine receptor expression profiles and expression pattern of ENT2, ENT3, and ENT4 were similar in cardiomyocytes isolated from ENT1-null adult mice compared with cardiomyocytes isolated from wild-type littermates (Rose et al., 2010). Quantitative RT-PCR was used to investigate mENT1-4 and mCNT1-3 transcripts in wild-type and ENT1-null mouse brain (Parkinson et al., 2011). This study showed that the most abundant transporter in wild-type brain was mENT1, while mENT2 was most abundant in the mENT1-null brain (Parkinson et al., 2011). Beside this difference, the NT expression patterns were similar between the wildtype and mENT1-null whole brain. This indicated that absence of mENT1 could be at least partially compensated by increased expression of mENT2 (Parkinson et al., 2011).

4. Nucleoside transporters at the blood-brain barrier and at the blood-cerebrospinal fluid barrier

A constant and well-controlled composition of the extracellular fluid in the central nervous system (CNS) is essential for efficient neuronal processing. To control the brain microenvironment, the endothelial blood-brain barriers (BBB) exists in all vertebrates, except for a few fish species (Bundgaard and Abbott, 2008). The BBB and the blood-cerebrospinal fluid barrier (BCSFB) are formed by brain endothelial cells (BECs) and choroid plexus (CP) epithelial cells, respectively (for a review see Redzic, 2011). The BBB and the BCSFB are not only anatomical barriers, but also dynamic tissues that express multiple transporters, receptors and enzymes.

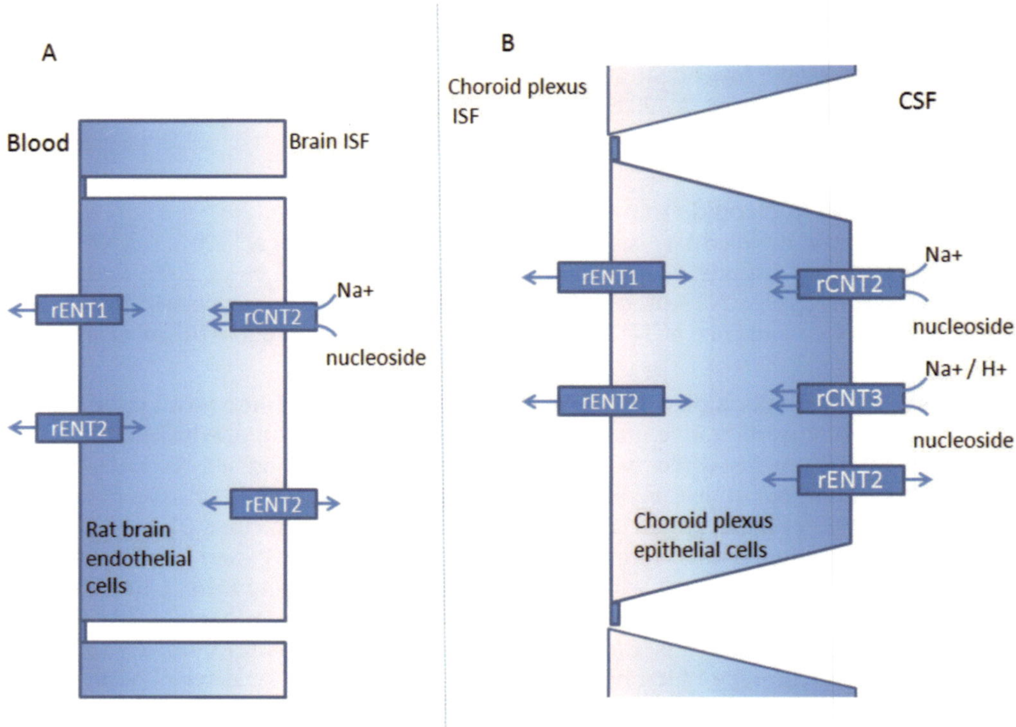

Fig. 2. A proposed distribution of rENTs and rCNTs in rat brain endothelial cells (A) and in rat choroid plexus epithelial cells (B). A model was proposed based on in vitro data, when rat brain endothelial cells and rat choroid plexus epithelial cells were grown as monolayers on permeable supports (Redzic et al., 2005, Redzic et al., 2006).

The two main functions of these barriers are to impede free diffusion between brain fluids and blood and to provide transport processes for essential nutrients, ions and metabolic waste products. Presence of tight junctions between adjacent brain endothelial cells or choroid plexus epithelial cells restrict paracellular diffusion across these cellular layers. Thus, hydrophilic molecules (like naturally occurring nucleosides) cannot readily enter brain ISF or CSF by simple diffusion and must be transferred across the layer by ENTs and CNTs located in these cellular layers. On the other hand, many synthetic nucleosides and some nucleobases are scarcely soluble in water and they are more soluble in lipids; such molecules can diffuse into lipid bilayers, but both the BBB and the BCSFB use ATP-driven transporters that mediate efflux of lipophilic molecules (Miller, 2010).

Adenosine transport across the BBB was investigated *in vivo*; efflux transport studies (brain intracellular fluid (ISF) to blood transport) and influx transport studies (blood to brain ISF transport) were performed following intracerebral and intracarotid injections of

[^{14}C]adenosine, respectively, together with a [^{3}H]vascular space marker (Isakovic et al., 2004). This study revealed that estimated BBB efflux clearance of [^{14}C] radioactivity after intracerebral injection of [^{14}C]adenosine was almost threefold higher than the estimated BBB influx clearance of radioactivity after intracarotid injection of this molecule (Isakovic et al., 2004). However, if the values of Vmax and Km calculated from this study plus the reported brain ISF adenosine concentration (Melani et al. 1999) are inserted into the Michaelis equation, an estimated velocity of BBB efflux transport *in vivo* was 100-fold lower than the reported rate of uptake of adenosine into neurones/glia (Lawrence et al. 1994) and the rate of phosphorylation by adenosine kinase inside the cells (Phillips and Newsholme 1979), which indicates that adenosine BBB efflux transport does not play an important role in adenosine homeostasis under resting physiological conditions. This study also revealed that most [^{14}C]radioactivity in plasma appeared with the HPLC peaks for adenosine metabolites adenine and hypoxanthine after the intracerebral injection of [^{14}C] adenosine, while negligible amounts appeared within the adenosine peak; this suggested that the brain capillary endothelial cells appear to act as an enzymatic barrier for adenosine, rapidly degrading this molecule (Isakovic et al., 2004). Using the same technique, the BBB efflux transport of other purines was studied *in vivo* after the intracerebral injection of radiolabelled purines; this study has revealed rapid BBB efflux clearance of hypoxanthine and adenine (Isakovic et al., 2002).

Rat brain endothelial cells (RBECs) were also grown as primary monocultures on permeable supports (filters); under those circumstances they developed transcellular electrical resistance that was sufficient to provide separate studies of cellular uptake with upper chamber as a donor and with lower chamber as a donor (Redzic et al., 2005). This study revealed that RBECs expressed rENT1, rENT2 and rCNT2 mRNA and protein; interestingly, rCNT2 was the most abundant at both transcript and protein level. Transcripts for rCNT1 and rCNT3 were either absent or of very low abundance. [^{3}H]adenosine transport data revealed that the cellular uptake of this nucleoside was sodium-dependent only when lower chamber was a donor. Sodium-independent uptake of adenosine was observed across both membranes, consistent with detection of both rENT1 and rENT2 proteins in these cells, but the pattern of inhibition by NBMPR suggested that rENT1 was confined to the membranes facing the upper chamber, whereas rENT2 was probably present in both membrane domains (Redzic et al., 2005). When RBEC are grown on permeable supports, the cellular membranes facing the lower and upper chambers display some of the characteristics of the *in vivo* basolateral (brain ISF-facing) and apical (blood-facing) membranes, respectively (Reichel et al. 2003). Therefore, findings from this study suggested that concentrative adenosine uptake at the BBB *in vivo* may be limited to the brain ISF-facing membrane, whereas transport *via* ENT1 occurs only on the opposite side. Such a pattern of nucleoside transporter distribution (presented in Figure 2A) combined with the detected rapid metabolism of adenosine in endothelial cells (Isakovic et al. 2004) may suggest that the role of the BBB is to remove adenosine from the brain ISF, rather than to mediate uptake of this purine nucleoside from the circulation.

Primary cultures of sheep CP epithelial cells (CPEC) were also grown as monolayers on permeable supports (Redzic et al., 2006) and these cells expressed some features typical of the CPEC *in situ;* they developed relatively high transepithelial electrical resistance which was accompanied by low paracellular permeability, a property that enabled the use of this model for studies of transcellular transport of radiolabelled adenosine. Transcellular permeability of these monolayers towards [^{14}C]adenosine was surprisingly low, but when adenosine intracellular metabolism was inhibited, there was more than a five-fold increase in the transcellular permeability for [^{14}C]adenosine, which indicated that intracellular phosphorylation of adenosine into nucleotides and/or its degradation into nucleobases that show different kinetic properties to adenosine might be the cause of low transcellular permeability. This study also applied HPLC analysis with simultaneous detection of radioactivity and revealed that [^{14}C] radioactivity which appeared in the acceptor chamber after the incubation of CPEC monolayers with [^{14}C]adenosine in the donor chamber, mostly was present as [^{14}C] hypoxanthine, which indicated that sheep CPEC in primary culture, similarly to the rat brain endothelial cells, act as an enzymatic barrier towards adenosine (Redzic et al., 2006). Uptake studies on this model revealed that [^{14}C]adenosine concentrative uptake was confined to the apical ('CSF') side of these cells, indicating uneven distribution of nucleoside transporters and a possible role in removing adenosine from the CSF.

A study on sheep CPEC in primary culture, grown on permeable supports, gave an insight on nucleobase transport and metabolism in the CPEC; it was revealed that uptake of [^{14}C]hypoxanthine by the apical side was partially Na^+-dependent and partially Na^+-independent, the latter process being partially mediated by ENT2. Hypoxanthine was metabolized inside the CPEC through the action of hypoxanthine-guanine phosphoribosyl transferase, producing nucleotides and the nucleoside inosine. Some hypoxanthine and inosine left CPEC through the opposite side of the cell. This might suggest that the uptake of hypoxanthine by the apical side of the sheep CPEC could serve two important functions *in vivo*, which was to provide material for local demands of the CPE for nucleotides through the salvage pathways, as well as to remove excess hypoxanthine to the CP interstitial fluid.

The same model was also used to grow primary cultures of rat CPEC; RT-PCR and Western blots of revealed the presence of rENT1, rENT2, rCNT2 and rCNT3, but not the pyrimidine-preferring rCNT1 (Redzic et al., 2005). Adenosine uptake by these cells showed a polarized distribution of Na^+-dependent transport of [^{14}C]adenosine at the apical cell surface that could be attributed to rCNT2 and/or rCNT3. Na^+-independent transport that was partially NBMPR-sensitive at the basolateral cell surface which could be attributed to the presence of rENT1 and rENT2 [91]. The remaining adenosine uptake at apical cell surfaces that was sodium-independent was NBMPR-insensitive, thus could be attributed to rENT2 (Figure 2B) (Redzic et al., 2005).

Expression of nucleoside transporters at transcript level and nucleoside uptake was studied in isolated portions of human lateral ventricle choroid plexuses that were obtained during neurosurgery (Redzic et al., 2010a). Quantitative RT-PCR revealed that transcripts for hENT1-3 and hCNT3 were present with mRNA for hENT3 being the most abundant. hCNT1 and hCNT2 transcripts were absent or present at very low abundance. Human CP samples took up radiolabelled inosine by both concentrative and equilibrative processes. However, the equilibrative uptake was mediated only by hENT2, while hENT1 transport activity was absent, which could suggested either that this protein was absent in the human CP or that it was confined to the basolateral side of the CP epithelium (which did not come in contact with uptake buffer in this study) (Redzic et al., 2010a).

Thus, several lines of evidences suggest that polarized distribution of nucleoside transporters at the BBB and in the CP epithelium, with CNTs located on sides facing brain extracellular fluids (ISF and CSF) and equlibrative transport across the opposite, blood facing side, may play an important role in the removal of nucleosides from brain fluids. Also, it appears that brain endothelial cells represent an enzymatic barrier towards at least some nucleosides and nucleobases; this enzymatic activity may further impede blood to brain transport.

5. Expression of NTs in neurons and astrocytes and the role of these transporters in nucleoside homeostasis in the brain

Adenosine concentration in the brain extracellular fluid (ECF) depends on three processes: (a) its formation in neurons (Zamzow et al., 2008, Parkinson et al. 2005) and transport from neurons across the plasma membrane to the ECF; (b) its formation extracellularly through the action of soluble or membrane bound ecto-nucleotidases on ATP that is released from astrocytes (Parkinson and Xiong, 2004) and uptake by astrocytes, a process that is normally followed by intracellular conversion to inosine and hypoxanthine (Zamzow et al., 2008). However, relative contributions of intracellular and extracellular formation are not clear. A classical view suggests that adenosine is mainly formed intracellularly as a consequence of ATP hydrolysis; cellular concentrations of ATP are manifolds higher than concentrations of adenosine (Fredholm et al., 2005), so a small increases in ATP degradation can cause a large increase in adenosine concentration. Once it is formed, intracellular adenosine leaves cells by facilitated diffusion via ENTs. There are several lines of evidences showing that neurons in primary culture, after being exposed to hypoxia / glucose deprivation released adenosine and inosine (Parkinson et al., 2005, Parkinson and Xiong, 2004) and also release these two nucleosides when they were treated with the glutamate receptor agonist N-methyl-D-aspartate (Zamzow et al., 2008, 2009), while dipyridamole, a non-selective ENT1/2 inhibitor in rat cells, inhibited this release.

A non-classical view suggests that adenosine is mainly formed extracellularly by a series of reactions catalyzed by ecto-nucleotidases following cellular release of ATP (Dunwiddie and Masino 2001). Evidences suggest that rat cortical astrocytes in primary cultures, when exposed to hypoxia, release adenosine and inosine, but that release was not blocked by dipyridamole, suggesting that transport across the plasma membrane did not play a role in this release (Parkinson and Xiong, 2004). Thus, it appears that in the brain both pathways for adenosine production are present, with neurons releasing mainly adenosine (as a product of ATP hydrolysis) and astrocytes releasing ATP that is hydrolysed extracellularly to adenosine (Parkinson et al., 2005). Furthermore, data suggest that adenosine that was produced by neurons was mainly taken up by astrocytes and metabolized intracellularly to hypoxanthine (Zamzow et al., 2008); hypoxanthine was then released in the ISF. The net effect of this process is that adenosine neuromodulatory action was time-limited, since adenosine was rapidly converted to nucleobase hypoxanthine, which has no effect in cell signaling.

A study that explored the role of neuronal equilibrative NTs in adenosine influx and efflux during cerebral ischemia has used mice with neuronal expression of hENT1 and wild type littermates to compare responses to in vitro and in vivo hypoxic / ischemic conditions (Zhang et al., 2011). Hypoxia / oxygen-glucose deprivation produced greater inhibition of excitatory neurotransmission in slices from wild type mice than from mice expressing hENT1. Presence of NBMPR abolished these differences, which altogether indicated that neuronal equilibrative NTs reduce hypoxia / ischemia-induced increase in extracellular adenosine concentrations (Zhang et al., 2011). This may suggest that that inhibition of neuronal adenosine transporters may beneficial for the treatment of cerebral ischemia.

A recent study has revealed that hypoxia and glucose deprivation can also affect expression of nucleoside transporters in rat astrocytes in primary culture. Those cells expressed rENT1, rENT2, rCNT1 and rCNT3; rCNT2 was present at transcript level but the protein could not be detected (Redzic et al., 2010b). Hypoxia and glucose deprivation (60 min) was accompanied by an increase in adenosine and ATP concentration in culture medium and caused a decrease in the expression of rENT1 in astrocytes; hypoxia and glucose deprivation followed by 1 h recovery period caused a decrease in the expression of rENT1 and rENT2 and a decrease in equilibrative cellular uptake of [^{3}H]adenosine by astrocytes (Redzic et al., 2010b). Astrocyte cultures that were subjected to 1h hypoxia and glucose deprivation that was followed by 1 h recovery period were less able to take up [^{3}H]adenosine by equilibrative mechanisms than cultures from the control group. That decrease in uptake ability could potentially increase ISF adenosine during ischemia (Redzic et al., 2010b).

6. Transport of anti-HIV drugs by human nucleoside transporters

Since the onset of the AIDS pandemic in 1981, infection with the human immunodeficiency virus (HIV) infection has spread exponentially throughout the world. HIV is neuro-invasive (with invasion occurring early in the course of the infection), neuro-virulent (causing a neuropathy, myopathy, myelopathy, and dementia), but it is not especially neurotrophic (Manji and Miller 2004). Several drugs are now available for treatment of HIV infection, including the following nucleoside analogues reverse transcriptase inhibitors: zidovudine (1-[(2R,4S,5S)-4-azido-5-(hydroxymethyl)oxolan-2-yl]-5-methyl-1,2,3,4-tetrahydropyrimidine-2,4-dione), also known as 3′-azido-3′-deoxythymidine (trade name Retrovir), abacavir [4-(2-amino-6-cyclopropylamino-9H-purin-9-yl)-1- cyclopent-2-enyl]methanol) (trade name Ziagen), stavudine (1-[(2R,5S)-5-(hydroxymethyl)-2,5-dihydrofuran-2-yl]-5-methyl-1,2,3,4-tetrahydropyrimidine-2,4-dione) also known as 2'-3'-didehydro-2'-3'-dideoxythymidine (trade name Zerit), lamivudine (4-amino-1-[(2R,5S)-2-(hydroxymethyl)-1,3-oxathiolan-5-yl]-1,2-dihydropyrimidin-2-one) also known as 2',3'-dideoxy-3'-thiacytidine (trade names Zeffix, Heptovir or Epivir), emitricitabine (4-amino-5-fluoro-1-[(2R,5S)-2-(hydroxymethyl)-1,3-oxathiolan-5-yl]-1,2-dihydropyrimidin-2-one), trade name Emtriva, zalcitabine (4-amino-1-[(2R,5S)-5-(hydroxymethyl)oxolan-2-yl]-1,2-dihydropyrimidin-2-one) also known as 2'-3'-dideoxycytidine (trade name Hivid) and didanosine (9-[(2R,5S)-5-(hydroxymethyl)oxolan-2-yl]-6,9-dihydro-3H-purin-6-one) also known as 2',3'-dideoxyinosine (trade name Videx). Potentially, all those nucleoside analogues could be used for the neuro-HIV treatment; however, their effect on HIV replication in the brain largely depends on its ability to enter the CNS and concentrations that they can achieve in the brain ECF and in the cytoplasm. Transport across the BBB largely depends on physico-chemical characteristics of a drug (polarity, lipophilicity, molecular weight) (for the role of lipophilicity in the BBB passage see Abbott et al., 2008 and Abbott et al., 2010). Based upon their measured CSF concentrations and therapeutic effects, these anti-HIV nucleosides are classified either as high CNS penetrating drugs (zidovudine and abacavir), intermediate CNS penetrating drugs (stavudine, lamivudine and emitricitabine) or low CNS penetrating drugs (zalcitabine and didanosine) (Letendre et al., 2008).The first drug that was approved for AIDS was zidovudine. Intracellularly, this drug is phosphorylated to azidothymidine triphosphate, which then inhibits reverse transcriptase and thus impedes viral replication. This drug was partially successful in controlling replication of HIV in the brain. NTs- mediated uptake across the BBB of zidovudine is low; however, because of its lipophilic nature, it passes the BBB by a simple diffusion and then enters the cells. Thus, it appears that distribution of zidovudine in the brain fluids largely do not depend on NT- mediated transport across the BBB and CPs (Thomas and Segal., 1997). However, *in vitro* studies confirmed that zidovudine, zalcitabine and didanosine are substrates for several nucleoside transporters (Table 2) (Baldwin et al., 2005, Yao et al., 2001).

RTI	Nucleoside transporter that mediate transport	Source
Zidovudine	hENT2, hENT3, hCNT1	Baldwin et al., 2005, Yao et al., 2001
Zalcitabine	hENT1-3, hCNT1, hCNT3	Baldwin et al., 2005, Yao et al., 2001
Didanosine	hENT2*, hENT3, hCNT2, hCNT3	Baldwin et al., 2005, Yao et al., 2001

Table 2. Transport of nucleoside analogues reverse transcriptase inhibitors (RTIs) by human nucleoside transporters. *The estimated Km value for hENT2 is 2.3 mM

Human ENT2, expressed in *Xenopus* oocytes, transports zidovudine, zalcitabine and didanosine (Yao et al., 2001). Human ENT3 (which is mainly located intracellularly) also transports these three nucleoside analogues, while hENT1 transports zalcitabine. hCNT1, which is pyrimidine nucleoside-selective, transports pyrimidine analogues zidovudine and zalcitabine, hCNT2, which is purine nucleoside-selective, transports purine analogue didanosine, while hCNT3, which is broadly selective, transports all three drugs (Smith et al., 2004, Smith et al., 2005).

7. Conclusion

Over the last two decades, seven separate human nucleoside transporters have been cloned and successfully produced as functional recombinant proteins in a heterologous expression system (*Xenopus Laevis* oocytes), which enabled their functional characterization. Findings from these studies provided the tools that were needed to better understand nucleoside transport in the brain under normal physiological conditions and under various pathophysiological conditions (e.g. ischemia / hypoxia) as well as to understand therapeutic potential of these processes. Molecular structure of equlibrative nucleoside transporters has been elucidated, but more data on clarification of concentrative nucleoside transporters molecular architecture are still needed. The roles of individual nucleoside transporters in cells that possess multiple transporter isoforms are still not being fully elucidated, which also applies to their roles in the brain. An important attempt to disentanglement the contributions of individual nucleoside transporters was done by a genetic knock-out approach, which produced mENT1-null mice. Such knowledge should provide important data required to produce nucleoside analogues reverse transcriptase inhibitors that are brain-accessible.

8. References

Abbott, J., Dolman, E., & Patabendige, K. (2008). Assays to predict drug permeation across the blood-brain barrier, and distribution to brain. *Current Drug Metabolism*, Vol.9, No.9,(November 2008), pp. 901-10, ISSN 1389-2002

Abbott, J., Patabendige, K., Dolman, E., Yusof, R., & Begley, J. (2010). Structure and function of the blood-brain barrier. *Neurobiology of Dis*ease, Vol.37, No.1, (January 2010), pp.13-25, ISSN 0969-9961

Alanko, L., Porkka-Heiskanen, T., & Soinila, S. (2006). Localization of equilibrative nucleoside transporters in the rat brain. *Journal of Chemical Neuroanatomy*, Vol.31,(April 2010), pp. 162-8, ISSN 0891-0618

Anderson, CM. Xiong, W. Young, JD., Cass, CE., & Parkinson, FE. (1996). Demonstration of the existence of mRNAs encoding the N1/cif and N2/cit sodium/nucleoside cotransporters in rat brain. *Molecular Brain Research*, Vol.42, No.2, (December 1996), pp. 358-61, ISSN 0169-328X

Anderson, CM., Xiong, W., Geiger, JD., Young, JD. Cass, CE., Baldwin, SA., & Parkinson, FE. (1999). Distribution of equilibrative, nitrobenzylthioinosine-sensitive nucleoside transporters (ENT1) in brain. *Journal of Neurochemistry*, Vol.73, No.2, (August 1999), pp. 867-73, ISSN 0022-3042

Anderson, CM.; Baldwin, SA.; Young, JD.; Cass, CE., & Parkinson, FE. (1999). Distribution of mRNA encoding a nitrobenzylthioinosine-insensitive nucleoside transporter (ENT2) in rat brain. *Molecular Brain Research*, Vol.70, No.2, (July 1999), pp. 293-7, ISSN 0169-328X

Bailey, A., Matthes, H., Kieffer, B., Slowe, S., Hourani, SM., & Kitchen, I. (2002). Quantitative autoradiography of adenosine receptors and NBTI-sensitive adenosine transporters in the brains and spinal cords of mice deficient in the mu-opioid receptor gene. *Brain Research*, Vol.943, No.1, (July 2002), pp. 68-79, ISSN 0006-8993

Baldwin, SA., Beal, PR., Yao, SY., King, AE., Cass, CE., & Young, JD. (2004). The equilibrative nucleoside transporter family, SLC29. *Pflugers Archiv European Journal of Physiology*, Vol.447, No.5, (February 2004), pp. 735-43, ISSN 0031-6768

Baldwin, SA., Yao, SY., Hyde, RJ., Ng, AM., Foppolo, S., Barnes, K., Ritzel, MW., Cass, CE., & Young, J.D. (2005). Functional characterization of novel human and mouse equilibrative nucleoside transporters (hENT3 and mENT3) located in intracellular membranes. *Journal of Biologycal Chemistry*, Vol.280, No.16, (April 2005), pp.15880-7, ISSN 0021-9258

Barnes, K., Dobrzynski, H., Foppolo, S., Beal, PR., Ismat, F., Scullion, ER., Sun, L., Tellez, J., Ritzel, MW., Claycomb, WC., Cass, CE., Young, JD., Billeter-Clark, R., Boyett, MR., & Baldwin, SA. (2006). Distribution and functional characterization of equilibrative nucleoside transporter-4, a novel cardiac adenosine transporter activated at acidic pH. *Circulation Research*, Vol.99, No.5, (September 2006), pp. 510-9, ISSN 0009-7330

Bundgaard, M., & Abbott, NJ.(2008). All vertebrates started out with a glial blood-brain barrier 4-500 million years ago. *Glia*, Vol.56, No.7, (May 2008), pp. 699-708, ISSN 0894-1491

Cai, G., Salonikidis, PS., Fei, J., Schwarz, W., Schülein, R., Reutter, W., & Fan H. (2005). The role of N-glycosylation in the stability, trafficking and GABA-uptake of GABA-transporter 1. Terminal N-glycans facilitate efficient GABA-uptake activity of the GABA transporter. *FEBS Journal*, Vol.272, No.7, (April 2005), pp. 1625-38, ISSN 1742-464X

Cass, CE., Young, JD., & Baldwin, SA. (1998). Recent advances in the molecular biology of nucleoside transporters of mammalian cells. *Biochemistry and Cell Biology*, Vol.76, No.5, (1998), pp. 761-70, ISSN 0829-8211

Che, M., Ortiz, DF., & Arias, IM. (1995). Primary structure and functional expression of a cDNA encoding the bile canalicular, purine-specific Na+-nucleoside cotransporter. *Journal of Biologycal Chemistry*, Vol.270, No.23, (Jun 1995), pp. 13596–9, ISSN 0021-9258

Choi, DS., Cascini, MG., Mailliard, W., Young, H., Paredes, P., McMahon, T., Diamond, I., Bonci. A., & Messing, RO. (2004). The type 1 equilibrative nucleoside transporter regulates ethanol intoxication and preference. *Nature Neuroscience,* Vol.7, No.8, (August 2004), pp. 855-61, ISSN 1097-6256

Crawford, CR., Patel, DH., Naeve, C., & Belt, JA. (1998) Cloning of the human equilibrative, nitrobenzylmercaptopurine riboside (NBMPR)-insensitive nucleoside transporter ei by functional expression in a transport-deficient cell line. *Journal of Biological Chemistry,* Vol.273, No.9, (February 1998), pp. 5288–93, ISSN 0021-9258

Dahlin, A., Xia, L., Kong, W., Hevner, R., & Wang, J. (2007). Expression and immunolocalization of the plasma membrane monoamine transporter in the brain. *Neuroscience,* Vol.146, No.3, (May 2007), pp. 1193-211, ISSN 0306-4522

Dunwiddie, TV., & Masino, SA. (2001). The role and regulation of adenosine in the central nervous system. *Annual Review of Neuroscience,* Vol.24, (March 2001), pp. 31-55, ISSN 0147-006X

Fredholm, BB., Chen, JF., Cunha, RA., Svenningsson, P., & Vaugeois, JM. (2005). Adenosine and brain function. *International Review of Neurobiology,* Vol.63, (2005), pp. 191-270, ISSN 0074-7742

Hendriks, M., Koudijs, BW., van Balkom, V., Oorschot, J., Klumperman, PM., Deen, P., & van der Sluijs P. (2004) Glycosylation is important for cell surface expression of the water channel aquaporin-2 but is not essential for tetramerization in the endoplasmic reticulum. *Journal of Biological Chemistry,* Vol.279, No.4, (January 2004), pp. 2975-83, ISSN 0021-9258

Geiger, JD., &Nagy, JI. (1984). Heterogeneous distribution of adenosine transport sites labelled by [3H]nitrobenzylthioinosine in rat brain: an autoradiographic and membrane binding study. *Brain Research Bulletin,* Vol.13, No.5, (November 1984), pp. 657-66, ISSN 0361-9230

Gerstin, KM., Dresser, MJ., Wang, J., & Giacomini, KM. (2000) Molecular cloning of a Na+-dependent nucleoside transporter from rabbit intestine. *Pharmaceutical Research,* Vol.17, No.8, (August 2000), pp. 906–10, ISSN 0724-8741

Govindarajan, R., Leung, GP., Zhou, M., Tse, CM., Wang, J., & Unadkat, JD. (2009). Facilitated mitochondrial import of antiviral and anticancer nucleoside drugs by human equilibrative nucleoside transporter-3. *American Journal of Physiology Gastrointestinal and Liver Physiology,* Vol.296, No.4, (April 2009), pp. G910-22, ISSN 0193-1857

Gray, JH., Owen, RP., & Giacomini, KM. (2004) The concentrative nucleoside transporter family, SLC28. *Pflugers Archive European Journal of Physiology,* Vol.447, No.5, (February 2004), pp. 728-34, ISSN 0031-6768

Griffiths, M., Beaumont, N., Yao, SYM., Sundaram, M., Boumah, CE., Davies, A., Kwong, FYP., Coe, I., Cass, CE., Young, JD., & Baldwin, SA. (1997a). Cloning of a human nucleoside transporter implicated in the cellular uptake of adenosine and chemotherapeutic drugs. *Nature Medicine,* Vol.3, No.1, (January 1997), pp.89–93, ISSN 1078-8956

Griffiths, M., Yao, SYM., Abidi, F., Phillips, SEV., Cass, CE., Young, JD., & Baldwin, SA. (1997b) Molecular Cloning and characterization of a nitrobenzylthioinosine-insensitive (ei) equilibrative nucleoside transporter from human placenta. *Biochemical Journal,* Vol.328, (December 1997), pp. 739–43, ISSN 0264-6021

Guillen-Gomez, E., Calbet, M., Casado, J., de Lacea, L., Soriano, E., Pastor-Anglada, M., & Burgaya, F. (2004). Distribution of CNT2 and ENT1 transcripts in rat brain: selective decrease of CNT2 mRNA in the cerebral cortex of sleep-deprived rats. *Journal of Neurochemistry,* Vol.90, No.4, (August 2004), pp. 883-93, ISSN 0022-3042

Hyde, RJ., Cass, CE., Young, JD., & Baldwin, SA. (2001) The ENT family of eukaryote nucleoside and nucleobase transporters: recent advances in the investigation of structure/function relationships and the identification of novel isoforms. *Molecular Membrane Biology*, Vol.18, No.1, (January-March 2001), pp. 53-63, ISSN 0968-7688

Isakovic, AJ., Abbott, NJ., & Redzic, ZB (2004). Brain to blood efflux transport of adenosine: blood-brain barrier studies in the rat. *Journal of Neurochemistry*, Vol.90, No.2, (July 2004), pp. 272-86, ISSN 0022-3042

Isakovic, AJ., Segal, MB., Milojkovic, BA., Dacevic, MP., Misirlic, ST., Rakic, ML., & Redzic, ZB. (2002). The efflux of purine nucleobases and nucleosides from the rat brain. *Neuroscience Letters*, Vol.318, No.2, (January 2002), pp. 65-8, ISSN 0304-3940

Jennings, LL., Hao, C., Cabrita, MA., Vickers, MF., Baldwin, SA., Young, JD., & Cass, CE. (2001). Distinct regional distribution of human equilibrative nucleoside transporter proteins 1 and 2 (hENT1 and hENT2) in the central nervous system. *Neuropharmacology*, Vol.40, No.5, (April 2001), pp. 722-31, ISSN 0028-3908

Jones, KW., & Hammond, JR. (1992). Heterogeneity of [3H]dipyridamole binding to CNS membranes: correlation with [3H]nitrobenzylthioinosine binding and [3H]uridine influx studies. *Journal of Neurochemistry*, Vol.59, No.4, (October 1992), pp. 1363-71, ISSN 0022-3042

King, AE., Ackey, MA., Cass, CE., Young, JD., & Baldwin, SA. (2006). Nucleoside transporters: from scavengers to novel therapeutic targets. *Trends in Pharmacological Sciences*, Vol.27, No.8, (August 2006), pp. 416-25, ISSN 0165-6147

Lawrence, AJ., Castillo-Melendez, M., & Jarrott, B. (1994) [^{3}H]adenosine transport in rat dorsal brain stem using a crude synaptosomal preparation. *Neurochemistry International*, Vol.25, No.3, (September 1994), pp. 221-6, ISSN 0197-0186

Lee, EW., Lai, Y., Zhang, H., & Unadkat, JD. (2006). Identification of the mitochondrial targeting signal of the human equilibrative nucleoside transporter 1 (hENT1): implications for interspecies differences in mitochondrial toxicity of fialuridine. *Journal of Biological Chemistry*, Vol.281, No.24, (June 2006), pp. 16700-6, ISSN 0021-9258

Leisewitz, AV., Zimmerman, EI., Huang, M., Jones, SZ., Yang, J., & Graves, LM. (2011). Regulation of ENT1 expression and ENT1-dependent nucleoside transport by c-Jun N-terminal kinase. *Biochemical and Biophysical Research Communication*, Vol.404, No1, (January 2011), pp. 370-5, ISSN 0006-291X

Letendre, S., Marquie-Beck, J., Capparelli, E., Best, B., Clifford, D., Collier, AC., Gelman, BB., McArthur, JC., McCutchan, JA., Morgello, S, Simpson, D., Grant, I., & Ellis, R.J. (2008). Validation of the CNS Penetration-Effectiveness rank for quantifying antiretroviral penetration into the central nervous system. *Archives of Neurology*, Vol.65, No.1, (2008), pp. 65-70, ISSN 0003-9942

Lu, H., Chen, C., & Klassen, C. (2004). Tissue distribution of concentrative and equilibrative nucleoside transporters in male and female mice. *Drug Metabolism and Disposition*, Vol.32, No.12, (December 2004), pp. 1455-61, ISSN 0090-9556

Mani, RS., Hammond, JR., Marjan, JM., Graham, KA., Young, JD., Baldwin, SA., & Cass, CE. (1998). Demonstration of equilibrative nucleoside transporters (hENT1 and hENT2) in nuclear envelopes of cultured human choriocarcinoma (BeWo) cells by functional reconstitution in proteoliposomes. *Journal of Biological Chemistry*, Vol.273, No.46, (November 1998), pp. 30818-25, ISSN 0021-9258

Manji, H., & Miller, R. (2004). The neurology of HIV infection. *Journal of Neurology Neurosurgery and Psychiatry*, Vol.75, Supp.1. (Mart 2004), i29-i35, ISSN 0022-3050

Melani, A., Pantoni, L., Corsi, C., Bianchi, L., Monopoli, A., Bertorelli, R., Pepeu, G., & Pedata, F. (1999) Striatal outflow of adenosine, excitatory amino acids, c-aminobutyric acid and taurine in awake freely moving rats after middle cerebral artery occlusion. Correlation with neurological deficit and histopathological damage. *Stroke*, Vol.30, No.11, (November 1999), pp. 2448–55, ISSN 0039-2499

Miller, DS. (2010). Regulation of P-glycoprotein and other ABC drug transporters at the blood-brain barrier. *Trends in Pharmacological Sciences*, Vol. 31, No.6, (Jun 2010), pp. 246-54, ISSN 0165-6147

Moss, FJ., Imoukhuede, PI., Scott, K., Hu, J., Jankowsky, JL., Quick, MW., & Lester, HA. (2009). GABA transporter function, oligomerization state, and anchoring: correlates with subcellularly resolved FRET. *Journal of General Physiolology*, Vol.134, No.6, (December 2009), pp. 489-521, ISSN 0022-1295

Nagai, K., Nagasawa, K., & Fujimoto, S. (2005). Transport mechanisms for adenosine and uridine in primary-cultured rat cortical neurons and astrocytes. *Biochemical and Biophysical Research Communication*, Vol.334, No.4, (September 2005), pp. 1343-50, ISSN 0006-291X

Nivillac, NM., Bacani, J., & Coe, IR. (2011). The life cycle of human equilibrative nucleoside transporter 1: From ER export to degradation. *Experimental Cell Research*, (March 2011), *In press*, ISSN 0014-4827

Paproski, RJ., Ng, AM., Yao, SY., Graham, K., Young, JD., & Cass, CE. (2008). The role of human nucleoside transporters in uptake of 3'-deoxy-3'-fluorothymidine. *Molecular Pharmacology*, Vol.74, No.5, (November 2008), pp. 1372-80, ISSN 0026-895X

Parkinson, FE., & Xiong, W. (2004). Stimulus- and cell-type-specific release of purines in cultured rat forebrain astrocytes and neurons. *Journal of Neurochemistry*, Vol.88, No.5, (March 2004), pp. 1305–12, ISSN 0022-3042

Parkinson, FE., Damaraju, VL., Graham, K., Yao, SY., Baldwin, SA., Cass, CE., & Young, JD. (2011). Molecular Biology of Nucleoside Transporters and Their Distributions and Functions in the Brain. *Current Topics in Medical Chemistry*, (March 2011), *In press*, ISSN 1568-0266

Parkinson, FE., Ferguson, J., Zamzow, CR., & Xiong, W. (2006). Gene expression for enzymes and transporters involved in regulating adenosine and inosine levels in rat forebrain neurons, astrocytes and C6 glioma cells. *Journal of Neuroscience Research*, Vol.84, No.4, (September 2006), pp. 801-8, ISSN 0360-4012

Parkinson, FE., Johansson, B., Lindström, K., & Fredholm, BB. (1996). Adenosine A1 and A2a receptors and nitrobenzylthioinosine-sensitive transporters in gerbil brain: no changes following long-term treatment with the adenosine transport inhibitor propentofylline. *Neuropharmacology*, Vol.35, No.1, (January 1996), pp. 79-89, ISSN 0028-3908

Parkinson, FE., Xiong, W., & Zamzow, CR. (2005). Astrocytes and neurons: different roles in regulating adenosine levels. *Neurological Research*, Vol.27, No.2, (2005), pp. 153-60, ISSN 0161-6412

Patel, DH., Crawford, CR., Naeve, CW., & Belt, JA. (2000) Cloning, genomic organization and chromosomal localization of the gene encoding the murine sodium-dependent, purine-selective, concentrative nucleoside transporter (CNT2). *Gene*, Vol.242, No.1-2, (January 2000), pp. 51–8, ISSN 0378-1119

Peng, L., Huang, R., Yu, AC., Fung, KY., Rathbone, MP., & Hertz, L. (2005). Nucleoside transporter expression and function in cultured mouse astrocytes. *Glia*, Vol.52, No.1, (October 2005), pp. 25-35, ISSN 0894-1491

Phillips, E., & Newsholme, EA. (1979). Maximum activities, properties and distribution of 5¢-nucleotidase, adenosine kinase and adenosine deaminase in rat and human brain. *Journal of Neurochemistry*, Vol.33, No.2, (August 1979), pp. 553–8, ISSN 0022-3042

Redzic, Z. (2011). Molecular biology of the blood-brain and the blood-cerebrospinal fluid barriers: similarities and differences. *Fluids and Barriers of the CNS*, Vol.8, No. 1, (January 2011), pp. 3

Redzic, ZB., Biringer, J., Barnes, K., Baldwin, SA., Al-Sarraf, H., Nicola, PA., Young, JD., Cass, CE., Barrand, MA., & Hladky, SB. (2005). Polarized distribution of nucleoside transporters in rat brain endothelial and choroid plexus epithelial cells. *Journal of Neurochemistry*, Vol.94, No.5, (September 2005), pp. 1420-6, ISSN 0022-3042

Redzic, ZB., Isakovic, AJ., Misirlic Dencic, ST., Popadic, D., & Segal, MB. (2006) Uneven distribution of nucleoside transporters and intracellular enzymatic degradation prevent transport of intact [^{14}C] adenosine across the sheep choroid plexus epithelium as a monolayer in primary culture. *Cerebrospinal Fluid Research*, Vol.29., No.3 (March 2006), pp.1, ISSN 1743-8454

Redzic, ZB., Malatiali, SA., Al-Bader, M., & Al-Sarraf, H. (2010b) Effects of hypoxia, glucose deprivation and recovery on the expression of nucleoside transporters and adenosine uptake in primary culture of rat cortical astrocytes. *Neurochemistry Research*, Vol.35, No.9, (September 2010), pp. 1434-44

Redzic, ZB., Malatiali, SA., Grujicic, D., & Isakovic, AJ. (2010a). Expression and functional activity of nucleoside transporters in human choroid plexus. *Cerebrospinal Fluid Research*, Vol. 7, No.2 (January 2010), ISSN1743-8454

Reichel, A., Begley, DJ., & Abbott, NJ. (2003) An overview of in vitro techniques for blood–brain barrier studies. *Methods in Molecular Medicine*, Vol.89, (2003), pp. 307–24, ISSN 1543-1894

Ritzel, MW., Ng, AM., Yao, SY., Graham, K., Loewen, SK., Smith, KM., Ritzel, RG., Mowles, DA., Carpenter, P., Chen, XZ., Karpinski, E., Hyde, RJ., Baldwin, SA., Cass, CE., & Young, JD. (2001). Molecular identification and characterization of novel human and mouse concentrative Na+-nucleoside cotransporter proteins (hCNT3 and mCNT3) broadly selective for purine and pyrimidine nucleosides (system cib). *Journal of Biological Chemistry*, Vol.276, No.4, (January 2001), pp. 2914–27, ISSN 0021-9258

Ritzel, MW., Yao, SY., Huang, MY., Elliott, JF., Cass, CE., & Young, JD. (1997). Molecular cloning and functional expression of cDNAs encoding a human Na+-nucleoside cotransporter (hCNT1). *American Journal of Physiology*, Vol.272, No.2, (February 1997), pp. C707–14, ISSN 0002-9513

Ritzel, MW., Yao, SY., Ng, AM., Mackey, JR., Cass, CE., & Young, JD. (1998) Molecular cloning, functional expression and chromosomal localization of a cDNA encoding a human Na+/nucleoside cotransporter (hCNT2) selective for purine nucleosides and uridine. *Molecular Membrane Biology*, Vol.15, No. (October-December 1998), pp. 203–11, ISSN 0968-7688

Rose, JB., Naydenova, Z., Bang, A., Eguchi, M., Sweeney, G., Choi, DS., Hammond, JR., & Coe, IR. (2010). Equilibrative nucleoside transporter 1 plays an essential role in cardioprotection. *American Journal of Physiology and Heart Circulatory Physiology*, Vol.298, No.3, (March 2010), pp. H771-7, ISSN 0363-6135

Slugoski, MD., Loewen, SK., Ng, AML., Smith, KM., Yao, SYM., Karpinski, E., Cass, CE., Baldwin, SA., & Young, JD. (2007) Residue mutations in transmembrane helix 8 of human concentrative Na^+/nucleoside cotransporter hCNT1 affect permeant selectivity and cation coupling. *Biochemistry, Vol.* 46, No. 6, (February 2007), pp. 1684-93, ISSN 0006-2960

Slugoski, M D., Smith, K M., Mulinta, R., Ng, AML., Yao, SYM., Morrison, EL., Lee, QOT., Zhang, J., Karpinski, E., Cass, CE., Baldwin, SA., & Young, JD. (2008) A conformationally mobile cysteine residue (Cys-561) modulates Na+ and H^+ activation of human CNT3. *Journal of Biological Chemistry,* Vol. 283, No. 36, (September 2008), pp. 24922-34, ISSN 0021-9258

Smith, KM., Ng, AM., Yao, SY., Labedz, KA., Knaus, EE., Wiebe, LI., Cass, CE., Baldwin, SA., Chen, XZ., Karpinski, E., & Young, JD. (2004). Electrophysiological characterization of a recombinant human Na+-coupled nucleoside transporter (hCNT1) produced in Xenopus oocytes. *Journal of Physiology,* Vol.558,(August 2004), pp. 807-23, ISSN 0022-3751

Smith, KM., Slugoski, MD., Cass, CE., Baldwin, SA., Karpinski, E., & Young, JD. (2007). Cation coupling properties of human concentrative nucleoside transporters hCNT1, hCNT2 and hCNT3. *Molecular Membrane Biology,* Vol.24, No.1, (January-February 2007), pp. 53-64, ISSN 0968-7688

Smith, KM., Slugoski, MD., Loewen, SK., Ng, AM., Yao, SY., Chen, XZ., Karpinski, E., Cass, CE., Baldwin, SA., & Young, JD. (2005). The broadly selective human Na+/nucleoside cotransporter (hCNT3) exhibits novel cation-coupled nucleoside transport characteristics. *Journal of Biolgycal Chemistry,* Vol.280, No.27, (July 2005), pp. 25436-49, ISSN 0021-9258

Tanaka, K., Xu, W., Zhou, F., & You, G. (2004). Role of glycosylation in the organic anion transporter OAT1. *Journal of Biological Chemistry,* Vol.279, No.15, (April 2004), pp. 14961-6, ISSN 0021-9258

Thomas, SA., & Segal, MB. (1997). The passage of azidodeoxythymidine into and within the central nervous system: does it follow the parent compound, thymidine? *Journal of Pharmacology and Experimental Therapeutics,* Vol.281, No.3, (Jun 1997), pp. 1211-8, ISSN 0022-3565

Torres, M., Delicado, EG., Fideu, MD., & Miras-Portugal, MT. (1992). Down-regulation and recycling of the nitrobenzylthioinosine-sensitive nucleoside transporter in cultured chromaffin cells, *Biochemica et Biophysica Acta,* Vol.1105, No.2, (April 1992), pp. 291-9,

Vialou, V., Balasse, L., Dumas, S., Giros, B., & Gautron, S. (2007). Neurochemical characterization of pathways expressing plasma membrane monoamine transporter in the rat brain. *Neuroscience,* Vol.144, No.2, (January 2007), pp. 616-22, ISSN 0306-4522

Visser, F., Sun, L., Baldwin, SA., Young, JD., & Cass, CE. (2007). Residues 334 and 338 in transmembrane segment 8 of human equilibrative nucleoside transporter 1 are important determinants of inhibitor sensitivity, protein folding and catalytic turnover. *Journal of Biological Chemistry,* Vol.282, No.19, (May 2007), pp. 14148-57, ISSN 0021-9258

Visser, F., Vickers, MF., Ng, AM., Baldwin, SA., Young, JD., & Cass, CE. (2002). Mutation of residue 33 of human equilibrative nucleoside transporters 1 and 2 alters sensitivity to inhibition of transport by dilazep and dipyridamole. *Journal of Biological Chemistry,* Vol.277, No.1, (January 2002), pp. 395-401, ISSN 0021-9258

Wang, J., Su, SF., Dresser, MJ., Schaner, ME., Washington, CB., & Giacomini, KM. (1997) Na+-dependent purine nucleoside transporter from human kidney: cloning and functional characterization. American Journal of Physiology, Vol.273, No.6, (December 1997), pp. F1058–65, ISSN 0363-6127

Yao, SY., Ng, AM., Sundaram, M., Cass, CE., Baldwin, SA., & Young, JD. (2001). Transport of antiviral 3'-deoxy-nucleoside drugs by recombinant human and rat equilibrative, nitrobenzylthioinosine (NBMPR)-insensitive (ENT2) nucleoside transporter proteins produced in Xenopus oocytes. Molecular Membrane Biology, Vol.18, No.2, (April-Jun 2001), pp. 161-7, ISSN 0968-7688

Yao, SY., Ng, AM., Vickers, MF., Sundaram, M., Cass, CE., Baldwin, SA., & Young, JD. (2002) Functional and molecular characterization of nucleobase transport by recombinant human and rat equilibrative nucleoside transporters 1 and 2. Chimeric constructs reveal a role for the ENT2 helix 5-6 region in nucleobase translocation. *Journal of Biological Chemistry*, Vol.277., No.28, (July 2002), pp. 24938-48, ISSN 0021-9258

Young, JD., & Jarvis, SM. (1983). Nucleoside transport in animal cells. *Bioscience Reports*, Vol.3, No.4, (April 1983), pp. 309-22, ISSN 0144-8463

Zamzow, CR., Bose, R., & Parkinson, FE. (2009). N-methyl-D-aspartate-evoked adenosine and inosine release from neurons requires extracellular calcium. *Canadian Journal of Physiology and Pharmacology*, Vol.87, No.10, (October 2009), pp. 850-8, ISSN 0008-4212

Zamzow, CR., Xiong, W., & Parkinson, FE. (2008) Adenosine produced by neurons is metabolized to hypoxanthine by astrocytes. *Journal of Neuroscience Research*, Vol. 86, No.15, (November 2008), pp. 3447–55, ISSN 0360-4012

Zhang, D., Xiong, W., Albensi, BC., & Parkinson, FE. (2011). Expression of human equilibrative nucleoside transporter 1 (hENT1) in mouse neurons regulates adenosine levels in physiological and hypoxic-ischemic conditions. *Journal of Neurochemistry*, (March 2011), *In press*, ISSN 0022-3042

Zhang, J., Visser, F., King, KM., Baldwin, SA., Young, JD., & Cass, CE. (2007) The role of nucleoside transporters in cancer chemotherapy with nucleoside drugs. *Cancer Metastasis Reviews*, Vol.26, No.1, (2007), pp. 85-110, ISSN 0167-7659

Zhang, Q., Hong, M., Duan, P., Pan, Z., Ma, J., & You G. (2008). Organic anion transporter OAT1 undergoes constitutive and protein kinase C-regulated trafficking through a dynamin- and clathrin-dependent pathway. *Journal of Biological Chemistry*, Vol.283, No.47, (November 2008), pp. 32570-9, ISSN 0021-9258

Zhou, M., Engel, K., & Wang, J. (2007) Evidence for significant contribution of a newly identified monoamine transporter (PMAT) to serotonin uptake in the human brain. *Biochemical Pharmacology*, Vol.73, No.1, (January 2007), pp. 147-54, ISSN 0006-2952

5

Interaction of Traditional Remedies Against HIV, Nutrients and ARVs

Eugenia Barros
CSIR Biosciences, Meiring Naudee Road, Brummeria, Pretoria
South Africa

1. Introduction

South Africa is home to the world's largest population of people living with HIV/AIDs (5.7 million) and Sub-Saharan Africa is heavily affected with 22.4 million people living with the disease. Access to highly active antiretroviral (ARV) drugs is limited and many patients even when they are on ARVs consult traditional healers for herbal remedies. These traditional remedies as well as natural health products are widely used by HIV-infected patients in Southern Africa and other parts of the world.

The limitations and uncertainties surrounding the effectiveness of ARVs in the treatment of HIV/AIDS have created a continuing search for new data on the possible drug-drug and drug-nutrient interactions. In this regard advances in the study of cytochrome P450, the enzyme system most commonly involved in drug metabolism, has provided mechanisms to investigate interactions of ARVs with natural health products and with nutrients in foods.

This chapter reviews some of the possible effects of certain foods of plant origin, including dietary supplements of herbal and botanical origin, indigenous foods and traditional medicines on the regulation of CYP450 enzyme activities, focusing on their possible interaction with ARV drugs. It also discusses future considerations surrounding the improvement of HIV/AIDS treatment management aiming at reducing resistance to ARV drugs and increase awareness of potential food-drug interactions that can render ARV treatment ineffective.

2. CYP450, ARVs and nutrition

The cytochrome P450 enzymes are the major catalysts in drug metabolism and one of the best characterized metabolic protein complexes (Wilkinson, 2005). Although in humans 57 CYP450 genes have been identified only a small number of the encoded proteins, mainly in the CYP1, CYP2 and CYP3 families, appear to contribute to the metabolism of clinically used drugs. CYP450 enzymes reduce or alter the pharmacologic activity of many drugs, attenuating its biological activity and facilitating or even accelerating its elimination from the body. They can also metabolize many chemicals present in the diet and in the environment (Wilkinson, 2005). The major site of CYP450 mediated metabolism is the liver but the enterocytes in the epithelium of the small intestine is also a potentially important site. The gastrointestinal track is the site where insoluble 'food/herb/natural products – drug complexes' can be formed that can result in reduced drug efficacy.

2.1 Antiretrovirals (ARVs)

The HIV virus uses three viral enzymes to replicate namely reverse transcriptase, protease and integrase. The current antiretroviral (ARV) drugs target the viral reverse transcriptase and the protease enzymes and are divided into four classes, nucleoside reverse transcriptase inhibitors (NRTIs), non-nucleoside reverse transcriptase inhibitors (NNRTIs) and HIV protease inhibitors (PIs); the fourth class of ARVs are the HIV fusion inhibitors that prevent virus-cell fusion and this way prevents infection of target cells (Cos et al., 2004). Some of the anti-HIV drugs that are in clinical use are shown in Table 1. Normally a cocktail is prepared by combining two nucleoside reverse transcriptase inhibitors with either one non-nucleoside transcriptase inhibitor or with one protease inhibitor in order to make a highly active ARV treatment (HAART) that has resulted in dramatic reductions of plasma virus levels (Anabwani & Navario, 2005). These ARV drugs are predominantly metabolized by the CYP450 enzymes in families CYP3A, 4, 5 and 7; the HIV protease inhibitors are also substrates for the drug transporter P-glycoprotein.

The activity of CYP3A may be inhibited/reduced or induced as a result of drug interactions and this may have serious clinical implications. To try and minimize the problem of drug interactions, the identification and classification of many of the CYP3A substrates including the inhibitors and inducers of major clinical importance are available to clinicians so that an appropriate dosage strategy is found for each drug (Wilkinson, 2005). Rifampicin, a common drug used to treat tuberculosis, and some anticonvulsants are examples of drugs that induce CYP3A; so when these drugs are taken concurrently with HIV-protease inhibitors, therapeutic failure may occur as there is a marked reduction of the drug in the plasma. A similar situation can occur with non-prescription products like St John's wort, used in alternative medicine, and a potent inducer of CYP3A (Wilkinson, 2005). In addition drug toxicity can also happen as a result of overlapping toxicities from drugs used to treat opportunistic infections and ARVs (Anabwani & Navario, 2005) as well as from drugs or traditional herbal medicines used to treat disorders associated with HIV-related problems like nausea, depression, insomnia, dermatological disorders, weakness and opportunistic infections (Mills, 2005b).

There are however instances where the inhibitory effect to CYP3A activity from a drug can be used for therapeutic advantage. This is the case of the ARV protease inhibitor, ritonavir, which is known to "significantly reduce CYP3A-mediated first-pass metabolism of certain inhibitors of HIV-encoded protease and substantially increases their levels in the plasma" (Wilkinson, 2005). This phenomenon has formed the basis of combining ritonavir with other protease inhibitors in the treatment of HIV-1 infection.

2.2 Traditional remedies and herbal medicines

Traditional medicines make use of the therapeutic power of plants and herbs and are widely used in Africa and in South Africa by traditional practitioners/healers, offering an alternative choice for the treatment of a variety of ailments and diseases. Some of the natural products and herbs that are used in traditional medicine are shown in Table2; some of their most common applications are also indicated.

Plant extracts known to have antimicrobial properties have been found to be synergistic enhancers when taken in combination with standard drugs. In some cases the synergistic properties were only found to be effective when plant antimicrobials were taken concurrently with standard drugs, enhancing the effect of the drug. Kamatou et al., (2006) reported on the effectiveness of two plants, *Salvia chamelaeagnea* and *Leonotis leonurus* against

Nucleoside reverse transcriptase inhibitors (NRTIs)			
Generic name	**Trade names**	**Availability in South Africa**	**Regimen in South Africa**
Didanosine	Videx, ddl, Sspen-Didanosine	Yes	Paediatric HIV infection regimen 2 Adult HIV infection regimen 2
Emtricitabine	Emtriva, FTC	No	Not available
Lamivudine	Epivir, 3TC, Cipla-Lamivudine, Aspen-Lamivudine	Yes	Paediatric HIV infection regimen 1 Adult HIV infection regimen 1
Stavudine	Zerit, d4T, Stavir, Aspen-Stavudine	Yes	Paediatric HIV infection regimen 1 Adult HIV infection regimen 1
Zalcitabine	Hivid, ddC	Yes	Not currently part of SA guidelines
Zidovudine	Retrovir, AZT, ZDV,Aspen-Zidovudine	Yes	Paediatric HIV infection regimen 2 Adult HIV infection regimen 2
Abacavir	Ziagen	Yes	Adult and paediatric HIV infection Used in combination with other NRTIs
Tenofovir	Viread	Yes	No guidelines available
Non-nucleoside reverse transcriptase inhibitors (NNRTIs)			
Generic name	**Trade names**	**Availability in South Africa**	**Regimen in South Africa**
Delavirdine	Rescriptor	Yes	Not frequently used
Nevirapine	Viramune	Yes	Adult HIV infection regimen 1
Efavirenz	Sustiva, Stocrin	Yes	Paediatric HIV infection regimen 1 Adult HIV infection regimen 1
Protease inhibitors (PIs)			
Generic name	**Trade names**	**Availability in South Africa**	**Regimen in South Africa**
Indinavir	Crixivan	Yes	No guidelines available
Nelfinavir	Viracept	Yes	No guidelines available
Ritonavir	Norvir	Yes	No guidelines available
Saquinavir	Invirase is a hard-gel capsule; Fortovase is a soft-gel capsule	Yes	No guidelines available
Amprenavir	Agenerase	Yes	No guidelines available
Atazanavir	Reyataz	Yes	No guidelines available
Fosamprenavir calcium	Lexiva	Yes	No guidelines available

Fusion inhibitors			
Generic name	**Trade names**	**Availability in South Africa**	**Regimen in South Africa**
Enfuvirtide	Fuzeon, T-20	No	Not available
Combinations of NRTIs, NNRTIs and PIs			
Combinations	**Trade names**	**Availability in South Africa**	**Regimen in South Africa**
Combination of NRTI	Abacavir + Lamivudine	Yes	No guidelines available
Combination of NRTI (Combivir, Avacomb, Aspen-Lamzid)	Zidovudine + Lamivudine	Yes	No guidelines available
Combination of NRTI	Abacavir + Zidovudine	Yes (less common)	No guidelines available
Combination of NRTI	Didanosine + Zidovudine	Yes (less common)	No guidelines available
Combination of NRTI	Stavudine + Lamivudine	Yes (less common)	No guidelines available
Combination NRTI + NNRTI	Tenofovir + Lamivudine + Efavirenz	Yes	Adult HIV infection 1st line regimen 1
Combination NRTI + NNRTI	Tenofovir + Lamivudine + Nevirapine	Yes	Adult HIV infection 1st line regimen 2
Combination NRTI + NNRTI	Stavudine + Lamivudine + Efavirenz	Yes	Adult HIV infection 1st line regimen 3
Combination NRTI + NNRTI	Stavudine + Lamivudine + Nevirapine	Yes	Adult HIV infection 1st line regimen 4
Combination NRTI + NNRTI	Zidovudine + Lamivudine + Efavirenz	Yes	Adult HIV infection 1st line regimen 5
Combination NRTI + NNRTI	Zidovudine + Lamivudine + Nevirapine	Yes	Adult HIV infection 1st line regimen 6
Combination of PIs (Kaletra, LPV/r)	Lopinavir + Ritonavir	Yes	Paediatric HIV infection regimen 1 Adult HIV infection regimen 2

Table 1. List of some of the anti-HIV drugs belonging to the four classes of ARVs in clinical use (Cos et al., 2004). The information relating to the drug availability and regimen in South Africa is from the South African Department of Health (www.doh.gov.za/docs/misc./hiv/manual/pharmacoloy_art.pdf)

Gram +ve bacteria when taken in combination than when they were taken individually. Aiyegon & Okoho (2009) reviewed the use of several bioactive plant products in combination with standard antibiotics demonstrating its application in antimicrobial chemotherapy. However they also cautioned on the possible problems related to toxicity and overdose as less concentration of the two products will be required when they are taken in combination.

Information on the systems whereby bioactive plant products are metabolized is not readily available; future studies should be encouraged to ensure that better results can be obtained from the combined use of medicinal plants and the drugs used in orthodox medicine. It is necessary to understand what kind of interactions are possible and how best to avoid them so that that the maximum benefits are derived from the substances people ingest with the least possible risk.

Plant	Common name	Applications and traditional uses	References
Allium sativum	Garlic	Anti-microbial and antispasmodic properties; antioxidant	Mills & Bone, 2000
Aspalathus linearis	Rooibos tea Rooibos' extracts	Healthy drink; help with stomach cramp and vomiting in infantile colic; antioxidant Alleviate dermatological problems e.g. eczema, skin allergies	Joubert et al., 2008
Athrixia phylicoides	Bush tea	Herbal tea; treatment of boils, acne, throat infections, infected wounds	Joubert et al., 2008
Catharanthus roseus	-	Treatment of many disorders including diabetes, malaria, inflammation and hypertension	van den Bout-van den Beukel et al., 2006
Cyclopia spp	Honeybush tea	Health booster; alleviate chronic catarrh and pulmonary tuberculosis	Joubert et al., 2008
Harpagophytum procumbens	Devil's claw	Pain killer, improves flexibility and mobility associated with rheumatic diseases	van den Bout-van den Beukel et al., 2006
Echinacea purpurea	Echinacea / Purple coneflower	Immune tonic; treatment of upper respiratory infections; anti-inflammatory	Barret, 2003
Hydrastis canadensis	Goldenseal root	Immune booster; antimicrobial ; anti-inflamatory	Sandhu et al., 2003
Hypoxis hemerocallidea	African potato	Antioxidant properties, treatment urinary infections, nervous disorders, cancer, HIV-AIDS	Mills et al., 2005a
Hypericum perforatum	St. John's wort	Treatment of depression	Lee et al., 2006
Sutherlandia frutescens	Cancer bush	Anti-viral activity including retroviruses Anti-inflammatory properties Treatment of stress related maladies	Mills et al., 2005a

Table 2. Some of the natural products and herbs used in traditional medicine with some of their most common applications

2.3 Nutrients in foods including indigenous foods and dietary supplements

In addition to drug-drug interactions observed when drugs are metabolized by the same CYP450 enzyme system interactions between foods and drugs have also been reported and have been responsible for drug dosage adjustments in order to maintain drug concentrations within its therapeutic window (Jang et al., 2004).

The various phases in which foods or dietary supplements may interact with co-administered drugs are during gastrointestinal absorption, distribution, metabolism and elimination (Jang et al., 2004). The metabolic phase is particularly important in food-drug interactions where the consumption of particular foods modulates the activity of a drug-metabolizing enzyme system, resulting in an alteration in the pharmacokinetics of the drugs metabolized by that system (Jang et al., 2004). Some foods and dietary supplements that contain complex mixtures of phyto-chemicals have the greatest potential to induce or inhibit the expression and activity of drug-metabolizing enzymes.

The interaction between HIV/AIDS and nutrition is particularly important as severe malnutrition impairs immune function and decreases resistance to infection. The immune cells depend on metabolic pathways that use various nutrients as critical cofactors for their actions and activities; during deficiencies of trace elements, of vitamins or when there is protein-calorie malnutrition, the individual defence mechanism is compromised. In developing countries micronutrient deficiencies are particularly common in HIV-infected individuals and several studies have shown that low serum levels of vitamin A poses a great risk for the rapid progression of the disease towards development of AIDS and then death (Anabwani et al., 2005).

In order to address nutrient deficiencies in HIV-infected persons, particularly in developing countries, the consumption of a varied diet using foods high in nutritional value including protein, micronutrients and phytochemicals that are available in their communities has been encouraged. For the most vulnerable communities the available foods are primarily indigenous foods. There is very little known about the nutrient composition of some of the indigenous foods and about the interaction of the specific nutrients with ARVs. More efforts are being made to identify and analyse specific nutrients of indigenous foods in an attempt to increase awareness of potential food-drug interactions and maximize effectiveness of ARVs.

Some of the traditional foods that are eaten in different parts of South Africa include pumpkin leaves with or without pumpkin seeds; amaranthus leaves; jugo beans; wild melon; bean mix made up of jugo beans, brown beans and maize; masonja made up of mopani and nuts; tihove made up of samp, nuts, cowpeas and beans; nyaka made up of wheat, sorghum, beans and peas; madumbe; corchorus; cleome and nightshade (T. Moroka, personal communication). In our laboratories we are in the process of evaluating plant food extracts from indigenous and traditional foods and remedies to determine the ability of these extracts to inhibit human CYP450 enzyme activities, especially CYP3A4, using *in vitro* assays. This study will contribute to the evaluation of the impact that these foods can have in HIV-infected individuals if consumed at the same time as the ARV drugs are taken.

2.4 Possible therapeutic failure or development of drug resistance

Drug-drug interactions have become an important issue in health care where drug resistance or treatment failure is always a concern. As dietary and nutrient supplementation strategies are considered in the treatment of HIV infection it aims to take advantage of the mixture of active compounds derived from plant/herb extracts and ARVs to produce the desired clinical effect. The same applies to the active ingredients in foods including indigenous foods; proper analysis should be done to determine the enzyme system by which these nutrients are metabolized and this way prevent any alteration in the pharmacokinetics of the ARVs.

Clinical studies using drugs and herbal medicines with the same metabolic route as ARVs have shown to have the potential to significantly interact with ARV metabolism through the modulation of hemethiolate-containing enzymes of the CYP450 system, in particular CYP3A4 activity. *Hypoxis hemerocallidea,* commonly known as African potato, and *Sutherlandia,* are two botanical supplements widely used in Sub-Saharan Africa that have been reported to potentially increase drug toxicity, viral resistance and treatment failure when used in conjunction with ARVs (Mills et al., 2005a).

The marked inhibitory effect of grapefruit juice with a number of orally administered drugs that are substrates to CYP3A4 was first reported by Bailey et al., (2003). Further investigations confirmed that due to its interaction with prescribed drugs where the peak of a drug level could be increased by a factor of three without any change in the half-life of the medication, grapefruit is contra-indicated in patients receiving drugs that are mainly metabolized by CYP3A4 (Jang et al., 2004). There are many other reports where treatment is rendered ineffective because of unknown interactions between nutrients and prescribed drugs and it is particularly important when the total drug absorption is altered (Bibi, 2008).

Drug toxicity also exists with drugs that are modulated by CYP1A2 when co-administered with CYP1A2 dietary supplements. Jan et al. (2004) reported a study done on patients taking certain drugs that are metabolized by CYP1A2 (acetaminophen, imipramine, theophylline, estradiol or warfarin). When these drugs were taken concurrently with CYP1A2 dietary supplements the patients' ability to metabolize the drugs was considerably lowered and could have resulted in drug toxicity. On the other hand when these drugs were taken concurrently with CYP1A2-inducing dietary supplements, the patients' ability to metabolize the drugs was greater causing them to be eliminated faster, resulting in reduced pharmaceutical activity (Jang et al., 2004). However for the purpose of this short review emphasis was placed on reports of drug-food interactions with drugs and foods that are modulated by the same CYP450 enzyme systems used by the commonly used ARVs in Africa.

A study of herb-drug interactions between five Malaysian medicinal plants and drugs metabolized by CYP2C9, CYP2D6 and CYP3A4 showed that *Orthosiphon stamineus, Mitragyna speciosa* and *Andrographis paniculta* were potential inhibitors of the three enzyme activities, suggesting that these medicinal plants should not be used simultaneously with these classes of drugs (Hanapi et al., 2010). Two other plants *Eurycoma longifolia* and *Mitragyna speciosa* showed no significant inhibition suggesting that they can be taken concurrently with ARVs. These tests were done using an *in vitro* assay system that contains recombinant human CYP450 enzyme; this is the same *in vitro* system that is being used in our laboratories as it is sufficiently robust to handle many samples at the same time (E. Barros, personal communication).

Rooibos (*Aspalathis linearis*) tea and honeybush (*Cyclopia intermedia*) tea are natural herbs indigenous to South Africa that have been widely used as herbal remedies for a wide range of ailments. The antioxidant properties of the teas and plant extracts from these two plants are important in boosting the human immune system; these antioxidants protect cells against oxidative damage by scavenging for free radicals. However the simultaneous intake of rooibos and honeybush with certain ARV drugs should be taken with caution due to the

Plant/herb name	Test system	Relevant chemical constituents (bioactive)	Effect on CYP3A4 enzyme system or P-gp	References
American Ginseng (*Panax quinquefolius*)	*In vitro*	Ginsenoside, propanaxatriol ginsenoside	Inhibition CYP3A4	van den Bout-van den Beukel et al., 2006
Asian Ginseng (*Panax ginseng*)	*In vitro*	Ginsenoside, propanaxatriol ginsenoside	Inhibition CYP3A4	van den Bout-van den Beukel et al., 2006
African potato (*Hypoxis hemerocallidea*)	*In vitro*	Hypoxoside which is converted into rooperol	Increase inhibition by 86% CYP3A4	Mills et al., 2005a, 2005b
Catharanthus roseus	*In vitro*	Ajmalicine and serpentine	Weak or no inhibitory effect CYP3A4	van den Bout-van den Beukel et al., 2006
Seville orange (*Citrus aurantium*)	*In vivo* *In vitro*	- -	Inhibition P-gp Inhibition CYP3A4	Tarirai et al., 2010
Devil's claw	*In vitro*	Harpagoside	Inhibition CYP3A4	van den Bout-van den Beukel et al., 2006
Echinacea	*In vitro*	Quercetin	Inhibition CYP3A4	van den Bout-van den Beukel et al., 2006
Eucalyptus oil (*Eucalyptus globules*)	*In vitro*	Cineole	Inhibition CYP3A4	van den Bout-van den Beukel et al., 2006
Evening primrose	*In vitro*	Linoleic acid, oleic acid, palmitic acid, stearic acid	Moderate inhibition CYP3A4	van den Bout-van den Beukel et al., 2006
Garlic	*In vitro* and *In vivo* Clinical studies *In vivo*	Alliin, allicin Garlic extracts Garlic extracts	Weak inhibition CYP3A4 Induction CYP3A4 and P-gp No significant inhibition of CYP3A4	Tarirai et al., 2010 Piscitelli et al., 2002 Markowitz et al., 2003
Ginger (*Zingiber officinale*)	Case report	Gingerols, zingiberene, shoagols,	Inhibition CYP3A4	van den Bout-van den Beukel et al., 2006
Ginkgo (*Ginkgo biloba*)	*In vitro*	Ginkgolic acids	Inhibition CYP3A4 and P-gp	van den Bout-van den Beukel et al., 2006

Goldenseal root (*Hydrastis canadensis*)	*In vitro* Clinical studies	Isoquinoline alkaloids	Inhibition CYP3A4 No effect on CYP3A4 nor P-gp	Sandhu et al., 2003 Lee et al., 2006
Grapefruit juice (*Citrus paradise*)	*In vivo* *In vitro* and *in vivo*	Naringenin; furanocoumarin bergamottin; Diosmin	Inhibition CYP3A4 Induction CYP3A4 and P-gp	Tarirai et al., 2010
Milk thistle (*Silybum marianum*)	*In vitro* Clinical studies	Isoprenoid dihydrosilybins, silymarin, sylibinins, taxifolin, apigenin,luteolin	Induction P-gp	Tarirai et al., 2010 van den Bout-van den Beukel et al., 2006
Rooibos tea	*In vivo*	Pinitol	Induction CYP3A	Matsuda et al.,2007
Soy (*Glyvine max*)	*In vitro*	Genistein, daidzen (phytoestrogen)	Inhibition CYP3A4 and P-gp	van den Bout-van den Beukel et al., 2006
St John's wort	*In vitro*	Hyperforin, hypericin, quercetin, isoquercetin, biflavonoids, naphthoadianthrones, catechins, tannins	Induction CYP3A4 and P-gp	Piscitelli et al.,2000 Mannel, 2004
Sutherlandia	*In vitro*	L-canavanine that is an arginine analogue	Near complete inhibition (96%) CYP3A4 Inhibition P-gp	Mills et al., 2005a van den Bout-van den Beukel et al., 2006
Cranberry juice (*Vaccinium macrocarpon*)	*In vitro*	Flavonoids (antioxidants)	Inhibition CYP3A4	van den Bout-van den Beukel et al., 2006
Valerian (*Valeriana officinalis*)	*In vitro*	Isovalerianic or valerenic acid	Inhibitor CYP3A4 and P-gp	van den Bout-van den Beukel et al., 2006

Table 3. Examples of plant and herbal products used with ARVs in the treatment of HIV-AIDs with reference to metabolism by CYP450 3A4 and/or P-glycoprotein (P-gp)

induction of CYP3A4 activity (Mashuda et al., 2007); they should be taken preferably at different times. Table 3 contains some examples of plant and herbal products used with ARVs in the treatment of HIV-AIDs with reference to metabolism by CYP450 3A4 and/or P-glycoprotein (P-gp).

The concurrent use of natural health products with ARVs is also widespread and there are varied reports on the level of interaction with certain natural health products resulting in changes in the efficacy of the ARV treatment. Natural health products are often complex mixtures containing organic compounds many of which can induce and/or inhibit the enzymatic pathways involved in the metabolism of ARV drugs (Lee et al., 2006).

St. John's wort, a well known natural health product, is commonly used by HIV-infected patients due to its antidepressant properties. One of its constituents, hyperforin, is a very active inducer of CYP3A4 activity and responsible for a reduction in drug activity. Mannel (2004) reported a case of a reduction in the activity of an ARV drug cocktail containing indinavir-lamivudine-stavudine when it was co-administered with St John's wort. A similar interaction of St John's wort was reported with the co-administration of two separate ARVs namely indinavir and nevirapine (Lee et al., 2006).

Garlic is another natural health product commonly used by HIV-infected patients where reports have shown different types of interactions with different ARVs. A decrease in the plasma concentration of fortovase, the soft gel formulation of saquinavir, was found in patients taking garlic while on fortovase treatment possibly due to induction of intestinal CYP3A4 and/or P-gp (Piscitelli et al., 2002). Another report of the concurrent intake of garlic supplements by an HIV-infected patient on ritonavir therapy suggested inhibition of garlic metabolism caused by ritonavir leading to potential garlic toxicity (Lee et al., 2006). Other *in vivo* and *in vitro* studies on the pharmacokinetic interactions of garlic with ARVs have reported either a slight reduction or no effect on CYP3A4 activity. The variation observed with the co-administration of garlic and the different ARVs are possibly due to the different garlic constituents present in the various garlic supplements.

Vitamins are another group of natural health products widely used by patients on ARV therapy. However evaluation of the pharmacokinetic interactions between vitamins and ARVs is very complex as not only there are many vitamins but there are also different combinations of vitamins, different doses and they can also be administered singly or in a multivitamin form. So vitamins tend to be evaluated singly. The two most commonly tested vitamins are Vitamin C and Vitamin E. A study of the interaction between Vitamin C and indinavir done on healthy people using a high dosage of Vitamin C (1000 mg/day) showed a reduction in the plasma concentration of indinavir. A variation was however observed in the level of bioavailable indinavir among the different individuals (Slain et al., 2005). This interaction would lead to treatment failure in HIV-infected individuals.

Goldenseal root was reported to cause a strong inhibition in the activity of CYP3A4 using *in vitro* studies (Lee et al., 2006), yet when clinical tests were done on the interaction between goldenseal and indinavir, no change was observed in the bioavailability of indinavir (Sandhu et al., 2003).

It is important to note that there is some variation on the results obtained for the *in vitro* and *in vivo* evaluations of the pharmacokinetic interactions among natural health products and ARVs and those obtained from clinical studies. One possibility could be the pharmacogenetic influence on the clinical studies that is absent in both *in vitro* and *in vivo* studies.

Although in most cases the pharmacokinetic interactions of ARVs with other products are done with a single ARV it is rare for an ARV therapy to include a single ARV; it normally contains combinations of two and most commonly three antiretroviral drugs. This makes the study of the interaction of these different combinations of ARV drugs with the different natural health products and complementary medicines a more complex task. It is however valuable to know the metabolic route of each natural health product and complementary medicine so that a better judgment can be made of what to take and when, to avoid treatment failure and worse still, to prevent the development of resistance to treatment by HIV-infected individuals. Tarirai et al. (2010) suggested that certain NHPs and complementary medicines could be administered either 2 hours before or 2 hours after the drug for which an interaction is known to exist.

There are some reports on the beneficial interaction between some natural health products in helping to reduce the progression of HIV/AIDS either by targeting the HIV virus replication or by alleviating the toxic effects associated with the intake of ARVs; more scientific and clinical data is however still needed. Antioxidants play an important part in maintaining a healthy immune system and controlling oxidative stress. The presence of oxidative stress in HIV-infected individuals is known to contribute to the progression of the disease. Although the role of plant-derived antioxidants including flavanoids and proanthocyanins in helping to reduce oxidative stress has been suggested in HIV-infected individuals there is not enough evidence to confirm this to be the case (Cos et al., 2004). While a dietary intervention with antioxidants could be considered as a cost-effective strategy in the HIV treatment the metabolic route of these plant derived antioxidant compounds need to be properly evaluated to prevent any pharmacokinetic interactions with ARV drugs.

While limited information is available on the pharmacokinetic interactions between natural health products and other complementary and alternative medicines with ARV drugs often healthcare providers and patients perceive their concurrent administration unlikely to be harmful. In addition physicians are often not aware of the patients' use of natural health products or complementary medicines and are therefore not able to discuss with the patient the best way to combine the use of conventional medicine with unconventional therapies, including herbal medicines.

An aspect that is particularly important in developing countries, where the level of malnutrition is very high, is the possible effect that fortified staple foods can have on HIV-infected individuals by the simultaneous intake of ARVs. A similar situation has been reported with the co-administration of certain antibiotics, like tetracyclines and fluoquinolones, which bind to the iron and calcium in foods and in dietary supplements (Tarirai et al., 2010). Awareness should also be made with the concurrent intake of certain fortified foods. Tuntipopipat et al. (2006) reported a reduction in the absorption of iron by a group of healthy females that consumed iron-fortified foods together with Chilli pepper. The iron was bound to capsaicin, the polyphenos that are found in Chilli (*Capsicum annum*). To avoid these types of interactions the intake of certain herbal preparations should be administered a couple of hours before or after the interacting drug. This approach will prevent the development of drug resistance that can be the result of reduced clinical efficacy of the drug.

In South Africa food fortification programmes have been implemented especially in schools in order to overcome some of the nutrient deficiencies including micronutrient deficiencies linked to poverty and malnutrition. These deficiencies are being addressed by the mandatory fortification of table salt with iodine and maize meal and bread flour with a vitamin mixture and mineral mixture (Vorster, 2010). The pharmacokinetic evaluations of fortified foods need to be included in future research to prevent treatment failure or development of resistance by any HIV-infected individuals.

2.5 Screening of natural health products and nutrients in foods for metabolism with CYP450 enzymes

CYP450 enzymes are biocatalytic enzymes crucial for the metabolisms of drugs and toxins. The CYP450 system is genetically determined and as such it varies among people. The polymorphic forms of CYP450 genes are responsible for the development of a significant number of adverse drug reactions (Ingelman-Sundberg, 2004). This constitutes an additional challenge for health practitioners to achieve the optimum level of a drug. There are some commercial tests available that can determine the individual's CYP450 activity based on the analysis of a blood-derived DNA sample. This test is available for CYP2D6 and CYP2C19 enzymes which cover about 25% of all drugs (Ingelman-Sundberg, 2004) but do not include CYP3A4, 5 and 7 enzyme families through which the currently used ARVs are metabolized. The pharmacogenetic profile of individuals on ARV treatment is an important factor in the evaluation of safety and risk of co-administered drugs with certain herbal/plant products; however this was outside the scope of this review.

CYP450 analysis of herbal and plant natural products commercially available as natural health products or complementary medicines was reported by Strandell et al., (2004) using *in vitro* inhibition assays. Extracts were prepared from these products and the level of inhibition of CYP3A4, 2D6 and 2C19 enzyme activities identified. Based on the levels of inhibition obtained for each of the products additional tests could be suggested including *in vivo* interaction studies. The screening of the active ingredients of 49 herbal species for the potential inhibition of CYP3A4 was reported by Lee et al., (2007) using a CYP HerboChip®. As these screening platforms become available it facilitates future research to determine the potential interactions between commonly used herbal medicines, natural foods and antiretroviral agents in order to prevent treatment failure and resistant HIV in HIV-infected individuals.

2.6 The way forward

Reliance on traditional herbal medicine by the majority of the population in Sub-Saharan Africa and the global increase in the use of natural products it will most probably contribute in an increase in the pharmacokinetic interactions between herbs and drugs; between natural ingredients found in foods, in natural health products or in complementary medicines and drugs; between drug and drug; and between herb and herb. As most of the herbs and natural products are categorized as foods it suggests that they did not have to follow the rigorous safety and efficacy regulations that are expected from prescription drugs including ARVs.

Knowledge of the potential interactions between drugs, ARVs and plant derived products is very limited and more research needs to be done to identify potential harmful interactions. The information generated needs to be documented and made available to traditional healers, health practitioners and also to the HIV-infected individuals so that they can understand the impact that those interactions can have on the development of drug resistance and treatment failure.

Caution should be exercised when evaluating the pharmacokinetic results of the plant extracts and herbal extracts since the extractions of the different constituents are not chemically standardized. Depending on the protocols used to extract the metabolic components of a particular plant a different result may be produced which in turn will generate a different outcome with the ARV drug concentrations. Moreover the same product that is available from a different 'brand' may produce a different result. While the production of drugs and other pharmaceutical agents have a defined chemical structure and molecular formula regardless of the manufacturer, there are many constituents in a particular plant extract. In addition their profiles are not only affected by the extraction method but can also be influenced by the plants' growing conditions, geographical location, part of the plant used, post-harvesting treatment and formulation among many other factors (Ngo et al., 2009). Although this process is very complex it should not deter from the implementation of a rigorous evaluation of the constituents in foods derived from plants so that appropriate corrective steps can be taken to address the concerns of individuals taking certain ARV medications concomitantly with certain foods.

The first step in the study of the pharmacokinetic interactions with ARV drugs should be to perform *in vitro* tests of the constituents of natural health products, complementary medicines, herbal products and indigenous foods. This approach allows the profiling of secondary metabolites of many natural products enabling the identification of any interactions in the modulation of CYP450 enzyme system before establishing the need to conduct more time-consuming and costly clinical studies. Furthermore the rigorous *in vitro* characterization of any dietary substance should be undertaken before embarking on a clinical drug-diet interaction study.

The way forward is therefore to make the healthcare givers, doctors, nurses and school dietitians aware of the possible food-drug interactions that occur through the formation of insoluble complexes in the gastrointestinal tract that can reduce the bioavailability of the co-administered ARV drugs.

3. Conclusion

Herbal medicines and other dietary supplements such as vitamins are commonly used as alternative medicines in Europe, America and Africa. In Africa herbal medicines are an integral part of the treatment regimen of most HIV-infected patients. However not enough information is available on the possible interactions between commonly used herbal medicines and antiretroviral agents. Furthermore many of the HIV-infected patients on antiretroviral therapy often do not report the concomitant usage of herbal medicines to their physicians; on the other hand not always the physicians are aware of the risk for herb-ARV interactions and therefore do not discuss the simultaneous intake of herbal medications with ARVs with their patients. Greater awareness and education is required to show that when herbal medicines and ARVs are metabolized by the same CYP450 enzymes significant drug interactions can occur. Those interactions can result in either induction or inhibition of the CYP450 enzymes that are involved in ARV metabolism. While induction could lead to subtherapeutic plasma levels of the ARV leading to possible therapeutic failure and enhanced risk of developing ARV drug resistance, inhibition could lead to high ARV plasma levels with the risk of possible serious side effects.

A contribution to the HIV-infected persons in developing countries is to continue to determine the CYP enzyme system used by the foods and remedies that they consume and this way try to reach an optimal plasma level of the ARVs in HIV-infected individuals. Although *in vitro* evaluations of the potential interactions of plant extracts from foods and herbs have been reported this represents only a small fraction of what is used by the different population groups in Africa including South Africa. The work that we have initiated covers a selection of indigenous foods and traditional medicines consumed by the resource poor communities in the region and it will contribute towards increased awareness of potential food-drug interactions; if the foods tested are found to be substrates for CYP450, especially CYP3A4, the potential interaction with some of the ARVs can be anticipated and the appropriate adjustments made to the ARV treatment; it will lead to a more effective ARV treatment and it will improve the quality of life of the people living with HIV/AIDS. Furthermore the knowledge being generated in this and similar studies will help prevent the development of drug resistance by people on HIV-treatment through the consumption of foods and food-related products that are modulated by the same CYP450 system of the ARVs.

4. References

Aiyegoro, O.A. & Okoh, A.I. (2009). Use of bioactive plant products in combination with standard antibiotics: Implications in antimicrobial chemotherapy. *Journal of Medicinal Plants Research*, Vol.3, No.13, pp. 1147-1152

Anabwani, G. & Navario, P. (2005). Nutrition and HIV/AIDS in sub-Saharan Africa: an overview. *Nutrition*, Vol.21, pp. 96-99

Bailey. D.G.; Dresser, G.K. & Bend, J.R. (2003). Bergamottin, lime juice and red wine as inhibitors of cytocrome P4503A4 activity: comparison with grapefruit juice. *Clinical Pharmacology and Therapeutics*, Vol.73, pp. 529-537

Bibi, Z. (2008). Role of cytochrome P450 in drug interactions. *Nutrition & Metabolism*, Vol.5, pp. 27, ISSN 1743-7075-5-27-37

Cos, P.; Maes, L.; Berghe, D.V.; Hermans, N.; Pieters, L. & Vlietinck, A. (2004). Plant substances as anti-HIV agents selected according to their putative mechanism of action. *J Nat Prod*, Vol.167, pp. 284-293

Fernandes, A.C.; Cromarty, A.D.; Albrecht, C. & van Rensburg, C.E. (2004). The antioxidant potential of *Sutherlandia* frutescens. J Ethnopharmacol, Vol.95, pp. 1-5

Hanapi, N.A.; Azizi, J.; Ismail, S. & Mansor, S.M. (2010) Evaluation of selected Malaysian medicinal plants on phase I drug metabolizing enzymes, CYP2C9, CYP2D6 and CYP3A4 *in vitro*. *Int J Pharmacol*, Vol. 6, pp. 494-499

Ingelman-Sundberg, M. (2004). Pharmacogenetics of cytochrome P450 and its applications in drug therapy: the past, present and future. *TRENDS in Pharmacological Sciences*, Vol.25, No.4, pp. 193-200

Lee, L.S.; Andrade, A.S.A. & Flexer, C. (2006). Interactions between natural health products and antiretroviral drugs: pharmacokinetic and pharmacodynamic effects. *Clinical Infectious Diseases*, Vol.43, pp. 1052-1059

Jang, E-H.; Park, Y-C. & Chung, W-G. (2004) Effects of dietary supplements on induction and inhibition of cytochrome P450's protein expression in rats. *Food and chemical toxicology*, Vol. 42, pp. 1749-1756

Joubert, E.; Gelderblom, W.C.A.; Louw, A. & de Beer, D. (2008). South African herbal teas: *Aspalathus linearis*, *Cyclopia* spp. and *Athrixia phylicoides* - A review. *J Ethnopharmacol*, Vol.119, pp. 376-412

Kamatou, G.P.P.; Viljoen, A.M.; van Vuuren, S.F. & van Zyl, R.L. (2006) In vitro evidence of antimicrobial synergy between Salvia chamelaeagnea and Leonotis leonurus. *South African Journal of Botany*, Vol.72, pp. 634-636

Lee, S.S.; Zhang, B.; He, M.L.; Chang, V.S.C. & Kung, H.F. (2007). Screening of active ingredients of herbal medicine for interaction with CYP450 3A4. *Phytotherapy Research*, Vo. 21, pp. 1096-1099

Mannel, M. (2004). Drug interactions with St John's wort: mechanisms and clinical implications. *Drug Saf*, Vol.27, pp. 773-797

Markowitz, J.S.; Devane, C.L.; Chavin, K.D.; Taylor, R.M.; Ruan, Y. & Donovan, J.L. (2003). Effects of garlic (Allium sativum L.) supplementation on cytochrome P450 2 D6 and

3A4 activity in healthy volunteers. *Clin Pharmacol Ther,* Vol.74, No.2, pp. 170-177

Matsuda, K.; Nishimura, Y.; Kurata, N.; Iwase, M. & Yasuhara, H. (2007) Effects of continuous ingestion of herbal teas on intestinal CYP3A in the rat. *Journal of Pharmacological Science,* Vol.103, pp.214-221

Mills, S. & Bone, K. (2000). Principles and practice of phytotherapy: modern herbal medicine. Edinburgh; New York: Churchill Livinsgtone

Mills, E.; Foster, B.C.; van Heeswijk, R.; Phillips, E.; Wilson, K.; Leonard, B.; Kosuge, K. & Kanfer, I. (2005a). Impact of African herbal medicines on antiretroviral metabolism. *AIDS,* Vol.19, pp. 95-97

Mills, E.; Cooper, C.; Seely, D. & Kanfer, I. (2005b). African herbal medicines in the treatment of HIV: *Hypoxis* and *Sutherlandia*. An overview of evidence and pharmacology. *Nutrition Journal,* Vol.4, pp.e19

Ngo, N.; Yan, Z.; Graf, T.N., Carrizosa, D.R.; Kashuba, A.D.M.; Dees, E.C.; Oberlies, N.H. & Paine, M.F.(2009). Identification of a cranberry juice product that inhibits enteric CYP3A-mediated first-pass metabolism in humans. Drug Metabolism and Disposition, Vol.37, pp.514-522

Piscitelli, S.C.; Burstein, A.H.; Chaitt, D.; Alfaro, R.M. & Falloon, J. (2000). *Lancet,* Vol.355, pp. 547-548

Piscitelli, S.C.; Burstein, A.H.; Weldon, N.; Gallicano, K.D. & Falloon, J. (2002). *Clin Infect Dis,* Vol.34, pp. 234-238

Roche, n.d. AmpliChip CYP450 Test. 2011-04-07. Available from: www.roche.com

Sandhu, R.S.; Prescilla, R.P.; Simonelli, T.M. & Edwards, D.J. (2003). Influence of goldenseal root on the pharmacokinetics of indinavir. *J Clin Pharmacol,* Vol.43, pp. 1283-1288

Slain, D.; Amsden, J.R.; Khakoo, R.A.; Fisher, M.A.; Lalka, D. & Hobbs, G.R. (2005). Effect of high-dosevitamin C on the steady-state pharmacokinetics of the protease inhibitor indinavir in healthy volunteers. *Pharmacotherapy,* Vol. 25, pp. 165-170

South African Department of Health. 2011-06-06. Available from: www.doh.gov.za/docs/misc/hiv/manual/pharmacology_art.pdf

Strandell, J.; Neil, A. & Carlin, G. (2004). An approach to the *in vitro* evaluation of potential for cytochrome P450 enzyme inhibition from herbals and other natural remedies. *Phytomedicine,* Vol.11, pp.98-104

Tarirai, C.; Viljoen, A.M. & Hamman, J. H. (2010). Herb-drug pharmacokinetic interactions reviewed. *Expert Opin. Drug Metab Toxicol,* Vol.6, No.12, pp. 1515-1538

Tuntipopipat, S.; Judprasong, K.; Zeder, C.; Wasantwisut, E.; Winichagoon, P.; Charoenkiatkul, S.; Hurrel, R. & Walczyk, T. (2006). Chilli, but not turmeric, inhibits iron absorption in young women from iron-fortified composite meal. *J Nutr,* Vol.136, No.12, pp. 2970-2974

Van den Bout-van den Beukel C.J.; Koopmans, P.P.; van der Ven, A.J.; De Smet, P.A. & Burger, D.M. (2006). Possible drug-metabolism interactions of medicinal herbs with antiretroviral agents. *Drug Metab Rev,* Vol.38, No.3, pp. 477-514

Vorster, H.H. (2010). The link between poverty and malnutrition: A South African perspective. *Health SA Gesondheid* Vol.15, pp. e1

Wilkinson, G.R. (2005). Drug metabolism and variability among patients in drug response. *N Engl J Med,* Vol.352, No.21, pp. 2211-2221.

Part 3

Opportunistic Microbial Infections

6

Syphilis in Men Infected with the Human Immunodeficiency Virus

Francisco Rodríguez-Gómez[1], Hortencia Cachay[1], David Chinchón[2], Enrique Jorquera[3] and Emilio Pujol[1]
[1]*Internal's Medicine Department, Hospital Juan Ramón Jiménez, Huelva,*
[2]*Department of Clinical Pathology*
[3]*Department of Dermathology/Hospital Juan Ramón Jiménez*
Spain

"He who knows syphilis, knows medicine"
Sir William Osler

1. Introduction

1.1 Historical perspectives

The origins of syphilis have been discussed for many centuries. Two main theories have been proposed: The new World or Columbian theory and the world or pre-Columbian theory. The Pre-Columbian theory purports that syphilis originated in central Africa and was introduced to Europe prior to the voyage by Columbus (Hudson, 1956). The former holds that syphilis was endemic in the part of the world now know as Haiti and was then acquired and carried to Europe by Columbus in the 1400s (Rothschild,2005). Bacteriological studies efforts the theory than the syphilis was introduced by Columbus to the Europe (Harper, 2008). In 1495 there was the first syphilis´s epidemic in Europe (Knell, 2004). John Hunter in 1767 inoculated matter from a patient whom believed to have gonorrhea onto into the prepuce and glans of a recipient, who traditionally is believed to be himself. Ten days after the inoculation, a chancre appeared, followed by signs of secondary syphilis. (Oriel, 1994).

It is now believed that the donor had both syphilis and gonorrhea, but Hunter was convinced that he had induced syphilis by inoculation of gonorrheal pus. In 1838 Philippe Ricord demonstrated conclusively that syphilis and gonorrhea were separate diseases on over 2500 human inoculations and he was the first to propose a scheme for the categorization of syphilis into primary, secondary, and tertiary stages, which is still used today. In 1905 Schaudinn y Hoffman demonstrated spirochetes in Giemsa-stained smears (Schaudinn, 1905), August von Wasermann devised a serum reaction test for syphilis (Wasermann, 1906). The treatments for syphilis included mercury, organic arsenical compounds (Sartin, 1995).In 1943 Mahoney (Mahoney, 1943) successfully treated the first four cases with penicillin (table 1).

1.2 Etiology

Treponema Pallidum is a member of the order *Spirochaetales,* family *Spirochaetaceae,* and genus *Treponema*. The pathogenic species are *T.pallidum* subsp. *pallidum* which causes venereal

1495	**A widespread syphilis epidemic had Spreads throught Europe (Knell, 2004).**
1767	John Hunter considerated that the disease to *Neisseria gonorrhoeae* and *T. pallidum* were the same (Oriel, 1994).
1838	Philippe Ricord: first to propose a scheme of syphilis into primary, secondary, and tertiary stages.
1859	Bazin: the term lues maligna was first used.
1896	Third International Congress of Dermatology: lues maligna was classified as the ulcerative form of secondary syphilis.
1897	Neisser and Haslund: clasic descriptions of lues maligna.
1905	Schaudinn y Hoffman: demostrated spirochetes in Giemsa-stained smears. (Schaudinn, 1905)
1906	Wasermann: first serologic test for syphilis. (Wasermann, 1906)
1943	Mahoney: first who successfully treated four cases of syphilis with penicillin. (Mahoney, 1943)
1988	Shulkin: first report HIV infected patient with lues maligna.

Table 1. Historical aspects of syphilis.

syphilis. *T.pallidum* subsp. *endemicum*, which causes endemic syphilis (bejel), T.subsp.*pertenue* which causes yaws, and *T.carateum*, which is the etiologic agent of pinta (Tramont,2010). The *T.pallidum* is a spirochete varying from 0.10 to 0.18 um in diameter and from 6-20 um in legth, making it invisible by light microscopy, for the visualization the Dark-field microscopy is generally used (Creigton, 1990).

T. pallidum, cannot be cultivated in vitro, although limited multiplication can be obtained in tissue cultures (rabbits are the laboratory animals most commonly used for maintaining virulent organism), for this reason is difficult to study and determine its metabolic, physical, and pathogenic features. There were few physiologic studies have previously shown that the organism has limited biosynthetic capabilities, requiring multiple nutrients from the host (Fraser, 1998). However, genomic sequencing has provided some insights by suggesting functional activities. This consists of a single circular chromosome of approximately 1,138,006 bases pairs, which places it close to the lowest end for the range of the bacteria. Unlike most pathogenic, its genome lacks apparent transponsable elements, suggesting that the genome is extremely conserved and stable. This is the likely explanation of why *T.pallidum* has remained exquisitely sensitive to penicillin for more than 70 year (Tramont, 2010).

1.3 Epidemiology

1.3.1 Transmission of disease

The primary mode of transmission is by sexual contact and the next common is transfer across the placenta (Singh, 1999). Kissing, blood transfusion, and accidental inoculation have also been reported as routes of transmission but are of minor importance today. The majority of infants with congenital syphilis are in uterus, but the newborn can also be infected by contact with an active genital lesion at the time of delivery (Fiumara, 1975).

Today, the acquisition of syphilis through transfused blood or blood products is now rare, at least in the developed world, because of the low incidence of disease, the requirement that all blood donors have a nonreactive non-treponemal blood test, and because *T.pallidum* cannot survive longer than 24 to 48 hours under the current conditions of blood bank storage (Tramond,2010).

Accidental direct inoculation can occur by needlestick or during handling of infected clinical material. Syphilis of the fingers is most common in medical personnel (Palfi, 2008).

1.3.2 Occurrence of the disease

In USA, prior to the penicillin age, the incidence in 1947 of primary and secondary syphilis was reported at 66.4 cases per 100,000 persons. Rates declined in 1956 to 3.9 cases per 100,000 persons due to availability of penicillin, changes in sexual behaviour, and public health measures (Nakashima, 1996). The most recent epidemic was noted in 1990, with reported rates for primary and secondary syphilis at 20 per 100 000 persons, although no simple factor can explain this trend, and important contributing factor is crack cocaine use and the exchange of illegal drugs for sex (Rolf, 1990) (Fig.1). In USA, the rates fell to 2.1 cases per 100 000 in 2000, rising to 3 cases per 100 000 in 2005 (86% men). Actually the syphilis is a health problem with a prevalence of 12 million cases per year in worldwide (Hook, 2004).

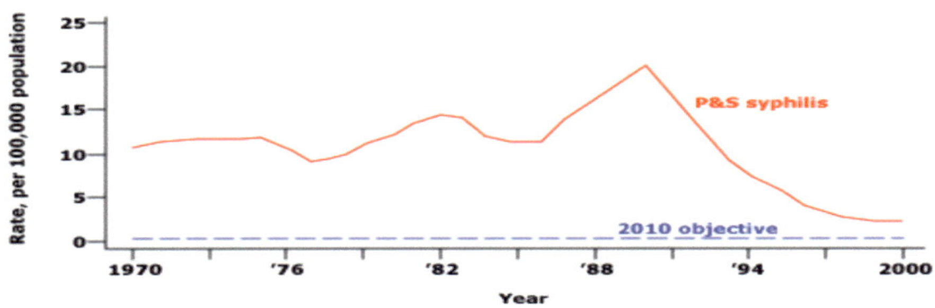

Fig. 1. Primary and Secondary Syphilis - Reported Rates: United States, 1970-2000 and the Healthy People Year 2010 Objective

Australia & New Zealand	10 000
North America	100 000
Eastern Europe & Central Asia	100 000
Western Europe	140 000
East Asia & Pacific	240 000
North Africa & the Middle East	370 000
Latin America & the Caribbean	3 million
sub-saharan Africa	4 million
South & Southeast Asia	4 million

Table 2. WHO estimates of number of new cases of Syphilis per year

1.3.3 Syphilis, HIV, and men who have sex with men (MSM)

Co-infection with syphilis and HIV is common due shared risk factors related to sexual behavior. In the USA, MSM have consistently represented the greatest single at risk group for HIV acquisition (Zetola, 2007). In Germany the rate is 75% (Ditzen, 2005). In Africa the prevalence of infection for HIV is 21% between MSM in comparation the 1-2% of general population (Wade, 2005). Some researchers have postulated that oral sex may now be more common among MSM since it is associated with a reduced frequency of HIV transmission; however, syphilitic transmission from oral lesions is highly probably.

1.4 Natural course of untreated syphilis

Descriptions of the natural history of untreated syphilis originate primarily from two large prospective studies and one study retrospective study. Boeck performed a prospective natural history of 1978 patients with early syphilis in 1891. His observations 20 years were then continued by Brusgaars, and this information was later termed the Oslo Study. Between 1949 and 1951, Gjestland undertook a follow up of 1404 of the original 1978 patients. The data were reviewed in 1955 and then recanalyzed in 1964 by Clark and Danbolt (Clark, 1964), the diagnoses were made clinically since neither serologic testing nor microscopy was available when the study began. The results indicate that approximately one-third of the patients developed tertiary manifestations of neurologic, cardiovascular, and gummatous (late benign) syphilis and that the probability of dying due to untreated syphilis was 17% and 8% in females (Table 3).

	%
Secondary syphilis	100
Cured alter secondary syphilis	60%
Tertiary syphilis	28%
Tertiary syphilis; Late benign syphilis	15% males 17% females
Tertiary syphilis; Cardiovascular syphilis	13,6% males, 7,6% females
Tertiary syphilis; Neurosyphilis	9,4% males, 5,0% females.
Mortality	17% males, 8% females.

Table 3. Clinical Manifestations of Untreated Syphilis

Rosahn retrospectively reviewed all autopsies at the Yale University School of Medicine from 1917 to 1941. Of 4000 autopsies of persons, 9.7% had evidence of syphilis, of them 77 patients with untreated syphilis and late anatomic lesions at autopsy (83% had cardiovascular complications, 9% had late benign lesions, and 8% had neurosyphilis (Rosahn, 1947). There was an increased overall mortality in syphilitic compared with nonsyphilitic populations.

1.5 Clinical manifestation

T.pallidum penetrates the intact mucous membrane or gains access through abraded skin, it enters the lymphatics and bloodstream and disseminates throughout the body. Clinical lesions appear when a concentration of approximately 10^7 organisms/mg of tissue is reached (Magnuson, 1956). The incubation period is directly proportional to the size of the inoculums (3-90 days approximately). In untreated cases, syphilis has traditionally been divided into the following stages: incubating, primary, secondary, early latent, late latent and late tertiary syphilis.

1.5.1 Primary syphilis

The classic primary chancre begins at the site of inoculations as a single, occasionally multiple, painless papule. The base is usually smooth; the borders are raised are raised and firm and have a characteristic cartilaginous consistency (Stokes, 1944). The size of the

chancre varies from 0.3 to 3.0 cm, multiples chancres can occur especially in persons who are inmunosuppresed as those coinfected with HIV (Chapel,1978&Rompalo,2001).
The localization, in men is the penis, more specifically the coronal sulcus and glans. Anorectal chancres are common in homosexual men (Horihan,2004). In women, the commonest locations of the lesions, in order of decreasing frequency, are the labia majora, labia minora, fourchette, and perineum. Regional lymphadenopathy consisting of moderately enlarged, firm, nonsuppurative, painless lymph nodes or satellite buboes usually accompanies the primary lesion (DiCarlo,1997).

1.5.2 Secondary syphilis

A rash of varying severity is the most common initial presenting symptom. This rash appears on the palms, soles, flanks, and arms and can range from macular to follicular and occasionally to pustular. Additionally up to 7% of patients may experience alopecia characterized by patchy hair loss of the scalp, beard, and lateral eyebrows, with is referred to as a moth-eaten appearance. Patients may also experience sore throats due to inflammatory involvement of the pharynx or the tonsils. Condiloma lata are found 5-22% of patients. Althoug the incidence of these effects is rare, syphilis can cause renal, ophthalmologic, hepatic, bone, and joint disease.

1.5.3 Latent (early and late) syphilis

Latent syphilis is a stage in which patients are seroreactive but asymptomatic. It occurs between the disappearance of secondary syphilis symptoms and the appearance of tertiary syphilis manifestations or therapeutic cure. About 90% of first relapses occur within 1 year , its defined early latent syphilis, and late latent syphilis is defined as occurring after 1 year (Gjestland, 1955).

1.5.4 Tertiary syphilis

Tertiary syphilis describes a broad range of manifestations but most commonly includes cardiovascular, gummatous, and/or neurological effects. Together, approximately 15% to 40% of individuals who are not treated will develop tertiary manifestations, with men at increased risk compared with women. Cardiovascular complications are the most common of the effects and typically present within 10 to 30 years of infection. They often involve the aortic arch and can lead to angina from coronary ostitis, aortic regurgitation, or aortic aneurysm. Gummas can present in any organ and can lead to complications, including ulcers of the skin, collapse of the palate or nasal septum, or organomegaly. It can develop any time after a year of infection, but incidence peaks at approximately 15 years.

1.6 Syphilis and HIV

The coinfection have shown no distinctive or unique clinical presentation or pathologic manifestations from those without concurrent HIV infection, they are at an increased risk to manifest a more protracted and malignant course, more constitutional symptoms, greater organ involvement, atypical and florid skin rashes, multiple genital ulcers in the 70% of patients (Rompalo,2010), 25% presented concomitant chancre during the secondary stage (Hutchinson, 1994), and a significant predisposition to develop symptomatic neurosyphilis (Tramont, 2010).

Stage of syphilis	Clinical manifestations	Percentage of cases	Incubation period
Primary	Chancre, regional lymphadenopathy		3 wk (3-90)
Secondary	Rash, condiloma latum, lymphadenopathy Constitutional symptoms(fever, malaise, weight loss) Mouth and throat (mucous patches, erosions, ulcer) Genital lesions (chancre, condyloma latum, mucous patch) Central nervou system Asymptomatic Symptomatic	90% 70% 35% 20% 8-40%	2-12 wk (2wk-6 mos)
Latent	Asymptomatic		Early,<1 yr; late,>1yr
Tertiary. Cardiovascular Syphilis	Aortic aneurisma, aortic regurgitation, coronary artery ostial stenosis		10-30 yr
Tertiary. Late neurosyphilis. Asymptomatic	Asymptomatic	31%	<2 yr
Tertiary. Late neurosyphilis. Acute syphilitic meningitis	Headache, meningeal irritation, confusion	1-2%	<2 yr
Tertiary. Late neurosyphilis. Meningovascular	Hemiplejia, seizures, aphasia.	10%	5-7 yr
Tertiary. Late neurosyphilis. General paresis	Changes in personality, affect, sensorium, intellect, insight, and judgment. Hiperactive reflexes, speech disturbances, Argyll Robertson pupils.		10-20 yr
Tertiary. Late neurosyphilis. Tabes dorsalis	Shooting or lightning pains into lower back or lower legs. Ataxia. Argyll Robertson pupils. Impotence. Blader disturbances. Fecal incontinence. Peripheral neuropathy. Romber sign. Cranial nerve involvement		15-20 yr
Tertiary. Gummatous Syphilis.	Monocytic infiltrates with tissue destruction of any organ	15%	1-46 yr (most cases 15 yr)

Table 4. Clinical phases of syphilis

1.6.1 Syphilis and HIV transmission

The two diseases can affect each other in a number ways. Studies epidemiologist showed that the syphilis increasing the likelihood of acquisition of HIV (Buchacz, 2004, Reynolds, 2006, Fleming 1999).

The acquisition and transmission of each other but syphilis also upregulates CCR5 coreceptor expression (Sellati, 2000) and causes local inmune activation, thereby further increasing likelihood of adquisition of HIV, the stimulation of syphilis infected patient immune system might induce replication of the virus (Quinn TC, 2000), decrease CD4 T cell counts and induce lymphocyte and CD4 apoptosis (Buchacz, 2004).
The pathogenic interaction between HIV and *T. pallidum* leading both to an immunodeficiency state may reduce the immunologic response to treponemal infection through a decrease in CMI, macrophage functional defects, and possibly immunomodulation of the humoral immunity response. Functional immunologic abnormalities may impair the host defense against syphilis, leading to more aggressive forms.
The serologic tests for syphilis may be modified, often resulting in extremely high titers (11% HIV-infected persons have a biologic false-positive serologic test result) and a failure to decrease in response to adequate treatment unless successfully treated with HAART.

	References
Genital ulcers can increase HIV transmision	Telzac, 1993.
T.pallidum induce the expression of CCR5 on macrophages in syphilitic lesions	Setalli, 2000
T.pallidum decreased CD4 T-cell counts and increased HIV viral load	Buchacz, 2004
Syphilis increased HIV transmission 2-to9-fold	Chesson, 2003
First six months after exposure of syphilis, represent the of greatest risk for HIV infection	Reynolds, 2006

Table 5. Syphilis and HIV transmission.

1.6.2 Clinical features of syphilis in HIV-infected patients

The majority of patients coinfected with HIV and syphilis have a primary syphilis similar to the population without HIV. However sometimes can show multiples chancres, larger and deeper and that heals more slowly (Hutchinson, 1994). The primary and secondary period overlap in 75% of cases (Rompalo, 2001). The signs of secondary syphilis can develop and succeed while chancres are still present. The rash may be more widespread and condylomata lata lesions more common than in patients without HIV.
Unusual cutaneous manifestations, particularly the malignant lues are not uncommon in HIV patients. Acute syphilitic meningitis, ocular manifestations and losing hearing are more common in HIV patients (Tramont, 2005). The progression of tertiary syphilis is faster in HIV patients (Hutchinson, 1994)

1.6.3 Diagnosis of syphilis in HIV-infected patients

1.6.3.1 Identification of T.pallidum (Lesion-Based Testing)

Direct fluorescent antibody test (DFA): A direct fluorescent antibody test can be performed on lesion exudate or tissue specimen. There are no differences in test performance characteristics among HIV-infected and non-infected patients.

Primary stage	• Multiple chancres • Chancres larger, deeper, and resolve more slowly • Atypical chancres appearing as abrasions or fissures
Secondary stage	• Coincident chancres with signs of secondary syphilis • Duration of rash may be slightly longer, and rash may be widespread • Atypical skin rashes, including papular, nodular, ulceronudular (lues maligna) • Reports of ocular syphilis, mainly uveitis. • Retinitis, papillitis, and cranial nerve abnormalities II, III, or V in association with syphilitic meningitis.
Tertiary syphilis; Late benign syphilis	• Several reports of gummas • One case of rapid progresion to gumma within several months of a chancre • Located in multiple organ systems including the brain
Tertiary syphilis; Cardiovascular syphilis	• Rare cases of rapidly developing aortitis reported
Tertiary syphilis; Neurosyphilis	• Progression to neurologic syphilis despite treatment of early syphilis • Reports of rapid progression to neurologic syphilis without long latency • Cases in patients with both normal and low CD4 counts • Clinical features include asymptomatic disease, meningitis, cranial nerve deficits, optic neuritis, myelitis, stroke, cerebral gummas

Table 6. Syphilis and HIV by stages. (Adapted from Syphilis. New York Department of Health AIDS Institute).

Darkfield microscopy: Examination of exudate from an ulcer base or a mucocutaneous lesion under darkfield microscopy can identify the spirochete (*T. pallidum*). This test is invalid for oral samples. There are no differences in test performance characteristics among HIV-infected and non-infected patients.

Silver stain: Spirochetes may be seen in biopsy specimens of suspicious lesions such as palmar macular rash or gummatous lesions. There are no differences in test performance characteristics among HIV-infected and non-infected patients.

1.6.3.2 Serology

The serology in patients co-infected syphilis and HIV are similar; however there are least differents in the serology but very important in the diagnostic (Table 7).

2. Case report and discussion

2.1 Case report

A 42-year-old homeosexual man with chronic infection for HIV from 2003, in stadium A2 without antiretroviral therapy consulted at the outpatient infection department at Juan Ramon Jimenez Hospital for fever of 38,5 ° C of three weeks of evolution, which the patient

	Reference
False positive non-treponemal antibody test (RPR/VDRL). In one study, 4% of HIV-infected patients tested had false-positive RPR results	Rompalo, 1992
Seroreactivity may be delayed or absent in HIV-infected patients. Rare cases have been reported of biopsy-proven secondary syphilis in HIV-infected patients with negative serology.	Tikjob, 1991
Higher mean serologic serum non-treponemal antibody levels than non-HIV-infected	Rolfs, 1997
Serum non-treponemal antibody levels may decline more slowly after treatment in HIV-infected patients than non-infected patients	Rolfs, 1997, Yinnon 1996.
Pro-zone reaction more commonly in HIV-infected persons	Schöfer, 1996

Table 7. Considerations for serology in HIV-infected patients.

relates to a "boil" perianal weeks before the beginning of the fever. On examination lymph nodes were palpable in the cervical, axillary and inguinal regions and skins lesions consisted of multiple erythematous present in his face, neck, trunk and extremities.

One week after came back by persistence of the fever and pain of the throat. The laboratory studies revelead the following: Hemograme, glucose, urea, creatinine and ions were normal, GPT 71 U/l, GOT 50U/l, GGT 212 U/l, phosphatase alkaline 149 U/l. His CD4 cell count was 315/mm3 and his HIV viral load of 102.718 copies/ml. The Acid-fast bacilli stains, bacterial, fungal cultures and Lowenstein's culture in urine were all negative. The abdominal ultrasound scan was normal. Before the persistence of the clinic in absence of diagnosis the hospitable for continue the study.

On examination, the patient was fever of 39 ° C with stable vital signs. In mucous oral was presented whitish plates, didn't show ulcerative lesions or thrush (fig.1), skins lesions in different stages in trunk (fig. 2, panel A,B), face and neck, consisting of stains, papules, pustules with center necrotic and ulcerative scabs. He had and inguinal lymph node of 1-2 cm, and cardiac, lung and abdominal examinations are benign. Neurologically, the patient was grossly intact without focal deficits.

The C reactive-protein was 3,9 mg/dl and the erhytrocyte sedimentation rate was 99 mm/hour. There were realized bacterial, fungal, mycobacterial culture and the blood detection of the antigen criptococo were normal. The Chest x-ray film was normal and the tomography thorax-abdominal didn't observe lesions in lung and in abdomen showed moderate enlargement hepatoesplenomegaly and lymphadenopathy in retroperitoneo, chains external ilíacas and inguinal approximately of 1,5 cm.

The histological examination of the ganglionar biopsy showed reaction granulomatous giants cells without necrotic debris (fig. 3, panel A), didn't observe acid-fast bacilli fast and the fungal culture was negative. The skin biopsy punch revelead infiltrated lymphocytes, histiocytes with extensive areas of necrosis and debris, (fig. 3, panel B), the culture of this one (conventional, fungi and mycobacterial) was negative. Warthin-Starry's stain was negative in both samples.

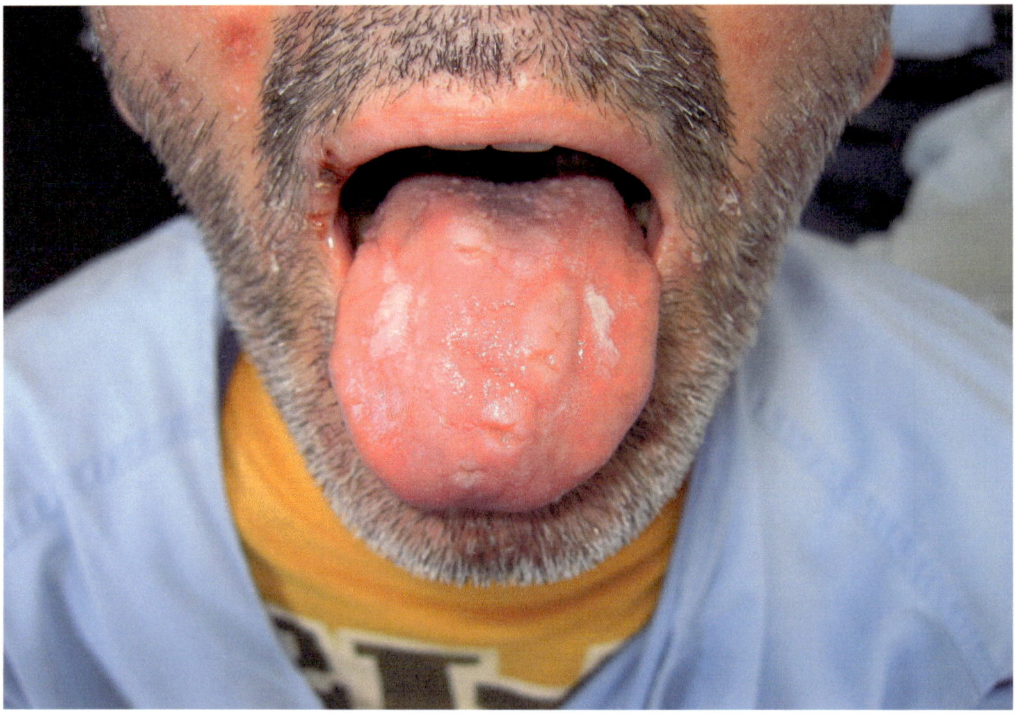

Fig. 2. Mucous patches confused with oral candidiasis.

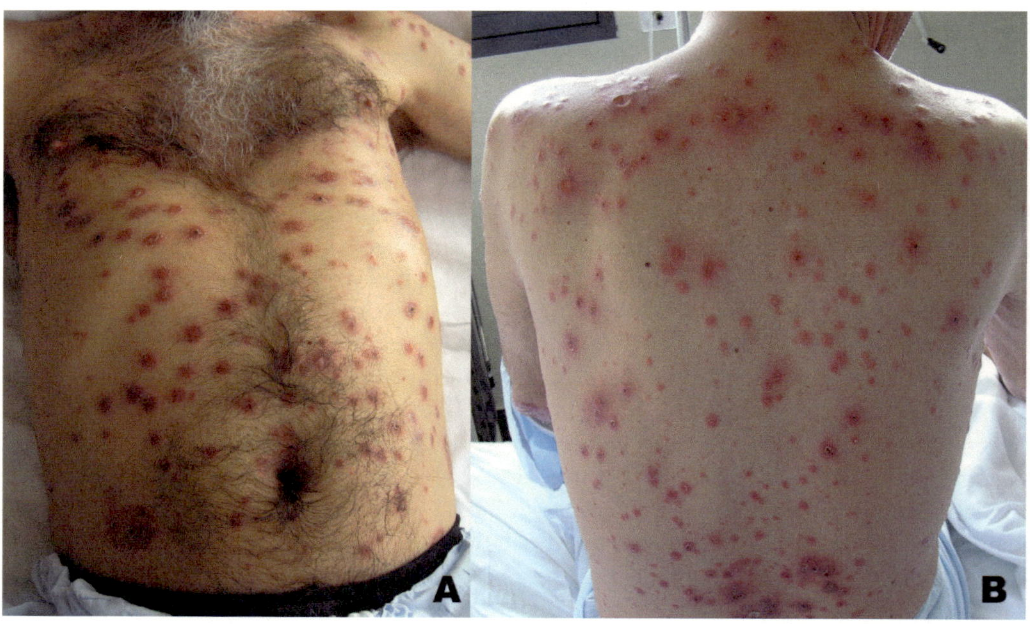

Fig. 3. Noduloulcerative lesions of the trunk. Disseminated ulceronodular rash is affecting the trunk and abdomen (A) and back (B). The lesions are papules, pustules, pustules with necrosis central and ulcerated.

Treatment began with nistatine for the muguet. The presence of long fever, skin lesions, hepatoesplenomegaly and ganglionar affectation with noncaseating granuloma, suspected infection for Bartonella beginning treatment with azitromicina (500 mg c/ 24 hours) with fever and decrease of the size of the inguinal lymphadenopathy. The serology's bartonella was negative <1/256 (IFI). The information together with the persistence of the fever and the skins lesions in a patient HIV forced us to reject the diagnosis of malignant Syphilis. The cerebrospinal fluid was without cell (VDRL negative).

Empirical treatment began with injection of intramuscular benzathine penicillin (2,4 million UI) in only dose, the fever defervesced over the next 24 hours, receiving in ambulatory regime two additional doses weekly. He didn't present Jarish-Herxheimer's reaction. There began antiretroviral treatment of high efficiency based on tenofovir 300mg with 200 mg of emtricitabina and efavirenz 600mg every 24 hours. He was discharged from the hospital with this therapy.

It was checked 10 days later in consultation being afebril and asymptomatic. The oral lesion had disappeared and the skins lesions ones were showing clear improvement. The syphilis serology showed a positive RPR titer 1/32, the immunoglobulin G was positive and the immunoglobulin M negative. The liver function test was normal three months after of the beginning the therapy. To six months RPR titer had descended to 1/4.

The rash approximately coincided months before with inconsistent condom use and several new sexual relationships.

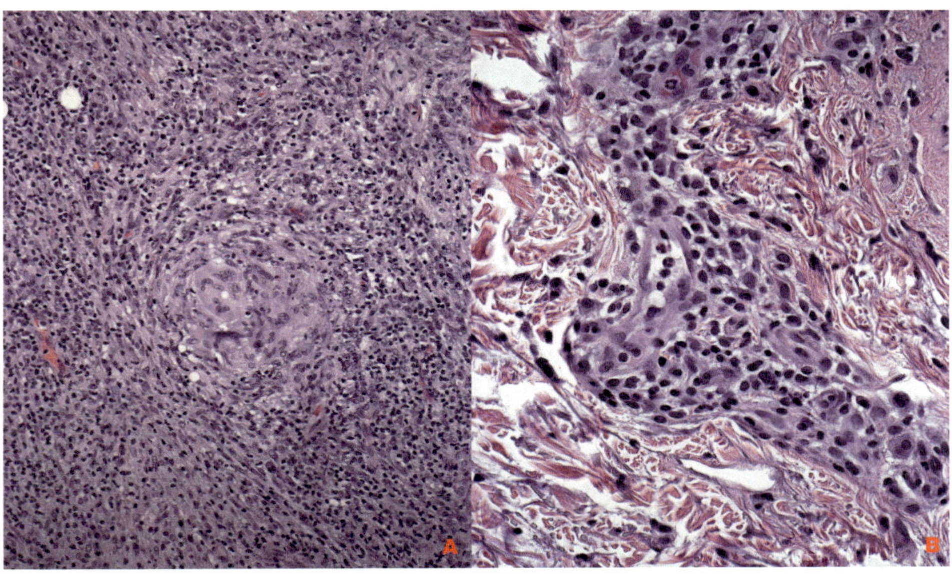

Fig. 4. A) Biopsy lymph node: Nodular growth without central necrosis with lymphoid and plasma cell, (H/E, original x 126). B) Biopsy skin: small base with moderately dense perivascular lymphocitic infíltrate and deep dermis (H&E, original x 252).

2.2 Discussion

2.2.1 Definition

Lues maligna was first described by Bazin (1859) and Dubuc (1864), who applied this term based on the bizarre clinical features and progressive course of this variant of syphilis.

During some decades, there was controversy about whether lues malignt was a severe variant of secondary syphilis or an early manifestation of tertiary syphilis; a question clarified by Haslund and Neisser in 1896-1897. In contrast to tertiary syphilis, the lesions of lues maligna are multiple, have a round or oval configuration, with no tendency to central healing, and exhibit a lamellated, brown-black rupioid crust. Moreover, the early onset of necrotic ulcers in the disease is in contrast to the later occurring gummas of tertiary syphilis. Neisser identified five clinical features of malignant syphilis:

• Short incubation period • Constitutional symptoms are pronounced • The skin and frequently the mucous membranes of the mouth and nose present multiple irregularity distributed lesions consisting of large pustules, ulcers, and rupioid ecthymatous lesions • The patient may have characteristics of the milder forms of the disease such as mucous membrane buccal patches, etc.
The skin lesions: • Pleomorphic • Papulopustules, beginning ulceration, deep ulceration, ulcers covered with crusts, healing lesions • Typically round or oval with a granulating base, and a lamellated, brown-black rupioid crust • The surrounding skin is little affected, showing only minimal erythema.

Table 8. Criteria required for malign lues diagnosis (Neisser, 1896).

Compatible gross and microscopic morphology
A high titer serologic test for syphilis Herxheimer reaction
Dramatic response to antibiotic therapy

Table 9. Criteria required for malign lues diagnosis (Fisher, 1969).

2.2.2 Risks factors for malignant lues

The risks factors for malignant lues are: constitutional symptoms. MSM, sex, syphilis previous. Shulkin proposed the HIV and the presence of opportunistic infections (Shulkin, 1988).

2.2.3 Incidence

The incidence of malignant lues in the cases of series were 0.36% (Haslund, 1987) in the age pre-HIV and 7.3% after of the co-infection (Schofer,1996).

2.2.4 Cases of ulceronodular syphilis in HIV patients

Shulkin published in 1988 the first case of malignant lues in British language. We checked the characteristics epidemiologist, diagnostic, evolutions and treatments in patients with co-infection ulceronodular syphilis-HIV from 1988 until 2010 (British and Spanish languages) including our case.

The total cases were 28 patients with mean age 33 years (R:18-61). There were twenty men and eight women. The risk factor most important was MSM in 45% of cases. The followed features are described in the next table.

2.2.5 Serology

The serology in patients with malignant syphilis is similar that the patients co-infected with syphilis-HIV presented high titles of non-treponemal antibody.

2.2.6 Treatment

The penicillin is the treatment of election. In the secondary syphilis (ulceronodular syphilis) the recommendation is only one dosis of Benzathine PCN 2.4 million UI, however there are other authors than recommended to additional two dosis of penicillin every one week to the initial treatment.

3. Conclusion

In the last years there was an increseased of cases of syphilis malign in relation with co-infection HIV. Early and targeted recognition and treatment of both diseases is essential to deterring continued trends in incidence and prevalence of this disease.

4. References

Baugh, R. & Musher, D. (2005). Secondary syphilitic lesions. Clin. Microbiology Rev, Vol x, N° 18:205-216.

Bazin, A. Lecon theorique et cliniques sur les syphilides: redigess par le fournier. Paris : Adrian Delahyare, 1859 :27,191.

Buchacz K, Petal P, Taylor M, Kerndt PR, Byers RH, Holmber SD, et al. Syphilis increases HIV viral load and decreased CD4 cell counts in HIV infected patients with new syphilis infections. AIDS 2004;18:2075-9.

Creigton, E.T. Darfield microscopy for teh detection and identification of Treponema Pallidum. Clinical Microbiology Reviews. 1999;vol12;2:188.

Chapel, T.A. 1978. The variability of syphilitic chancres. Sex. Trans. Infect. 5:68-70.

Chapel, T.A. 1980. The signs and symptoms of secondary syphilis. Sex. Transm. Dis. 7:161-164.

Clark EG, Danbolt N. The Oslo study of the natural course of untreated syphilis. Med Clin North Am. 1964;48:613-621.

Chesson HW, Pinkerton SD, Voight R, Counts GW. HIV infections and associated costs attributable to syphilis coinfection among African Americans. Am J Public Health. 2003;93(6):943-948.

de Carvalho NS, Mello GR, Castro GR, Telles FQ, Reggiani C, Piazza MJ.Malignant syphilis in an HIV seropositive woman. Int J Gynaecol Obstet. 2008 Sep;102(3):297-8.

DiCarlo RP, Martin DH. The clinical diagnosis of genital ulcer disease in men. Clin Infect Dis 1997;25:292-8.

Don PC, Rubinstein R, Christie S. Malignant syphilis (lues maligna) and concurrent infection with HIV. Int J Dermatol. 1995;34:403-7.

Fernández-Guarino M, Aldanondo Fernández de la Mora I, González García C, Harto Castaño A, Moreno Izquierdo R, Jaén Olasolo P. Malignant syphilis in patients with human immunodeficiency virus (HIV). Actas Dermosifiliogr. 2006 Jul-Aug;97(6):400-3.

Fiumara NJ. Syphilis in newborn clildrem. Clin Obstet Gynecol 1975;18:183-9.

Fraser CM, Norris SJ, Weinstock GM, et al. Complete genome sequence of *Treponema pallidum*, the syphilis spirochete. Science 1998;281:375-88.

Fisher DA, Chang LW, Tuffanelli DL. Lues Maligna. Arch Dermatol 1969 ;99 :70-73.

Gjestland, T. 1955. The Oslo Study of untreated syphilis: an epidemiologic investigation of the natural course of syphilis infection based upon a restudy of the Boeck-Bruusgaard material. Acta Derm. Venereol. 35(Suppl.34):1-368.

Hall C, Klausner J, Bolan G. Managing syphilis in the HIV-infected patient. Curr Infect Dis Rep. 2004;6:72-81.

Haslund A. Syphilis maligna. Archiv für Dermatologie und Syphilis. 1897;38:345-92.

Harper KN, Ocampo PS, Steiner BM, et al. On the origin of the treponematoses: a phylogenetic approach. PloS Negl Trop Dis 2008;2:e148.

Hook EW, Peeling RW. Syphilis control-a continuing challenge. N Eng J Med 2004;351(2):122-4.

Hourihan, M., H. Wheeler, R. Houghton, and B.T. Goh. 2004. Lessons from the syphilis outbreak in homosexual men in east London. Sex. Transm. Infect. 80:509-512.

Hudson, E. H. 1956. Treponematosis. Current Lit. Vener. Dis.,Spec. Issue,p.56.

Hutchinson CM, Hook EW III, Shepherd M , Verley J, Rompalo AM. Altered clinical presentation of early syphilis in patients with human immunodeficiency virus infection. Ann Intern Med. 1994;121(2):94-100.

Jepsen, O.B., K.H. Hougen, and A. Birch-Andersen. 1968. Electron microscopy of *Treponema pallidum* Nichols. Acta Pathol. Microbiol. Scand.74:241-258.

Karp G, Schlaeffer F, Jotkowitz A, Riesenberg K. Syphilis and HIV co-infection. Eur J Intern Med. 2009 Jan;20(1):9-13.

Knell RJ. Syphilis in renaissance Europe: rapid evolution of an introduced sexually transmitted disease? Proc Biol Sci 2004;271(suppl4):S174-6.

Lynn W, Lightman S. Syphilis and HIV: a dangerous combination. Lancet Infect Dis. 2004;4:456-466.

Magnuson HJ, Thomas EW, Olansky S, et al. Inoculation syphilis in human volunteers. Medicine (Baltimore). 1956;35:33-42.

Mahoney, J.F., R. C. Arnold, and A. D. Harris. 1943. Penicillin treatment of early syphilis. Am. J. Public Health 33:1387-1391.

Nakashima, A. K., R. T. Rolfs, M. L. Flock, P. Kilmarx, and J.R. Greenspan. 1996. Epidemiology of syphilis in the United States, 1941-1993. Sex. Transm. Dis. 23:16-23.

Neisser A. Malignant syphilis. Br J Dermatol. 1897;9:11-26.

Oriel, J.D. 1994. The scars of venus. Springer-Verlag, London, England.

Palfi Z, Ponyai K, Varkanyo V, et al. Primary syphilis of the finger. Dermatology. 2008:217:252-253.

Passoni LF, de Menezes JA, Ribeiro SR, Sampaio EC.Lues maligna in an HIV-infected patient. Rev Soc Bras Med Trop. 2005 Mar-Apr;38(2):181-4.

Pleimes M, Hartschuh W, Kutzner H, Enk AH, Hartmann M.Malignant syphilis with ocular involvement and organism-depleted lesions. Clin Infect Dis. 2009 Jan 1;48(1):83-5.

Pérez-Pérez L, Cabanillas M, Ginarte M, Sánchez-Aguilar D, Toribio J.Malignant syphilis in an HIV-infected patient. Actas Dermosifiliogr. 2007 Jun;98(5):351-4.

Prasad PV, Paari T, Chokkalingam K, Vijaybushanam V. Malignant syphilis (leus maligna) in a HIV infected patient. Indian J Dermatol Venereol Leprol. 2001 Jul-Aug;67(4):192-4.

Reynolds SJ, Risbud AR, Shepar ME, Romapalo AM, Ghate MV, Godbole SV, et al. High rates of syphilis among STI patients are contributing to the spread of HIV-1 in India. Sex Transm Inf 2006;82:121-6.

Romero-Jiménez MJ, Suárez Lozano I, Fajardo Picó JM, Barón Franco B.Malignant syphilis in patient with human immunodeficiency virus (HIV): case report and literature review. An Med Interna. 2003 Jul;20(7):373-6.

Rompalo AM, Cannon RO, Quinn TC, et al. Association of biologic false-positive reactions for syphilis with human immunodeficiency virus infection. J Infect Dis 1992;165:1124-1126.

Rompalo AM, Lawlor J, Seaman P, et al. Modification of syphilitic genital ulcers manifestations by coexistent HIV infection. Sex Transm Dis. 2001;28:448-454.

Rosahn, P. D. 1947. Autopsy studies in syphilis. J. Vener. Dis. Infect.21 (Suppl.)

Rolfs RT, Joesoef MR, Hendershot EF, et al. A randomized trial of enhanced therapy for early syphilis in patients with and without human immunodeficiency virus infection. The syphilis and HIV Study Group. N Engl J Med 1997;337:307-314

Rolfs, R. T., M. Goldberg, and R.G. Sharrar. 1990. Risk factors for syphilis:cocaine use and prostitution. Am. J. Public Health. 80:853-857.

Rothschild BM. History of Syphilis. Clinical Infectious Diseases 2005;40:1454-63.

Sartin, J.S., and H. O. Perry. 1995. From mercury to malaria to penicillin: the history of the treatment of syphilis at the Mayo Clinic. J. Am. Acad. -261 Dermatol. 32:255.

Schaudinn, F.N., and E. Hoffman. 1905. Vorlaufiger Bericht uber das Vorkommen von Spirochaeten in syphilitischen Krankheits produkten und bei Papillomen. Arbeiten K Gesundheits.22:527-534.

Sharma VK, Kumar B. Malignant syphilis or syphilis simulating malignancy. Int J Dermatol. 1991 Sep;30(9):676.

Sellati TJ, Wilkinson DA, Sheffield JS, Koup RA, Radolf JD, Norgard MV. Virulent *Treponema pallidum*, lipoprotein, and synthetic lipopeptides induce CCR5 on human monocytes and enhance their susceptibility to infection by human inmunodeficiency virus tipe 1. J Infect Dis 2000;181:283-293.

Singh AE, Romanowski B. Syphilis: review with emphasis on clinical, epidemiologic, and some biologic features. Clin Microbiol Rev 1999;12:187-209.

Stokes, J. H., H. Beerman, and N.R. Ingraham. 1944. Modern clinical syphilology. The W. B. Saunders Co.,Philadelphia,Pa.

Syphilis. New York Department of Health AIDS Institute: www. hivguidelines.org

Schöfer H, Imhof M, Thoma-Greber E, et al. Active syphilis in HIV infection: A multicentre retrospective survey-The German AIDS Study Group. Genitourin Med 1996;72:176-181.

Telzac EE, Cahisson MA, Bevier PJ, et al. HIV-1 seroconversion in patients with and without genital ulcer disease. Ann Intern Med 1993;119:1181-1186.

Tosca A, Stavropoulos PG, Hatziolou E, Arvanitis A, Stavrianeas N, Hatzivassiliou Stratigos JD. Malignant syphilis in HIV-infected patients. Int J Dermatol. 1990 Oct;29(8):575-8.

Tramont EC. *Treponema pallidum* (syphilis). In : Mandell GL, Bennett JE, Dolin R, ed. Principles and practice of infectious diseases. 7th ed. Orlando. FL: Churchill Livingstone, 2010:3035-3053.

Tikjob G, Russel M, Petersen CS, et al. Seronegative secondary syphilis in a patient with AIDS: Identification of *Treponema pallidum* in biopsy specimen. J Am Acad Dermatol 1991;24:506-508.

Tucker JD, Shah S, Jarell AD, Tsai KY, Zembowicz A, Kroshinsky D.Lues maligna in early HIV infection case report and review of the literature. 2-4. Sex Transm Dis. 2009 Aug;36(8):51

Wassermann, A., A. Neisser, and C. Bruck. 1906. Eine serodiagnostische Reaktion bei Syphilis. Dtsch. Med. Wochenschr.32:745-746.

WHO. World Health Organization - Trends in sexually transmitted infections and HIV in the European Region 1980-2005;2006.

Witkowski JA, Parish LC. The great imitator: malignant syphilis with hepatitis.

Clin Dermatol. 2002 Mar-Apr;20(2):156-63.

Yinnon AM, CouryDoniger P, Polito R, et al. Serologic response to treatment of syphilis in patients with HIV infections. Arch Intern Med 1996;156:321-325.

Zetola NM, Klausner JD, Kerndt PR,et al. Syphilis and HIV infection: An uptodate. Clin Infect Dis. 2007;44:1222-1228.

7

Rifamycin Use in HIV-Infected Patients with Tuberculosis

Aline Bergesch Barth, Eric Free Egelund and Charles Arthur Peloquin
University of Florida
United States

1. Introduction

One-third of the world's population is latently infected with mycobacterium tuberculosis (MTb).(Raviglione et al., 1995; 2010c) Of those infected a 5% to 10% chance exists during that person's lifetime for the disease to become active.(Corbett et al., 2003) Patients who are immunocompromised have a much greater risk of experiencing active tuberculosis. Patients who have contracted human immunodeficiency virus (HIV) have a 10% chance yearly of developing active disease. Tuberculosis (TB) is the most common opportunistic infection in patients with HIV.(2010a) A person with HIV is 20-30 times more likely to develop active tuberculosis than a person without the virus. (2010b) The World Health Organization (WHO) states that tuberculosis is the leading infectious killer in HIV-positive patients worldwide, killing one out of every four patients.

Guidelines recommend treating both infections concurrently as this has shown an increased probability of survival versus sequential therapy.(2010a; Abdool Karim et al., 2010) Unfortunately, several problems arise when combining therapy. Both disease states require multidrug regimens for long durations of time. TB is generally treated for nine or more months in patients with dual disease states, while HIV is treated for a lifetime. Not only does the combination of regimens lead to multi-way drug interactions, but to overlapping side effects, the immune reconstitution inflammatory syndrome (IRIS), and subsequently an increased difficulty on the part of the patient to adhere to the complicated regimens, which ultimately may result in viral or bacterial resistance.

The current recommendations for treating tuberculosis in HIV patients are the same as treatment in patients without HIV: an initial two month phase of isoniazid, pyrazinamide, ethambutol and rifampin or rifabutin followed by an extended four month phase of isoniazid and one of the rifamycins. In HIV patients the duration may be substantially longer. While each of the rifamycins have significant Cytochrome P450 (CYP450) interactions, rifabutin is considered to have the least among the three and therefore the best choice to be used in treating tuberculosis in HIV patients. (Piscitelli and Gallicano, 2001) Rifabutin is not available in many parts of the world which need it most, specifically low-resource countries (e.g., many sub-Saharan Africa nations). Also, many of the antiretrovirals which are necessary to treat AIDS are not available.

With multiple drug interactions, overlapping toxicities, and an unknown pharmacokinetic response in individual patients, clinicians are often at a disadvantage in making treatment decisions. Monitoring of serum concentrations could help elucidate sub- or supratherapeutic concentrations of not only the rifamycins but co-administered HIV medications, leading to a more optimal dosing of medications, reduced toxicities, and a decreased likelihood of drug resistance. In this chapter we will discuss the co-pathophysiology of HIV and TB, the interactions among the rifamycins and HIV medications, and how therapeutic drug management (TDM), also known as therapeutic drug monitoring, may aid the clinician in making informed clinical decisions.

2. Interrelated pathophysiology

The specific pathways by which TB and HIV impact each other have yet to be fully elucidated. (Patel et al., 2007) CD4+ T-helper cells in the body activate macrophages which engulf MTb. In an immunocompetent patient alveolar macrophages undergo apoptosis to destroy MTb. With HIV infection macrophages are prevented from initiating apoptosis. Alternatively, TB-infected macrophages express tumor necrosis factor-alpha (TNF-α) which leads to an increase in HIV replication. As HIV replication increases, TB is no longer well contained. The clinical course of TB accelerates which may lead to extrapulmonary involvement. In short, the combination of the two disease states begins a vicious cycle which ultimately leads to an increased risk of mortality.

3. The rifamycins

The first rifamycins were isolated in 1957 from the bacterium *Streptomyces mediterranei* (now *Amycolatopsis rifamycinica*).(Margalith, 1960) Since their discovery they have been used in the treatment of numerous diseases including: methicillin-resistant *Staphylococcus aureus* (MRSA), leprosy, Legionnaires' disease, and, of course, TB. The rifamycins currently available for treatment of TB are rifampin, rifabutin, and rifapentine. They are considered the most important drugs for the treatment of TB due to their potent sterilizing effect on MTb. Briefly, the sterilizing effect is the ability of a TB drug to prevent post-treatment relapses. Regimens without a rifamycin or not using a rifamycin for at least six months have increased rates of treatment failure.(Okwera et al., 1994; Jindani et al., 2004) A meta-analysis by Khan et al. reported that patients using regimens with a rifamycin for only two months were much more likely to experience relapse than those patients on a regimen consisting of a rifamycin for at least eight months.(Khan et al., 2010) The rifamycins act by inhibiting the DNA dependent RNA polymerase encoded by the *rpoB* gene. The rifamycin binds to the β-subunit and blocks the synthesis of the RNA chain. Importantly, the drugs do not inhibit the mammalian enzyme. In regards to the rifamycin family, rifampin is the fastest absorbed with the highest bioavailability, while rifapentine has the slowest absorption and a half-life Intermediate (~13.19h) (1998) between the short half-life of rifampin (~2.46h) (2004 Jan) and the long terminal elimination half-life of rifabutin (~45h)(2010 Jan).

3.1 Rifampin

Rifampin has been used in the treatment of TB for nearly half a century. Along with isoniazid, rifampin is considered the cornerstone for successful treatment. However, rifampin's potent inductive effects on many hepatic and intestinal enzymes as well as the drug transporter, P-glycoprotein, generate many drug interactions. With regards to HIV treatment, rifampin interacts with the non-nucleoside reverse transcriptase inhibitors (NNRTIs), the protease inhibitors (PIs), the integrase inhibitors (e.g., raltegravir), and the entry inhibitors (e.g., maraviroc). Ideally, rifabutin is substituted for rifampin in HIV patients. Unfortunately, rifabutin is not available in most resource-poor countries who cannot afford the newer rifamycin. Also, unlike rifampin, rifabutin is not available in a multidrug capsule (e.g., Rifater®: rifampin, isoniazid, pyrazinamide) which aids adherence. Thus, drug interactions between rifampin and HIV medications must be managed. In this chapter we will limit our discussion to rifampin's interactions with the NNRTIs and the PIs as these are the most commonly used medications for HIV treatment.

3.1.1 Rifampin & the PIs

Due to its inhibitory effects on CYP enzymes, ritonavir is generally prescribed at a low dose with a second PI (also known as ritonavir "boosting"). (King et al., 2004; Burger et al., 2006b) As rifampin's inductive effects are especially strong with the PIs, only two formulations approach therapeutic concentrations when given concomitantly with rifampin: lopinavir and saquinavir, both of which must be administered with substantial doses of ritonavir. (Maartens et al., 2009)

The standard dose of lopinavir-ritonavir is 400/100 mg given twice daily. When administered with the standard 600 mg dose of rifampin, Bertz et al. noted a substantial reduction in C_{max} (45%), AUC (75%) and C_{min} (99%). (Bertz R, 2001) Building upon this observation, La Porte et al. performed a study with 32 healthy volunteers to compare the pharmacokinetics of the standard lopinavir-ritonavir dose given without rifampin with two dose-adjusted regimens: 800/200 mg twice daily and 400/400 mg twice daily of lopinavir/ritonavir with rifampin. (la Porte et al., 2004) Lopinavir concentrations were markedly higher in the adjusted regimens, when compared to the reported data for standard doses. However, the authors could not demonstrate that the adjusted regimens were equivalent to lopinavir-ritonavir without rifampin. This may be due to rifampin's inductive effects, or limitations of the study (e.g., small sample size). Regardless, the study indicates that super-boosted lopinavir-ritonavir may be an option for co-infected patients when alternative regimens are unavailable. The C_{max}, $AUC_{0\text{-}12}$, and C_{min} for lopinavir during therapy composed by lopinavir-ritonavir 400/400 mg after 10 and 24 days, respectively, were: 12.3 and 11.5 mg/liter; 102.9 and 100.7 mg*h/liter; 5.2 and 5.9 mg/liter. The lopinavir C_{max}, $AUC_{0\text{-}12}$ and C_{min} for the lopinavir-ritonavir 800/200 mg regimen after days 10 and 24 were: 12.9 and 13.8 mg/liter; 111.8 and 104.5 mg*h/liter and 6.5 and 5.1 mg/liter, respectively. Of note, the authors point out that 31% of the patients stopped treatment with the adjusted regimens due to side effects, primarily elevated liver function tests (LFTs). In patients co-infected with HIV and TB who must receive the medications for a greater amount of time and/or additional potential hepatotoxic drugs these side effects may be exacerbated.

In a study of ten healthy volunteers, rifampin reduced the concentration of atazanavir significantly for both 300 and 400 mg doses given BID. (Acosta et al., 2007) A larger study with 71 healthy volunteers revealed that ritonavir was not able to overcome rifampin's induction. The following proportions of atazanavir-ritonavir were analyzed: 300/100 mg, 300/200 mg and 400/200 mg, in combination with 600 mg of rifampin. (Burger et al., 2006b) These dosage regimens were compared with the administration of just atazanavir 400 mg or with the combination atazanavir-ritonavir 300/100 mg. The comparisons showed significant reductions in C_{max} and AUC. However, the reductions in C_{min} were the most significant: around 60% for the regimens when compared with just atazanavir 400 mg and greater than 90% for the three regimens when compared to the combination atazanavir-ritonavir 300/100 mg. The obtained atazanavir C_{min} were: 15.9 ng/mL (300/100/600 mg-atazanavir/

ritonavir/rifampin), 40.6 ng/mL (300/200/600 mg-atazanavir/ritonavir/rifampin) and 74.4 ng/mL (400/200/600 mg-atazanavir/ritonavir/rifampin). Another study from Mallolas and collaborators confirmed these results. (Mallolas et al., 2007) The researchers performed a study in patients with HIV to verify the feasibility of a regimen with 600 mg of rifampin combined with 300/100 of atazanavir-ritonavir. The study had to be interrupted because of very low concentrations of atazanavir. The median reductions in C_{max}, AUC, and C_{min} for the three patients that completed the treatment were 48, 64, and 100%, respectively.

In a study of 22 patients co-infected with TB and HIV, Ribera et al. found that saquinavir was reduced substantially in the presence of rifampin. (Ribera et al., 2007) Patients were treated with the standard TB regimen of rifampin, isoniazid, pyrazinamide, and with or without ethambutol for two months. Ethambutol and pyrazinamide were then dropped from the regimen and once-daily antiretroviral (ART) added. ART consisted of 1600 mg saquinavir, and 200 mg ritonavir along with didanosine and lamivudine. The saquinavir pharmacokinetic parameters C_{max}, $AUC_{0\text{-}24}$, and C_{min} were reduced by 35%, 40% and 49%, respectively. The obtained saquinavir C_{max}, $AUC_{0\text{-}24}$, C_{min} were 2.1 µg/mL, 13.6 µg*h/mL and 0.06 µg/mL, respectively. The authors concluded that twice-daily administration of saquinavir or higher doses might result in therapeutic concentrations, but it is unknown what doses would be necessary. A study of 30 co-infected HIV/TB patients given 400 mg saquinavir and 400 mg ritonavir plus two NRTIs suggests that these doses are able to maintain therapeutic concentrations of rifampin and the PIs; however, the study had a substantial attrition rate with ten patients dropping out during TB therapy and another fifteen patients dropping when ART was added. (Rolla et al., 2006)

Hepatotoxicity is one of the primary concerns facing clinicians when using a saquinavir-containing regimen with the rifamycins. A 2009 two-period crossover study consisting of 28 healthy volunteers received either 600 mg rifampin once daily or 1000/100 mg saquinavir-ritonavir twice daily for two weeks. (Schmitt et al., 2009) Volunteers then received all three drugs for two weeks. All patients in the arm who initially received rifampin and subsequently received saquinavir-ritonavir experienced elevations in their alanine aminotransferases (ALTs) from 11 to 70 times the upper limit of normal, prompting an early termination of the study.

In a study of six HIV patients, ritonavir (100mg - BID) was not able to overcome the induction caused by rifampin (300 mg – half of the normal dose) in indinavir (800 mg - BID) metabolism. An 87% reduction in the indinavir concentration and a 94% reduction in ritonavir concentration was verified 12 hours after the last dose. (Justesen et al., 2004) This study detected a C_{max} of 10,116 ng/mL and C_{min} of 112 ng/mL (both quantified 4 days after rifampin administration). The AUC was not calculated.

In short, ritonavir's effect on overcoming the induction caused by rifampin is variable according to the co-administered PI and the dosage schemes have to be carefully chosen in order to achieve therapeutic drug concentrations. Also, it is important to consider the possible hepatotoxicity which may occur with increased dosing.

3.1.2 Rifampin & the NNRTIs

Efavirenz is primarily metabolized by CYP2B6 and to a lesser extent by CYP3A4 and CYP2A6 to inactive metabolites. (Kwara et al., 2010; Rakhmanina and van den Anker, 2010) As rifampin is a potent inducer of CYP2B6, concern exists regarding efavirenz concentrations when the two are given concurrently, considering that subtherapeutic efavirenz concentrations could lead to treatment failure and resistance. This hypothesis was based on previous studies where reduced efavirenz concentrations caused treatment failure. In a study performed by Marzolini and collaborators virological failure was associated with low plasma concentrations in 50% of the patients on efavirenz (C_{min}<1000 μg/L) while CNS toxicity was three times more frequent in patients with high efavirenz concentrations (C_{min}>4000 μg/L). (Marzolini et al., 2001) The drug concentrations were determined between 8 and 20 hours post dose and the concentrations varied from 125 to 15,230 μg/L. The drug is administered at bedtime because of its side effects, therefore it is difficult to determine the real C_{min}. Efavirenz CNS toxicity occurs in approximately 20-40% (Gazzard, 1999) of patients, manifesting as light-headedness, feeling faint, dizzy, "out of control," or restless.

Attempting to avoid sub-therapeutic concentrations, an increase in the efavirenz dosage from 600 mg to 800 mg has been recommended when concomitant treatment with rifampin is necessary (2004). A trial with 24 patients showed a reduction of efavirenz (600 mg) C_{max}, AUC and C_{min} of around 24, 22, and 25%, respectively, in the presence of rifampin. (Lopez-Cortes et al., 2002) The obtained C_{max}, AUC and C_{min} for efavirenz 600 mg in presence of rifampin, were 2.32 mg/L, 28.3 mg*h/L and 0.63 mg/L, respectively. However, the concentrations achieved with the combination of rifampin and efavirenz 800 mg are equivalent to values obtained with efavirenz 600 mg without rifampin. No improvement in virological efficacy with concomitant administration of rifampin and efavirenz 800 mg in relation to efavirenz C_{min} and virological efficacy has been proven. (Manosuthi et al., 2005; Lopez-Cortes et al., 2006; Manosuthi et al., 2006)

Moreover, the use of a higher dose may increase the risk for experiencing side effects, especially in patients from specific ethnic groups. African-Americans, Hispanics and Asians tend to have higher efavirenz concentrations than Caucasians. (Burger et al., 2006a; Ramachandran et al., 2009; Kwara et al., 2010)

It is not clear if body weight is related to efavirenz plasma concentration or clearance, considering that studies have found contradictory results. Additional studies are needed regarding the impact of body weight, especially in patients weighing more than 60 kg. (Manosuthi et al., 2009b) What effect sex may play is contradictory as well. While some studies have found that females have higher plasma concentrations than males, other studies show no difference. (Gounden et al., 2010)

Pharmacogenomics studies have been performed to elucidate the source of variability on efavirenz plasma concentrations. The effect of CYP2B6 polymorphisms on efavirenz concentrations was investigated in several studies. The polymorphism CYP2B6 516 G>T (CYP2B6*6) has the most data. The 516 T/T genotype was associated with lower efavirenz clearance, a longer half-life (~48 hours), and CNS toxicity. (Tsuchiya et al., 2004; Arab-Alameddine et al., 2009) Thus, while efavirenz may be affected only mildly by the rifamycins the effects of certain covariates, specifically the role of pharmacogenetics, needs to be resolved.

The concomitant administration of nevirapine with rifampin is known to reduce the exposure of nevirapine, affecting pharmacokinetic parameters such as C_{max}, AUC, and C_{min}. Despite this reduction various studies show drug concentrations to be within therapeutic range. (Ribera et al., 2001; Autar et al., 2005; Matteelli et al., 2009) However, a small study by Ramachandran et al. noted that 8 out of 13 patients had blood concentrations under the C_{min} (3 μg/mL). (Ramachandran et al., 2009) They proposed the use of a higher dose (300 mg) for providing therapeutic drug concentrations to those patients; however, the study was composed of a small number of patients and conducted in a short period of time. The effect of rifampin on nevirapine's concentrations seems to decrease over time when nevirapine is used chronically with anti-TB drugs. Matteelli et al. conducted a study with 16 co-infected patients receiving HIV and TB treatment. (Mattelli et al., 2004) A reduction in the AUC of nevirapine by 25.6% was detected after four weeks of TB treatment while patients experienced a reduction of only 7.5% after 10 weeks. The C_{max}, AUC, and C_{min} of nevirapine after 4 weeks were 4.8 µg/mL, 43.7 µg*h/mL and 3.2 µg/mL, respectively.

Manosuthi and collaborators conducted a study comparing the use of efavirenz or nevirapine with rifampin.(Manosuthi et al., 2009a) They found that the levels (C_{min}) of efavirenz (600 mg) are less affected by rifampin than the levels of nevirapine (400 mg). The mean C_{min} for week six were 4.27 mg/L (efavirenz) and 5.59 mg/L (nevirapine), and for week twelve: 3.54 mg/L (efavirenz) and 5.6 mg/L (nevirapine).

3.2 Rifabutin

Several medium-sized studies suggest that rifabutin may be as effective as rifampin for TB treatment. (Felten, 1987; Gonzalez-Montaner et al., 1994; McGregor et al., 1996) Schwander et al. first compared rifabutin to rifampin in co-infected HIV patients and found rifabutin to be as effective in the treatment of TB. Additionally, rifabutin treated patients in the study experienced earlier sputum conversion than their rifampin counterparts.

Two issues arise with the use of rifabutin in AIDS patients. The first involves intermittent dosing and the second is in regards to drug interactions. In the pharmacokinetic sub-study of Tuberculosis Trials Consortium (TBTC) Study 23, patients were treated with twice-weekly rifabutin and isoniazid. (Weiner et al., 2005) Eight of the 102 patients involved in the study developed rifamycin resistance with seven of these experiencing low serum concentrations of rifabutin. As with rifampin, due to the possibility of MTb developing resistance, highly intermittent dosing is not recommended in this patient population.

As previously mentioned, rifabutin has less of an inductive effect on enzymes than rifampin (~40% less). (Burman et al., 1999) For this reason rifabutin is the preferred rifamycin for use in HIV patients when available. While less potent than rifampin and rifapentine, rifabutin still has several significant interactions with medications used to treat HIV or concomitant infections. Further complicating treatment with rifabutin is the fact that it is a CYP3A4 substrate itself, leading to interactions with CYP inducers and inhibitors. For HIV patients requiring either a PI- or NNRTI-based therapy this poses substantial difficulty in finding a good therapeutic regimen.

3.2.1 Rifabutin & the PIs

Due to the potential of lopinavir-ritonavir to increase the serum concentrations of rifabutin the current recommendation by the CDC is to lower the dose of rifabutin from 300 mg thrice weekly to 150 mg thrice weekly or every other day when given together. There is recent evidence to suggest that this recommendation should be reconsidered.

A pharmacokinetic study by Boulanger et al. measured the drug concentrations of rifabutin and lopinavir-ritonavir as well as the rifabutin metabolite, 25-desacetyl rifabutin, in HIV positive patients with active tuberculosis. (Boulanger et al., 2009) When rifabutin was administered at 150 mg thrice weekly in combination with lopinavir-ritonavir a majority of the patients had C_{max} values below the normal range (0.3 to 0.9 ug/ml). PK-PD simulations by the authors suggested that when the two medications are administered together, rifabutin should be given daily, and that doses as high as 450 mg daily would be needed to achieve free drug plasma concentrations at or above the minimum inhibitory concentration (MIC) for part of the dosing interval. The obtained rifabutin C_{max} and AUC_{0-24} were 0.23 µg/mL and 2.97 µg*h/mL, respectively. It should be noted that one patient developed rifamycin resistance during the study.

A second study by Khachi et al. reported similar results. (Khachi et al., 2009) The authors monitored concentrations of an antiretroviral regimen containing lopinavir-ritonavir (400/100 mg) in combination with rifabutin 150 mg. Of the five patients studied, rifabutin levels were below target in all five patients (0.10 to 0.37 ug/ml). Two patients were reported to "deteriorate clinically" and had their rifabutin increased to 300 mg three times a week. Additionally, lopinavir-ritonavir concentrations were below targeted concentrations in two patients. While both studies are limited in scope due to small sample sizes, ten and five patients respectively, they indicate the need for a larger study to determine appropriate dosing.

Darunavir and tipranavir result in increased rifabutin concentrations while rifabutin decreases their concentrations. (2004) The CDC recommends decreasing the dose of rifabutin by 75% to 150 mg every other day or 150 mg thrice weekly. However, these daily primarily reflect data from healthy volunteers, who tend to have more profound increases in rifabutin and 25-desacetyl-rifabutin concentrations than HIV-infected patients. As noted above, daily rifabutin doses, perhaps starting with 150 mg, may be preferred. This requires additional study. The remaining PIs (amprenavir, fosamprenavir, atazanavir, and indinavir) increase the AUC of rifabutin from 200 to 250% (again, primarily in healthy volunteers), while rifabutin does not appreciably alter any of their pharmacokinetics with the exception of indinavir. Indinavir is recommended to be increased to 1000 mg every 8 hours while rifabutin should be decreased to 150 mg daily or 300 mg three times per week.

Finally, saquinavir is contraindicated with rifabutin use unless boosted by ritonavir. When rifabutin is used with unboosted saquinavir there is an approximate 40% increase in rifabutin AUC and a subsequent 40% decrease in saquinavir AUC.(2007 Jul.) Dosing is then recommended at 150 mg every other day or thrice weekly. All of these recommendations reflect mean changes, mostly from healthy volunteers, and results in individual HIV-infected patients may be substantially different.(Gallicano et al., 2001)

3.2.2 Rifabutin & the NNRTIs

All of the NNRTIs are reported to interact with rifabutin to some degree. Delavirdine is contraindicated with rifabutin use due to an increase in rifabutin's AUC (over 200%) and a decrease in delavirdine's (80%)(2004). When rifabutin is prescribed with a PI boosted regimen, etravirine should be avoided because of the reduction in its concentration. (2008 Jan) This leaves efavirenz and nevirapine as the two NNRTIs which work best with rifabutin.

When efavirenz is given the AUC of rifabutin is decreased substantially, necessitating a dose of 450 to 600 mg. Studies explored three times weekly dosing regimens; daily dosing with rifabutin 450 to 600 mg also would be acceptable with efavirenz (2004). The same is true of nevirapine regarding cell counts, but with a dose of 300 mg daily or thrice weekly for rifabutin. Again, three times weekly rifabutin may not be sufficient in all or even most patients, given the demonstrated risk of acquired rifamycin resistance in HIV-infected patients receiving intermittent rifabutin regimens.

3.3 Rifapentine

Rifapentine is the latest rifamycin to be developed. A cyclopentyl derivative of rifampin, rifapentine has a longer half-life than rifampin and a 2 to 4-fold lower MIC.(Birmingham et al., 1978; Vital Durand et al., 1986) Unfortunately, rifapentine also inherited rifampin's strong enzyme-inducing properties. Thanks to its extended half-life, rifapentine has been tested for intermittent dosing in the hopes of increasing patient compliance. Use of rifapentine is primarily reserved for the four month continuation phase of TB treatment, but is being studied for possible initial therapy. As with rifampin and rifabutin problems arose with highly intermittent dosing. TBTC Study 22 compared once-weekly rifapentine and isoniazid with twice-weekly rifampin and isoniazid in co-infected HIV/TB patients. (Vernon et al., 1999) HIV positive patients in the once-weekly rifapentine arm had higher rates of relapse than HIV positive patients in the twice-weekly rifampin arm. Four of the five patients who relapsed had acquired rifamycin monoresistance.

4. Immune Reconstitution Inflammatory Syndrome (IRIS)

In addition to drug interactions another common problem associated with co-infected patients which bears mentioning is the immune reconstitution inflammatory syndrome, otherwise known simply as IRIS.(Jevtovic et al., 2005; Tappuni, 2011) IRIS most commonly occurs when ART is added to a patient's regimen already being treated for TB. IRIS may occur anywhere from days to months following addition of ART. Symptoms are broad and may range from a mild fever to renal failure. Respiratory distress, expanding intracranial lesions and meningitis, lymphadenopathy, and skin lesions may develop also.

The exact mechanism of IRIS is not completely known. Researchers believe that when ART begins to reduce HIV's viral load the body's immune system gradually recovers. This recovery leads to the immune system's "awareness" of TB. The body overreacts to MTb antigens, releasing inflammatory cytokines and causing the aforementioned symptoms. Risk factors identified include: extrapulmonary TB, African-American race (one study), and early initiation of ART following TB therapy.(Breen et al., 2004; Burman et al., 2007)

Steroids are most often used as initial treatment of IRIS. Some clinicians recommend prednisone 1 mg/kg/day or dexamethasone 8 to 16 mg/kg/day divided twice daily. (Sexton, 2011) Clinicians should initiate steroids on a case-by-case basis and be cautious about their use. Studies are mixed in regards to the mortality benefit of steroids and one study reported an increased incidence of Kaposi's Sarcoma. (Hakim et al., 2000; Elliott et al., 2004; Sharma et al., 2008) Other drug treatments which have been tried, but have little information regarding their use are: the non-steroidal anti-inflammatories (NSAIDs), the TNF-α inhibitor, pentoxifylline, and thalidomide. (Marais et al., 2009) However, information regarding their efficacy is scarce.

5. Pediatrics

A relatively small amount of literature exists regarding rifamycin pharmacokinetics for young patients with HIV and TB. Schaaf et al. examined 54 pediatric patients, aged three months to 13 years, receiving rifampin, 21 of which had HIV. (Schaaf et al., 2009) In the study a majority of HIV positive and HIV negative patients experienced concentrations below what is considered the normal two hours C_{max} range (8-24 ug/ml). While there was a trend for HIV positive patients toward a lower rifampin C_{max}, no significant difference existed between the two groups.

Ren et al performed a study with 30 children aged seven months to four years and divided them in two groups. (Ren Y, 2008) One group composed of 15 HIV positive children without TB received lopinavir and ritonavir in a 4:1 ratio without rifampin. The second group of 15 HIV positive children with TB were treated with an increased concentration of ritonavir to achieve 1:1 ratio of lopinavir-ritonavir ("super boosted" lopinavir). There was a reduction of the C_{max} and $AUC_{0\text{-}12}$ in the group that received additional ritonavir. However, there was no difference in the C_{min} between both groups. The lopinavir C_{max}, $AUC_{0\text{-}12}$, and C_{min} obtained for the regimen with rifampin were: 10.5 mg/L, 80.9 mg*h/L and 3.94 mg/L, respectively.
The same researchers used population pharmacokinetic analysis to characterize the pharmacokinetic interactions and to examine the data from the Ren study.(Elsherbiny et al., 2010) The adjustment of ritonavir to an equal proportion of the PI's (that is, 1:1) was not able to entirely overcome the inductive effect that rifampin has over lopinavir. One of the reasons, as the authors point out, can be the fact that children aged one to four have more pronounced enzymatic activity, eliminating the lopinavir. However, the predicted trough concentrations by the model are over 1 ug/ml, indicating that with the additional ritonavir concentrations of lopinavir will be efficacious. More studies are necessary to verify the safety and efficacy of this combination. Studies also are needed regarding the use of rifabutin and rifapentine in the pediatric setting as data are limited.

6. Therapeutic drug management

Due to the extensive drug interactions, the overlapping side effects, and the length of treatment, a patient co-infected with TB and HIV has a more difficult time adhering to his or her regimen than patients with either disease state alone. TDM offers clinicians the ability to make a more informed therapeutic decision. Several studies have shown TDM to be of benefit in the TB patient. (Peloquin, 2002b) TDM for HIV medications has been studied in a series of small trials. Because most such trials have several additional variables, it is difficult to achieve statistical significance in these settings. However, it remains true that PIs are competitive, reversible inhibitors, so their continued presence is required for continued activity. Also, patients with HIV may have other opportunistic infections and experience malabsorption which can affect the concentration of TB drugs. (Kotler DP et al., 1984; Gillin JS et al., 1985; Peloquin, 2002b) TDM could be a useful tool to monitor the concentration in those patients. In a review of eight trials Kredo et al. reported that routine use of TDM is not warranted but TDM use in treatment-naïve patients initiated on a PI containing regimen may improve virological efficacy. (Kredo et al., 2009)
In addition TDM may prove useful in determining which patients are experiencing malabsorption. Few studies have expressly looked at the malabsorption of anti-TB medications in HIV patients, and data are still accumulating, but evidence points toward the disease state negatively affecting concentrations of TB medications. A retrospective study of 21 HIV/TB patients by Holland et al. demonstrates this effect. Out of 21 patients, 18 had two-hour concentrations of at least one drug (either, isoniazid, a rifamycin, or both) below the recommended range. (Holland et al., 2009) Current guidelines list TDM as an option for clinicians but further research in the area is needed. (CDC, 2007)
TDM is recommended by many clinicians when both TB and HIV are treated concomitantly, especially when PIs and NNRTIs are used. However, TDM is not a substitute for clinical evaluation or directly observed treatment, but is useful to verify inadequate dose administration, or help solve drug-drug interaction problems. (Peloquin, 2002a)

7. Conclusion

Patients co-infected with HIV and TB have a difficult time adhering to their medication regimens due to many reasons. Even in those patients who are fortunate enough to receive appropriate treatment adherence is difficult. In addition to overlapping side effects and the possibility of IRIS, the drug regimens are lengthy and involve many drug interactions.

Drug interactions between the rifamycins and the PIs and NNRTIs are varied and not easily quantified. Often, concentrations are unique to the individual in whom the interactions take place. One solution to this problem is to either use and/or develop new medications that have fewer interactions. While studies are underway with new (as well as older) anti-TB drugs a set timeline for their arrival is unknown. Additionally, a majority of patients reside in resource-poor settings where economics (or political or military strife) inhibit optimal care.

Until new and improved regimens are developed a reasonable solution is to monitor the concentrations of HIV and anti-TB medications and alter the doses when warranted to achieve therapeutic success, i.e., TDM. TDM has been used in TB patients for many years and is considered a valuable tool by many clinicians in the successful treatment of their patients.

8. References

1998. Rifapentine (Priftin) [package insert]. Kansas City, KA: Hoechst Marion Roussel.

2004. Updated Guidelines for the Use of Rifamycins for the Treatment of Tuberculosis Among HIV-Infected Patients Taking Protease Inhibitors or Nonnucleoside Reverse Transcriptase Inhibitors In: Control CDC, editor.: Morbidity and Mortality Weekly Report.

2010a. Treatment of tuberculosis: guidelines for national programmes. In, 4th ed. Geneva: World Health Organiazation.

2011b WHO TB/HIV Facts 2011. Available on the World Wide Web at http://www.who.int/tb/challenges/hiv/factsheet_hivtb_2011.pdf

2010c. WHO global tuberculosis control report 2010. Summary. Cent Eur J Public Health 18:237.

2004 Jan Rifampin (Rifadin)[package insert]. Bridgewater, NJ: Aventis Pharmaceuticals.

2007. Jul. Invirase® (saquinavir) [package insert] In: Pharmaceuticals R, editor. Nutley, NJ: Roche Pharmaceuticals.

2008 Jan. Intelence™ (etravirine) [package insert]. Raritan, NJ: Tibotec Therapeutics.

2010 Jan. Rifabutin (Mycobutin) [package insert]. New York, NY: Pfizer.

Abdool Karim Q, Abdool Karim SS, Baxter C, Friedland G, Gengiah T, Gray A, Grobler A, Naidoo K, Padayatchi N, El-Sadr W. 2010. The SAPIT trial provides essential evidence on risks and benefits of integrated and sequential treatment of HIV and tuberculosis. S Afr Med J 100:808-809.

Acosta EP, Kendall MA, Gerber JG, Alston-Smith B, Koletar SL, Zolopa AR, Agarwala S, Child M, Bertz R, Hosey L, Haas DW. 2007. Effect of concomitantly administered rifampin on the pharmacokinetics and safety of atazanavir administered twice daily. Antimicrob Agents Chemother 51:3104-3110.

Arab-Alameddine M, Di Iulio J, Buclin T, Rotger M, Lubomirov R, Cavassini M, Fayet A, Decosterd LA, Eap CB, Biollaz J, Telenti A, Csajka C. 2009. Pharmacogenetics-based population pharmacokinetic analysis of efavirenz in HIV-1-infected individuals. Clin Pharmacol Ther 85:485-494.

Autar RS, Wit FW, Sankote J, Mahanontharit A, Anekthananon T, Mootsikapun P, Sujaikaew K, Cooper DA, Lange JM, Phanuphak P, Ruxrungtham K, Burger DM. 2005. Nevirapine plasma concentrations and concomitant use of rifampin in patients coinfected with HIV-1 and tuberculosis. Antivir Ther 10:937-943.

Bertz R LW, Hsu A, et al. 2001. Effects of gender, race, age and weight on the pharmacokinetics of lopinavir after single-dose Kaletra. In: 2nd International Workshop on Clinical Pharmacology of HIV Therapy. Noordwijk, the Netherlands.

Birmingham AT, Coleman AJ, Orme ML, Park BK, Pearson NJ, Short AH, Southgate PJ. 1978. Antibacterial activity in serum and urine following oral administration in man of DL473 (a cyclopentyl derivative of rifampicin) [proceedings]. Br J Clin Pharmacol 6:455P-456P.

Boulanger C, Hollender E, Farrell K, Stambaugh JJ, Maasen D, Ashkin D, Symes S, Espinoza LA, Rivero RO, Graham JJ, Peloquin CA. 2009. Pharmacokinetic evaluation of rifabutin in combination with lopinavir-ritonavir in patients with HIV infection and active tuberculosis. Clin Infect Dis 49:1305-1311.

Breen RA, Smith CJ, Bettinson H, Dart S, Bannister B, Johnson MA, Lipman MC. 2004. Paradoxical reactions during tuberculosis treatment in patients with and without HIV co-infection. Thorax 59:704-707.

Burger D, van der Heiden I, la Porte C, van der Ende M, Groeneveld P, Richter C, Koopmans P, Kroon F, Sprenger H, Lindemans J, Schenk P, van Schaik R. 2006a. Interpatient variability in the pharmacokinetics of the HIV non-nucleoside reverse transcriptase inhibitor efavirenz: the effect of gender, race, and CYP2B6 polymorphism. Br J Clin Pharmacol 61:148-154.

Burger DM, Agarwala S, Child M, Been-Tiktak A, Wang Y, Bertz R. 2006b. Effect of rifampin on steady-state pharmacokinetics of atazanavir with ritonavir in healthy volunteers. Antimicrob Agents Chemother 50:3336-3342.

Burman W, Weis S, Vernon A, Khan A, Benator D, Jones B, Silva C, King B, LaHart C, Mangura B, Weiner M, El-Sadr W. 2007. Frequency, severity and duration of immune reconstitution events in HIV-related tuberculosis. Int J Tuberc Lung Dis 11:1282-1289.

Burman WJ, Gallicano K, Peloquin C. 1999. Therapeutic implications of drug interactions in the treatment of human immunodeficiency virus-related tuberculosis. Clin Infect Dis 28:419-429; quiz 430.

CDC. 2007. Managing Drug Interactions in the Treatment of HIV-Related Tuberculosis. In: Control CfD, editor.

Corbett EL, Watt CJ, Walker N, Maher D, Williams BG, Raviglione MC, Dye C. 2003. The growing burden of tuberculosis: global trends and interactions with the HIV epidemic. Arch Intern Med 163:1009-1021.

Elliott AM, Luzze H, Quigley MA, Nakiyingi JS, Kyaligonza S, Namujju PB, Ducar C, Ellner JJ, Whitworth JA, Mugerwa R, Johnson JL, Okwera A. 2004. A randomized, double-blind, placebo-controlled trial of the use of prednisolone as an adjunct to treatment in HIV-1-associated pleural tuberculosis. J Infect Dis 190:869-878.

Elsherbiny D, Ren Y, McIlleron H, Maartens G, Simonsson US. 2010. Population pharmacokinetics of lopinavir in combination with rifampicin-based antitubercular treatment in HIV-infected South African children. Eur J Clin Pharmacol 66: 1017-1023.

Felten MK. 1987. Is rifabutin needed in South Africa for the treatment of tuberculosis? S Afr Med J 72:578-579.

Gallicano K, Khaliq Y, Carignan G, Tseng A, Walmsley S, Cameron DW. 2001. A pharmacokinetic study of intermittent rifabutin dosing with a combination of ritonavir and saquinavir in patients infected with human immunodeficiency virus. Clin Pharmacol Ther 70:149-158.

Gazzard BG. 1999. Efavirenz in the management of HIV infection. Int J Clin Pract 53:60-64.

Gillin JS, Shike M, Alcock N, Urmacher C, Krown S, Kurtz RC, Lightdale CJ, SJ. W. 1985. Malabsorption and mucosal abnormalities of the small intestine in the acquired immunodeficiency syndrome. Ann Intern Med 102:619-622.

Gonzalez-Montaner LJ, Natal S, Yongchaiyud P, Olliaro P. 1994. Rifabutin for the treatment of newly-diagnosed pulmonary tuberculosis: a multinational, randomized, comparative study versus Rifampicin. Rifabutin Study Group. Tuber Lung Dis 75:341-347.

Gounden V, van Niekerk C, Snyman T, George JA. 2010. Presence of the CYP2B6 516G> T polymorphism, increased plasma Efavirenz concentrations and early neuropsychiatric side effects in South African HIV-infected patients. AIDS Res Ther 7:32.

Hakim JG, Ternouth I, Mushangi E, Siziya S, Robertson V, Malin A. 2000. Double blind randomised placebo controlled trial of adjunctive prednisolone in the treatment of effusive tuberculous pericarditis in HIV seropositive patients. Heart 84: 183-188.

Holland DP, Hamilton CD, Weintrob AC, Engemann JJ, Fortenberry ER, Peloquin CA, Stout JE. 2009. Therapeutic drug monitoring of antimycobacterial drugs in patients with both tuberculosis and advanced human immunodeficiency virus infection. Pharmacotherapy 29:503-510.

Jevtovic DJ, Salemovic D, Ranin J, Pesic I, Zerjav S, Djurkovic-Djakovic O. 2005. The prevalence and risk of immune restoration disease in HIV-infected patients treated with highly active antiretroviral therapy. HIV Med 6:140-143.

Jindani A, Nunn AJ, Enarson DA. 2004. Two 8-month regimens of chemotherapy for treatment of newly diagnosed pulmonary tuberculosis: international multicentre randomised trial. Lancet 364:1244-1251.

Justesen U, Andersen A, Klitgaard N, Brøsen K, Gerstoft J, Pedersen C. 2004 Pharmacokinetic interaction between rifampin and the combination of indinavir and low-dose ritonavir in HIV-infected patients. Clin Infect Dis 38:426-429.

Kappelhoff BS, van Leth F, MacGregor TR, Lange J, Beijnen JH, Huitema AD. 2005. Nevirapine and efavirenz pharmacokinetics and covariate analysis in the 2NN study. Antivir Ther 10:145-155.

Khachi H, O'Connell R, Ladenheim D, Orkin C. 2009. Pharmacokinetic interactions between rifabutin and lopinavir/ritonavir in HIV-infected patients with mycobacterial co-infection. J Antimicrob Chemother 64:871-873.

Khan FA, Minion J, Pai M, Royce S, Burman W, Harries AD, Menzies D. 2010. Treatment of active tuberculosis in HIV-coinfected patients: a systematic review and meta-analysis. Clin Infect Dis 50:1288-1299.

King JR, Wynn H, Brundage R, Acosta EP. 2004. Pharmacokinetic enhancement of protease inhibitor therapy. Clin Pharmacokinet 43:291-310.

Kotler DP, Gaetz HP, Lange M, Klein EB, PR. H. 1984. Enteropathy associated with the acquired immunodeficiency syndrome. Ann Intern Med 101:421-428.

Kredo T, Van der Walt JS, Siegfried N, Cohen K. 2009. Therapeutic drug monitoring of antiretrovirals for people with HIV. Cochrane Database Syst Rev:CD007268.

Kwara A, Ramachandran G, Swaminathan S. 2010. Dose adjustment of the non-nucleoside reverse transcriptase inhibitors during concurrent rifampicin-containing tuberculosis therapy: one size does not fit all. Expert Opin Drug Metab Toxicol 6:55-68.

la Porte C, Colbers E, Bertz R, Voncken D, Wikstrom K, Boeree M, Koopmans P, Hekster Y, Burger D. 2004. Pharmacokinetics of adjusted-dose lopinavir-ritonavir combined with rifampin in healthy volunteers. Antimicrob Agents Chemother 48:1553-1560.

Lopez-Cortes LF, Ruiz-Valderas R, Ruiz-Morales J, Leon E, de Campos AV, Marin-Niebla A, Marquez-Solero M, Lozano F, Valiente R. 2006. Efavirenz trough levels are not associated with virological failure throughout therapy with 800 mg daily and a rifampicin-containing antituberculosis regimen. J Antimicrob Chemother 58: 1017-1023.

Lopez-Cortes LF, Ruiz-Valderas R, Viciana P, Alarcon-Gonzalez A, Gomez-Mateos J, Leon-Jimenez E, Sarasanacenta M, Lopez-Pua Y, Pachon J. 2002. Pharmacokinetic interactions between efavirenz and rifampicin in HIV-infected patients with tuberculosis. Clin Pharmacokinet 41:681-690.

Maartens G, Decloedt E, Cohen K. 2009. Effectiveness and safety of antiretrovirals with rifampicin: crucial issues for high-burden countries. Antivir Ther 14: 1039-1043.

Mallolas J, Sarasa M, Nomdedeu M, Soriano A, Lopez-Pua Y, Blanco JL, Martinez E, Gatell JM. 2007. Pharmacokinetic interaction between rifampicin and ritonavir-boosted atazanavir in HIV-infected patients. HIV Med 8:131-134.

Manosuthi W, Kiertiburanakul S, Sungkanuparph S, Ruxrungtham K, Vibhagool A, Rattanasiri S, Thakkinstian A. 2006. Efavirenz 600 mg/day versus efavirenz 800 mg/day in HIV-infected patients with tuberculosis receiving rifampicin: 48 weeks results. AIDS 20:131-132.

Manosuthi W, Sungkanuparph S, Tantanathip P, Lueangniyomkul A, Mankatitham W, Prasithsirskul W, Burapatarawong S, Thongyen S, Likanonsakul S, Thawornwa U, Prommool V, Ruxrungtham K. 2009a. A randomized trial comparing plasma drug concentrations and efficacies between 2 nonnucleoside reverse-transcriptase inhibitor-based regimens in HIV-infected patients receiving rifampicin: the N2R Study. Clin Infect Dis 48:1752-1759.

Manosuthi W, Sungkanuparph S, Tantanathip P, Mankatitham W, Lueangniyomkul A, Thongyen S, Eampokarap B, Uttayamakul S, Suwanvattana P, Kaewsaard S, Ruxrungtham K. 2009b. Body weight cutoff for daily dosage of efavirenz and 60-week efficacy of efavirenz-based regimen in human immunodeficiency virus and tuberculosis coinfected patients receiving rifampin. Antimicrob Agents Chemother 53:4545-4548.

Manosuthi W, Sungkanuparph S, Thakkinstian A, Vibhagool A, Kiertiburanakul S, Rattanasiri S, Prasithsirikul W, Sankote J, Mahanontharit A, Ruxrungtham K. 2005. Efavirenz levels and 24-week efficacy in HIV-infected patients with tuberculosis receiving highly active antiretroviral therapy and rifampicin. AIDS 19:1481-1486.

Marais S, Wilkinson RJ, Pepper DJ, Meintjes G. 2009. Management of patients with the immune reconstitution inflammatory syndrome. Curr HIV/AIDS Rep 6: 162-171.

Margalith D. 1960. [Dr. Jacob SEIDE (1900-1960)]. Harofe Haivri Heb Med J 2:171-172.

Marzolini C, Telenti A, Decosterd LA, Greub G, Biollaz J, Buclin T. 2001. Efavirenz plasma levels can predict treatment failure and central nervous system side effects in HIV-1-infected patients. AIDS 15:71-75.

Matteelli A, Saleri N, Villani P, Bonkoungou V, Carvalho AC, Kouanda S, Sanou MJ, Simpore J, Monno L, Carosi G, Regazzi M, Dembele M. 2009. Reversible reduction of nevirapine plasma concentrations during rifampicin treatment in patients coinfected with HIV-1 and tuberculosis. J Acquir Immune Defic Syndr 52:64-69.

McGregor MM, Olliaro P, Wolmarans L, Mabuza B, Bredell M, Felten MK, Fourie PB. 1996. Efficacy and safety of rifabutin in the treatment of patients with newly diagnosed pulmonary tuberculosis. Am J Respir Crit Care Med 154:1462-1467.

Okwera A, Whalen C, Byekwaso F, Vjecha M, Johnson J, Huebner R, Mugerwa R, Ellner J. 1994. Randomised trial of thiacetazone and rifampicin-containing regimens for pulmonary tuberculosis in HIV-infected Ugandans. The Makerere University-Case Western University Research Collaboration. Lancet 344:1323-1328.

Patel NR, Zhu J, Tachado SD, Zhang J, Wan Z, Saukkonen J, Koziel H. 2007. HIV impairs TNF-alpha mediated macrophage apoptotic response to Mycobacterium tuberculosis. J Immunol 179:6973-6980.

Peloquin C. 2002a. Therapeutic drug monitoring in the treatment of tuberculosis. Drugs 62:2169-2183.

Peloquin CA. 2002b. Therapeutic drug monitoring in the treatment of tuberculosis. Drugs 62:2169-2183.

Piscitelli SC, Gallicano KD. 2001. Interactions among drugs for HIV and opportunistic infections. N Engl J Med 344:984-996.

Rakhmanina NY, van den Anker JN. 2010. Efavirenz in the therapy of HIV infection. Expert Opin Drug Metab Toxicol 6:95-103.

Ramachandran G, Hemanth Kumar AK, Rajasekaran S, Kumar P, Ramesh K, Anitha S, Narendran G, Menon P, Gomathi C, Swaminathan S. 2009. CYP2B6 G516T polymorphism but not rifampin coadministration influences steady-state pharmacokinetics of efavirenz in human immunodeficiency virus-infected patients in South India. Antimicrob Agents Chemother 53:863-868.

Raviglione MC, Snider DE, Jr., Kochi A. 1995. Global epidemiology of tuberculosis. Morbidity and mortality of a worldwide epidemic. JAMA 273:220-226.

Ren Y NJ, Egbers C, Eley BS, Meyers TM, Smith PJ, Maartens G, McIlleron HM. 2008. Effect of rifampicin on lopinavir pharmacokinetics in HIV-infected children with tuberculosis. J Acquir Immune Defic Syndr 47:566-569.

Ribera E, Azuaje C, Lopez RM, Domingo P, Curran A, Feijoo M, Pou L, Sanchez P, Sambeat MA, Colomer J, Lopez-Colomes JL, Crespo M, Falco V, Ocana I, Pahissa A. 2007. Pharmacokinetic interaction between rifampicin and the once-daily combination of saquinavir and low-dose ritonavir in HIV-infected patients with tuberculosis. J Antimicrob Chemother 59:690-697.

Ribera E, Pou L, Lopez RM, Crespo M, Falco V, Ocana I, Ruiz I, Pahissa A. 2001. Pharmacokinetic interaction between nevirapine and rifampicin in HIV-infected patients with tuberculosis. J Acquir Immune Defic Syndr 28:450-453.

Rolla VC, da Silva Vieira MA, Pereira Pinto D, Lourenco MC, de Jesus Cda S, Goncalves Morgado M, Ferreira Filho M, Werneck-Barroso E. 2006. Safety, efficacy and pharmacokinetics of ritonavir 400mg/saquinavir 400mg twice daily plus rifampicin combined therapy in HIV patients with tuberculosis. Clin Drug Investig 26:469-479.

Schaaf HS, Willemse M, Cilliers K, Labadarios D, Maritz JS, Hussey GD, McIlleron H, Smith P, Donald PR. 2009. Rifampin pharmacokinetics in children, with and without human immunodeficiency virus infection, hospitalized for the management of severe forms of tuberculosis. BMC Med 7:19.

Schmitt C, Riek M, Winters K, Schutz M, Grange S. 2009. Unexpected Hepatotoxicity of Rifampin and Saquinavir/Ritonavir in Healthy Male Volunteers. Arch Drug Inf 2:8-16.

Sexton D, Pien, BC. 2011. Immune Reconstitution Inflammatory Syndrome. In: Basow DS, editor. Waltham, MA: UpToDate.

Sharma A, Makrandi S, Modi M, Marfatia Y. 2008. Immune reconstitution inflammatory syndrome. Indian J Dermatol Venereol Leprol 74:619-621.

Stohr W, Back D, Dunn D, Sabin C, Winston A, Gilson R, Pillay D, Hill T, Ainsworth J, Pozniak A, Leen C, Bansi L, Fisher M, Orkin C, Anderson J, Johnson M, Easterbrook P, Gibbons S, Khoo S. 2008. Factors influencing efavirenz and nevirapine plasma concentration: effect of ethnicity, weight and co-medication. Antivir Ther 13:675-685.

Tappuni AR. 2011. Immune reconstitution inflammatory syndrome. Adv Dent Res 23:90-96.

Tsuchiya K, Gatanaga H, Tachikawa N, Teruya K, Kikuchi Y, Yoshino M, Kuwahara T, Shirasaka T, Kimura S, Oka S. 2004. Homozygous CYP2B6 *6 (Q172H and K262R) correlates with high plasma efavirenz concentrations in HIV-1 patients treated with standard efavirenz-containing regimens. Biochem Biophys Res Commun 319:1322-1326.

Vernon A, Burman W, Benator D, Khan A, Bozeman L. 1999. Acquired rifamycin monoresistance in patients with HIV-related tuberculosis treated with once-weekly rifapentine and isoniazid. Tuberculosis Trials Consortium. Lancet 353:1843-1847.

Vital Durand D, Hampden C, Boobis AR, Park BK, Davies DS. 1986. Induction of mixed function oxidase activity in man by rifapentine (MDL 473), a long-acting rifamycin derivative. Br J Clin Pharmacol 21:1-7.

Weiner M, Benator D, Burman W, Peloquin CA, Khan A, Vernon A, Jones B, Silva-Trigo C, Zhao Z, Hodge T. 2005. Association between acquired rifamycin resistance and the pharmacokinetics of rifabutin and isoniazid among patients with HIV and tuberculosis. Clin Infect Dis 40:1481-1491.

8

Reversal Reaction as a Manifestation of Immune Reconstitution Inflammatory Syndrome

Vinicius Menezes, Anna Maria Sales, José Augusto Nery, Ximena Illarramendi, Alice Miranda, Maria Clara Galhardo and Euzenir Sarno
Leprosy Laboratory, Oswaldo Cruz Institute, Oswaldo Cruz Foundation
Evandro Chagas Clinical Research Institute, Oswaldo Cruz Foundation
Brazil

1. Introduction

Leprosy is a chronic infectious disease cause by the *Mycobacterium leprae*. The disease is found worldwide, especially, in countries situated in tropical and subtropical regions. According to the reports of the World Health Organization (WHO) the global registered prevalence of leprosy at the beginning of 2010 stood at 211,903 cases, whereas the number of new cases detected during 2009 was 244,796 (World Health Organization [WHO], 2010). Although there has been a declining trend in prevalence and detection of new cases, leprosy is still a public health problem in Brazil. In 2009, the prevalence rate of the disease was 1.99 per 10,000 habitants and 37,610 new cases of leprosy were detected in the entire country (Brazilian Ministry of Health, 2011). On the other hand, the Human deficiency Virus (HIV) infection is one of the greatest health problems of the world due to its pandemic nature and high morbidity and mortality rates. In the absence of treatment, the Acquired immunodeficiency syndrome (AIDS) usually leads to premature death. The World Health Organization estimates that 33.3 million people were living with HIV in the end of 2009 around the globe and 2.6 million people became HIV infected in 2009 (Joint United Nations Programme on HIV/AIDS [UNAIDS], 2010). In Brazil, the AIDS epidemic has been maintained stable in the last few years. In 2009, the incidence rate was 20.1 per 100,000 habitants and 38,538 new cases of AIDS were registered in the country (Brazilian Ministry of Health, 2010). Although the prevalence rate of coinfected individuals has never been estimated neither in Brazil nor worldwide, leprosy and the HIV infection seem to overlap in a number of countries, mainly in Africa and Asia continents.

As observed with others Mycobacterial infections, it has been speculated that HIV and *Mycobacterium leprae* coinfection could exacerbate the pathogenesis of leprosy lesions and/ or could lead to increased susceptibility of leprosy. However, up to date, HIV infection has not seemed to modify the epidemiology and the natural course of leprosy (Ustianowski et al., 2006). In contrast, initiation of anti-retroviral treatment has been reported to be associated with activation of sub-clinical *M. leprae* infection and exacerbation of existing leprosy lesions (Menezes et al., 2009).

It is well known that highly active anti-retroviral therapy (HAART) in HIV patients is associated with dramatic reduction of HIV viral load and subsequent increase in CD4 T lymphocytes and immune function. While the recovery of the immune system results in clinical benefits and decrease in the incidence of opportunistic diseases and death, a subset of patients experience clinical deterioration after HAART is initiated. This phenomenon is termed immune reconstitution inflammatory syndrome (Muller et al., 2010). This entity describes a collection of different inflammatory disorders which is associated with paradoxical worsening of symptoms and signs related to sub-clinical or preexisting infectious as well as of non infectious processes following HAART introduction (Hirsch et al., 2004). IRIS seems to result from dysfunction of some aspects of the immune system that affect the restoration of pathogen specific immune response and/ or immune regulation (French, 2009). The immunopathology of IRIS is poorly understood but it seems to be highly determined by the provoking pathogen. In this way, inflammation in Mycobacterial infections is often associated with characteristics of a TH1 immune response (French et al., 2009). The sudden clinical deterioration associated with IRIS can be at times fatal and needs prompt intervention (Murdoch et al., 2007). The incidence of IRIS is not well know but it has been described ranging from less than 10% to more than 50%(Muller et al., 2010).

Some evidences suggest that antiretroviral therapy can accelerate the onset of leprosy symptoms. In a retrospective cohort study, Sarno et al has demonstrated that in those individuals who initiated HAART the length of time covered up to leprosy diagnosis was significantly shorter than in those not receiving HAART (p=0,01) (Sarno et al., 2008). In another study, in the Amazon region of Brazil, seven patients out of 25 presented leprosy as manifestation of IRIS (Talhari et al., 2010). One study, in French Guyana, has observed that the incidence of leprosy was higher in HIV patients receiving HAART for less than 3 months than in HIV untreated patients (13 against 0,7 per 1,000 person-year, p=0,02) (Couppié et al., 2009). Another study, in India, has found a high incidence of leprosy of 5.22 per 1,000 person-year in HIV patients on HAART (Vinay et al., 2009). Several case reports of leprosy associated with IRIS have been published in the literature (Martiniuk et al., 2007; Chow et al., 2009), including one of histoid leprosy case (Bumb et al., 2010).

Currently, it is widely accepted that the reconstitution of the immune function observed in HIV patients on HAART can trigger leprosy reaction. Leprosy reactions are immune-inflammatory events that complicate the disease. The frequency of reaction has been reported to range from 2.6% to 20% of PB patients (Becx-Bleumink & Berhe, 1992) and from 15% to 60% of MB cases (Bwire R & Kawuma HJ, 1994; Nery JAC et al., 1998). It is broadly accepted that reaction is the result of a shift in the patient´s level of inflammation and/or cell- mediated immunity which, in turn, leads to accelerated nerve damage and serious physical disabilities (Sarno et al., 2008). It is frequently observed during multidrug therapy (MDT), but it may be developed before or after leprosy treatment. These reactional states are classified as type 1 (Reversal Reaction) or Type 2 (Erithema Nodosum Lepromatosum) reaction depending on the clinical characteristics of the acute episode and its immune background. Strong evidences currently indicates that reversal reactions are the result of an enhancement of cellular immunity and delayed hypersensitivity to *M. leprae* antigens, but both the precipitating factors and the physiopathological mechanisms involved remain ill-defined (Scollard et al., 2006). Reversal reaction is clinically characterized by the worsening of previous leprosy lesion or appearance of new infiltrated, erythematous plaques. It may be accompanied by neuritis or systemic symptoms such as fever, malaise, arthralgia, or edema.

Since HAART for AIDS treatment has become available in countries where leprosy is endemic, around 41 cases of leprosy reaction associated to IRIS have been described in the literature (Tables 1 and 2) (Pavie et al., 2009). It is worth to notice that the majority of the patients were paucibacillary (65,8%) and most of them (90,2%) developed reversal reaction with only 4 cases of Erythema nodosum leprosum published (Tables 1 and 2). The mean time that patients developed reaction after initiation of HAART was 18.95 (4-172) weeks (median:8, Mode:8, standard deviation:31,1)(Tables 1 and 2). Twenty three (56.09%) of the cases were from Brazil (Pereira et al., 2004; Visco-Comandini et al., 2004; Trindade et al., 2005; Talhari et al., 2007; Caruso et al., 2007; Batista et al., 2008; Deps et al., 2008 & Menezes et al., 2009), 13 (31.7%) from India (Narang et al., 2005; Singal et al., 2006; Kharkar et al., 2007; Kar et al., 2009 &Vinay et al., 2009), 3 (7.31%) from Haiti (Couppié et al., 2004 & Pavie et al., 2009), 1 (2.43%) from Uganda(Lawn et al., 2003) and 1(2.43%) from French Guiana(Couppié et al., 2004). Thirty one (75.6%) patients were man and 10 (27.3%) women. Twelve (27.3%) cases presented neuritis associated to reaction (Tables 1 and 2).

References	Leprosy/ Reaction Types	Weeks on HAART	CD4 Cell/µl		Viral load/Ml	
			HIV	IRIS	HIV	IRIS
(Lawn et al., 2003)	BT + RR	4	10	70	120,000	1,000
(Couppie et al., 2004)	BB + RR	6	87	257	19,000	650
	BT + RR + N	8	130	278	40,701	68
	BT + RR + N	12	31	171	62,700	50
(Pereira et al., 2004)	BT +RR	8	73	270	NA	NA
	BT +RR	24	35	100	NA	NA
(Visco-Comandini et al., 2004)	BT + RR	8	7	90	NA	NA
(Narang et al., 2005)	BT + RR	8	125	280	150,000	1,750
(Trindade et al., 2005)	BB+ RR	24	87	NA	<80	NA
	BB+ RR+N	4	223	NA	NA	NA
	BT+ RR	8	430	NA	NA	NA
	I +RR	8	NA	NA	<400	NA
(Singal et al., 2006)	BL + RR+N	4	108	224	NA	NA
(Kharkar et al., 2007)	BT + RR	12	299	504	NA	NA
	BT + RR	8	114	184	NA	NA
(Talhari et al., 2007)	BT + RR+N	12	92	426	NA	8,300
(Caruso et al., 2007)	BT+ RR	16	NA	57	NA	< 80
(Batista et al., 2008)	BT + RR+N	8	14	172	21,300	69,000
	BT + RR+N	8	104	235	NA	<80
(Deps et al., 2008)	BT + RR	10	33		6,310	NA
	BT + RR	4	170		9,230	NA

Table 1. Characteristics of 21 cases of leprosy reactions associated with immune reconstitution inflammatory syndrome published in literature until 2008:
Abbreviations: BT= Tuberculoid borderline; BB= Borderline borderline; BL= Lepromatous borderline; RR= Reversal reaction; N= Neuritis; NA= Not available.

References	Leprosy/ Reaction Types	Weeks on HAART	CD4 Cell/µl		Viral load/Ml	
			HIV	IRIS	HIV	IRIS
(Menezes et al., 2009)	BT+ RR	4	142	499	300	<80
	BB+ RR	4	37	200	53,000	2,200
	BT+ RR	8	NA	226	NA	<80
	BT+ RR	10	62	226	NA	<80
	BT+ RR + N	4	85	190	5,700,000	140
	BB+ RR	8	179	271	39,000	<80
	BB+ RR	4	160	140	77,204	4,880
	BT+ RR	16	76	215	180,000	<80
	BB+ RR	4	NA	408	NA	<80
	BT+ RR	16	NA	171	14,000	<80
(Kar et al., 2009)	BT+RR	7	125	333	NA	NA
(Pavie et al., 2009)	MB+RR+N	40	25	110	100,000	<80
(Vinay et al., 2009)	MB+ENL	172	177	892	NA	NA
	MB+RR+N	32	75	170	NA	NA
	PB+RR+N	24	85	251	NA	NA
	MB+ENL	8	99	99	NA	NA
	MB+ENL	112	124	239	NA	NA
	MB+ENL+N	16	31	144	NA	NA
	PB+RR	64	331	374	NA	NA
	PB+RR	20	174	436	NA	NA

Table 2. Characteristics of 20 cases of leprosy reactions associated with immune reconstitution inflammatory syndrome published in literature in 2009. Abbreviations: BT= Tuberculoid borderline; BB= Borderline borderline; BL= Lepromatous borderline; RR= Reversal reaction; N= Neuritis; ENL= Erithema nodosum lepromatosum; NA= Not available.

In the present series, the highest casuistic published so far, 12 cases of leprosy reaction as manifestation of IRIS are thoroughly described in order to establish clinical and immunological parameters of definition.

2. Subjects and methods

2.1 Study design and inclusion criteria

The Leprosy Laboratory and the Evandro Chagas Clinical Research Institute (IPEC), FIOCRUZ, Rio de Janeiro, have been evaluating coinfected HIV/*M. leprae* patients since 1989. Both institutions are reference centers in Rio de Janeiro for these diseases and so far, a total of 100 patients have been followed.

For the purpose of this study, we have reviewed the charts of all patients coinfected with *M. leprae* and HIV who were referred to the Leprosy laboratory/Fiocruz and the IPEC between 1997 and 2010. Inclusion criteria were based on the definition criteria proposed by French et al (French et al., 2004). Thus, reversal reaction as a manifestation of IRIS was defined as the presence of reaction any time during the first 6 months of HAART associated to decrease >1 log in HIV-1 viral load. In addition, it was defined in HAART naïve patients with no previous laboratory tests data (Viral load or CD4 lymphocytes count), if reaction was present during the first 6 months after initiation of HAART associated to undetectable HIV-1 viral load.

Since the introduction of HAART for AIDS treatment by the Brazilian government in 1997 until the year of 2010, 33 patients had leprosy reaction under HAART, 12 of which were diagnosed with IRIS and were grouped into the case series presented in the present study. Case reports of 10 of these patients have been published (Menezes et al., 2009) but additional data was obtained and as they are part of the cohort studied they were maintained to compose the present case series.

2.2 Definitions and clinical routine

All patients followed the clinic routine dermatological and neurological evaluation. For diagnostic purposes, skin biopsies were obtained by punch. Samples were routinely processed, paraffin embedded, and stained with hematoxylin and eosin (H&E) and Wade's modification of the Ziehl-Nielsen method for detection of acid-fast bacilli (2 sections of each staining). Slit skin smears were obtained from six body sites (one from each earlobe, one from each elbow, one from a lesion and one from the contra-lateral knee). The smears were stained for acid-fast bacilli (AFB) by Ziehl-Neelsen techniques. The bacilloscopic index (BI) was calculated using the Ridley & Jopling logarithmic scale (Ridley & Jopling, 1966), based on analysis of 100 fields. The lepromin test was measured 30 days after the intradermal injection of 0.1 mL of heat-killed *M. leprae* in the anterior forearm. The result was either scored as negative if <5 mm, or positive if ≥5 mm. Leprosy was then diagnosed and classified according to Ridley-Jopling criteria(Ridley & Jopling, 1966). The diagnosis of reversal reaction was histophatologically defined on the presence of epithelioid cells granuloma. In this study we identified two main patterns of reversal reaction depending on the severity of the tissue inflammatory changes (Ridley 1969):

- mild acanthosis and exocytosis; well developed cohesive epithelioid granulomas intermingled with few lymphocytes; blood vessels, arrector pili muscles, adnexa and nerve bundles; sparse multinucleated cells and small foci of red blood cell extravasation.
- Exuberant changes as moderate to severe acanthosis, spongiosis and exocytosis; epithelial apoptosis and basal epidermal erosion; severe dermal inflammatory infiltration, including granulomas dissociated by marked edema or centered by necrosis, as well as numerous giant cells and red blood cell extravasation.

All the patients were treated for leprosy with multidrug therapy. Reversal reaction was treated following recommendations of the Brazilian Ministry of Health, with a daily morning dose of prednisone, starting with 1mg/kg for 1 month, followed by a 10mg/month progressive reduction.

Diagnosis of HIV infection followed the Brazilian Ministry of Health regulations, which include the performance of two tests; the immune-enzymatic method (ELISA) plus immune-fluorescence or Western Blot (National STD/AIDS program of Brazil, 2008). The CD4 cell count and viral load were determined around the time of HIV diagnosis and again around the time of leprosy diagnosis (defined as the first time the patient visited a health center with signs of leprosy). HAART was started at CD4 cell count of less than or equal to 200 cells/μL or if an opportunistic infection was diagnosed (National STD/AIDS program of Brazil, 2008). To control the HIV infection, the patients were submitted to periodical clinical evaluation and routine laboratory tests. The exchange of information related to the evolution of both infections is a routine at the Units, and remained under the responsibility of the professionals involved in the study.

2.3 Data collection and statistical analysis

Pertinent data were collected from the patient charts at both institutions. All analysis were performed using SPSS 16.0. The difference of the CD4 lymphocytes count and HIV viral load before and at the onset of reversal reaction associated with IRIS was analysed by the Wilcoxon test.

2.4 Ethical concerns

The study was approved by the ethics committee of the Oswaldo Cruz Institute and the IPEC.

3. Results

Among the total 33 patients experiencing leprosy reversal reaction under HAART, 12 (36.3%) met the predetermined IRIS criteria. Demographic, clinical and laboratory data of these 12 patients are presented in Table 3 (Figure 1). Ten patients were initially diagnosed with HIV infection. Significantly, HAART induced reaction in nine patients who had not been diagnosed with leprosy. All but one patient received standard treatment for reaction with a daily oral dose of prednisone. Five patients needed prolonged use of prednisone for up to 12 months (Table 3).

Case	Age/Sex	Leprosy/ reaction types	Lesion number/ complication	Lepromin test (mm)	BI	Time in prednisone (months)
1	48/M	BT/RR	2/ none	12	0	0
2	33/F	BB/RR	>20/ ulcer	10	0.5	9
3	39/M	BT/RR	>10/ulcer	6	0	12
4	34/M	BT/RR	>20/none	0	0	8
5	28/M	BT/RR + N	>20/none	0	0	10
6	46/M	BB/RR	1/none	12	0.57	11
7	22/M	BB/RR	>20/none	0	2.25	
8	28/M	BT/RR	1/ulcer	9	0	6
9	22/F	BB/RR	2/none	0	0.5	2
10	54/M	BT/RR	>20/none	0	0	0
11	27/M	BT/RR	>20/ulcer	NA	0	6
12	M	BB/RR	>10/none	10	0.57	9

Table 3. Clinical and epidemiological data of 12 patients with defined IRIS.BT= Borderline Tuberculoid, BB= Borderline Borderline, RR= reversal reaction; N=Neuritis

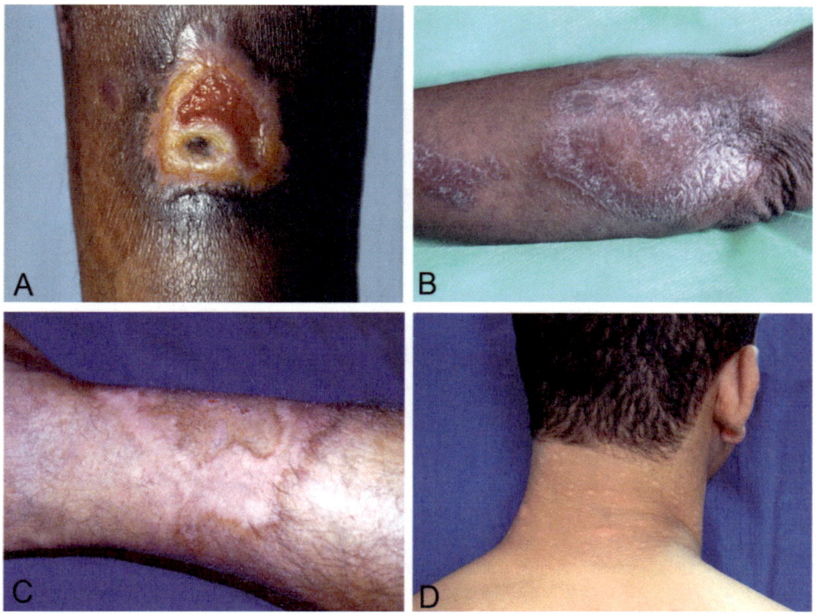

Fig. 1. Clinical pattern of reversal reaction skin lesions.
1A - Clean, ulcerated plaque with well-defined borders. 1B - Infiltrated and erythematous plaques with a scaly surface and irregular borders. 1C – Erythematous, queloid-like plaque with small central ulcerations. 1D - Disseminated urticariform lesions of various sizes.

The clinical or laboratory findings of all patients showed immune suppression prior to reversal reaction diagnosis. However, only 5 patients had opportunistic infection, namely pneumocistosis, esophageal candidiasis, neurotoxoplasmosis and disseminated tuberculosis. Moreover, by the time reaction occurred during HAART treatment, most of the patients had an increase of the CD4/CD8 T lymphocyte rate, mainly due to increase of CD4 cell count mean of 204.5 cells/μL (92-446cells/μL) (Table 4) (Figure 2). Nine patients had an undetectable viral load when reaction developed and three had a mean viral load reduction of 2.4 log (1.4 - 4.6 log) (Table 4) (Figure 2). All patients were treated for HIV with regimens containing two nucleoside reverse transcriptase inhibitors in combination with a protease inhibitor (8.33%), a boosted protease inhibitor (33.33%), or a nonnucleoside reverse transcriptase inhibitor (58.33%) (Table 4). The mean time the patients presented reversal reaction after starting HAART was 7.8 weeks (Table 4).
All patients presented erythematous infiltrated plaques and were in the borderline spectrum of leprosy. Four patients had complicated ulcerated lesions (figure 1A & 1C) (Table 3). The histopathological features observed in all the skin biopsies were fulfilled the patterns described for the diagnosis of reversal reaction with tissue severity (figure 3), ranging from heavy infiltration, foci of necrosis and extensive involvement of the epidermis (figure 3C & 3D), to moderate cellular infiltration with well-formed granulomas (figure 3A & 3B) (Table 5). There was evidence of fragmented acid-fast bacilli in 6 skin biopsies (Table 5). Two samples (cases 1 and 11) showed unusually extensive multinucleated cells permeating the granulomas (Table 5). The biopsy of patient 2 had heavy dermal edema and marked inflammatory infiltration, including some polymorphonuclear leukocytes and many foci of necrosis. Initially, these features led to a mistaken diagnosis of *erythema nodosum leprosum*.

After a clinical and histopathological review, reversal reaction superimposed to a multibacillary background was established.

Case	HAART regimen	Weeks on HAART	CD4 Cell/μl HIV	CD4 Cell/μl IRIS	Viral load/Ml HIV	Viral load/Ml IRIS
1	AZT+3TC+NFV	4	142	499	300	<80
2	AZT+ DDI+EFVZ	4	37	200	53,000	2,200
3	AZT+ DDI+EFVZ	8	NA	226	NA	<80
4	D4T+ 3TC+ NVP	10	62	226	NA	<80
5	D4T+3TC+LPV/ RTV	4	85	190	5,700,000	140
6	AZT+3TC+LPV/ RTV	8	179	271	39000	<80
7	TDF+ 3TC+ATV/ RTV	4	160	140	77,204	4880
8	AZT+ 3TC+EFVZ	16	76	215	180,000	<80
9	AZT+3TC+LPV/ RTV	4	NA	408	NA	<80
10	D4T+ 3TC + EFVZ	16	NA	171	14000	<80
11	AZT+3TC+EFVZ	12	03	173	407,800	<80
12	AZT+3TC+EFVZ	4	125	571	321,560	<80

Table 4. Laboratory data of the 12 patients with reversal reaction and defined IRIS Abreviations: NA= not available. AZT= Zidovudine; 3TC= Lamivudine; D4T= Stavudine; DDI= Didanosine; TDF: Tenofovir, NVP= Nevirapina; EFVZ= Efavirenz, NFV= Nelfinavir; ATV/RTV= Atazanavir/ Ritonavir; LPV/RTV= Lopinavir/Ritonavir.

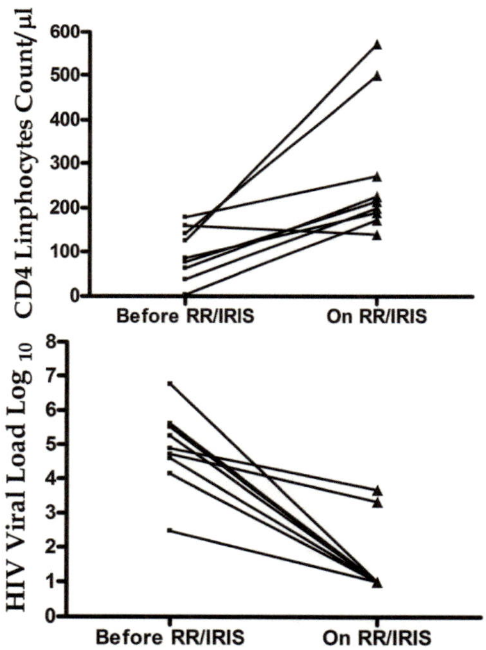

Fig. 2. Longitudinal analysis of CD4 lymphocytes count and HIV viral load before and at the onset of reversal reaction/IRIS. The mean increase of the CD4 cells count and the mean decrease of the HIV viral load were significant (p=0,007 and p=0,003, respectively).

Case	AFB (ILB)	Giant cells [a]	Granuloma lymphocyte	necrosis [b]	Severeness
1	0	+++	20%	+	Severe
2	2.6	++	20%	++	Severe
3	0	+	15%	+	Severe
4	1	-	30%	+	Severe
5	3	-	20%	-	Mild
6	0	+	30%	-	Mild
7	2.8	+	20%	-	Mild
8	0	+	20%	-	Mild
9	0	+	20%	++	Severe
10	1.9	++	19%	+	Severe
11	0	+++	25%	++	Severe
12	1	++	20%	-	Severe

Table 5. Histopathological data of the 12 patients with reversal reaction and defined IRISpatients. In relation to control. Symbols: a) + = few, ++ = several, +++ = many, -=not observed; b) + = little, ++ = moderate, -=not observed.

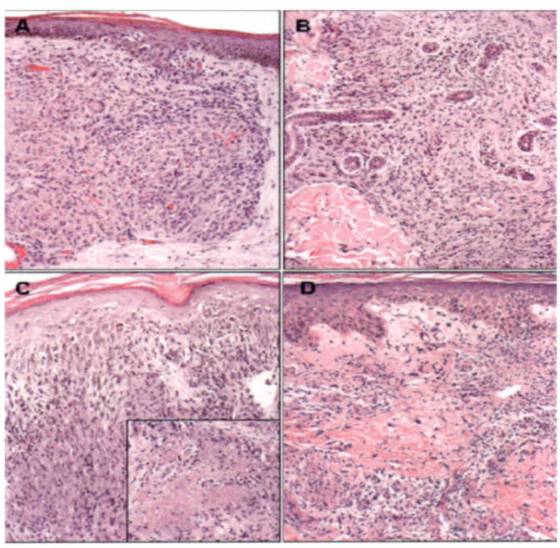

Fig. 3. Histopathological patterns of skin lesions in IRIS patients
A. Epidermis with intraepithelial lymphocytes and apoptosis; dermis showing cohesive tuberculoid granulomas with multinucleated giant cells in RR (pat. 6); *B.* Angled epithelioid granuloma dissociating adnexa in RR(pat. 5); *C, D.* Severe epidermal changes, dermal edema, and epithelioid granulomas with foci of necrosis (inset) in RR type D (pat. 9 and 2, respectively; H&E, original magnification, X200).

4. Discussion

As observed in the present case series, in the HAART era, leprosy reaction associated with IRIS appears to be a frequent event in coinfected patients. The 36% reversal reaction rate in coinfected patients undergoing HAART is similar to that estimated for tuberculosis as a manifestation of IRIS (French., 2009). Interestingly, HAART triggered reversal reaction in 88% of the patients not previously known to have leprosy. As likewise seen in the literature (Table 1 and 2), most of the present IRIS cases associated to leprosy had the predominantly borderline-tuberculoid form. The borderline forms are considered the most unstable in that the immunological capability of the patient to restrain the infection is only partial. During reversal reaction, high amounts of inflammatory cytokines such as interferon gamma and tumor necrosis factor are produced, reflecting the immune activation characteristics of skin lesions with a tuberculoid pattern (Nery et al., 2000).

Although the moment of infection for either HIV or leprosy is difficult to establish, most of the patients were first diagnosed with HIV. In the present case series the period of time elapsed between HAART introduction and leprosy reaction was variable but similar to previously described in the literature, which ranges from 4 to 24 weeks (Hirsch et al., 2004). In HIV negative individuals, reversal reaction usually occurs during the initial months of multidrug therapy. As recently reported, the diagnosis of leprosy is associated with improved immune status in HIV infected individuals (Sarno et al., 2008). The appearance of clinical signs of *M. leprae* infection in the form of reversal reaction observed in this series and in published case reports is not a manifestation of immune suppression but rather of immune reconstitution. This is further supported by the presence of a positive lepromin test in some of the multibacillary patients.

Among the risks factors associated to the development of IRIS, male gender (Shelburne et al., 2005), young age (Ratnam et al., 2006), and immune suppression (Shelburne et al., 2005; Ratnam et al., 2006) were also observed in the present series. Other risk factors, such as short interval between initiating treatment for opportunistic infection (OI), a rapid fall in HIV-1 RNA after HAART, and being ART naïve at the time of OI diagnosis were observed in most of the patients(Shelburne et al., 2005). Additional significant predictors include a lower baseline CD4 cell percentage, a lower CD4 cell count at ART initiation, and a lower CD4 to CD8 cell ratio at baseline were observed in a few cases (Ratnam et al., 2006). In the same way, a higher baseline CD8 cell count is associated with IRIS as CD8 cell counts represent the presence of immune activation[29, 36, 37] (Ratnam et al., 2006) (Robertson et al., 2006) (Cianchetta-Sivori et al., 2007). In a case control study, the nadir CD4 T count of less than 100 cells was independently predictive of development of IRIS as well as the absolute drop in viraemia positively correlated with increasing risk for IRIS (Manabe et al., 2007). In this series, 5 cases had less than 100 CD4+ cells/μL.

Absolute CD4 T cell increase was observed in most patients, but in 1 patient a cell count decrease was observed. As recently described, absolute CD4 T cell increase is not present in all cases of IRIS (French et al., 2004; Shelburne et al., 2006). Approximately 10% of IRIS complicated MAC infection occurred in the absence of an increase of CD4 T cells count(Manabe et al., 2007). Robertson *et al* suggested to remove an increase CD4 cell count as a sole criterion of IRIS, because CD4 lymphocyte plasma levels do not necessary reflect function(Robertson et al., 2006). Immune responses may be restored before a rise in plasma CD4 cell count is detected. They proposed that an increase in CD4 T cell count should be viewed as supportive of diagnosis rather than required for it.

Manabe *et al* suggested that the use of the most potent regimens (boosted protease inhibitors [BPIs] and/or non-nucleoside reverse transcriptase inhibitors [NNRTIs]) is an independent risk factor for the development of IRIS (Manabe et al., 2007). In particular, the use of BPIs was associated with IRIS. All of the patients but one, in the present series, were using either one or more of these drugs. In addition, HAART induced reduction of 2.5 logs RNA levels has shown the highest risk of IRIS (Manabe et al., 2007). In the present study, a similar log reduction was observed in the cases with viral load data.

The pathogenesis of IRIS remains speculative. Current theories involve the combination of underlying antigen burden, the degree of immune restoration, as well as the host genetic susceptibility (Price et al., 2001). According to Murdoch, the antigenic stimulus can be intact, "clinically silent" organism or dead or dying organism and their residual antigens (Murdoch et al., 2007). A common feature of the cases of IRIS is that clinical presentation of the opportunistic infection is often atypical compared with that usually observed in HIV-1 infected patients (French et al., 2004). On the other hand, the pathogenesis of reversal reaction is still not completely understood. Restoration of the *M. leprae* specific immune response has been claimed, but convincing data are lacking. During reversal reaction, high amount of inflammatory cytokines are produced reflecting the immune reactivation of the skin lesions with tuberculoid pattern (Sampaio et al., 1995; Krutzik et al., 2005).

Among the various risk factors described for reversal reaction are concomitant infections, immunization, and pregnancy (Nery JA et al., 1998). In addition, in the present case series, HAART triggered reversal reaction in 88% of the patients not previously known to have leprosy. Different from initially expected HIV infection *per se* did not modify the course of the disease, but immune restoration by HAART does appear to worsen reversal reaction. In the present series, some patients had numerous lesions and ulcers and needed extended corticoid therapy, demonstrating a more intense inflammatory process. Such pattern could explain the profound scars left by the reversal reaction lesions that are not observed in non HIV patients. This type of presentation with numerous skin lesions and ulcerations is more usually seen in type II leprosy reactions which are more frequent in multibacillary patients and was never referred in the context of IRIS. On the other hand, patients with tuberculoid forms which display strong cellular response to *M. leprae,* usually have neuritis. Surprisingly, only one patient in this series was diagnosed with neuritis. The histological findings observed in all patients were typical of reversal reaction (Ridley & Radia,1981) even in those presenting AFB+ biopsies. Disorganized and disperse granulomas could be seen in some cases, thus rending difficult to classify those patients according to the leprosy spectrum (cases 2, 5 and 9). The presence of necrosis only occurred in severe reactions, either in small foci or causing liquefaction of the granuloma, followed by fibrosis as in case 3, leaving profound scars. In some other cases, however, the granulomas take typical tuberculoid characteristics, with cohesive epithelioid cells surrounded by a lymphocytic halo. The presence of low number of AFB has already been described in borderline tuberculoid lesions (Ridley & Jopling, 1966).

Treatment of complications due to IRIS in other coinfections is frequently necessary to minimize short-term morbidity but in the long-term follow-up, outcome appears to be good (Murdoch et al., 2007; Riddell et al., 2007). In the present series the patients were treated with prednisone as standard for reversal reaction, and had a favorable evolution in spite of the severity of disease or the need of a short extension of the use of corticoids. Prednisone is the drug of choice for treating reversal reaction because it reduces nerve edema, exerts an immunosuppressive effect, and decreases post-inflammatory scar formation (Naafs 1996; Andersson et al., 2005). Thus, no modification of the standard therapy for reversal reaction is needed in case of IRIS in leprosy patients.

5. Conclusions

The present is the largest case series of reversal reaction associated with IRIS in coinfected patients described in the literature. In countries like Brazil, where both epidemics overlap and HAART has been broadly administered, leprosy reaction associated to IRIS is prone to occur. It might be posited, therefore, that the appearance of clinical signs of *M. leprae* infection in HIV-infected individuals is not a manifestation of immunosuppression but rather of immune reconstitution. In the present series, the patients treated with prednisone as standard reversal reaction therapy had a favorable evolution despite disease severity. Thus, the results of this study clearly indicate that no modification of the standard reversal reaction therapy appears necessary in the case of leprosy patients with IRIS. However, there is still need of prospective studies to evaluate the association of leprosy reactions and IRIS in order to better characterize the pathology and immunology of the coinfection.

6. Acknowledgment

We would especially like to thank Dr. Mariza Morgado and Dr. Thais Porto Amadeu.

7. References

Andersson AK, Chaduvula M, Atkinson SE, Khanolkar-Young S, Jain S, Sunnetha L, Suneetha S & Lockwood DN. Effects of prednisolone treatment on cytokine expression in patients with leprosy type 1 reactions. *Infection and Immunity*, Vol. 73, No.6,(June 2005), pp.3725-3733, ISSN: 0019-9567.

Batista MD, Porro AM, Maeda SM, Gomes EE, Yoshioka MCN, Enokihara MMSS & Tomimori J.(2008). Leprosy reversal reaction as immune reconstitution inflammatory syndrome in patients with AIDS. *Clinical infectious disease*, Vol.46, No.6, (March 2008), e56-60, ISSN:1537-6591.

Becx-Bleumink M & Berhe D. (1992). Ocurrence of reaction, their diagnosis and management in leprosy patients treated with multidrug therapy; experience of leprosy control program of the All-Africa leprosy and rehabilitation Training Center (ALERT) in Ethiopia. *International journal of leprosy and other mycobacterial disease*, Vol. 60, No.2, (June 1992), pp. 173-184, ISSN:0148-916X.

Brazilian Ministrry of Health, 2010. Boletim epidemiólogicos AIDS/DST: versão preliminar. Brazilian Ministry of Health. Retrieved from http://www.aids.gov.br/sites/default/files/publicacao/2010/boletim2010_preliminar_pdf_34434.pdf

Brazilian Ministry of Health. (2011). Distribuição da hanseníase no Brasil, In: *Portal Saúde*, 03/13/2011, Available from: http://portal.saude.gov.br/portal/saude/profissional/visualizar_texto.cfm?idtxt=31200.

Bumb RA, Ghiya BC, Jakhar R & Prasad N. (2010). Histoid leprosy in a HIV positive patient takin cTARV. *Leprosy review*, Vol. 81, No. 3, (September 2010), pp. 221-223, ISSN:0305-7518.

Bwire R & Kawuma HJ. (1994). Type 1 reactions in leprosy, neuritis and steroid therapy: the impact of the human immunodeficiency virus. *Transactions of the royal society of tropical medicine and hygiene*, Vol. 88, No.3, (May 1994), pp. 315-316, ISSN:0035-9203.

Caruso RL, Fernandes RM, Serra MS, Lima RB & Martins CJ. (2007). Atypical reversal reaction in a borderline leprosy patient co-infected with HIV. Anais Brasileiros de Dermatologia, Vol.82, No.6, (November 2007), pp. 553-557, ISSN:0365-0596.

Cianchetta-Sivori M, Raso S, Fernandez-Guerrero M, Gorgolas M, Garcia R. (2007). Do CD8(+)CD25(+) cells predict immune reconstitution syndrome in HIV-positive patients who begin HAART? *AIDS*, Vol.21, No.17, (November 2007), pp.2347-2349, ISSN: 0269-9370.

Chow D, Okinaka L, Souza S, Shikuma C & Tice A. (2009). Hansen´s disease with HIV: a case of immune reconstitution disease. *Hawaii Medical Journal*, Vol.68, No.2, (March 2009), pp. 27-29, ISSN:0017-8594.

Couppié P, Abel S, Voinchet H,Roussel M, Hélénon R, Huerre M, Sainte-Marie D & Cabié A. Immune reconstitution inflammatory syndrome associated with HIV and leprosy. *Archives of Dermatology*, Vol.140, No.8,(August 2004),pp.997-1000, ISSN:0096-5359

Couppié P, Domergue V, Clyti E, Guedj ME, Vaz T, Sainte-Marie D, Marty C & Nacher M. (2009). Increased incidence of leprosy following HAART initiation: a manifestation of the immune reconstitution disease. *AIDS*, Vol.23, No.12, (July 2009), pp. 1599-1600, ISSN: 0269-9370.

Deps PD, Gripp CG, Madureira BP, Lucas EA. (2008). Immune reconstitution syndrome associated with leprosy: two cases. *International Journal of STD & AIDS*, Vol.19, No.2, (February 2008), pp.135-136, ISSN:0956-4624.

French MA, Price P, Stone SF. Immune restoration disease after antiretroviral therapy. *AIDS*, Vol. 18, No. 12,(August 2004), pp.1615-1627, ISSN: 0269-9370.

French MA. (2009). Immune reconstitution inflammatory syndrome: a reappraisal. Clinical infectious disease, Vol.48, No 1, (January 2009), pp.101-107, ISSN: 1058-4838.

Hirsch HH, Kaufmann G, Sendi P, Battegay M. (2004).Immune reconstitution in HIV-infected patients. *Clinical Infectious Disease*, Vol. 38, No 8, (April 2004), pp.1159-1166, ISSN: 1058-4838.

Joint United Nations Programme on HIV/AIDS, 2010. *Global report: Unaids report on the global AIDS epidemic 2010*.UNAIDS. Retrieved from http://www.unaids.org/globalreport/

Kar HK, Sharma P &Bhardwaj M. (2009). Borderline tuberculoid leprosy with upgrading type 1 reaction in a HIV seropositive patient, after antiretroviral therapy: an immune reconstitution inflammatory syndrome. *Leprosy review*, Vol.80, No.1, (March 2009), pp.85-88, ISSN: 0305-7518.

Kharkar V, Bhor UH, Mahajan S, Khopkar U. (2007). Type I lepra reaction presenting as immune reconstitution inflammatory syndrome. *Indian Journal of Dermatology, Venereology and Leprology*, Vol. 73, No.4 , (July 2007),pp.253-256, ISSN:0378-6323.

Krutzik SR, Tan B, Li H, Ochoa MT, Liu PT, Sharfstein SE, Graeber TG, Sieling PA, Liu YJ, Rea TH, Bloom BR & Modlin RL.(2005). TLR activation triggers the rapid differentiation of monocytes into macrophages and dendritic cells. *Nature Medicine*, Vol.11, No. 6,(June 2005), pp.653-660, ISSN:1078-8956.

Lawn SD, Wood C, Lockwood DN. Borderline tuberculoid leprosy: an immune reconstitution phenomenon in a human immunodeficiency virus-infected person. *Clinical Infectious Disease*,Vol.36, No 1,(January 2003), e5-6, ISSN:1537- 6591.

Manabe YC, Campbell JD, Sydnor E, Moore RD. (2007). Immune reconstitution inflammatory syndrome: risk factors and treatment implications. *Journal of Acquired Immune Deficiency Syndrome*, Vol.46, No.4, (April 2007), pp.456-462, ISSN:1525-4135.

Martiniuk F, Rao SD, Rea TH, Glickman MS, Giovinazzo J, Rom WN, Cabrera A & Levis WR. (2007). Leprosy as immune reconstitution inflammatory syndrome in HIV-positive persons. *Emerging infectious disease,* Vol.13, No.9, (September 2007), pp. 1438-1439, ISSN:1080-6059.

Menezes VM, Sales AM, Illarramendi X, Miranda A, Morgado MG, Gutierrez-Galhardo MC, Sarno EM & Nery JAC (2009). Leprosy reaction as a manifestation of immune reconstitution inflammatory syndrome. *AIDS,* Vol.23, No.5, (March 2009), pp.641-643, ISSN:0269-9370.

Muller M, WAndell S, Colebunders R, Attia S, Furrer H &Egger M (2010). Immune reconstitution inflammatory syndrome in patients starting antiretroviral therapy for HIV infection: a systematic review and meta-analysis. *Lancet infectious disease,* Vol.10, No.4, (April 2010), pp. 251-261, ISSN:1473-3099.

Murdoch DM, Venter WD, Van Rie A, Feldman C (2007). Immune reconstitution inflammatory syndrome (IRIS): review of common infectious manifestations and treatment options. *AIDS Research Therapy,* Vol. 4, No.9, (May 2007), pp.1-10, ISSN:1742-6405.

Naafs B. Bangkok Workshop on Leprosy Research. Treatment of reactions and nerve damage. *International Journal of Leprosy and Other Mycobacterial Diseases,* Vol. 64, No.4 supplement, (December 1996), S21-28, ISSN: 0148-916X.

Narang T, Dogra S, Kaur I. (2005). Borderline tuberculoid leprosy with type 1 reaction in an HIV patient--a phenomenon of immune reconstitution. *International Journal of Leprosy and Other Mycobacterial Diseases,* Vol.73, No.3,(September 2005), pp.203-205, ISSN:0148-916X.

National STD/AIDS program of Brazil, 2008. *Recomendações para terapia anti-retroviral em adultos e adolescentes infectados pelo HIV: 2008* (7th edition), Brazilian Ministry of Health, ISBN:978-85-334-1352-8, Brasília.

Nery JAC, Vieira LM, de Matos HJ, Gallo ME & Sarno EN. (1998). Reactional states in multibacillary Hansen disease patients during multidrug therapy. *Revista do Instituto de medicina tropical de São Paulo,* Vol. 40, No. 6, (November 1998), pp. 363-370, ISSN:0036-4665.

Nery JA, Sampaio EP, Galhardo MC,Perissé AR, Vieira LM, Salles AM & Sarno EN. (2000). *M. leprae*-HIV co-infection: pattern of immune response in vivo and in vitro. *Indian Journal of Leprosy,* Vol.72, No.2, (April 2000),pp.155-167, ISSN:0254-9395.

Pavie J, de Castro N, Molina JM & Flageul B. (2010). Severe perheral neuropathy following HAART initiation in a HIV-infected patient with leprosy. *Journal of the international association of physicians in AIDS care,* Vol.9, No. 4, (July 2010), pp. 232-235, ISSN:1545-1097.

Pereira GA, Stefani MM, Araujo Filho JA, Souza LC, Stefani GP, Martelli CM. (2004). Human immunodeficiency virus type 1 (HIV-1) and Mycobacterium leprae co-infection: HIV-1 subtypes and clinical, immunologic, and histopathologic profiles in a Brazilian cohort. *American Journal of Tropical Medicine and Hygiene,*Vol.71, No.5, (November 2004), pp.679-684, ISSN:0002-9637.

Price P, Mathiot N, Krueger R, Stone S, Keane NM, French MA. (2001). Immune dysfunction and immune restoration disease in HIV patients given highly active antiretroviral therapy. *Journal of Clinical Virology,* Vol. 22, No.3, (October 2001), pp.279-287, ISSN:1386-6532.

Sampaio EP, Caneshi JR, Nery JA, Duppre NC, Pereira GM, Vieira LM, Moreira AL, Kaplan G & Sarno EM. (1995). Cellular immune response to Mycobacterium leprae infection in human immunodeficiency virus-infected individuals. *Infection and Immunity*, Vol.63, No. 5, (May 1995), pp.1848-1854, ISSN:0019-9567.

Ratnam I, Chiu C, Kandala NB, Easterbrook PJ. (2006) Incidence and risk factors for immune reconstitution inflammatory syndrome in an ethnically diverse HIV type 1-infected cohort. *Clinical Infectious Disease*, Vol. 42, No.3, (February 2006), pp.418-427, ISSN:1058-4838.

Riddell JT, Kaul DR, Karakousis PC, Gallant JE, Mitty J, Kazanjian PH. *Mycobacterium avium* complex immune reconstitution inflammatory syndrome: long term outcomes. *Journal of Translational Medicine*, Vol.5, N0. 50, (October 2007), pp.1-7.ISSN:1479-5876.

Ridley DS, Jopling WH. (1966). Classification of Leprosy according to immunity. A five group system. *International Journal of Leprosy and Other Mycobacterial Disease*, Vol.34, No.3, (July 1966), pp.255-273, ISSN: 0148-916X.

Ridley DS. (1969). Reactions in leprosy. *Leprosy Review*, Vol.40, No.2, (April 1969), pp.77-81, ISSN: 0305-7518.

Ridley DS, Radia KB. The histological course of reactions in borderline leprosy and their outcome. *International Journal of Leprosy and Other Mycobacterial Diseases*, Vol. 49, No.4, (December 1981), pp.383-392, ISSN: 0148-916X.

Robertson J, Meier M, Wall J, Ying J, Fichtenbaum CJ. (2006). Immune reconstitution syndrome in HIV: validating a case definition and identifying clinical predictors in persons initiating antiretroviral therapy. *Clinical Infectious Disease*, Vol.42, No.11, (June 2006), pp.1639-1646, ISSN:1058-4838.

Sarno EN, Illarramendi X, Nery JA, Sales AM, Gutierrez-Galhardo MC, Penna MLF, Sampaio EP, Kaplan G.(2008) HIV-*M. leprae* interaction: can HAART modify the course of leprosy? *Public Health Reports* 2008,Vol.123, No. 2, (March 2008), pp.206-212, ISSN:0033-3549.

Scollard DM, Adams LB, Gillis TP, Krahenbuhl JL, Truman RW & Williams DL (2006). The continuing Challenges of Leprosy. Clinical Microbiology Reviews, Vol.19, No.2, (April 2006), pp.338-381, ISSN:0893-8512.

Shelburne SA, Visnegarwala F, Darcourt J, Graviss EA, Giordano TP, White AC Jr & Hamill RJ.(2005). Incidence and risk factors for immune reconstitution inflammatory syndrome during highly active antiretroviral therapy. *AIDS*, Vol.19, No.4,(March 2005), pp. 399-406, ISSN: 0269-9370.

Shelburne SA, Montes M, Hamill RJ. (2006). Immune reconstitution inflammatory syndrome: more answers, more questions. *Journal of Antimicrobial Chemotherapy*, Vol. 57, No.2, (February 2006), pp.167-170, ISSN:0305-7453

Singal A, Mehta S, Pandhi D. (2006).Immune reconstitution inflammatory syndrome in an HIV seropositive leprosy patient. *Leprosy Review*, Vol. 77, No.1, (March 2006),pp.76-80, ISSN: 0305-7518.

Talhari C, Machado PR, Ferreira LC, Talhari S. (2007). Shifting of the clinical spectrum of leprosy in an HIV-positive patient: a manifestation of immune reconstitution inflammatory syndrome? *Leprosy Review*, Vol.78, No.2, (June 2007), pp.151-154, ISSN:0305-7518.

Talhari C, Mira MT, Massone C,Braga A, Chrusciak-Talhari A, Santos M, Orsi AT, Matsuo C, Rabelo R, Nogueira L, Ferreira LCL, Ribeiro-Rodrigues R & Talhari S. (2010). Leprosy and HIV coinfection: a clinical, pathological, immunological and therapeutic study of a cohort from a Brazilian referral center for infectious disease. *Journal of Infectious disease*, Vol. 202, No. 3, (August 2010), pp. 345-354, ISSN:0022-1899.

Trindade MA, Manini MI, Masetti JH, Leite MA, Takahashi MD & Naafs B. (2005). Leprosy and HIV co-infection in five patients. Leprosy review, Vol. 76, No. 2, (June 2005), pp. 162-166, ISSN: 0305-7518.

Ustianowski AP, Lawn SD, Lockwood DN (2006). Interactions between HIV infection and leprosy: a paradox. *Lancet Infectious Disease*,Vol.6, No 6, (June 2006), pp.350-360, ISSN:1473-3099.

Vinay K, Smita J, Nikhil G & Neeta G. (2009). Human Immunodeficiency Virus and Leprosy coinfection in Pune, India. *Journal of clinical microbiology*, Vol. 47, No. 9, (September 2009), pp.2998-2999, ISSN:0095-1137.

Visco-Comandini U, Longo B, Cuzzi T, Paglia MG, Antonucci G. (2004).Tuberculoid leprosy in a patient with AIDS: a manifestation of immune restoration syndrome. *Scandinavian Journal of Infectious Disease*, Vol.36, No.11-12, (December 2004), pp.881-883, ISSN:0036-5548.

World Health Organization, 2010. *Global leprosy situation, 2010.* Weekly epidemiological record, Vol.85, No. 35 (August, 2010) pp. (337-348), ISSN 0049-8114.

Part 4

Laboratory Diagnosis

9

The HIV Seronegative Window Period: Diagnostic Challenges and Solutions

Tamar Jehuda-Cohen
SMART Biotech Ltd. Rehovot Israel; and Bio-Medical Engineering, Technion Israel Institute of Technology, Haifa
Israel

1. Introduction

1.1 The phenomenon of the HIV seronegative window period

An exposure of an individual for the first time, to an infectious agent or any other foreign antigen, usually leads to recognition of the foreign antigen by the cells of the immune system (priming) followed by the generation of antibodies that specifically react with the foreign antigen. The process of generating detectable levels of antibodies against a new antigen/pathogen usually requires ~7 days following the initial exposure and infection.

In HIV infection there is a longer time lapse between infection and seroconversion. This time is termed the seronegative window period (WP). If an HIV antibody test is performed during the WP the result will be negative. However, the infected person is infectious and could potentially transmit HIV to others during this time. People taking an HIV test are advised, if the result is negative for HIV specific antibodies, to return for follow-up testing in 2-3 months.

The initial indications to the possible existence of a WP came from case reports where HIV seronegative individuals transmitted infection to others, by both the blood (blood transfusion, shared needles, medical practice), and the sexual routes (both homosexual and heterosexual). Pooling all those reported cases, coupled with mathematical modelling, has led the CDC to estimate the WP to be ~3 month (the time it takes 95% of the population to seroconvert following an HIV infection). This phenomenon, while considered as part of the "norm" in HIV infections, is actually quite surprising, as HIV is a very strong immunogen, and eventually it elicits high levels of a broad spectrum of antibodies against both envelope and core antigen. Clearly this WP is a major obstacle in the path of early and complete detection of HIV infection, and it is this challenge and the different solutions to it that are the focus of this chapter. However, when trying to overcome this hurdle, it behoves us to try and understand the immunological enigma of the WP, and its causes; as understanding the roots of the problem is usually a major part of the solution.

1.2 Using the monkey model of AIDS to study the HIV seronegative window period

1.2.1 The monkey model of HIV infection

The monkey model of AIDS, i.e. the Simian immunodeficiency virus (SIV) in monkeys, has been used for research of the different aspects of the HIV infection and its pathological sequllea, including the interactions between the immune system and the virus at different

stages of the infection. There are two main groups of monkeys in this model – those who are natural hosts of SIV, and those who can be experimentally infected by it. The African monkeys (Sooty Mangabeys) are among the natural hosts for SIV (they develop high viral titres but do not show any signs of SIV related disease throughout their life).
When virus from Sooty Mangabeys (or other African monkeys) is transmitted to naïve Asian monkeys (e.g. Macaques) it leads to an SIV infection with an infection course and pathological sequella similar to that of HIV in humans. Thus this serves as a good animal model for studying HIV infection and AIDS. The time to seroconversion in the Asian monkeys is similar to that observed and estimated in humans. Of course, unlike in natural infection, the length of the WP can be accurately measured in experimental infections. Studying the immune response against SIV in the Asian rhesus macaques, who upon experimental infection with SIV develop disease and clinical symptoms remarkably similar to human HIV-1 infection, could shed some light on the WP as part of the common course of the HIV infection and maybe on the longer seronegative state too.

1.2.2 The seronegative WP in SIV infection

Most of the young Sooty Mangabeys remain seronegative for 2-3 years, eventually seroconverting. As the seroconversion age range coincides with sexual maturity, the dogma has been that these monkeys become infected via the sexual route. However, there have been several reports indicating that they might be infected throughout the seronegative early years of their lives (Jehuda-Cohen et al. 1991; Villinger et al. 1991) and potentially even from birth (Jehuda-Cohen et al. 1991; McClure et al. 1991). If infection occurs in utero or at birth, then the seroconversion upon sexual maturity could be attributed to "new" SIV stimulus or re-infection, which would change the immunological state and lead to stimulation and generation of a measurable antibody response. One possible model for explaining the whole phenomenon could be some form of peripheral tolerance to SIV induced by the in-utero exposure, which would be "broken" when similar but not the same antigen enters the system via the sexual route. Interestingly, in a colony of several dozens of seronegative magabeys, which were kept, as adults, in a separate, seronegative colony for over 8 years, an alpha male sero-converted, for reasons yet to be determined. This could suggest that these natural hosts of SIV may have been infected for a long time and thus had a very long WP (Villinger F. personal communications).
In experimentally infected Asian monkeys, a seronegative window period of more than several weeks is more rare. However, there has been cases of low dose infections where the monkeys remained in a seronegative state for months and years (unpublished data). We have also reported a prolonged seronegative state in macaque babies following infection in-utero or soon after birth (Jehuda-Cohen et al. 1991).

1.2.3 Exposed seronegative (ESN) individuals from high risk groups

Some individuals residing in very high risk populations have been reported to remain seronegative for many years in spite of repeated exposures to the virus. While this WP has been known to be highly variable, the precise mechanisms that give rise to this long seronegative WP have yet to be defined. It is not clear whether the 'exposed seronegative' [NIH workshop 2010 on ESN] is a unique phenomenon, separate from the common seronegative WP, or it could be viewed as the far extreme end of a possible spectrum of the length of that WP. In any case, it has been reasoned that delineation of the mechanisms underlying this phenomenon could provide important clues for effective vaccine formulations.

While studies of these cohorts of ESN people are of interest, they do not shed any light on the early immunological events following the HIV infection, as we see in the ESN only the end result (G. Shearer, personal communications). The SIV infected nonhuman primates, might be able to provided a valuable model to study this issue too.

There have now been several reports that a small but significant number of these rhesus macaques when experimentally infected with repeated low doses of SIV intra-rectally or intra-vaginally become highly resistant to infection with a dose of challenge virus that otherwise leads to 100% infection of this species. Of importance is the finding that these highly resistant rhesus macaques neither sero-converted nor developed any detectable SIV specific cellular immunity (Ansari A. personal communications).

1.2.4 Immunological findings of the early stages of infection

The mechanisms underlying the seronegative WP are complex and studying them is encumbered by the fact that we do not have a way to identify those who are in the eclipse period. Thus we are left with three main routs to study this very critical time in the HIV infection, i.e. its onset: 1. Set up large scale studies where fresh blood samples, from HR cohorts, are collected longitudinally for months and years, so that when there is a seroconversion, it is possible to have, retrospectively, good samples (e.g. cryo-preserved cells) to study those early days in the HIV-human-natural setup. 2. To run the immunological and virological studies on samples from the acute phase of the infection and the early days post seroconversion. 3. To use the monkey model of AIDS, in which the time of SIV experimental infection is known, and the virus, its dose, the route of infection, the rate and type of repeat exposures/infections can all be controlled.

The first option is extremely expensive and labour intensive, and rarely attempted, as the vast majority of the samples processed for PBMC etc, will be of those who will remain seronegative through out the study. There has been much work published using the 2nd route (Myron S. Cohen 2007; Margoli 2009), albeit they offer us a view into the post active viremia stage, leaving us in the dark as to the earliest days post infection. Such studies (Tomaras and Haynes 2009) have revealed that there is early destruction of B cell generative microenvironment, and that this might be one of the causes for a delay in protective anti HIV antibody responses (Richman et al. 2003; Davis et al. 2009; Stacey et al. 2009) and other parameters of antibody response (Tomaras et al. 2008). Polyclonal cell activation in early HIV infection and loss of gut germinal centres have been observed (Levesque et al. 2009). These findings of B cell depletion have been confirmed in acute human HIV infected individuals (Marovich M. personal communications). A rapid cytokine storm in acute HIV infection might also contribute to the lack of an appropriate maturing antibody response (Stacey et al. 2009).

Using the SIV model, it has been reported during acute infection, that there is not only a major depletion of CD4+ T cells but also a major depletion of B cells (Titanji et al. 2010). In a study comparing the early immune response to two different SIV strains, with different pathological outcomes, it was shown that: early systemic immune activation, T cell proliferation, and a more prominent and broader array of cytokine/chemokine responses facilitate SIV replication, and may play a key role in persistence of infection, and the progression to AIDS (Xu et al. 2011). This immune activation and SIV proliferation also leads to a fast depletion of T cells.

2. Potential causes and effectors of the length of the WP

Before we look into the potential effectors of its length, we should remember that, in fact, any WP in HIV infection is an enigma as HIV has very strong immunogenic structures, which eventually elicit a strong immune response against it. The CDC states that the length of the WP for HIV varies from country to country and from population to population, as it is affected by geographical, social, genetic and other factors, all of which affect the immune system of the host.

One such example would be the WP in pregnant women. Pregnancy has been purported to induce an altered immune state and some data suggests that certain infections may have worse presentations and outcomes during pregnancy (Landers et al. 1997). Following experimental HIV vaccination in Brazil, anti-HIV-1 immune response was the strongest in intravenous drug users (IDU) group and the weakest in pregnant women. A comparative analysis between pregnant women cohorts from different regions of Brazil indicated an even lower response for the southern population (Bongertz et al. 1998). So, unrecognized HIV infection just prior or during pregnancy may result in higher rates of prenatal transmission (Patterson et al. 2007). In addition, presence of parasitic worms is generally associated with immune suppression. A study on the impact of helminthes on the response to immunization in pregnant women and children in Uganda has shown that infection with helminthes has suppressive effects on the immune response (Elliott et al. 2007). General immune suppression in MSM would be another example, and in that population a very long WP has been reported (Imagawa et al. 1989; Gupta et al. 1992). Viral genotypes and clades (Andersson et al. 2005), social and environmental factors, and genetics, could also play a role in determining the HIV WP.

Studies in the SIV (monkey) model of AIDS were part of the research that enabled an understanding of some of the underlying viral and immunological mechanisms that lead to the seronegative yet infected stage of the infection. It has been discovered that the immune system "sees" the virus at the onset of the infection, gets primed by it, but due to specific immune suppression it does not lead to seroconversion (Powell et al. 1991; Jehuda-Cohen et al. 1994). Only several weeks or months later, when there are high levels of virus in the blood, antibodies are finally produced by the immune system at detectable levels in the blood. In a study among individuals who were at high risk for HIV, a similar suppression of antibody production was found leading to a seronegative state in spite of an HIV infection (Jehuda-Cohen et al. 1990).

Upon infection, the HIV seems to home to the lymphoid tissues, of which the leading one is the gut mucosal tissue. At that time there would be no, or almost no, virus detected in the blood. A link has been proposed between the time of active viremia in the blood reaching certain levels, and the time of seroconversion (Busch et al. 1995). The time between the infection and the active viremia reaching detectable levels in the blood is called the eclipse period. There has been reports of low, intermittent levels of detectable levels of virus in the blood (Fiebig et al. 2003) for weeks, until eventually the infection changes to an active viremia leading, usually, to constant measurable levels of virus in the blood, and to seroconversion.

3. Ways to shorten the window period and the time of "no-detection"

3.1 Better detection of antibodies

The WP has been a major concern in both the blood banks (and other tissue transplants) and in the diagnostic arena. While the detection of HIV specific antibodies in the plasma has remained the gold standard for diagnosis, there has been much pressure to develop methods which could shorten the period of no-detection. The initial steps taken where to enable the detection of IgM antibodies in addition to the IgG antibodies, thus bringing to the market the 3rd generation assays for HIV specific antibodies. (The 1st and 2nd generation assays detected only HIV specific IgG). This, together with increased sensitivity has shortened the WP, yet the confirmation by Western blot kept the confirmed diagnosis delayed as before (Owen et al. 2008).

3.2 Detection of virus in the blood

The second approach was to address the issue of no-detection via the detection of the active viremia in the blood which precedes the seroconversion. Thus, methods which detect the presence of the virus in the blood (p24 antigen, viral RNA, or pro-viral DNA) have enabled the detection of the infection 7-12 days, respectively, prior to seroconversion. This improved detection has enabled the detection of RNA, prior to seroconversion in 0.3% of 14,005 frequently tested MSM in Seattle STD clinic (represents 20% of all HIV infections detected), (Stekler et al. 2009); and in 0.08% of 21,222 STD clinic patients in New York City (represents 9% of all HIV infections detected), (Shepard et al, MMWR in press).
Linear regression analysis of the detectable part of the active viremia stage led to an estimation that the "beginning" of the active viremia in the blood was 10 days prior to the virus reaching detectable levels in the blood. Thus the total length of the active viremia prior to seroconversion was estimated at 22 days (Busch et al. 2005). The detectable part of the active viremia prior to seroconversion i.e. the virus positive yet antibody negative plasma is called the "acute stage" of the HIV infection. The part of the active viremia which is not detectable, and the period prior to the active viremia, when the virus reside in the mucosal membranes of the gut (Brenchley and Douek 2008; Mestecky et al. 2009), in lymph nodes (Pantaleo et al. 1994; Schacker 2008), macrophages in the lung and other tissues (Orenstein 2001), is termed the eclipse period.

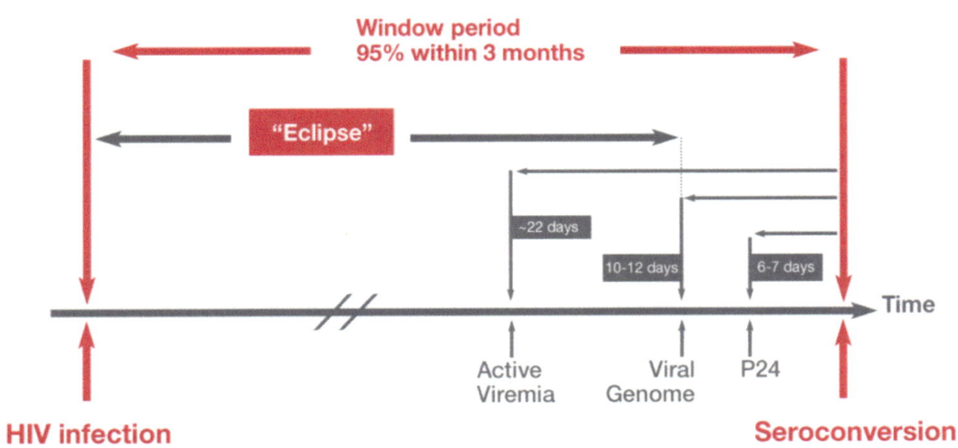

Fig. 1. Time line from HIV infection to seroconversion.

3.3 Dealing with the root of the problem

Since the mechanisms underlying the seronegative WP include specific immune suppression, other factors affecting the immune state of the person could affect the length of the WP. Such conditions include pregnancy, parasitic infections and other co-infections, MSM relationships, hemodialysis, and others. The variability in the length of the WP also means a variable length for the eclipse period, i.e. the period in which the HIV infection is totally missed by all the currently available assays in plasma. Thus the optimal way to solve the WP problem would be to be able to overcome the immune suppression and lead to antibody production, in-vitro, soon after the initial HIV infection and immune priming in-vivo.

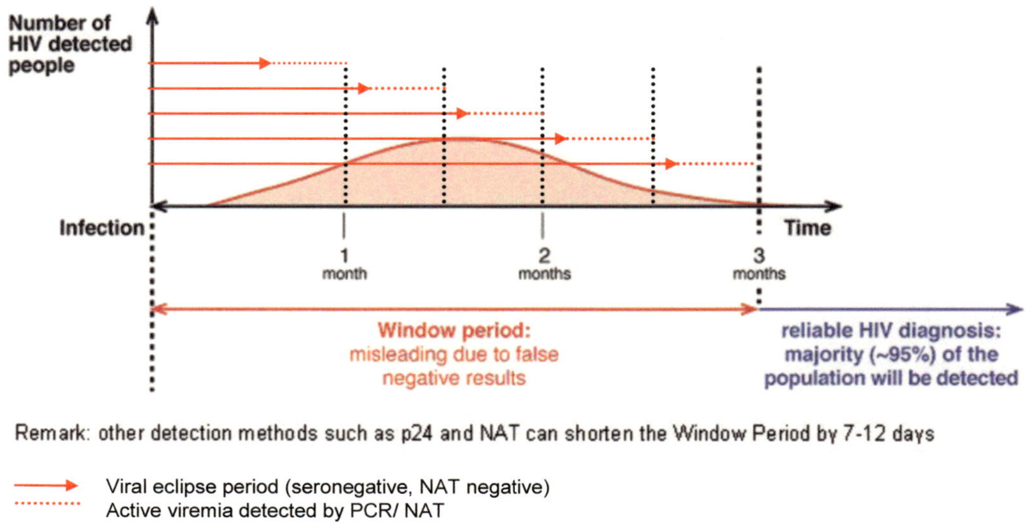

Fig. 2. An illustration of the statistical distribution of the length of the seronegative WP in a population, and the relative length of the viral eclipse period.

4. The Stimmunology concept and the SMARTube HIV

Since the immune system "sees" the virus, and its lymphocytes, both T and B cell, get primed by it within minutes of infection, tapping into these early events could enable the detection of HIV infection within days. A method was developed to enable the process which has been initiated in-vivo (specific cell priming) to be completed in-vitro, by leading to cell proliferation and differentiation and to HIV specific antibody production, in the case of an HIV infection. The stimulation in-vitro is designed to overcome the immune suppression in-vivo and to provide the lymphocytes in the blood sample a strong stimuli to produce antibodies in culture.

This unique and innovative technology (called Stimmunology) has been shown to enable the detection of HIV infection within a week after exposure, several weeks or months prior to seroconversion. Detecting infection via the specific antibodies in the blood is routinely used in any clinical laboratory and seropositivity to HIV is considered the gold standard in diagnostics. The sample used in these assays can be serum or plasma with or without pre-stimulation.

The embodiment of Stimmunology into a simple to use product is the SMARTube™, which requires one ml. fresh whole blood. Blood, when introduced to the SMARTube, is stimulated so as to enhance the synthesis of HIV specific antibody, and the differentiation of HIV primed B cells to antibody producing cells. The resulting plasma, enriched with antibodies via the tissue culture step, is called SMARTplasma. SMARTube accelerates antibody production bringing the antibody levels, in the SMARTplasma, across the regular ELISA testing's detection threshold, leading to earlier, better and more complete detection and diagnosis of the HIV infection.

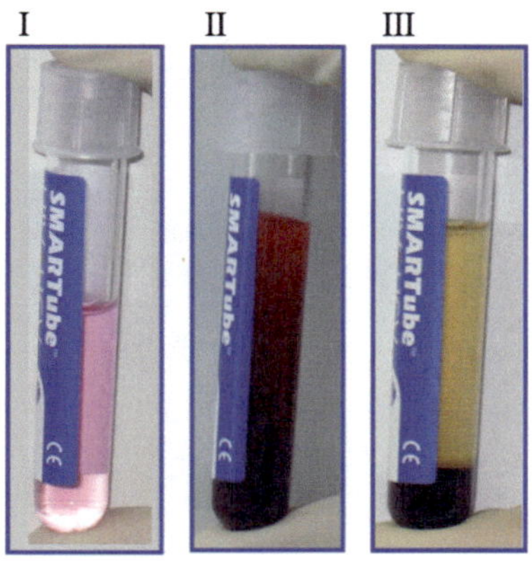

I SMARTube™ before use

II SMARTube™ containing 1 ml of whole blood sample-time 0.

III SMARTube™ after incubation.

Fig. 3. Getting SMARTplasma from fresh whole blood by incubation in the SMARTube for 3-5 days in a 37°C, 5%CO_2 incubator.

5. SMARTube enables detection of antibodies prior to seroconversion

Comparative laboratory studies were conducted in different populations and different geographical locations, testing plasma and SMARTplasma in parallel, from the same blood sample, using locally approved diagnostic kits. The confirmation of an initial antibody positive test results (of plasma and/or SMARTplasma) was done following the local guidelines and algorithms; thus differentiating between true antibody positive samples and false positive ones.

In China, among 653 IDU 149 were confirmed seropositive (antibody positive in plasma) and 2 (1.3% additional HIV positives) additional individuals were confirmed antibody positive in SMARTplasma, enabling detection of the HIV infection prior to seroconversion [Dr. Wang Y. personal communications]. In a parallel study, conducted using 2000 low risk individuals from the blood donors of Beijing blood bank, no additional positives were found using the SMARTube, showing no adverse effect on specificity. It was further documented that when testing SMARTplasma there was a marked reduction in the rate of false positive readings, in both diagnostic kits used [Qui W. personal communications] When blood donors from a high prevalence, high incidence population (Kenya) were tested for HIV infection, there was a high rate (4%) of missed HIV infections, detectable by the antibody diagnostic kits only after incubation of the blood samples in the SMARTube (Mumo et al. 2009). Viral testing was done on the seronegative WP samples detected using SMARTube , and virus was detected in ~50% of the SMARTplasma positive seronegative. This further confirms the fact that the SMARTube is not dependent on detectable levels of virus in the blood in order to enable the detection of very early infection, i.e. with it HIV infection can be detected even in the viral eclipse period.

An immigrant group, coming from a high risk country into Israel, where the risk was through sexual transmission, was also tested (Novikov and Jehuda-Cohen 2009). In both waves of immigration additional HIV antibody positive infected individuals were detected. In the first wave of 285 tested, 8 of the 15 infections were in the WP, while in the second wave of the 537 tested, 2 of the 28 infections were in the WP. The difference between the two populations was that the first population had been exposed to high prevalence and high risk of HIV only for one year, which explains the lower prevalence and the higher number of the infections being recent ones, with many still in the seronegative WP. The second population was exposed to HIV for several years, leading to a higher prevalence but a lower number of new infections which were missed by current serology.

Country	Population studied	Total tested	ST negative		ST positive*	
			Serology negative	Serology positive*	Serology negative	Serology positive*
High Risk						
Israel	*Immigrants from high risk areas, high risk population first wave*	285	270	0	8	7
	Immigrants from high risk areas, high risk population 2nd wave	537	519	0	2	26
Mexico	*Very high risk population, multiple, current exposures*	200	175	0	5	20
Kenya	*Screening of high risk population*	555	513	0	14	28
	Adult blood donors	513	447	0	21	45
	Youth blood donors	332	310	0	10	12
	Seronegative Pregnant women	20	8	0	5	7
China	*High risk population (IVDU), Sichuan District*	653	502	0	2	149
South Africa	*Blood donors from high risk population*	90	85	0	2	3
Russian Federation	*Discordant couples, high risk population, Blood donors,*	24	18	0	1	5
Hungary	*Routine Laboratory tests*	41	40	0	0	1
	National AIDS center	203	55	0	1	147
Romania	*Routine Private Laboratory tests*	200	200	0	0	0
Low Risk						
China	*Low risk population, Beijing Blood Bank*	2000	2000	0	0	0
Russian Federation	*Low risk population, Blood donors*	25	25	0	0	0
Israel	*Low risk population, Blood donors*	1500	1500	0	0	0
* Positive = confirmed by repeat testing.						

Table 1. Increase in HIV antibody levels, using the SMARTube, led to earlier detection of HIV infection (i.e. detection of seronegative, yet infected, individuals)

In Russia, 25 discordant couples were tested using the SMARTube. Five were seropositive on both plasma and SMARTplasma, however there was an infected person who tested positive only when using SMARTplasma (Olshansky 2008). Viral load was 900,000, i.e. that person was not only HIV infected and still in the WP, but also very infectious, and missed by current serology. When the SMARTube was incorporated into routine laboratory use, within the first 300 samples tested, the confirmed diagnosis of one patient was achieved, using SMARTube, 4-6 weeks prior to complete seroconversion in plasma (Bicbulatova et al. 2010).

In South Africa, in a high prevalence and incidence area, a cross sectional comparative study showed full concordance between the confirmed antibody positive results in plasma and in SMARTplasma. In a prospective study, several hundred individuals were followed, monthly for up to 9 months, to measure the rate of new infections by seroconversions. In several individuals, antibodies were detected in SMARTplasma 1-4 months prior to plasma seroconversion [Sexton C. personal communications].

It is important to note, that while the incubation of the blood in the SMARTube increases the levels of the HIV specific antibodies in infected individuals, it does not adversely affect the diagnostic specificity. On the contrary, the SMARTube has been found to decrease the false positive rate on the routinely used diagnostic kits, thus increasing the specificity of the kit in the tested population (Mumo et al. 2009; Novikov and Jehuda-Cohen 2009, and unpublished data). There are several mechanisms which contribute to this phenomena, one of them being that while increasing the specific signal (HIV antibodies) the plasma itself is diluted 1:5 (1ml of blood, i.e. ~0.5ml plasma, put into 2ml of SMART solution), thus decreasing "noise" and leading to a decrease of as high as 100% in the false positive rate.

In addition, the use of the SMARTube enables the laboratory to get, and provide, a more confirmed negative result. Currently, using plasma, those who were seronegative, yet in the WP, (i.e. actually infected) are falsely recorded as negative. One cannot differentiate between those who are truly HIV negative and those who are HIV infected yet still in the WP - they all give the same 'negative reading' on the assays used. When using the SMARTube, the WP samples test positive, thus making the antibody negative results confirmed negative (see Fig.4).

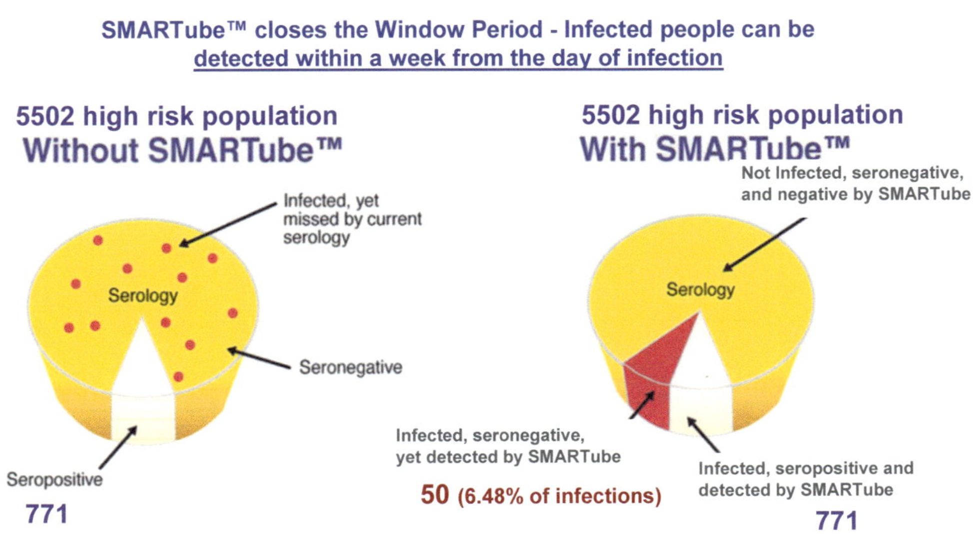

Fig. 4. Consolidated results from laboratory clinical data in different studies using SMARTplasma (following incubation in the SMARTube) in parallel to regular plasma

6. The importance of early detection of HIV infection

6.1 Infection at the seronegative WP is infectious

Over the course of the HIV epidemic, there have been reports in literature of individual who tested negative for antibodies yet were infected and infectious, leading to the infection of others. Long term seronegative yet infected state has been reported, especially once more sensitive methods for detecting the virus were developed (Imagawa et al. 1989; Ensoli et al. 1990; Gupta et al. 1992).

Incomplete detection of potentially infectious blood units (Ling et al. 2000), and other donated organs (e.g. sperm, kidney, bone marrow) can transmit HIV infection to the recipients. Thus the need to shorten the window period, by as much as possible, has been an important goal of the health systems around the world. The importance of blood safety and of transplanting organs which are free of HIV (and HCV and others) infection have been major engines in the introduction of viral (RNA) testing into blood screening and into organ donors' testing. The cost of NAT testing of the single, individual, organ donor is acceptable. The cost at the blood bank level had to be dramatically reduced, and this was done by testing the blood in pools of 16, 24, 40 and more blood units/pooled test. The gain by the pooled testing, and the loss of sensitivity due to the pooling has been the topic of many studies and reviews, and is not in the scope of this chapter.

6.2 Infectious blood and blood products from donors at the seronegative WP and the viral eclipse

The transmission of HIV via blood transfusions was markedly reduced by the introduction of NAT testing to the blood banks, yet there have been several cases of HIV transmitted through a blood donation, in the USA, in spite of the testing for both antibodies and viral RNA (limit of detection 150 copies/ml). Such cases are termed HIV breakthrough cases (Delwart et al. 2004). In some cases one WP blood donation infected two recipients (Taylor et al. 2002). In Germany, in 2007, a 67 year old man got HIV from a screened blood donation

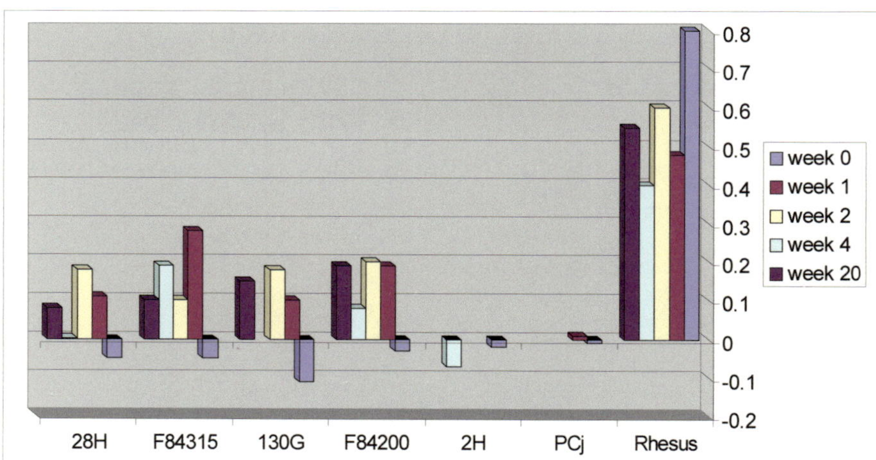

Fig. 5. SIV-reactive antibodies following Stimmunology - detection in the first week of infection (28H, F84315, 130G, and F84200 were transfused. 2H and Pcj were negative controls. Rhesus is a seropositive monkey).

(Schmidt et al. 2009). In Singapore, it has been reported that a blood transfusion was the source of an HIV infection. The authors state that the blood donation and transfusion of blood components occurred in Singapore, where blood donation testing for HIV is similar to US protocols, including anti-HIV-1 and anti-HIV-2 EIAs and an HIV-1 p24 antigen EIA (Ling et al. 2000). In another report two infections were caused by a blood donation in 2002 (Phelps et al. 2004). The donor was an adolescent repeat donor who tested HIV antibody positive in May 2002, and the previous donation (3 months earlier) must have been during the seronegative WP and at the eclipse of the virus too.

A study in monkeys (SIV) to address the question of infectiousness of blood from seronegative monkeys (sooty mangabeys), yet positive for SIV antibodies after cell activation in-vitro showed 100% infectivity as 4/4 of the naïve macaques, transfused with the seronegative mangebeys' blood, seroconverted 1-3 moths following the transfusion (Jehuda-Cohen et al. 1991). At the same study, it was possible to compare the WP using plasma versus the detection of antibodies following the Stimmunology process. All 4 transfused monkeys (Fig. 5.) had detectable levels of SIV antibodies following the stimulation process at the first bleed, one week post-transfusion (3-11 weeks earlier).

6.3 Organs from donors at the seronegative WP and the viral eclipse – transmitted infection

The relevance of the following cases, reported in literature, and mentioned here as examples, is not in their number and prevalence but rather for the light they shed on the WP, which even during the viral eclipse could be infectious, and thus of a major diagnostic concern.

In a report of a liver transplant, which transmitted HCV (Ahn and Cohen 2008) the authors summarize cases of HIV transmission through solid organ transplantation between 1985-1987. This problem was much more pronounced then, when only antibody testing (1st and 2nd generation) was available. However, shortening of the seronegative WP by more sensitive ELISA, and by 3rd generation ELISA, and adding the viral RNA testing (for a 10-12 days shorter WP), did not solve the problem completely (CDC 1987; Simonds et al. 1992; Mitra 2004).

Two related cases of infectious donations are described from a cornea donor during the pre seroconversion window (Najioullah et al. 2004). HIV was transmitted via a kidney transplant from a cadaveric donor (Borchi et al. 2010). In 2007, it was reported that, four transplant recipients in Chicago have contracted HIV and hepatitis C virus from an organ donor (Grady 2007). The organ donor tested negative for both viruses, both in antibody and in viral genome testing and apparently the donor was still in the seronegative WP and the viral eclipse period and thus the infection was missed. Following this case estimation of the window period between infection and detection by ELISA assay and NAT testing for HIV, hepatitis B virus, and hepatitis C virus was published (Singer et al. 2008). The CDC reported a case of infection via a kidney transplant in NYC in 2009 (CDC 2011). The donor was in the seronegative WP. Another kidney transplant HIV infection has just been reported this year by the USA health administration.

6.4 Individuals at the early stages of infections are the most infectious

Statistical analysis of epidemiological data indicates that the majority of new infections are transmitted from the small % of individuals who are in the early stages of the infection and that the acute infections are the most infectious (Pilcher et al. 2001; Pilcher et al. 2004; Wawer et al. 2005). An analysis of HIV-1 Transmission, by stage of infection, indicated that primary infection was estimated to be 26 times more infectious than asymptomatic infection. High infectiousness during primary infection was estimated to last for 3 months after seroconversion. Thus we have 4-5 months of very high infectiousness, with 25-40% of that time the infection is in the seronegative WP (Hollingsworth et al. 2008). In 2007, it was reported, based on a North American urban study, that primary/early infection, representing <10% of the samples, disproportionately accounted for approximately half (49%) of onward transmission events" (Brenner et al. 2007).

Recent primate data demonstrate marked enhanced infectiousness of viral variants isolated from acutely infected macaques compared with viruses isolated from animals in the chronic phase of disease. These data are supported by phylogenetic analyses of recently transmitted cases in humans, implying that individuals with Primary HIV infection (PHI) may contribute disproportionately to onward transmission at a population level (Hamlyn 2010).

Other studies have shown that those who are unaware of the sero-status are 3.5 times more infectious than those who are aware (Marks et al. 2006). The CDC has reported that the high proportion of MSM unaware of their HIV infection continues to be a serious public health concern, because these MSM account for the majority of estimated new HIV transmissions in the United States (CDC 2010). One can only stipulate, on the effect of false negative results given to individuals who suspected infection for reasons best known to them. A false negative result could remove the final deterrent from behaviors which could set them at risk of HIV transmission. False-negative, WP, people do not take precautions or listen to preventive guidelines.

6.5 Pregnant women in the WP, a missed opportunity to treat and save the babies

The problem of the seronegative WP is especially critical in pregnant women. On one hand, the infection, which could have been transmitted close to the time of pregnancy, could have a longer WP due to the general slight immune suppression induced to preserve the fetus. On the other hand, there is usually a one time chance to save the fetus from infection, reducing the risk of mother-to-child-transmission from 28-30% to 1-2%, by giving the mother a short course of ARV during pregnancy and child birth (Cooper et al. 2002; WHO 2006). That chance is during the initial (and sometimes only) visit to the doctor or antenatal clinic. However, the provision of ARV is contingent on the expecting mother testing antibody positive, thus excluding from the treatment those who are in the WP at the time of testing (Dao et al. 2007). Thus the efficacy of the PMTCT programs, which include HIV testing to all pregnant women and ARV to all those who are HIV seropositive, depends, among other factors, on overcoming the seronegative WP to get early and complete detection of the infected mothers (Workowski and Berman 2010).

In a study conducted among very high risk pregnant women in Kenya, antibodies were detected in SMARTplasma 2.5-5 months (mean time between last seronegative and first seropositive sample) prior to detection in plasma (Mumo et al. 2009).

The long WP in pregnant women could have, in some rare cases, another ramification - missed infections in the new-born. Babies born to seronegative mothers, even from a high risk population, are not suspected to be infected. However, children born to (seronegative yet infected) mothers in the WP could get infected. This phenomenon has been documented in monkeys (SIV) and in unique case reports in HIV (Jehuda-Cohen et al. 1991; Jehuda-Cohen et al. 1992).

In Botswana, there is a state wide PMTCT program. In 2007 nearly all pregnant women (>95%) had antenatal care and delivered in hospital, and ~80% of pregnant women were tested for HIV (Creek et al. 2007), and by 2007 91% of seropositive pregnant women received ARV (NACA 2007; 2008). However, the rate of MTCT has not been reduced to the expected level of 1-2% and remains at ~4%. It is thought that some of the unresolved MTCT are partially due to missed infections due to the WP.

Patient ID	Sample date	1st Ab test Plasma	1st test SMART plasma	Repeat Ab test Plasma	Repeat Ab test SMART plasma	p24 Ag	SMART plasma WB	Seroconversion after SMART plasma +Pos result (mid-point)
ML1232	0	0.469	**2.457**		**2.325**	**1.914**	pos	
	3 Months	0.350						
	5 Months	**18.750**						4 Months
ML1326	0	0.450	**2.871**		**3.700**	0.677	ND	
	4 Months	**6.125**						2 Months
	10 Months	**10.181**						
ML1356	0	0.137	**1.579**		1.733	0.484	Ind	
	4 Months	0.044						
	6 Months	**6.187**		**8.150**				5 Months
TDD164	0	0.931	**5.650**	0.817	**4.667**	0.486	pos	
	5 Months	**1.375**		**1.767**				2.5 Months
	10 Months	**11.800**						
	12 Months	**11.031**						
ML1324	0	0.656	**1.607**		**2.300**	**2.263**	pos	
	2 Months	0.425						**Lost**

Ab test - Ab ELISA test; P24 Ag - ELISA test for p24 antigen; WB - Western Blot; Pos - positive; Ind. - indeterminate; Lost - lost to follow-up. Results are presented as a ratio Signal/Cut off

Table 2. Follow up HIV antibody testing of Kenyan pregnant women from high risk population (ELISA O.D. readings are presented as a Signal/Cut off ratio)

Blood samples	Date of birth	Date of first SIV-seropositive sample	ELISA Ab titer	Supernatant fluid following Stimmunology (cutoff 0.120)	PCR results	RT activity by the co-culture assay
Mother 1 (FHe)	7/82	-	>1:10	0.28±0.03	+	18.711
Infant 1.1 (FYb)	8/86	11/88	1:8000	0.97±0.03	+	35.253
Infant 1.2 (FVj)	6/88	3/89	1:2000	0.68±0.05	+	22.498
Mother 2 (FOe)	1/83	-	>1:10	0.22±0.01	+	15.966
Infant 2.1 (FRi)	7/88	3/90	1:4000	0.89±0.04	+	24.595
Negative control	-	-	>1:10	0.01±0.01	-	452
Positive control	-	-	1:4000	0.76±0.05	+	31.211

Table 3. Results of sera and Stimmunology enhanced samples from two SIV-seronegative female monkeys with seropositive infants

6.6 Earlier detection could lead to earlier treatment

Test and Treat programs are being evaluated around the world. Treating as early as possible is both for the benefit of the infected individual (e.g. better prognosis, a potential for cure) and of society (as ARV reduces the viral load, and thus the risk of transmission to others). There are contradicting voices regarding implementation of Test & Treat to all seropositive individuals, regardless of how long they have been infected. However, with regard to treating early and acute infections, there is a consensus that it is beneficial both for the individual and the society. PHI refers to the initial phase (up to 6 months following acquisition) of infection characterized by a transient period of massive unchecked viral replication with consequent destruction of memory CD4 T-cells (Douek et al. 2002). There are some large scale studies on going to evaluate the benefits of ARV at the PHI state as part of the Test and Treat approach. Until these provide concrete proof for the benefit to both the individual and society (and in that order), the current world policy for treatment only after CD4 <350/ml would most probably not change (WHO 2010).

The goal of early intervention is to preserve immune function which is ordinarily lost, enhance rapid viral control, and limit the size of the HIV reservoir, with the aim of attenuating long-term outcome (May et al. 2007). Studies regarding the effect of HIV on the brain in the early stages of HIV infection have been recently published. One demonstrated that several markers of inflammation were higher in acutely infected people (Valcour V 2011). These changes were found as early as the second and third of four 'Feibig stages' prior to seroconversion (Fiebig et al. 2003). In another study HIV injury to the brain, affecting its structure, were seen as early as 2 months post infection. The early initiation of ART was supported by preliminary results showing a lesser effect in people on HIV treatment (Rangin et al. 2011).

Intuitively, the earlier that intervention can be initiated following HIV acquisition, the more enhanced will be the anticipated effect on outcome. Although much of the early immunological work has focused on acute infection (Rosenberg et al. 2000; Kaufmann et al. 2004), a more recent study (Hecht et al. 2006) comparing early intervention (<14 days) with later (2 weeks to 6 months) identified immunological benefit in both groups although enhanced outcome was only seen with earlier intervention.

It is also of interest to note that while viral testing is an important tool for the detection of an acute HIV infection, it does not serve as the stand alone diagnostic assay and the recommendations are that when acute HIV infection is diagnosed by a positive viral test (such as HIV RNA or p24 antigen) coupled with a negative HIV antibody test, a confirmatory HIV antibody test should be performed over the next 3 months to confirm seroconversion (DHHS and OARAC 2011). Thus, the ability to detect HIV specific antibodies, at the acute phase, by using the SMARTube could play an important role in providing immediate confirmation of HIV diagnosis by specific antibody assays.

6.7 A potential value of initiating treatment early

In 2007, it was stated that based on the measurements of decay of the HIV reservoir in patients who initiated antiviral therapy early in infection, the half-life of this latent viral reservoir was estimated to be 4.6 months. With this, it was projected that it will take up to 7.7 years of continuous therapy to completely eliminate latently infected resting CD4+ T cells in infected individuals who initiate antiviral therapy early in HIV infection (Chun et al. 2007). This and other studies have led to the initiation of the experimental Test and Treat programs.

6.8 Measured potential benefits of early treatment

6.8.1 Increase in life expectancy due to early treatment

Recently it has been estimated that an expanded HIV test and treat program in Washington DC will increase life expectancy of HIV-infected patients but will have a modest impact on HIV transmission over the next 5 years and is unlikely to halt the HIV epidemic (Walensky et al. 2010). In another paper (Bendavid et al. 2010) it was predicted that early treatment, when compared to the status quo, universal testing and treatment, was associated with a life expectancy gain of ~12.0 months of life, and ~35.3% fewer infections over a 10-year time horizon. Their results support the notion that universal testing and treatment could have significant mortality benefits. A recent estimate from South Africa suggest that ART may prolong life expectancy of infected individuals by 12.5 years (Walensky et al. 2009).

6.8.2 Reduction in community viral load

San Francisco Department of Public Health reported that as 'community viral load' (the amount of virus in the blood of all HIV-infected individuals tested in San Francisco) declined from 2005 to 2008 because of drug treatment and increased awareness, the number of new infections in the city also dropped (Das et al. 2010). Similar results were presented for a study of IDU in Vancouver (Wood et al. 2009). Recently it was reported that when treatment was expanded to IDU with HIV throughout British Columbia, new HIV diagnoses in that group dropped by around 50%.

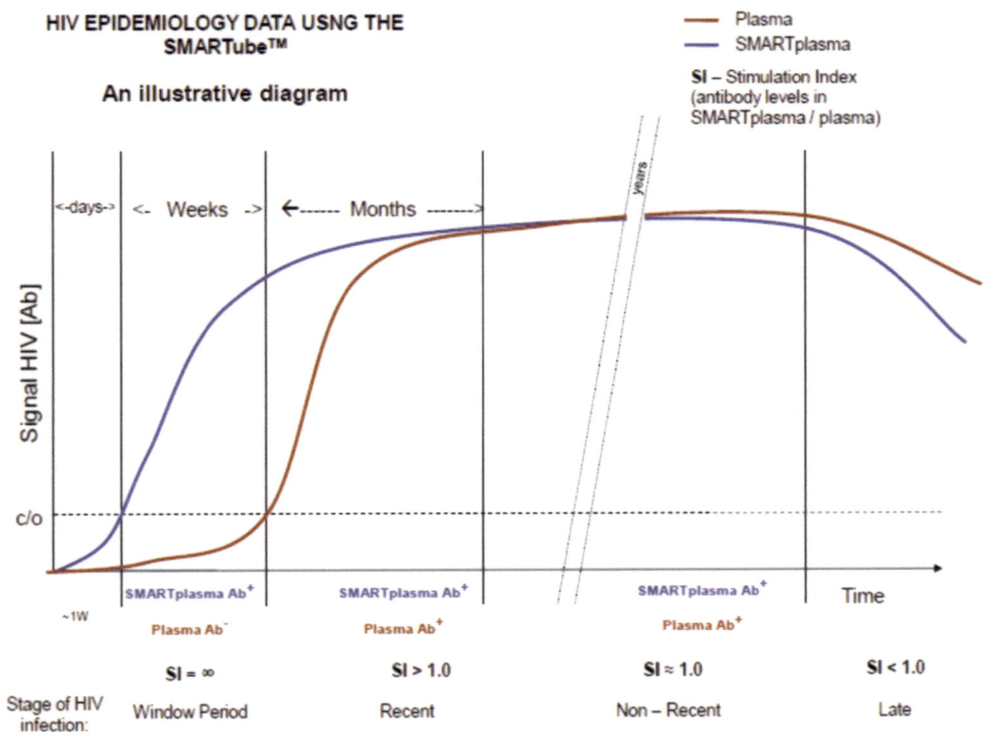

Fig. 6. Detecting very early (WP) HIV infection and differentiating recent from non-recent seropositive infections by using the SMARTube and comparing the levels of HIV antibodies in SMARTplasma versus plasma - An illustrative diagram

6.8.3 Reduced rate of transmission

Recently results were published (Granich et al. 2009) showing that test-and-treat program could eliminate HIV transmission, defined as an incidence below one case per 1,000 people per year, within a decade. This was supported by a report based on independent studies in Canada (Check Hayden). In the United States, treating HIV infection aggressively before symptoms appear could help to control the spread of the disease (Hamlyn 2010). These findings could have an effect on the WHO ARV treatment policies in the future.

The initial stage, acute HIV infection, has a short duration (measured in weeks to months), is difficult to diagnose, and is associated with high levels of viremia (Dieffenbach and Fauci 2009). The large amount of virus in most newly infected individuals renders them highly infectious to others (Pinkerton 2008). Thus these primary and early infections should be the ones that early treatment is focused on. The challenge is to detect the infection early, and also to be able to differentiate between recent and non recent infection once diagnosed. The SMARTube offers a unique tool to enable both detection of infection within a week and the differentiation of recent from non-recent infection.

7. What is the length of the seronegative WP?

7.1 Statistical estimation guiding public health institutions

The WP is a general HIV phenomenon, that is, antibodies are not produced against HIV within a week or so of infection. The current epidemiological-diagnostic WP is estimated to be 8-10 weeks (and >95% of the infected individuals will seroconvert within 3 months) (CMA 1995; CDC 2001; Branson et al. 2006; Workowski and Berman 2010). Thus, there is an underlying mechanism of initial specific immune suppression which would affect the length of the WP, and which varies pending genetic, environmental, and immunological background.

The length of the WP should not be confused with the length of the active viremia which precedes the Seroconversion (Fiebig et al. 2003). The estimated time "0" of that active viremia stage (Busch et al. 1995), has nothing to do with the time of infection. There has been reported cases where virus has been detected 10-14 days post infection due to blood or organ donation which was in the WP. However, the duration of the WP in the donor, as well as the duration of the WP in the more common routes of infection (e.g. sexual, IDU) and "natural doses" of inoculums (Hladik and McElrath 2008) are generally unknown and cannot be derived from the transfusion and transplantation cases.

7.2 Estimating the length of the WP using the SMARTube

Classically, as time of infection is mostly unknown, the time of seroconversion is calculated, based on the median between the last seronegative and the first seropositive sample. Since with the SMARTube detection of HIV specific antibodies can be achieved within days of infection, the time of infection can be better estimated (the median between the last SMARTplasma negative and SMARTplasma positive results for HIV specific antibodies). This, coupled with the time of seroconversion, it can offer a tool for calculating the length of the seronegative WP in a given population.

In some cases the time of infection can be statistically estimated in a population based study, when there is migration at a given time point from a low risk area and life style to a high risk area and life style. With the aid of the SMARTube, and given the defined, relatively short, time of exposure to HIV in that immigrant population, the length of the WP in such a population was estimated (Novikov and Jehuda-Cohen 2009). The variables shown in table 4 include the number of infectious days (IP) within the 365-day stay in the refugee camp, defined here to range between 183-304 days. Furthermore, the time interval for performance of the blood tests ranged between 0-90 days (TP) of arrival in Israel. A window-period of 15 days, was assumed for any viral infection prior to humoral immune responses. These variables were run in calculations used to determine the WP length while assuming a ratio of 1, 50 or 90% of infections due to internal sexual contacts. All in all the length of the "mean" WP was estimated to be 160 days (>5 moths).

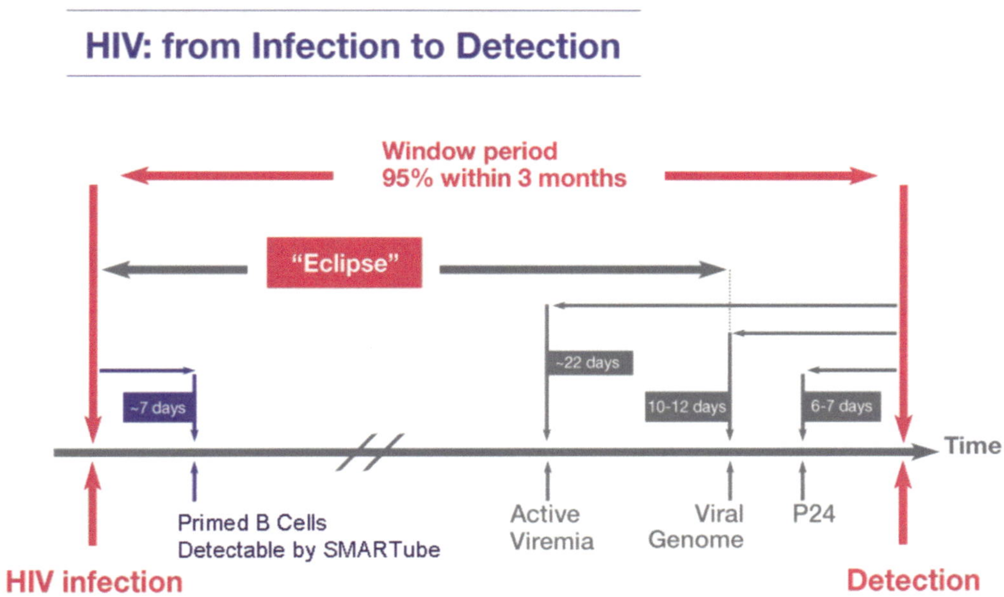

Fig. 7. The time line from infection to detection, and the contribution of the SMARTube, which enables detection during the window period, as soon as there are primed B cells in the blood.

Infectious period (IP)	Testing period (TP)	Calculated window period length (days)					
		Percent of internal contacts					
		1%	SD	50%	SD	90%	SD
183	30	119.5	20.2	110.2	19.9	80.3	17.5
183	90	148.4	20.4	139.2	20.5	111.5	17.9
243	30	154.1	26.7	141	26.1	102.1	24.5
243	90	182.3	27.5	167.8	28	132.6	24.2
304	30	188.1	33.8	171.9	34.4	122.6	29.2
304	90	215.6	34.4	199.4	34.9	153.9	30.1

Table 4. Calculation of HIV window period lengths based on SMARTplasma versus plasma HIV antibody results.

Some follow up studies were conducted testing individuals who tested seronegative in the initial screening. A total of 16 new infections were identified, all of which were SMARTplasma positive, only 5 of them were plasma positive, i.e. 11 of those 16 new infections, were SMARTplasma positive in a blood sample, prior to seroconversion. Of those 11 individuals who were identified during the seronegative WP, 9 were followed until seroconversion. All those 9 (100%) SMARTplasma positive, yet seronegative for HIV antibodies, seroconverted within 1 to 5 months from the time of first SMARTplasma positive, yet seronegative sample. From these studies it can be concluded that the SMARTube™ enables the detection of HIV antibodies (and thus HIV infection), weeks and months prior to seroconversion.

8. Conclusions

The seronegative WP is an important factor in diagnosing the HIV infection, understanding its immunological- pathological sequella, monitoring the transmission and spread of HIV, and controlling the HIV epidemic. An important key to all the above is being able to detect the infection within days, and thus study the earliest possible interactions between the virus and the immune system. This earliest possible detection needs to be independent of the state of viremia, the location of the virus in the tissues, and seroconversion. A method which enables the detection of the initial, early stage, HIV primed B cells, has been developed which could open a window of opportunity to understand the HIV infection better and thus overcome its challenges to man and society.

9. Acknowledgment

The author is grateful to O. Serok, S. Gorodin, S. Suliman, M. Bar, for their technical and scientific assistance in preparing the manuscript. This chapter would not have been possible without the support of Y. Serok and D. Feinstein, who deserve many thanks. A special acknowledgment to A. Ansari and S. Peel for fruitful scientific discussion on this intriguing issue of the seronegative window period.

10. References

Ahn, J. and S. M. Cohen (2008). "Transmission of human immunodeficiency virus and hepatitis C virus through liver transplantation." Liver Transpl 14(11): 1603-8.

Andersson, S., O. Larsen, et al. (2005). "Human immunodeficiency virus (HIV)-2-specific T lymphocyte proliferative responses in HIV-2 -infected and in HIV-2-exposed but uninfected individuals in Guinea-Bissau. "British Society for Immunology, Clinical and Experimental Immunology 139: 483–489.

Bendavid, E., M. L. Brandeau, et al. (2010). "Comparative effectiveness of HIV testing and treatment in highly endemic regions." Arch Intern Med 170(15): 1347-54.

Bicbulatova, L. N., E. V. Drobunina, et al. (2010). "Diagnostic importance of the SMARTube™ test in detection of antibodies to HIV. " HIV / AIDS, blood borne hepatitis and tuberculosis collection. International Conference of Development of Research and Supervision of Infectious Diseases, St. Petersburg, Russia.

Bongertz, V., C. I. Costa, et al. (1998). "HIV specific humoral immune response in Rio de Janeiro, Brazil. The HEC/Fiocruz AIDS Clinical Research Group." Mem Inst Oswaldo Cruz 93(3): 391-8.

Borchi, B., S. Ambu, et al. (2010). "Case report: HIV infection from a kidney transplant." Transplant Proc 42(6): 2267-9.

Branson, B. M., H. H. Handsfield, et al. (2006). "Revised recommendations for HIV testing of adults, adolescents, and pregnant women in health-care settings." MMWR Recomm Rep 55(RR-14): 1-17; quiz CE1-4.

Brenchley, J. M. and D. C. Douek (2008). "HIV infection and the gastrointestinal immune system." Mucosal Immunol 1(1): 23-30.

Brenner, B. G., M. Roger, et al. (2007). "High rates of forward transmission events after acute/early HIV-1 infection." J Infect Dis 195(7): 951-9.

Busch, M. P., S. A. Glynn, et al. (2005). "Relative sensitivities of licensed nucleic acid amplification tests for detection of viremia in early human immunodeficiency virus and hepatitis C virus infection." Transfusion 45(12): 1853-63.

Busch, M. P., L. L. Lee, et al. (1995). "Time course of detection of viral and serologic markers preceding human immunodeficiency virus type 1 seroconversion: implications for screening of blood and tissue donors." Transfusion 35(2): 91-7.

CDC (1987). "Leads from the MMWR. HIV human immunodeficiency virus infection transmitted from an organ donor screened for HIV antibody--North Carolina." Jama 258(3): 308-9.

CDC (2001). "Revised guidelines for HIV counseling, testing, and referral." MMWR Recomm Rep 50(RR-19): 1-57; quiz CE1-19a1-CE6-19a1.

CDC (2010). "Prevalence and awareness of HIV infection among men who have sex with men --- 21 cities, United States, 2008." MMWR Morb Mortal Wkly Rep 59(37): 1201-7.

CDC (2011). "HIV Transmitted from a Living Organ Donor --- New York City, 2009." MMWR Morb Mortal Wkly Rep 60(10): 297-301.

Check Hayden, E. (2010). "Seek, test and treat' slows HIV." Nature 463(7284): 1006.

Chun, T. W., J. S. Justement, et al. (2007). "Decay of the HIV reservoir in patients receiving antiretroviral therapy for extended periods: implications for eradication of virus." J Infect Dis 195(12): 1762-4.

CMA (1995). "Consensus statement regarding the HIV "window period"." Can Commun Dis Rep 21(24): 213-5.

Cooper, E. R., M. Charurat, et al. (2002). "Combination antiretroviral strategies for the treatment of pregnant HIV-1-infected women and prevention of perinatal HIV-1 transmission." J Acquir Immune Defic Syndr 29(5): 484-94.

Creek, T. L., R. Ntumy, et al. (2007). "Successful introduction of routine opt-out HIV testing in antenatal care in Botswana." J Acquir Immune Defic Syndr 45(1): 102-7.

Dao, H., L. M. Mofenson, et al. (2007). "International recommendations on antiretroviral drugs for treatment of HIV-infected women and prevention of mother-to-child HIV transmission in resource-limited settings: 2006 update." Am J Obstet Gynecol 197(3 Suppl): 42-55.

Das, M., P. L. Chu, et al. (2010). "Decreases in community viral load are accompanied by reductions in new HIV infections in San Francisco." PLoS One 5(6): e11068.

Davis, K. L., E. S. Gray, et al. (2009). "High titer HIV-1 V3-specific antibodies with broad reactivity but low neutralizing potency in acute infection and following vaccination." Virology 387(2): 414-26.

Delwart, E. L., N. D. Kalmin, et al. (2004). "First report of human immunodeficiency virus transmission via an RNA-screened blood donation." Vox Sang 86(3): 171-7.

DHHS and OARAC (2011). Panel on Antiretroviral Guidelines for Adults and Adolescents. Guidelines for the use of antiretroviral agents in HIV-1-infected adults and adolescents.

. D. o. H. a. H. Services.

Dieffenbach, C. W. and A. S. Fauci (2009). "Universal voluntary testing and treatment for prevention of HIV transmission." Jama 301(22): 2380-2.

Douek, D. C., J. M. Brenchley, et al. (2002). "HIV preferentially infects HIV-specific CD4+ T cells." Nature 417(6884): 95-8.

Elkins, D. (2008). "Blood-supply crisis strikes Canada: Sudden 40% drop is unprecedented." Retrieved 29 October,2010, from http://www.canadianmedicinenews.com/2008/10/blood-supply-crisis-strikes-canada.html.

Elliott, A., M. Kizza, et al. (2007). "The impact of helminths on the response to immunization and on the incidence of infection and disease in childhood in Uganda: design of a randomized, double-blind, placebo-controlled, factorial trial of deworming interventions delivered in pregnancy and early childhood." Clin Trials 4(1): 42-57.

Ensoli, F., V. Fiorelli, et al. (1990). "Proviral sequences detection of human immunodeficiency virus in seronegative subjects by polymerase chain reaction." Mol Cell Probes 4(2): 153-61.

Fiebig, E. W., D. J. Wright, et al. (2003). "Dynamics of HIV viremia and antibody seroconversion in plasma donors: implications for diagnosis and staging of primary HIV infection." Aids 17(13): 1871-9.

Grady, D. (2007). Four transplant recipients contract HIV, New York Times.

Granich, R. M., C. F. Gilks, et al. (2009). "Universal voluntary HIV testing with immediate antiretroviral therapy as a strategy for elimination of HIV transmission: a mathematical model." Lancet 373(9657): 48-57.

Gupta, P., L. Kingsley, et al. (1992). "Low prevalence of HIV in high-risk seronegative homosexual men evidenced by virus culture and polymerase chain reaction." Aids 6(2): 143-9.

Hamlyn, E., Jones, V.,Porter, K.,Fidler, S. (2010). "Antiretroviral treatment of primary HIV infection to reduce onward transmission." Curr Opin HIV AIDS 5(4): 283-90.

Hecht, F. M., L. Wang, et al. (2006). "A multicenter observational study of the potential benefits of initiating combination antiretroviral therapy during acute HIV infection." J Infect Dis 194(6): 725-33.

Hladik, F. and M. J. McElrath (2008). "Setting the stage: host invasion by HIV." Nat Rev Immunol 8(6): 447-57.

Hollingsworth, T. D., R. M. Anderson, et al. (2008). "HIV-1 transmission, by stage of infection." J Infect Dis 198(5): 687-93.

Imagawa, D. T., M. H. Lee, et al. (1989). "Human immunodeficiency virus type 1 infection in homosexual men who remain seronegative for prolonged periods." N Engl J Med 320(22): 1458-62.

Jehuda-Cohen, T., J. D. Powell, et al. (1991). "Transmission of retroviral infection by transfusion of seronegative blood in nonhuman primates." J Infect Dis 163(6): 1223-8.

Jehuda-Cohen, T., J. D. Powell, et al. (1994). "Evidence for simian immunodeficiency virus-specific IgM and IgG response in peripheral blood mononuclear cells of serum enzyme-linked immunosorbent assay-negative nonhuman primates." J Acquir Immune Defic Syndr 7(6): 539-50.

Jehuda-Cohen, T., B. A. Slade, et al. (1990). "Polyclonal B-cell activation reveals antibodies against human immunodeficiency virus type 1 (HIV-1) in HIV-1-seronegative individuals." Proc Natl Acad Sci U S A 87(10): 3972-6.

Jehuda-Cohen, T., F. Villinger, et al. (1991). "Presence of SIV antibodies in the sera of infants born to SIV-seronegative monkeys." J Acquir Immune Defic Syndr 4(2): 204-5.

Jehuda-Cohen, T., A. Vonsover, et al. (1992). "'Silent' HIV infection among wives of seropositive HIV carriers in the Ethiopian community in Israel." Scand J Immunol Suppl 11: 81-3.

Kaufmann, D. E., M. Lichterfeld, et al. (2004). "Limited durability of viral control following treated acute HIV infection." PLoS Med 1(2): e36.

Landers, D. V., B. Martinez de Tejada, et al. (1997). "Immunology of HIV and pregnancy. The effects of each on the other." Obstet Gynecol Clin North Am 24(4): 821-31.

Levesque, M. C., M. A. Moody, et al. (2009). "Polyclonal B cell differentiation and loss of gastrointestinal tract germinal centers in the earliest stages of HIV-1 infection." PLoS Med 6(7): e1000107.

Ling, A. E., K. E. Robbins, et al. (2000). "Failure of routine HIV-1 tests in a case involving transmission with preseroconversion blood components during the infectious window period." Jama 284(2): 210-4.

Margoli, D. M. (2009). "Mucosal and Innate Immune Responses, and Viral Reservoirs in Tissues and Cells During Acute HIV-1 Infection." Center for HIV/AIDS Vaccine Immunology (CHAVI).

Marks, G., N. Crepaz, et al. (2006). "Estimating sexual transmission of HIV from persons aware and unaware that they are infected with the virus in the USA." Aids 20(10): 1447-50.

May, M., J. A. Sterne, et al. (2007). "Prognosis of HIV-1-infected patients up to 5 years after initiation of HAART: collaborative analysis of prospective studies." Aids 21(9): 1185-97.

McClure, H. M., D. C. Anderson, et al. (1991). "Maternal transmission of SIVsmm in rhesus macaques." J Med Primatol 20(4): 182-7.

Mestecky, J., Z. Moldoveanu, et al. (2009). "Mucosal immunology of the genital and gastrointestinal tracts and HIV-1 infection." J Reprod Immunol 83(1-2): 196-200.

Mitra, C. (2004). "Human immunodeficiency virus infection in a renal transplant recipien." The Indian J Nephrol 14(1): 25-27.

Mumo, J., A. Vansover, et al. (2009). "Detecting seronegative-early HIV infections among adult versus student Kenyan blood donors, by using Stimmunology." Exp Biol Med (Maywood) 234(8): 931-9.

Myron S. Cohen, J. A. A. a. R. S. (2007). "Host Immune Responses to HIV-1 Acute HIV-1 Infection - Acute HIV-1 Infection prospective cohort study." Center for HIV/AIDS Vaccine Immunology (CHAVI).

NACA (2007). National AIDS Coordinating Agency (2007) 2008 Progress Report of the National Response to the UNGASS Declaration of Commitment on HIV/AIDS, Ministry of State President, National AIDS Coordinating Agency, December 2007.

NACA (2008). "National AIDS Coordinating Agency October to December 2007 National AIDS Council Report, BHRIMS February 2008."

Najioullah, F., V. Barlet, et al. (2004). "Failure and success of HIV tests for the prevention of HIV-1 transmission by blood and tissue donations." J Med Virol 73(3): 347-9.

Novikov, I. and T. Jehuda-Cohen (2009). "HIV type 1 infection among Ethiopian immigrants to Israel: enhanced in vitro antibody stimulation for estimating the length of the window period." AIDS Res Hum Retroviruses 25(2): 165-74.

Olshansky, A. (2008). "Possibility of SMARTube application for optimization of hepatitis C and HIV-infection diagnosis." VIII International Conference «Viral hepatitis: problems of epidemiology, diagnostics, treatment & prevention, Moscow, Russia.

Orenstein, J. M. (2001). "The macrophage in HIV infection." Immunobiology 204(5): 598-602.

Owen, S. M., C. Yang, et al. (2008). "Alternative algorithms for human immunodeficiency virus infection diagnosis using tests that are licensed in the United States." J Clin Microbiol 46(5): 1588-95.

Pantaleo, G., C. Graziosi, et al. (1994). "Role of lymphoid organs in the pathogenesis of human immunodeficiency virus (HIV) infection." Immunol Rev 140: 105-30.

Patterson, K. B., P. A. Leone, et al. (2007). "Frequent detection of acute HIV infection in pregnant women." Aids 21(17): 2303-8.

Phelps, R., K. Robbins, et al. (2004). "Window-period human immunodeficiency virus transmission to two recipients by an adolescent blood donor." Transfusion 44(6): 929-33.

Pilcher, C. D., J. J. Eron, Jr., et al. (2001). "Sexual transmission during the incubation period of primary HIV infection." Jama 286(14): 1713-4.

Pilcher, C. D., H. C. Tien, et al. (2004). "Brief but efficient: acute HIV infection and the sexual transmission of HIV." J Infect Dis 189(10): 1785-92.

Pinkerton, S. D. (2008). "Probability of HIV transmission during acute infection in Rakai, Uganda." AIDS Behav 12(5): 677-84.

Powell, J. D., D. P. Bednarik, et al. (1991). "Regulation of immune activation/retroviral replication by CD8+ T cells." Ann N Y Acad Sci 636: 360-2.

Rangin, A., Y. Wu, et al. (2011). "Injury to the Brain Is Evident Early in HIV Infection." 8th Conference on Retroviruses and Opportunistic Infections (CROI 2011), Boston.

Richman, D. D., T. Wrin, et al. (2003). "Rapid evolution of the neutralizing antibody response to HIV type 1 infection." Proc Natl Acad Sci U S A 100(7): 4144-9.

Rosenberg, E. S., M. Altfeld, et al. (2000). "Immune control of HIV-1 after early treatment of acute infection." Nature 407(6803): 523-6.

Schacker, T. (2008). "The role of secondary lymphatic tissue in immune deficiency of HIV infection." Aids 22 Suppl 3: S13-8.

Schmidt, M., K. Korn, et al. (2009). "First transmission of human immunodeficiency virus Type 1 by a cellular blood product after mandatory nucleic acid screening in Germany." Transfusion 49(9): 1836-44.

Simonds, R. J., S. D. Holmberg, et al. (1992). "Transmission of human immunodeficiency virus type 1 from a seronegative organ and tissue donor." N Engl J Med 326(11): 726-32.

Singer, A. L., L. M. Kucirka, et al. (2008). "The high-risk donor: viral infections in solid organ transplantation." Curr Opin Organ Transplant 13(4): 400-4.

Stacey, A. R., P. J. Norris, et al. (2009). "Induction of a striking systemic cytokine cascade prior to peak viremia in acute human immunodeficiency virus type 1 infection, in contrast to more modest and delayed responses in acute hepatitis B and C virus infections." J Virol 83(8): 3719-33.

Stekler, J. D., P. D. Swenson, et al. (2009). "HIV testing in a high-incidence population: is antibody testing alone good enough?" Clin Infect Dis 49(3): 444-53.

Taylor, C., T. H. Price, et al. (2002). "Possible HCV transmission from blood screened by pooled nucleic acid testing." Transfusion 42(9): 9S-9S.

Titanji, K., V. Velu, et al. (2010). "Acute depletion of activated memory B cells involves the PD-1 pathway in rapidly progressing SIV-infected macaques." J Clin Invest 120(11): 3878-90.

Tomaras, G. D. and B. F. Haynes (2009). "HIV-1-specific antibody responses during acute and chronic HIV-1 infection." Curr Opin HIV AIDS 4(5): 373-9.

Tomaras, G. D., N. L. Yates, et al. (2008). "Initial B-cell responses to transmitted human immunodeficiency virus type 1: virion-binding immunoglobulin M (IgM) and IgG antibodies followed by plasma anti-gp41 antibodies with ineffective control of initial viremia." J Virol 82(24): 12449-63.

Valcour V, S. N., Chalermchai T, Marovich M, Lerdlum S, Suttichom D, Charnnarong N, Jagodzinski L, Michael N, Ananworanich J & RV254/SEARCH 010 Study Group (2011). "HIV Brain Viral and Inflammatory Signature during Acute Infection." 18th Conference on Retroviruses and Opportunistic Infections (CROI 2011). Boston.

Villinger, F., J. D. Powell, et al. (1991). "Detection of occult simian immunodeficiency virus SIVsmm infection in asymptomatic seronegative nonhuman primates and evidence for variation in SIV gag sequence between in vivo- and in vitro-propagated virus." J Virol 65(4): 1855-62.

Walensky, R. P., A. D. Paltiel, et al. (2010). "Test and treat DC: forecasting the impact of a comprehensive HIV strategy in Washington DC." Clin Infect Dis 51(4): 392-400.

Walensky, R. P., L. L. Wolf, et al. (2009). "When to start antiretroviral therapy in resource-limited settings." Ann Intern Med 151(3): 157-66.

Wawer, M. J., R. H. Gray, et al. (2005). "Rates of HIV-1 transmission per coital act, by stage of HIV-1 infection, in Rakai, Uganda." J Infect Dis 191(9): 1403-9.

WHO (2006). "Antiretroviral drugs for treating pregnant women and preventing HIV infection in infants: towards universal.

access. Recommendations for a public health approach .HIV/AIDS Programme,World Health Organization.

WHO (2010). Antiretroviral therapy for HIV infection in adults and adolescents: recommendations for a public health approach - 2010 rev.

Wood, E., T. Kerr, et al. (2009). "Longitudinal community plasma HIV-1 RNA concentrations and incidence of HIV-1 among injecting drug users: prospective cohort study." Bmj 338: b1649.

Workowski, K. A. and S. Berman (2010). "Sexually transmitted diseases treatment guidelines, 2010." MMWR Recomm Rep 59(RR-12): 1-110.

Xu, H., X. Wang, et al. (2011). "Early Divergent Host Responses in SHIVsf162P3 and SIVmac251 Infected Macaques Correlate with Control of Viremia." PLoS One 6(3): e17965.

10

Pearls and Pitfalls of HIV-1 Serologic Laboratory Testing

Jiasheng Shao[1], Yunzhi Zhang[1], Yi-Wei Tang[2] and Hongzhou Lu[1]
[1]*Department of Infectious Diseases*[1]*, Shanghai Public Health Clinical Center, Fudan University, Shanghai*
[2]*Departments of Pathology and Medicine, Vanderbilt University Medical Center, Nashville,*
[1]*People's Republic of China*
[2]*TN, USA*[2]

1. Introduction

1.1 Case 1

A 45-year-old single man presents to a primary care unit with complaints of 'having a prostate problem". He wants to find out whether he has the same condition because his father and elder brother have the same problem. He tells doctors that he has always been in good health except for urinary symptoms. Approximately 1 year ago, he paid a medical visit due to a sore throat. When the patient is asked more closely about other symptoms besides the sore throat, he said that skin rash, coughs, malaise are included. He was prescribed a course of antibiotics and spent a week at home before returned to work. However, it took almost 2 weeks to recover fully. The patient accepts routine HIV testing and other tests specific for STIs are also obtained on the basis of his history. The patient is tested with the standard blood test. He is told that the HIV test results are negative when he returns for follow-up 2 weeks later. He comments that after being made aware of his personal risks, he convinced his wife to be tested (who is negative); because they both had other sex partners with an unknown sex and drug use history during their separation. Although family members and alleged partners, including spouses, should not be notified of a specific person's tests result, the CDC recommends as part of partner services that they should be independently encouraged to have HIV testing as part of routine care (CDC, 2008).

1.2 Case 2

A 21-year-old man comes to the outpatient clinic with complaints of 'burning while urinating' for the past 3 days. Symptoms such as fevers, flank pain, or penile discharge have been denied. He had several sexual partners over the past 6 months. He uses condoms with his casual partners but prefers not to do so with his primary partner. He attributes his present symptoms to condom breakage during sexual intercourse with a casual partner. He tells that he has sex only with men, but denies use of injection drugs. He has never been tested for HIV. Reasons for previously declining are that he 'is usually careful' and, besides, 'Magic Johnson has it and he looks good.' After some discussion, the patient states that he

has had blood drawn at emergency department visits at other hospitals in the past several years. However, he did not return for the test results and assumed that because he was not contacted about the results, all tests, including any for HIV, must be negative. However, he states that he is unemployed and frequently stays with friends at different locations. The patient initially declines HIV screening. He has a family member who works at the local health department and is very concerned that this person would have access to his results if he tested positive. State laws require that positive confirmatory HIV test results be reported to the surveillance division of the respective health department. However, access to test results is restricted to a very few individuals who have signed confidentiality agreements. Additionally, as noted after being reassured about test confidentiality, the patient agrees to screening. His rapid HIV test is reactive. This result was confirmed by follow-up testing. Linkage of patients newly diagnosed HIV positive to further care is very important and relatively brief interventions can be effective (Craw, JA., et al., 2008).
On the basis of other laboratory indices, such as CD4 count and viral load, it appears that the patient has been infected for many years.

1.3 Case 3

A 16-month-old boy presented with prolonged fever and oral candidiasis for the past 6 month. He was a term infant delivered by cesarean section without complications. He was breast-fed for the first 6 days of life and then switched to bottle-feeding. At one month of age, he developed oral candidiasis and was treated with mycostatin, but no effect was observed. Subsequently, he was hospitalized due to prolonged fever and cough and diagnosed with Pseudomonas aeruginosa infection by sputum culture. His cytomegalovirus and adenovirus IgM antibody tests were positive. Ultrasound examination of the abdomen revealed hepatosplenomegaly. His mother was HIV antibody positive one week before delivery, which was subsequently confirmed by a Genetic System HIV-1 Western-blot. Her CD4+ cell count was $212/mm^3$ and viral load was 1.6×10^6 copies/ml. The boy had a rapid HIV-1/2 antibody test performed twice in serum at age 5- and 7-month, which were negative. The Abbott rapid test was repeated at age 7- and 8-month during his hospitalization and the results remained negative; however, HIV-1/2 antibody was detected in his serum by an enzyme-linked immunosorbent assay (TNA-Abb, Dainabot Co., Tokyo, Japan) at the time of readmission when he was 7-mo old. HIV-1 Western-blot was performed in plasma at the Shanghai Centers for Disease Control and prevention, which revealed the presence of a single HIV gp120 band. His HIV viral loads ranged from 1.5 to 2.2×105 copies/ml in plasma during his hospitalization (Zhang, YZ., et al., 2008).

1.4 Case 4

A 26-year-old woman presents to a community-based facility because she suspects that she is pregnant. She has not had a menstrual period for 2 months. She has been married for 5 years, but has no child. The pregnant test is positive. The patient has a family history of sickle cell disease, and she asks about the diseases that she and her unborn child will be screened for as part of the initial prenatal evaluation. The patient was informed of the various screening tests routinely included in the initial prenatal evaluation. Although an HIV test is included in the general consent for obstetric care, she declines. She remarks that she has been monogamous for 5 years and had a negative test 'back then.' She reports having had some marital difficulties 'like all couples,' but she is not concerned about contracting HIV because she 'has never used drugs and is not gay.' Besides, her husband 'would kill me if I ever gave him something'. After the patient spent time discussing her reasons for declining testing and these concerns were addressed by the provider, she realized that she was not being singled out for an HIV test and agreed to screening. The result of the rapid HIV test was negative. She breathes a sigh of relief and discloses that some of her marital problems were due to her husband's infidelity.

2. Discussion and comments

It is estimated currently that 21% of HIV cases in the United States are undiagnosed (Campsmith, ML., et al., 2010). Recent studies showed that missed opportunity visits, i.e., when HIV screening is not included as a routine part of the appraisal or is not offered when it should have been, are very common
(Althoff, KN., et al., 2010; Duffus, WA., et al., 2009). In addition, there will always be a new generation of individuals at risk for HIV acquisition. Screening should be offered regardless of perceived behavioral risk, and the opportunity should not be lost to educate those who test negative. To redirect local health jurisdictions in taking a broader approach to HIV testing in their communities, the CDC published revised recommendations for routine HIV testing in healthcare settings in 2006 (Branson, BM., et al., 2006). These recommendations include routine screening of 13- to 64-year-old patients. However, it may be prudent to screen beyond the recommended older age limit if history suggests continued sexual activity. All patients being screened should be asked about specific behaviors associated with increased risk such as sexual practices, including multiple partners, condom use, and use of performance-enhancing medications and about injection drug use (Adimora, AA., et al., 2003). The CDC further recommends that routine screening take place in all healthcare facilities and institutions, unless prevalence of undiagnosed HIV infection in the patient population has been documented to be <0.1%. If such data are unavailable, routine screening should occur until it has been prospectively established that diagnostic yield is <1 per 1000 patients screened. When a yield of < 1 per 1000 is present, routine screening is no longer warranted and targeted testing should be used. Other recommendations for routine screening include any patient initiating treatment for tuberculosis (Taylor, Z., et al. 2005), because of the increased incidence of coinfection and the requisite modification to HIV therapy in case of coinfection in developing countries (Jiang, XY., et al., 2008). Any patient seeking treatment for an STD should be screened at each visit for a new complaint. Testing should be performed whether the patient is known or suspected to have specific behavioral risks for HIV infection. Repeat screening of persons not likely to be at high risk for HIV should be based on clinical judgment. Individuals at high risk for HIV should be screened at least annually. Indications of high risk include (1) injection drug users and their sex partners, (2) persons who exchange sex for drugs or money, (3) sex partners of HIV-infected individuals, (4) men who have sex with men (MSM), (5) heterosexuals who themselves or whose sex partners have had more than 1 sex partner since their most recent HIV test. Any identified risk exposure within the past 3-6 months should prompt rescreening within the next 3-6 months. If risk behavior continues, periodic testing in 3-6 months is recommended.
A meta-analysis of 11 independent findings (6 comparing HIV-aware persons with independent groups of unaware individuals; 5 comparing seroconverters before and after learning status) demonstrated that HIV-infected individuals were likely to reduce unprotected anal or vaginal intercourse after learning their positive serostatus. After

adjusting data to focus on partners not already infected, the analysis showed a 68% reduction in reports of unprotected anal or vaginal intercourse (Marks, G., et al. 2005). This is important because greater than 80% of HIV cases diagnosed in the United States are among individuals who report sexual exposure (CDC, 2010).

The cost-effectiveness of routine HIV screening has also been demonstrated. Recently, published papers concerning the cost-effectiveness of HIV screening concluded that even when the prevalence of HIV infection in specific populations is substantially lower than 1%, screening for HIV is cost-effective relative to other established screening programs (Farnham, PG., et al., 2008). Sanders indicated that screening was also cost-effective in comparison with other commonly accepted screening programs, even when the known population prevalence of HIV was substantially lower than 1% (Sanders, GD., et al., 2005).

Immediately after infection occurs, there is a rapid rise in plasma viremia with the virus being disseminated widely in the body. During the period from initial infection to complete seroconversion (referred to as primary HIV infection), routine tests for HIV antibody are unable to detect the new infection (Fiebig, EW., et al., 2003). This high concentration of the virus has important public health implications because the HIV diagnosis could be missed, and it is a period of extreme infectiousness
(Wawer, MJ., et al. 2005).

It has been shown that the majority of seropositive patients do not present with symptoms suggestive of HIV infection. Because of their nonspecific nature, it requires a high index of suspicion to associate the symptoms of acute retroviral syndrome (ARS) with primary HIV infection. The signs and symptoms of ARS can develop within days or occur up to weeks after initial exposure. Although these can last from a few days to more than 10 weeks, symptom duration is usually less than 2 weeks (Hecht, FM., et al., 2002). Fever, fatigue, rash, and pharyngitis are the most common symptoms of ARS. Other symptoms include lymphadenopathy, myalgia, headache, arthralgia, aseptic meningitis, weight loss, depression, night sweats, gastrointestinal distress, and oral or genital ulcers. Differential diagnosis includes infectious mononucleosis, secondary syphilis, acute hepatitis A or B, roseola or other viral exanthems, and toxoplasmosis. The occurrence and severity of symptoms during primary HIV infection correlate with the rapidity of clinical and immunologic decline. The nonspecific nature of these symptoms poses a major challenge for diagnosis, and emphasizes the need to obtain an accurate history of possible HIV exposure. For example, primary HIV infection should be considered in any patient with possible exposure presenting with fever of unknown cause (Pincus, JM., et al., 2003). This was especially pronounced in episodic care settings, such as STD clinics, emergency departments and urgent care facilities. The implementation of rapid testing for routine screening can substantially reduce the number of individuals who fail to learn test results, and minimize the expenses allocated to locate persons identified as HIV infected.

3. HIV testing with rapid technology

With the rapid test, as with the standard (conventional) HIV test, the provider should recommend testing, provide information about the test and an explanation of the window period, and give the patient an opportunity to decline or opt out of HIV testing; guides are available online (http://www.cdc.gov/hiv/topics/research/respect-2/counseling/pdf/RESPECT2StandardTestingCounselingProtocol.pdf). A number of US Food and Drug

Administration (FDA)-approved rapid HIV testing products are available (http://www.cdc.gov/hiv/topics/testing/rapid/rt-comparison.htm).

Providers who will be administering the test should be trained, either by the manufacturer or the local health department, in how to use the product available at their facilities. Rapid testing is done in a single session, so a patient should be assessed for their readiness to receive results on the same day. Positive rapid test results are preliminary and must be confirmed by Western blot or direct immunofluorescence assay before a diagnosis of HIV infection is established. However, negative results are considered conclusive and follow-up is not generally required (CDC, 2004).

As previously stated, because of the same-day availability of the results, rapid testing is very suitable for patients who are unlikely to return for their results. It is also the test of choice when an immediate treatment decision needs to be made (e.g., untested woman in labor, occupational or sexual exposure). In order to reduce the mortality, morbidity, and transmission among groups most affected (http://www.cdc.gov/hiv/topics/surveillance/resources/slides/mortality/index.htm), it is important to understand and address the reasons for late testing for HIV. Persons diagnosed with AIDS concurrently or soon after (e.g., 3 or fewer years) receiving their initial HIV test results continue to represent a significant number of missed opportunities for diagnosis and prevention. Although there has been a steady increase in the CD4 counts of infected individuals at initial presentation, a large North American data set found that the average remained below 350 cells/µL, whereas 500 cells/µL is the lower threshold for treatment initiation recommended by the US Department of Health & Human Services HIV treatment guidelines, as of December 2009 (http://www.aidsinfo.nih.gov/contentfiles/AdultandAdolescentGL.pdf). Data from 34 states showed that 38.3% of people who tested positive had progressed to AIDS 1 year or less after initial diagnosis of their HIV infection, and 45% had an AIDS diagnosis within 3 years (Shouse, RL., et al., 2009).

The percentage of individuals with AIDS occurring within 3 years after diagnosis increased with age, ranging from 22.7% in adolescents (13-19 years old) to 63.2% in those older than 60 years of age. Racial disparities were also noted (42.6% whites; 42.9% multiple/unknown race; 46.1% black/African American; 46.1% American Indian/Alaskan native; 48.4% Hispanic/Latino, and 50.4% Asian). A greater proportion of adolescent boys/men (46.9%) compared with adolescent girls/women (41.5%) developed AIDS within 3 years.

Possible reasons for late testing include stigma and homophobia as well as lack of access to testing facilities. Individuals may not seek HIV testing because they do not consider themselves at risk. Also, healthcare providers may not recognize the risk factors for HIV infection or the signs and symptoms of ARS, i.e., the signs and symptoms of primary HIV infection.

4. HIV serologic testing for men who have sex with men (MSM)

National HIV Behavioral Surveillance (NHBS) system estimates and monitors risk behaviors and collects data from metropolitan areas. According to the 2008 NHBS report, nearly 1 in 5 MSM were infected with HIV and 44% were unaware of their serostatus (CDC, 2010), 19% of MSMs were HIV infected, with the highest rates of prevalence among blacks (28%) followed by Hispanics (18%) and whites (16%). Increasing age and lower levels of income and education also were associated with higher prevalence rates. Poverty is also recognized as an important risk factor for HIV infection, and a greater proportion of MSM with no health

insurance and those who had not visited a healthcare provider during the preceding year were unaware of their infection; 55% of those unaware of their infection were not tested during the preceding 12 months.
HIV prevalence was highest among black MSM < 30 years of age. However, the majority of young black and Hispanic MSM in each age group were unaware of their HIV infection. Thus, available data suggest that HIV prevalence among MSM remains high; many HIV infected MSMs are unaware of their serostatus; and minority MSM are disproportionately affected by HIV. The NHBS data underscore the specific need for increased HIV testing efforts directed toward all MSM, especially minorities. It has been demonstrated that about 25% of individuals testing HIV positive and 33% of those testing negative did not return for results of standard testing (Kendrick, SR., et al., 2005).

5. HIV serologic testing for children

Most children were infected with HIV-1 through vertical transmission of the virus. The route of HIV-1 can occur in utero, at the time of labor and delivery, and breastfeeding. Before treatment or interventions to prevent transmission were available, the rate of MTCT of HIV-1 in the United States was approximately 25%. And now, both clinical and laboratory-based methods for the diagnosis of HIV-1 infection in children have been developed. Laboratory-based methods include both immunologic and virological assays. Evaluations of clinical staging systems for the diagnosis of HIV-1 infection in children in sub-Saharan Africa, especially in young infants, have suggested limited sensitivity (Jones, SA., et al., 2005). Laboratory-based methods for the diagnosis of HIV-1 infection can be divided into 2 groups: immunologic and virological. The former includes (1) Detection of HIV-1 Antibodies, (2) Enzyme-Linked Immunosorbent Assays, (3) Rapid Tests which is to detection of IgG antibodies against HIV-1, (3) Semi-quantitative Antibody Assays, (4) Western Blot Assays, (5) Indirect Immunofluorescence Assays, (6) Analysis by Flow cytometry. Virological assay includes HIV-1 Culture, HIV-1 DNA Assays, HIV-1 RNA Assays and p24 Antigen Assays (Read, JS, 2007).
Rapid HIV tests provide results in min, use minimal laboratory equipment, and have been widely used especially in resource-poor settings since their introduction. However, false-negative results have happened, especially when the tests are used in infants. The case showed above demonstrates that the rapid HIV antibody test can result in false-negative results in infants. There are at least two possible explanations for the child's negative rapid HIV-1 antibody results. First, the primary antibody production has been suppressed by the presence of maternal IgG antibodies (Karlsson, MC., et al., 1999).
Secondly, mothers living with HIV were highly immunosuppressed; therefore, the low level of maternally-derived circulating HIV-1 IgG was only detected by HIV-EIA and Western blot. While the antigen components used in the rapid assay merit further investigation, our data indicate that the HIV rapid assay test is not reliable in screening for HIV infection in infants aged <18 months. Due to passive transfer of maternal antibody during pregnancy, infants born to HIV-infected mothers remain antibody-positive into the second year of life, even if they are not infected. For this reason, standard HIV antibody tests cannot reliably confirm HIV infection in infants until after maternal antibodies have disappeared. Tests that can diagnose pediatric HIV infection accurately during the first year of life include HIV-PCR assays, HIV culture, and repeat p24 antigen tests (Shah, I. et al., 2006). The sensitivity and the specificity of an HIV DNA PCR at birth have been estimated to be 50% and 99%,

respectively. The sensitivity of the test improves dramatically in the first weeks of life and reaches a sensitivity of 90% or better when used in infants who are older than 1-mo of age. Two negative tests by PCR or viral culture after 3-mo of age would indicate that a child is not infected and would be more useful than screening serology. Although HIV DNA PCR and HIV RT-PCR are important tests in this clinical situation, they must be interpreted carefully. Several studies demonstrate a high sensitivity for both tests; however, specificities vary among reports. Also, HIV PCR testing should be repeated at regular, defined intervals, preferably lasting until the HIV antibody status of the infant is resolved (Sahni, AK., et al., 2005). HIV RNA amplification assays may be better at detecting HIV-infected infants than DNA PCR. In a cohort study, qualitative nucleic acid sequence-based amplification (NASBA) assay was shown to be highly specific and more sensitive than DNA PCR. NASBA results from infected children were compared with DNA PCR results from the same blood samples taken during the first 3 mo of life from HIV-infected and uninfected children. Sensitivity, specificity, and predictive values were calculated. The conclusion was that qualitative RNA assays (including RT-PCR) may be useful for diagnosing and excluding perinatal HIV infection in children after the first week of life for such purposes as initiating antiretroviral therapy and other treatment, resolving parental uncertainty, determining timing of transmission, and providing endpoints for intervention trials. Infants born to HIV-infected mothers are at great risk of becoming infected with HIV during labor and delivery. HIV is present in breast-milk, and the risk of transmission during breast-feeding depends on several factors including infant age, pattern of breast-feeding, breast-feeding duration, breast health, maternal viral load, and maternal immune status. HIV rapid assay may not be sensitive enough for testing HIV antibodies in infants who are less than 18-mo old. Other sensitive assays, including fourth-generation EIA as well as nucleic acid amplification-based assays should be used.

6. HIV serologic testing for pregnant women

Major successes have been achieved in prevention of (mother-to-child transmission) MTCT of HIV-1 in the United States; the MTCT rate has decreased to less than 2% with antiretroviral treatment of HIV-1–infected pregnant women and, for women who do not yet require treatment of their HIV-1 infection, with the use of the following efficacious interventions to prevent transmission: antiretroviral prophylaxis, cesarean section before labor and before rupture of membranes, 12 and complete avoidance of breastfeeding.

The CDC recommends that all pregnant women receive universal HIV testing as early as possible during prenatal care, with repeat testing in the third trimester in certain circumstances, such as those exhibiting signs or symptoms of infection, those with high-risk behaviors, and those living in or receiving care in areas with a high incidence or prevalence of HIV (identifies 1 HIV infection for every 1000 pregnant women tested). The screening preferably should occur at the first obstetric visit, after the patient has been informed that an HIV test will be performed unless declined (the opt-out screening model). Permission for HIV testing should be included as part of the general consent for healthcare. Clinicians should provide pregnant women with appropriate information in regard to HIV infection, risk factors, and reasons for testing, and transmission risk to ensure an informed decision about screening. Reasons for declining HIV testing should be addressed. If a woman has an unknown test history during prenatal care or undocumented serostatus at labor and delivery, she should be screened at the time of labor or immediately postpartum with a rapid HIV test, unless testing is declined. The majority of women with undocumented HIV testing or serostatus have few or no prenatal care visits. Rapid point-of-care testing during labor has been shown to be effective and accepted, with acceptance rates of 86% among those approached for testing during labor and delivery (Jamieson, DJ., et al., 2007).

The HIV test result of an expectant mother should be documented in her chart as well as in the medical record of her newborn. After appropriate maternal consent is given, maternal and pediatric healthcare providers should both be aware of the mother's HIV serostatus. This is necessary so that appropriate prophylaxis and testing of an HIV-exposed infant can occur, as well as proper management of any potential complications. It is important for pregnant women to know their serostatus as early as possible in the course of pregnancy to prevent transmission to infants and partners (Mofenson, L., et al., 2006; 55).

In 2005, approximately 92% of all HIV/AIDS cases in children younger than 13 years of age were due to vertical (mother-to-child) transmission. In the United States, the use of combination antiretroviral therapy during pregnancy has reduced the transmission rate from approximately 20%-30% to < 2%. Transmission to fetuses and infants can also be prevented through antiretroviral therapy, cesarean delivery, and avoiding breast-feeding. Transmission to partners and others can be prevented by changing previous risk behaviors, such as no or inconsistent condom use and by reducing viral load through antiretroviral treatment.

All patients, including all pregnant women, should be given the option to decline HIV testing. However, the clinician should discuss the reasons for declining testing and document the decision in the medical record. Risks for HIV and reasons for testing should be thoroughly reviewed. A woman may decline HIV testing for many reasons: She may not believe that she is at risk for HIV. Fear also may be influencing her decision, whether it is fear of being HIV positive, fear of discrimination if positive, or fear of partner retribution. Often, women think that they are not at risk for HIV due to a poor understanding of HIV and its risk factors. Women may also be unaware of their partners' HIV or STD risk, which also influences HIV transmission (Witte, SS., et al., 2010).

Other reasons for refusing HIV screening include scheduling conflicts; concerns over cost; health insurance; confidentiality; and other reasons, such as having a previous negative test. Identified issues should be addressed as fully as possible by the provider, with the intent of overcoming barriers and alleviating specific concerns about screening. HIV testing should continue to be recommended at subsequent prenatal visits if this has been refused in earlier visits. However, refusing HIV testing should never affect the level or quality of prenatal care provided to the patient.

7. References

Adimora, AA., Schoenbach, VJ. & Martinson, FE. (2003). Concurrent partnerships among rural African Americans with recently reported heterosexually transmitted HIV infection. Journal of Acquired Immune Deficiency Syndromes, Vol.34, No.4, pp.423-429, ISSN 1525-4135

Althoff, KN., Gange, SJ. & Klein, MB. (2005). Late presentation for human immunodeficiency virus care in the United States and Canada. Clinical Infectious Diseases, Vol. 50, No.11, pp.1512-1520, ISSN 1058-4838

Branson, BM., Handsfield, HH. & Lampe, MA. (2006). Centers for Disease Control and Prevention (CDC). Revised recommendations for HIV testing of adults, adolescents, and pregnant women in health-care settings. Recommendations and Reports: Morbidity and Mortality Weekly Report, Vol. 55, No.11, pp (RR14).1-17, ISSN 1545-8601

Campsmith, ML., Rhodes, PH.. & Hall, HI. (2010). Undiagnosed HIV prevalence among adults and adolescents in the United States at the end of 2006. Journal of Acquired Immune Deficiency Syndromes, Vol.47, No.5, pp.619-624, ISSN 1525-4135

Centers for Disease Control and Prevention. HIV surveillance reports. Diagnoses of HIV infection and AIDS in the United States and dependent areas, 2008. Page last updated: June 14, 2010. Available from: http://www.cdc.gov/hiv/topics/surveillance/resources/reports Accessed October 28, 2010

Centers for Disease Control and Prevention (CDC). (2004). Protocols for confirmation of reactive rapid HIV tests. Morbidity and Mortality Weekly Reports, Vol. 53, pp.221-222, ISSN 1545-8601

Centers for Disease Control and Prevention (CDC). (2010). Prevalence and awareness of HIV infection among men who have sex with men -21 cities, United States, 2008. Morbidity and Mortality Weekly Reports, Vol.59, pp.1201-1207, ISSN 1545-8601

Centers for Disease Control and Prevention (CDC). (2008). Recommendations for partner services programs for HIV infection, syphilis, gonorrhea, and chlamydial infection. Recommendations and Reports: Morbidity and Mortality Weekly Report, Vol. 57(RR-9), pp.1-83, ISSN 1545-8601

Craw, JA., Gardner, LI. & Marks, G. (2008). Brief strengths-based case management promotes entry into HIV medical care: results of the Antiretroviral Treatment Access Study-II. Journal of Acquired Immune Deficiency Syndromes, Vol. 47, No.11, pp.597-606, ISSN 1525-4135

Duffus, WA., Weis, K. & Kettinger, L. (2009). Risk-based HIV testing in South Carolina health care settings failed to identify the majority of infected individuals. AIDS Patient Care and STDS, Vol.23, No.5, pp.339-345, ISSN 1087-7449

Farnham, PG., Hutchinson, AB. & Sansom, SL. (2008). Comparing the costs of HIV screening strategies and technologies in health- care settings. Public Health Reports, Vol. 123 (suppl3), pp.51-62, ISSN 0033-3549

Fiebig, EW., Wright, DJ. & Rawal, BD. (2003). Dynamics of HIV viremia and antibody seroconversion in plasma donors: implications for diagnosis and staging of primary HIV infection. AIDS, Vol.17, No.13, pp.1871-1879, ISSN 1473-5571

Hecht, FM., Busch, MP. & Rawal, B. (2002). Use of laboratory tests and clinical symptoms for identification of primary HIV infection. AIDS, Vol.16, No.8, pp.1119-1129, ISSN 1473-5571

http://www.cdc.gov/hiv/topics/research/respect-2/counseling/pdf/RESPECT2StandardTestingCounselingProtocol.pdf

http://www.cdc.gov/hiv/topics/testing/rapid/rt-comparison.htm

http://www.cdc.gov/hiv/topics/surveillance/resources/slides/mortality/index.htm

http://www.aidsinfo.nih.gov/contentfiles/AdultandAdolescentGL.pdf

Jamieson, DJ., Cohen, MH. & Maupin, R. (2007). Rapid human immunodeficiency virus-1 testing on labor and delivery in 17 US hospitals: the MIRIAD experience. American Journal of Obstetrics and Gynecology, Vol.197 (suppl3), pp.S72-S82, ISSN 0002-9378

Jiang, X., Lu, H. & Zhang Y. (2008). A cross-sectional study of HIV and tuberculosis coinfection cases in mainland China. Southern Medical Journal, Vol.101, No.9, pp.914-917, ISSN 0038-4348

Jones, SA., Sherman, GG. & Coovadia, AH. (2005). Can clinical algorithms deliver an accurate diagnosis of HIV infection in infancy? Bulletin of World Health Organization, Vol.83, No.7, pp.559–560, ISSN 0042-9686

Karlsson, MC., Wernersson, S. & Diaz de Stahl T. (1999). Efficient IgG-mediated suppression of primary antibody responses in Fcgamma receptor-deficient mice. Proceeding of the National Academy of Science of United States of America, Vol.96, No.5, pp.2244-2249, ISSN 1091-6490

Kendrick, SR., Kroc, KA. & Withum, D. (2005). Outcomes of offering rapid point-of-care HIV testing in a sexually transmitted disease clinic. Journal of Acquired Immune Deficiency Syndromes, Vol.38, No.2, pp.142-146, ISSN 1525-4135

Marks, G., Crepaz, N. & Senterfitt, JW. (2005). Meta-analysis of high-risk sexual behavior in persons aware and unaware they are infected with HIV in the United States: implications for HIV prevention programs. Journal of Acquired Immune Deficiency Syndromes, Vol.39, No.4, pp.446-453, ISSN 1525-4135

Mofenson, L., Taylor, AW. & Rogers, M. (2006). Achievements in public health: reduction in perinatal transmission of HIV infection -United States, 1985-2005. Morbidity and Mortality Weekly Report, Vol.55, pp.592-597, ISSN 0149-2195

Pincus, JM., Crosby, SS. & Losina, E. Acute human immunodeficiency virus infection in patients presenting to an urban urgent care center. Clinical Infectious Diseases, 2003; 37:1699-1704

Read, JS. (2007). Diagnosis of HIV-1 infection in children younger than 18 months in the United States. Pediatrics, Vol.120, No.6, pp.1547-1562, ISSN 0031-4005

Sahni, AK., Gupta, RM. & Jena, J. (2005). Early detection of HIV-1 in infants by PCR. Indian Journal of Pathology and Microbiology, Vol.48, No.1, pp.49-52, ISSN 0974-5130

Sanders, GD., Bayoumi, AM. & Sundaram, V. (2005). Cost-effectiveness of screening for HIV in the era of highly active antiretroviral therapy. The New England Journal of Medicine, Vol.352, No.6, pp.570-585, ISSN 1533-4406

Shah, I. (2006). Efficacy of HIV PCR techniques to diagnose HIV in infants born to HIV infected mothers–an Indian perspective. Journal of Association of Physicians of India, Vol.54, pp.197-199, ISSN 0004-5772

Shouse, RL., Kajese, T. & Hall, HI. (2009). Late HIV testing-34 states, 1996-2005. Morbidity and Mortality Weekly Report, Vol.58, pp.661-665, ISSN 1545-8601

Taylor, Z., Nolan, CM. & Blumberg, HM. (2005). American Thoracic Society, Centers for Disease Control and Prevention, Infectious Diseases Society of America. Controlling tuberculosis in the United States: recommendations from the American Thoracic Society, CDC, and the Infectious Diseases Society of America. Recommendations and Reports: Morbidity and Mortality Weekly Report, Vol.54 (RR12), pp.1-81, ISSN 1545-8601

Wawer, MJ., Gray, RH. & Sewankambo, NK. (2005). Rates of HIV-1 transmission per coital act, by stage of HIV-1 infection, in Rakai, Uganda. Journal of Infectious Diseases, Vol.191, No.9, pp.1403-1409, ISSN 1528-8366

Witte, SS, El-Bassel, N. & Gilbert, L. (2010). Lack of awareness of partner STD risk among heterosexual couples. Perspectives on Sexual and Reproductive Health, Vol.42, No.1, pp.49-55, ISSN 1931-2393

Zhang, YZ., Wang, J. & Wilson, GJ. (2008). Negative results of a rapid antibody test for HIV in a 16-month-old infant with AIDS. Annals of Clinical and Laboratory Science, Vol.38, No.3, pp.293-295, ISSN 1550-8080

11

Surgical Pathology in HIV Infection in the Era of Antiretroviral Therapy

Mónica Belinda Romero-Guadarrama
Hospital General De México,
O.D., Medicine School National Autonomous University of Mexico (Unam)
Mexico City

1. Introduction

The natural history of infection with human immunodeficiency virus (HIV) has changed with the introduction of antiretroviral therapy (Fischl et al 1987), these drugs have the ability to inhibit viral replication and immune recovery of infected patients (Lalezari et al 1999). This has resulted in reduced mortality and morbidity caused by this viral infection (Mellors et al 1996). The human immunodeficiency viruses have extraordinary structural and evolutionary complexity since its original identification and description for over 25 years. Nine subtypes are known and three different subtypes, a total of 12, with subtype C HIV-1 responsible for more than half of infections in the world. The molecular and genetic study of HIV reflects the enormous and increasing variability of these organisms (Hue et al 2005).

The HIV viruses are highly variable and are adapted to the selective pressure of antiretroviral drugs, hence antiviral treatments, which started 19 years ago have selected strains with resistance mutations that complicate or invalidate the continuity of certain treatments and sometimes of all.

The geographical distribution and the percentage in the distribution of transmission pathways of the disease have changed over the past 25 years that have elapsed since the start of the epidemic (CDC, 2002). AIDS is an emerging disease in countries of the former Soviet Union, China, and sub-Saharan countries, the number of children and adults who are being infected is higher, producing a characteristic accelerating effect of prolonged epidemics. The AIDS program of the United Nations estimates that by the end of 2005, the total number of people worldwide living with HIV-/-AIDS was 40.3 million, 64% are in sub-Saharan Africa (WHO, 2005). In Europe 294,571 cases were reported in late 2004, 18.6% were women and 3.7% were children. The main transmission groups in Europe are injecting drug users (38.1%), homosexual contacts (29.5%), and heterosexual contacts (20%), although these parameters are not evenly distributed across the continent. While there has been an overall decrease of 6.7% over the previous year 2004 (HIV EURO 2005). In Mexico, the first case was diagnosed in 1983 and currently the largest number of cases (38.400) live in Mexico City, that is 17% of all HIV cases in the country for 2010. The age of onset is 15 to 49 years, 87% are men and 13% are women. The main route of infection is homosexual practice. In this country, AIDS is the third leading cause of death nationally among men 25 to 34 years and the sixth among women in this age group (http: // www. aid-sida-org/estadistic05.htlm).

The clinical presentation of AIDS varies from one geographic area to another according to the most prevalent transmission groups.
The purpose of this chapter is to conduct a general review of infectious agents and neoplasmas associated with some viral agents in the era of antiretroviral treatment of HIV-infected patients in specimens obtained by biopsy, surgical resection, or cytology material.

2. HIV infection

HIV infects several human cell types such as macrophages and glial cells, but its real target cell is the lymphocyte CD4+ and the following pathogenic processes divided into three periods can be disthinguished.
Primary infection during which the virus spreads to lymphoid organs. It is characterized by high levels of viremia and lasts between two and six weeks, patients have nonspecific symptoms. A few days after the initial infection occurs, they produce large amounts of viruses in activated lymphocytes from the lymph nodes, causing inflammation in the nodal lymphoid tissue. The first reaction of immunity against infection is provided by CD8+ cytotoxic lymphocytes, or CTL, which lyse infected cells that present viral antigens on their surface. The virus is never removed during primary infection, since it maintains a residual viral replication, which is detected in plasma or lymph nodes. Escape mutants seem to evade, by mutation in certain epitopes, the immune pressure of helper T lymphocytes and memory cells, there by escaping destruction CTL (Stremlau et al 2004). A few weeks after infection, there is a significant depletion of CD4+ cells in the digestive tract, long before CD4+ levels in blood are altered. One explanation for this activity in the gastrointestinal tract could be because cells in this area have the co-receptor CCR5, which is used by HIV to infect cells. (Pierson et al 2002)
The second period is the chronic asymptomatic infection, the average duration of this phase is 10 years, it is characterized by stable levels of CD4+ with a tendency to decrease progressively, the viral load drops and may be undetectable, but the virus continues its replication in the lymphoid tissue. The causes of decline in CD4+ cells during this phase of infection are only partially known. The increase in viral load and decreased CD4+ during this phase correlate inversely, but sometimes describe curves of complex kinetics that suggest the presence of multiple factors that influence the lysis of infected lymphocytes and the production of new virus particles. CD8+ lymphocytes remain slightly increased during this phase, indicating the existence of cytotoxic reactions against the virus and viral antigens are detected in follicular dendritic cells. Viral sub-populations become more heterogeneous.
Advanced HIV infection or AIDS. At this stage of the disease, the individual develops opportunistic infections, as CD4+ lymphocyte counts are lower than 200/µl viral replication is accelerated, the activity of anti-HIV CTL declines, and lymphoid morphology is destroyed. Lymphoid tissue degeneration may be due to replication of the virus, or may be an indirect consequence of chronic immune stimulation. Neurological tropism of the infection is observed and produced viruses are less sensitive to neutralizing antibodies.

3. Opportunistic infections

Among the most common opportunistic infections in Mexico and Spain are tuberculosis, Pneumocystis carinii pneumonia and esophageal candidiasis (Secretariat of the National Plan on AIDS 2005). While the introduction of new triple therapies have increased survival of patients infected with HIV, AIDS remains a disease with high mortality rate. Most

opportunistic infections occur as reactivation of latent infections that reappears when the immune system can no longer control them. The current frequency of opportunistic infections varies in different regions and have declined due to active antiretroviral therapy (HAART) (Kaplan et al 2000). From 15 to 30% of non treated HIV-infected patients develop pneumonia during the course of the disease caused by *Pneumocystis jiroveci*. Today opportunistic infections are less common in patients who respond to treatment with HAART. Among infections not associated with AIDS are some that appear in the general population, and have a higher incidence in patients with HIV infection, such as pneumococcal pneumonia, oropharyngeal candidiasis, or herpes zoster. A list of viral, bacterial, and fungal microorganisms that occur in patients with AIDS exists. These can even occur in patients with antiretroviral treatment and immune imbalance. (Table 1).
There are differences in the prevalence and incidence of some diseases that can be attributed to the characteristics of the population, climate, endemic diseases, to standards of hygiene, and medical care availability and pharmacology, as well as to socioeconomic and cultural factors.

Opportunistic infections in HIV patients
Helminthic and Protozoal Infections:
Cryptosporidiosis or isosporiasis (enteritis)
Toxoplasmosis (CNS Infection or pneumonia)
Fungal Infections
Pneumocystosis (pneumonia or Disseminated Infection)
Candidiasis (esophageal, tracheal, or pulmonary)
Cryptococcosis (CNS Infection)
Coccidioidomycosis (Disseminated)
Histoplasmosis (Disseminated)
Bacterial Infections
Mycobacteriosis ("atypical" Mycobacterim eg avium intracellulare, Disseminated or extrapulmonary; M. tuberculosis, pulmonary or extrapulmonary)
Salmonella Infections, Disseminated
Viral Infections
Cytomegalovirus (pulmonary, intestinal, retinitis or CNS infections)
Herpes simplex virus (localized or disseminated)
Varicella zoster virus (localized or disseminated)
Progressive multifocal leukoencephalopathy

Table 1.

3.1 Description of opportunistic microorganisms

3.1.1 Mycoses

Fungal infections are common in patients with HIV infection. Morbidity and mortality are influenced by antiretroviral treatment because of the close relationship between the degree of immunodeficiency, the frequency, and severity of fungal infections.

The advent of HAART and new antifungal agents, such as voriconazole and caspofungin, have decreased the incidence of fungal infections associated with HIV. Although, the causal agent can be clinically suspected, samples can be collected from some body fluids and other sites for the diagnosis, as for example puncture-/-aspiration of abscesses, puncture of cerebrospinal fluid, and from bile, pericardial, pleural, peritoneal, liquids. Bone marrow aspiration, nails, sputum, biopsies of deep tissues or skin, urine and blood. In tissues, the opportunistic organism can be suspected but to know the etiological agent, cultures must be made. (Romani 2004)

Fungal Yeasts: Candida and Cryptococcus Genera.

Candidiasis is the most common fungal infection in these patients, the most common clinical presentation of oropharyngeal candidiasis and vaginal candidiasis in women, occurs with greater frequency and severity than in the rest of the population and they are recurrent. Usually the diagnosis is clinical, by positive culture or visualization of the yeast through Gram staining. In the cervico-vaginal smears. Candida sp. can be morphologically suspected by the presence of yeasts and spores in the cellular smears and observing abundant inflammatory infiltration of polymorphonuclear cells. When the patient presents oropharyngeal candidiasis and dysphagia, diagnosis can be made by endoscopy and biopsy. Finally, invasive candidiasis is uncommon in AIDS patients, but, when present, bronchial or pulmonary candidiasis is observed in the final stages of the disease. (Whiteway et al, 2004).

Cryptococcus neoformans is a worldwide distributed yeast of, spherical shape produced by a single budding unique and posesses a mucopolysacharide capsule that confers virulence. Depending on the capsular polysaccharides four serotypes named A, B, C, and D have been described. According to these serotypes, there are two varieties: C. neoformans (serotypes A and D), which is the most common in patients with AIDS and C. vargatti neoformans (serotypes B and C). Exposure to the organism is frequent and the route of entry is the respiratory tract. The most common clinical form is meningoencephalitis and two-thirds of patients course with extrameningeal dissemination C. neoformans may disseminate widely to the skin, liver, spleen, adrenals and bones. The fungi induce a chronic granulomatous reaction comprising macrophages, lymphocytes, and foreign body-type giant cells. Suppuration also may occur, as well as a rare granulomatous arteritis of the circle of Willis. The diagnosis is made in the positive culture of cerebrospinal fluid or blood (Fig.1).

When evaluating the cerebrospinal fluid cytology, it is possible to observe the characteristics of encapsulated yeasts. The capsule does not stain with standard dyes, making it necessary to use china ink or Mayer's mucicarmine. The sensitivity of the test can reach 75%. Cryptococcosis is higher among HIV-infected persons with fewer than 100 $CD4^+$ lymphocytes/μl (Eisenman et al 2007).

Aspergillus sp

The incidence of invasive aspergillosis in patients infected with HIV is very low due to the spread of highly active antiretroviral therapy (HAART). Risk factors include neutropenia and steroid therapy. Aspergillus fumigatus is the most common species to cause disease, and it produces severe invasive infections in immunocompromised individuals. The usual location is the lung. Diagnosis is difficult because the isolation of Aspergillus sp from respiratory secretions has little value: when respiratory symptoms and pulmonary infiltrates are present, the value of Aspergillus sp. isolation from respiratory secretions increases. The detection of antigens such as galactomannans by ELISA or beta-1-3 glucan is more valuable. Another diagnostic test with a great potential is the polymerase chain reaction (PCR).

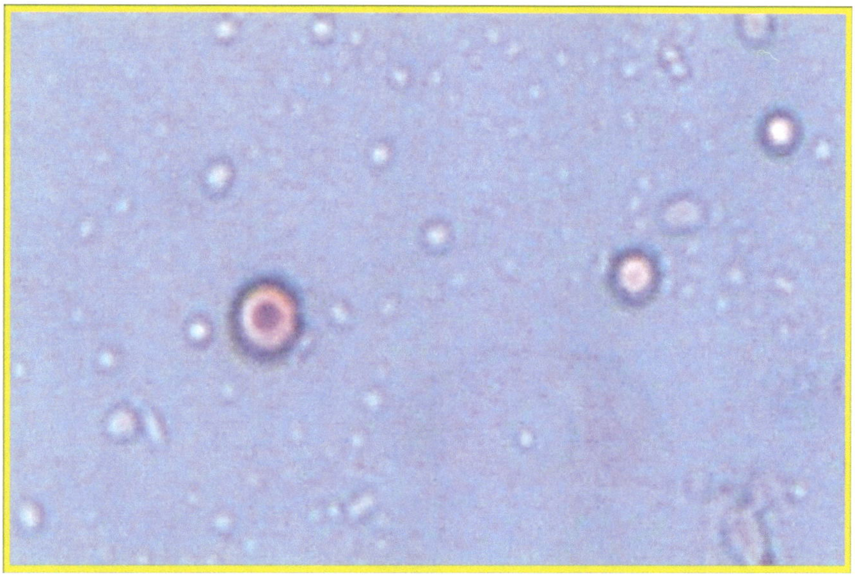

Fig. 1. Cryptococcus neoformans in cerebrospinal fluid. (40X China ink)

Morphology: Colonizing aspergillosis (aspergilloma) usually implies growth of the fungus in pulmonary cavities with minimal or no invasion of the tissues. Invasive aspergillosis is an opportunistic infection that is confined to immunosuppressed hosts. The primary lesions are usually in the lung, but widespread hematogenous dissemination with involvement of the heart valves and brain is common. Definitive diagnosis requires histological demonstration of hyphae in tissue and can be more evident if special stains such as periodic acid-Schiff and silver stains are performed, but the fungus must be isolated from sterile samples.

Sporothirx schenckii.

Sporotrichosis is an uncommon infection. The most common form of infection is cutaneous inoculation by contaminated sharps objects and clinical diagnosis is facilitated by the typical lymphocutaneous lesions. Recommended tests for diagnosis should be a skin biopsy and analysis of the purulent material. The pulmonary, musculoskeletal, and other less common forms occur in patients with cellular immunosuppression. The diagnosis is clinical, morphological, and through cultures.

Histoplasma capsulatum.

This microorganism is distributed in the American continent, but in Africa there is a variant of the disease caused by H. capsulatum, variety duboisii. It is a dimorphic fungus and produces common endemic mycosis in HIV-positive patients. The primary infection occurs by conidia inhalation. There are three clinical forms: acute primary infection, pulmonary cavity and acute disseminated infection, which is the most frequent in AIDS patients. The diagnosis is made by culture of respiratory, bone marrow samples, or by biopsy of lymph node, liver, lung, or skin (Fig.2). Methenamine-silver and PAS stainings are useful for its detection in biological fluids and tissues. It in tissue from patients with AIDS, abundant organisms in macrophages can be observed, in general there is no chronic granulomatous reaction. (Isenberg, 2004)

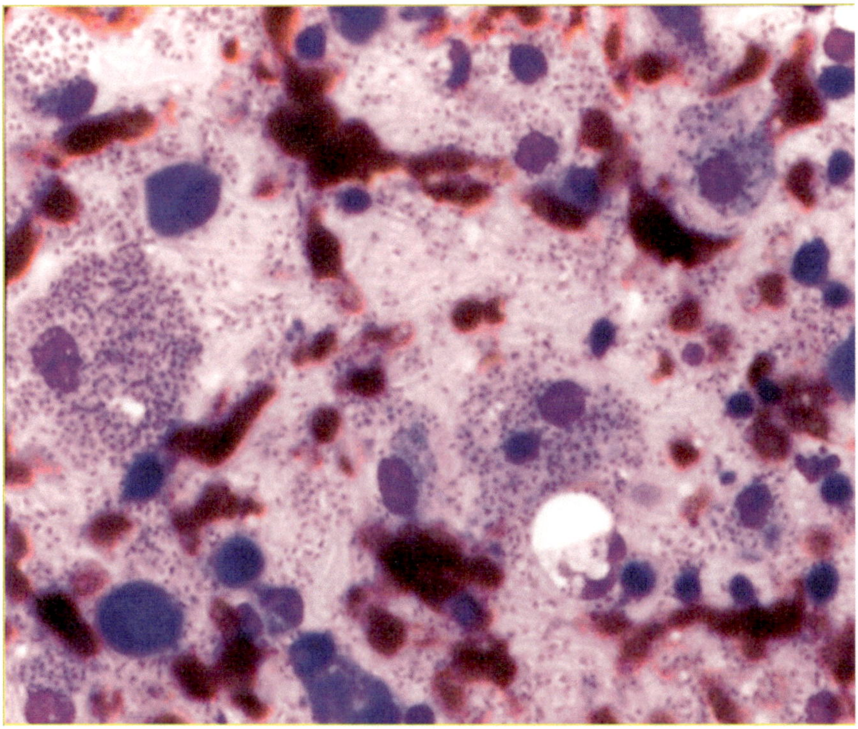

Fig. 2. Histoplasmosis in macrophages in a cervical lymph node. Aspiration biopsy. (PAS stain 40X)

Coccidioides immitis.
It is the causal agent of coccidioidiomicosis. It is a dimorphic fungus and is found in temperate areas of the American continent. The disease is acquired by inhalation of arthroconidia or cutaneous inoculation. There are three clinical forms: cutaneous, asymptomatic, and the disseminated form. The disseminated form was common before the era of HAART in endemic areas. The diagnosis is based on direct examination and culture of sputum, blood, broncho-alveolar lavage, skin and others. In tissue, spherules with endospores are observed and, as in other mycoses, special stains must be performed to identify the organism.
Blastomyces dermatitidis
This is a dimorphic fungus. Its natural habitat is the North American continent, although cases have been reported in Africa, Asia, and Europe. The initial infection is pulmonary, when there is hematogenous spread, it may affect the skin, bones, genitourinary and central nervous systems. In a fresh examination of sputum, skin lesions, or biopsy material characteristic yeast-like elements can be observed that allow for the presumptive diagnosis.
Other dimorphic fungi that occur in HIV patients in specific regions, such as Brazil and China, are Paracoccidioides brasiliensis and Penicillium marneffei, respectively (Patrick, 2003).

3.1.2 Virus infections

Cytomegalovirus.
The diagnosis of cytomegalovirus (CMV) must to rely on laboratory tests. Among the diagnostic tests used are: serological diagnosis, which a little use in HIV-positive patients.

Latex agglutination, or ELISA methods are recommended. Direct detection of the virus or its antigens. Cytological and histological techniques have insufficient sensitivity. However, it is the method of choice for CMV gastrointestinal involvement. If an immunohistochemical technique is used, it can improve the specificity. When there is lung disease, cytopathic changes can be observed in cells obtained from bronchial lavage or sputum. The culture is the gold standard for its specificity for the diagnosis of active infection.

Cytomegalovirus affection caused widespread disease and caused severe damage to the eyes and the gastrointestinal tract, chorioretinitis appeared in 25% of patients with HIV before the advent of HAART, but the condition has declined dramatically (Gerner, et al 1990). The condition of the gastrointestinal tract is observed in 5 to 10% of cases and manifests as ulcerative esophagitis. Detection in biopsies has a positive predictive value, but due to insufficient sensitivity of the samples are should be taken with the diagnosis through this route, ideally tissue should be used, being PCR the most sensitive technique for the diagnosis (Gleaves et al 1984).

Herpes simplex virus and varicella-zoster virus.

The diagnosis of infections with herpes simplex virus (HSV) and varicella zoster virus is basically through clinical criteria, but the severity of some cases or atypical clinical presentation warranted to confirm the diagnosis with laboratory tests (Ashley 1989).

The samples for diagnosis of viral infection are obtained by scraping and taking smears of mucocutaneous lesions, but also by biopsies and respiratory samples.

The affection caused by the herpes simplex virus is manifested by mucocutaneous ulcers in lips, esophagus, external genitals and perianal region. It is possible to see the cytopathic effect on a smear of the mucocutaneous ulcer (Fig. 3)

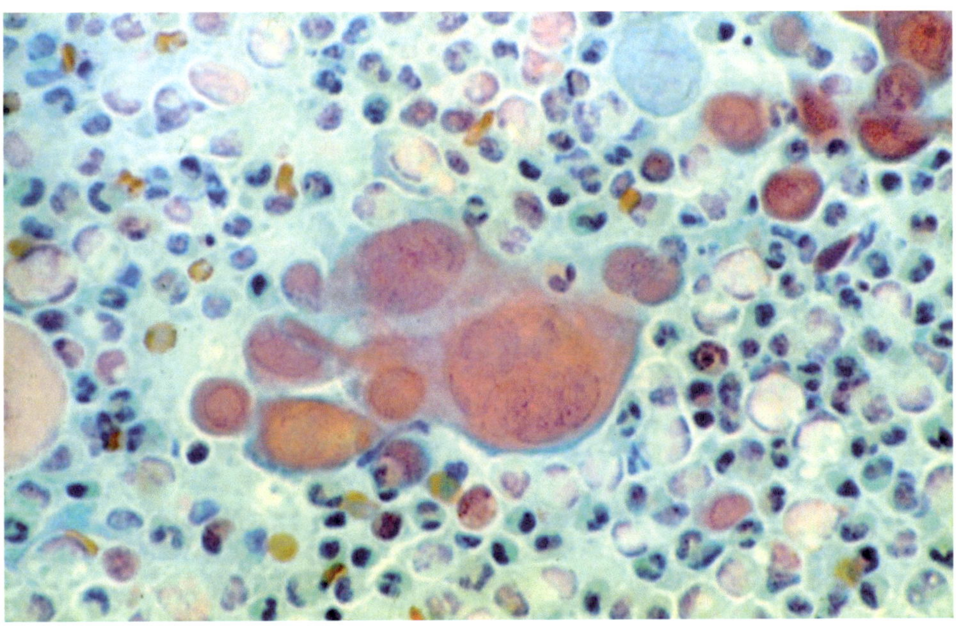

Fig. 3. Herpex simplex virus with cell inclusions or cytophatic effect in perianal region. (40X Papanicolaou stain)

Amplification by PCR is the method of choice for the diagnosis of central nervous system infections in the case of infection with varicella zoster virus. (Gerson et al 1991)
JC polyomavirus.
Compared to other opportunistic infections, new antiretroviral therapies have not had much impact on the occurrence of progressive multifocal leukoencephalopathy. It is possible to observe this complication even in patients virologically stable and the prognosis remains unfavorable. The diagnosis is clinical, supplemented by imaging studies and, at times, with histopathologic examination. Virological diagnosis is restricted to few laboratories and to the use of molecular techniques and electron microscopy.
The samples for the diagnosis are obtained from cerebrospinal fluid biopsies or from autopsies of patients who died from the disease (Athur et al 1989).

3.1.3 Mycobacterial infections: Mycobacterium tuberculosis and non tuberculous mycobacteria

The diagnosis of tuberculosis in HIV-infected patients may be difficult for many reasons, for the multiple atypical clinical and radiological presentations, negative value of the PPD cutaneous reaction, less sensitive bacilloscopies, and on the other hand by the appearance of multidrug-resistant M. tuberculosis strains, possible malabsorbtion, and the disturbing interaction between protease inhibitors and rifampicin. Besides the infection caused by tuberculosis mycobacteria (M.tuberculosis and M. bovis), infection caused by non-tuberculous mycobacteria are frequent in AIDS patientes. Of these the mycobacteria of the avium-intracellulare complex, which constitute the most important pathogen group, where disseminated disease was one of the most common opportunistic infections in these patients. Treatment with antiretrovirals has greatly decreased the disseminated disease mainly in the United States. Diagnosis is made in the following samples: simple or spontaneous sputum tissues (lymphoid tissue biopsies or lung) in sterile liquid such as pleura, pericardium and urine (Pfyffer et al 2003). Molecular biology techniques increases diagnostic sensitivity. In the tissue numerous acid-fast bacilli in alveolar macrophages or tissue are identified, and chronic granulomatous reaction in patients with advanced disease is absent (FTAA and Telent, 1997) (Fig. 4 and Fig. 5).
Other bacterial infections in HIV patients are syphilis caused by Treponema pallidum that causes ulcerative lesions and papules in the genital and anorectal areas.
Biopsy specimens of tissue or lymph node involvement may reveal the presence of treponema, which are apparent with the help of special stains for bacteria or by direct immunofluorescence. (Musher et al 1990).
Some antiretroviral drugs cause other diseases, such as, lipodystrophy and immune reconstitution syndrome, the clinical manifestations are mainly cutaneous (Mudroch et al 2008)
More than half of the manifestations of immune reconstitution syndrome occur in the skin. It has been reported that 10 to 25% of patients starting antiretroviral treatment suffer from this syndrome 90 days later (Rodwell, et al 2008). The most common diagnoses are folliculitis for any reason, reactivation of herpes virus infections, and molluscum contagiosum. Fungal infections, such as ringworm infections of the body and head, as well as systemic mycoses caused by Cryptoccocus (Lehloenya and Mentjes 2006).
It is important to take into account the latter cutaneous manifestations in patients with AIDS.

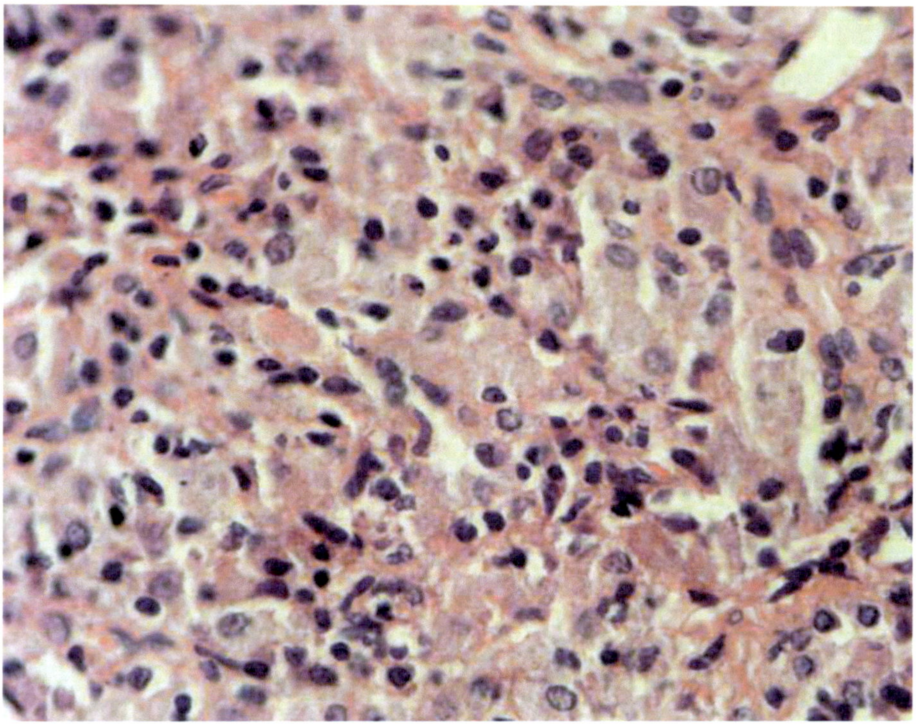

Fig. 4. Lymph node histologic section with histiocytes and lymphocytes in a patient with atypical Mycobacterium. (H-E 10X)

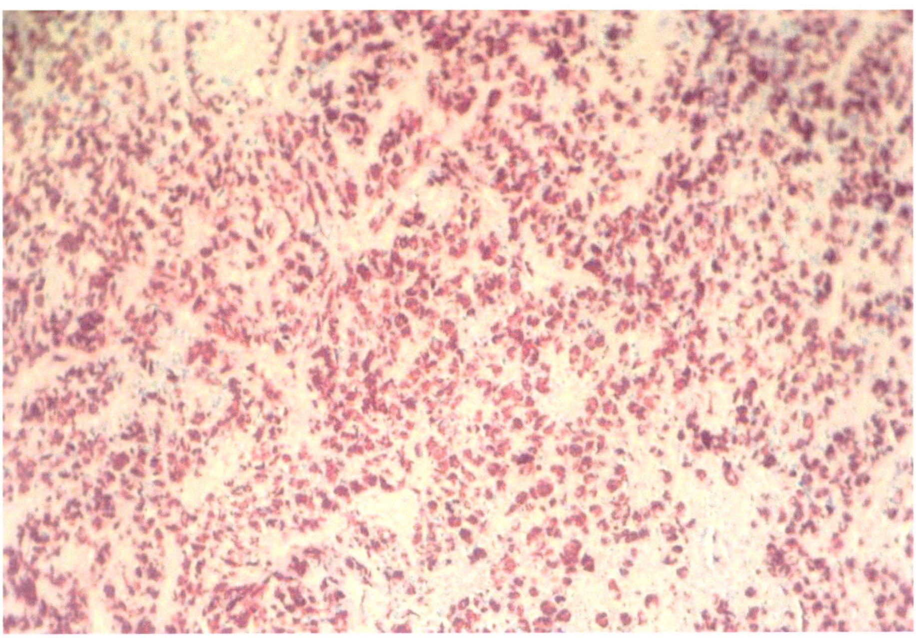

Fig. 5. Sheets of foamy macrophages are seen, which are packed with Mycobacterium demonstrated with acid-fast stains (10X)

4. Neoplasms

The common malignancies in HIV patients are associated with oncogenic DNA viruses like Epstein-Barr virus, Human Herpes virus 8, and human papilloma virus, related to non-Hodgkin and Hodgkin lymphomas, Kaposi's sarcoma, and squamous cell carcinomas such as cervical and anal carcinomas (Table 2).

Lymphoid neoplasms and neoplastic lesions in patients with HIV.
Kaposi sarcoma: cutaneous
and extracutaneous (lung, liver, gastrointestinal tract, lymph node involvement)
Hodgkin lymphoma
Non-Hodgkin's lymphoma immunophenotype B.
B lymphoma diffuse large cells (immunoblastic morphologic variant)
Primary lymphoma of the central nervous system.
B lymphoma serous cavities.
Plasmablastic lymphoma.
Burkitt lymphoma
B-cell lymphoma, marginal zone MALT
Linfoplasmacitoide lymphoma
Plasma cell neoplasms.
Lymphomas T.
Anaplastic lymphoma.
Specific peripheral T cell lymphoma
Lymphoma T / NK nasal type.
And more rarely others.
Non-neoplastic lesions that may mimic lymphoma in patients with HIV.
Multicentric Castleman disease.
CD 8 lymphocytosis syndrome
Lymphoid interstitial pneumonitis and other
epithelial tumors.
Squamous cell carcinoma of varying degrees of differentiation of the uterine cervix.
Squamous cell carcinoma of anus.
Squamous cell carcinoma of oral cavity

Table 2.

4.1 Kaposi sarcoma

Kaposi sarcoma (KS) is the most common malignancy in these patients, affecting homosexual individuals, but can be seen in any patient with HIV (Mitsuyasu 1990). In recent years, various studies have suggested that the herpes virus HHV-8 plays an important role in the pathogenesis of epidemic, endemic, African, and immunosuppressed Kaposi's sarcoma. It has also been observed in lymphomas cavities (Engels et al 2003). The incidence of KS has declined in recent years with the use of HAART; in most patients it presents with skin lesions, lymph node involvement and less commonly, oral mucosal or gastrointestinal tract lesions. In over 50% of patients with cutaneous KS, visceral involvement can be detected, such as small intestine and colon. Other affected organs are lung, lymph nodes, liver, heart, and brain.

Histologically, KS lesions are characterized by a proliferation of spindle cells forming vascular channels and expressing markers for endothelial cells and smooth muscle cells (Fig 6). Another change observed is the presence of chronic inflammatory infiltrate. It is believed that the injuries can come from a primitive mesenchymal precursor cell vascular channel. In the pathogenesis of KS, it is believed that spindle cells produce pro-inflammatory and angiogenic factors (Ganem 2006). Clinically, KS is more aggressive in HIV patients than in the sporadic form of the disease.

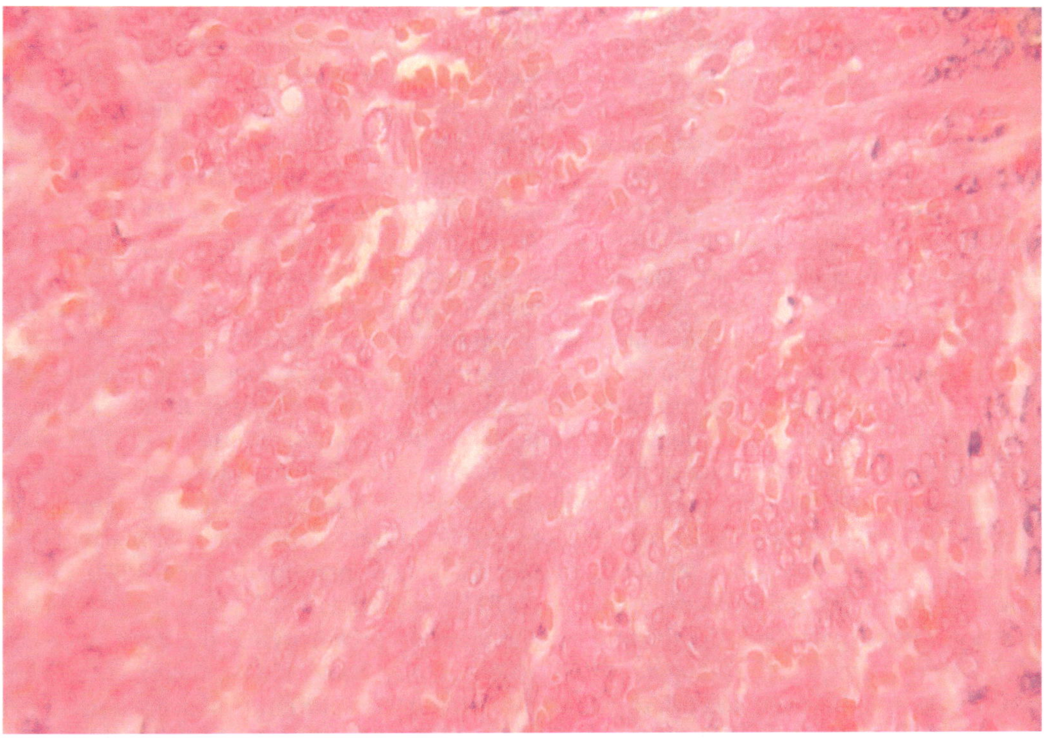

Fig. 6. Kaposi Sarcoma proliferation of spindle cells and vascular channels (H-E10X)

4.2 Lymphomas in HIV patients

The first cases of non-Hodgkin lymphoma (NHL) in patients with HIV infection were reported in homosexual subjects in 1982 and the first multicenter study of NHL in patients with HIV infection was published in 1984 (Ziegler et al 1984).

4.3 Non-Hodgkin lymphomas

In recent years we have recognized certain subtypes of uncommon NHL that appears almost exclusively in patients with HIV infection, such as primary effusion lymphoma, other types of lymphomas have peculiar clincopathological characteristics possibly as a result of immunosuppression. (Goedert et al 1998) These include Hodgkin lymphoma (HL), diffuse large B cell lymphomas, plasmablastic lymphoma (Selik and Rabkin 1998). Other lymphomas described in these patients in which no increased incidence has been described are: MALT-type marginal zone B lymphoma of the digestive tract, lymphoplasmacytoid lymphoma, chronic lymphocytic leukemia, solitary bone and extramedullary plasmacytoma, and immature T lymphomas (lymphoma/ lymphoblastic leukemia) and mature such as the perpheral unespecific T lymphoma, and in our country the nasal type lymphoma T / NK (Gonzalez et al 1998) (Tirelli et al 1995). Other hematological malignancies often described with variable frequencies are some leukemias myeloblastic and chronic myeloproliferative syndromes. Among non-neoplastic lymphoid processes are the multicentric Castleman disease, the CD 8 lymphocytosis syndrome, lymphoid interstitial pneumonitis and the polymorphous polyclonal lymphoproliferative disease B. (Table 2).

Lymphomas in patients with HIV infection are heterogeneous and often result from complex and sequential interaction of several factors (Knowles 1999; Baiocchi1999), such as chronic antigenic activation of B lymphocytes, where maintained stimulation and proliferation of B lymphocytes can be induced by the HIV infection itself, but other mechanisms exist mostly viral, as well as the continuous production of cytokines in response to infection by HIV. High serum concentration are detected of the following interleukins: IL-6, IL-10, and IL-12; it is though that these cytokines are relevant in the polyclonal expansion phase of B lymphocytes. Another factor associated is dysregulation of cytokines and of costimulatory networks, and oncogenic viruses infection.

Of the viruses that have been associated with neoplasmas , there are two implicated in the genesis of NHL, that is, the (EBV) and the human herpes virus type 8 (HHV-8). All viruses with oncogenic capacity share the feature of being in the organism either in their latent stage or as a chronic infection. The mechanisms by which the EBV participates in the genesis of lymphomas is as follows. In normal subjects, when they become infected with EBV they undergo seroconversion during the first decade of life. Primary infection is usually asymptomatic and the virus persists along the whole life. It enters the host by infecting B lymphocytes through the CD 21 (receptor of CD 3d) and persists in latent form after DNA adopts an extra-chromosomal (episome) circular shape (Anagnastopoulos et al 1999). In this stage, nine proteins and two non-coding small RNA, known as EBER 1 and 2, of unknown function can be expressed. Combination of the different proteins yield the three types of EBV latency (Lyons and Liebowitz, 1998), where EBNA 2 and LMP-1 (latent membrane protein- 1) are the most important considereing their transforming capacity exert on B lymphocytes. According to the presence of protein EBNA-2, two types of EBV are identified with different transforming activity. The most active is type 1 (Anagnastopulos et al 1999). In lymphomas, there is only one variant of the EBV, usually type 1 in the diffuse large B cell lymphomas, and type 2 in Burkitt´s lymphoma (Ometto et al 1997). The finding of viral episomes of a single type or clones in a given lymphoma indicates that the virus was present in the tumor cells at the start, and that it is probable relevant in its pathogenesis (Lyons and Liebowitz, 1998).

Factors that contribute to the development of the NHL act in stages and successively. After the initial stage of increased B lymphocytes proliferation follows one of oligoclonal B expansions, genetic alteration are introduced that conclude in a lymphoma (Gaidano et al 1998). When expressed in B lymphocytes, LMP-1 aggregates to the cell membrane and, just like CD 40, reacts with TNF (tumor necrosis factor) associated factors (TRAF), which translate the signal and activate the NK-kb transcriptional factor (Rickinson 1998). Binding of protein LMP-1 with TRAF (TNF associated factors) is the major determinant of the

transforming activity of B lymphocytes and as substances implicated in tumor invasion and in metastases (ICAM-1-LFA-3, metalloproteinases, among others). EBV infection is only one step in NHL genesis in HIV patients. In Burkitt´s lymphoma, EBV is present in a third of cases it has a type 1 latency, rarely LMP-1 protein is positive, since activation of C-MYC usually suppresses this protein (Gaidano et al 1998, 1997). In diffuse large B cell lymphomas, EBV is present in 80% of tumors and generally EBNA-2 and LMP-1 are positive.
The human herpes virus type 8 (HHV-8) has received increasing attention in the last years, it was described in Kaposi´s sarcoma (KS), but it has been constantly found in a special type of B lymphoma, i.e., in the primary lymphoma of cavity, where it is thought to have a direct etiological role (Cesarman et al 1995). This virus induces latent infection in peripheral B lymphocytes, immortalizes these cells in vitro, and induces development of NHL in humans.
It is believe that their presence in KS and LPC is needed but not enough for the pathogenesis, and other factors associated to inflammation are needed to develop malignancy (Mesri, 1999).
The virus could adopt a latency stage in CD19+B lymphocytes, it has been identified in normal tissues such as the gastrointestinal mucosa, lymph nodes and spleen. Its presence has been described in multicentric Castleman´s disease, in angio-immunoblastic lymphadenopathy, and in plasmablastic lymphomas (Luppi et al 1999).

4.4 Genetic alterations

These occur as posterior events to the polyclonal proliferation of lymphocytes B, they affect most frequently: c-MYC (re-arrangement and translocation in 50-75% of occasions, and point mutatuions in the second exon), P53(non-sense point mutations or at 16-375 of lymphomas), RAS (variable incidence of point mutations), and BCL-6 (rearrangements).
Molecular alterations affect differently the diverse types of NHL, HIV-infected patients with neoplasms have higer frequency of unstability of DNA microsatellites, which indicates that they have defficient DNA repair mechanisms (Simonelli et al 2003).
Changes in the incidence of lymphomas have been observed and marked decrease in primary lymphomas of the central nervous system has been confirmed. Incidence of systemic lymphomas has also varied, although there is no consensus among the different research groups (Skies and Crosby 2003).
The most frequent NHL varieties are the diffuse large B cell lymphoma, the Burkitt lymphoma, the plasmablastic and the primary effusion lymphomas.
Morphologically lymphomas in HIV patients are similar to those described in patients without viral infection. Diffuse large B cell lymphoma, without further specification, is defined as a heterogeneous group of lymphoid neoplasms of B cells with a diffuse growth pattern. According to current WHO classification (Swerdlow et al 2008), it is classified by morphological appearance in the following varieties: centroblastic, immunoblastic and anaplastic. Immunoblastic variant is more common in patients with HIV and is characterized by large cells, abundant cytoplasm and evident nucleoli center, about 90% of the cells must have these features to be called immunoblastic (Fig 7).
They are classified by their expression to different immunohistochemical markers such as CD 5 positive, those originated from the germinal center when tumor cells express CD10 and/or bcl6, and in non-germinal center originated when they do not express CD 10 (Hans et al 2003). Characterstically, they always express B markers such as: CD 19, CD 20 and CD 79a

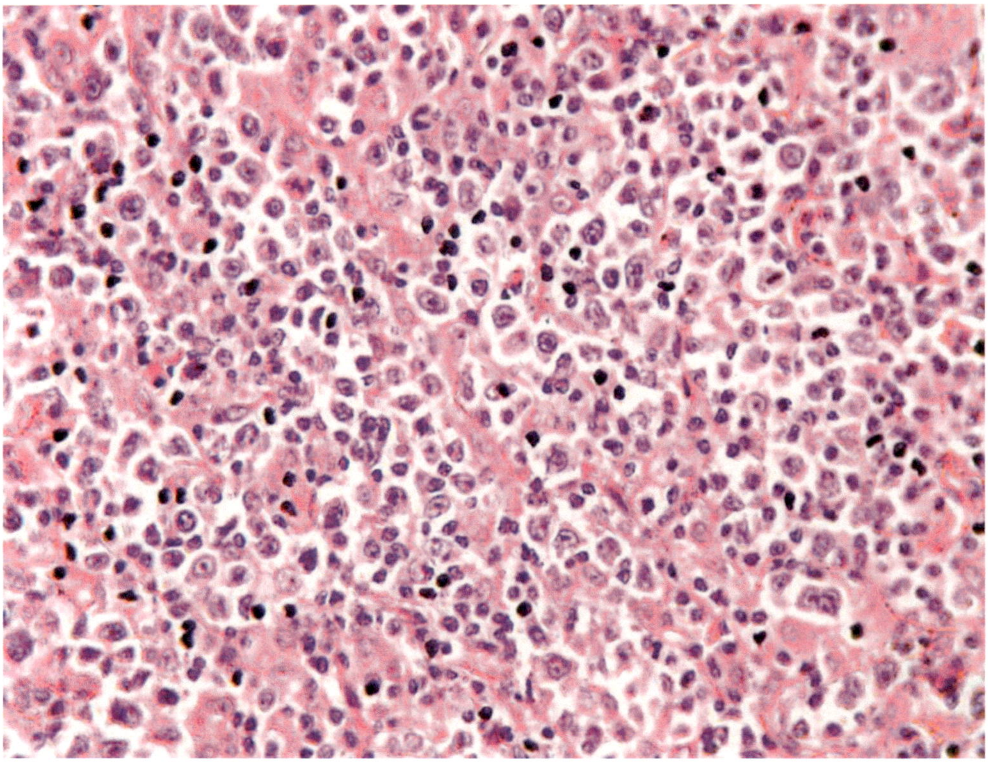

Fig. 7. Large B cell lymphoma (H-E 10X)

The plasmablastic lymphoma is characterized by diffuse proliferation o large cells that resemble immunoblasts, but the tumor cells have the immunophenotype of plasmatic cells. It was originally described in the oral cavity but can occur at any site. The express CD 138, CD 38, MUM-1 and Eber.

Primary effusion lymphoma is a large B cell neoplasm that occurs in the serose tissues without a palpable tumor mass. Co-infection with the EBV can be observed and it is the lymphoma most strongly associated with the HHV-8. The most affected sites are the pleural, pericardial and peritoneal cavities. According to phenotype, they express pan-B markers.

The Burkitt lymphoma associated to HIV generally occurs in lymph node and is characterized by the presence of monotonous o uniforme tumor cells with small nucleoli and fine and dispersed chromatine; cells are medium-sized and the classical "starry sky" pattern is observed quite frequently, characterized by the presence of abundant marcrophages with apoptotic cells. Through immunophenotype they are positive to pan B, CD 10, bcl 6, CD-38, and CD-43 markers. They depict a high cellular proliferation index (100%) and do not express TdT or bcl 2. (Swerdlow et al 2008).

Other lymphomas may also occur in patients with HIV, and one of the common extranodal sites is the gastrointestinal tract where the above mentioned types of lymphoma can occur, as well as small lymphocyte lymphomas such as the MALT-type B-cell lymphoma of the marginal zone (Ho- Yen et al 2007).

T lineage lymphomas are rare and have been, reported in isolated cases of patients with HIV. In a series of nose, palate and oropharynx lymphomas in a hospital in Mexico City, two male homosexual patients 54 years of age were found with nasal typeT/NK lymphoma, as known this is a lymphoma with certain regional characteristics and widely associated with EBV. (Romero et al 2008)(Figs 8 and 9), other peripheral T lymphomas may be present in these patients, clinically they tend to infiltrate skin and bone marrow more frequently but there is little information on treatment outcomes in the era of HAART (Arzoo et al 2004).

4.5 Hodgkin lymphoma

The Hodgkin lymphoma (LH) in HIV-infected patients can be seven-times more frequent that in healthy individuals, particularly in Europeans and Northeamericans (Tirelli et al 1995; Knowles et al 1988). Diagnostic criteria for LH are the same for either HIV or healthy individuals. However the most frequent subytype in HIV patients comprises the most unfavorable variants such as mixed cellularity and depletion of lymphocytes of the clasical HL($p<0.01$), other features published are the abundance of a proliferation of the fibrohistiocyte stroma and a higher perecentage of Reed-Sternberg cells (Ree et al 1991; Bellas et al 1996).

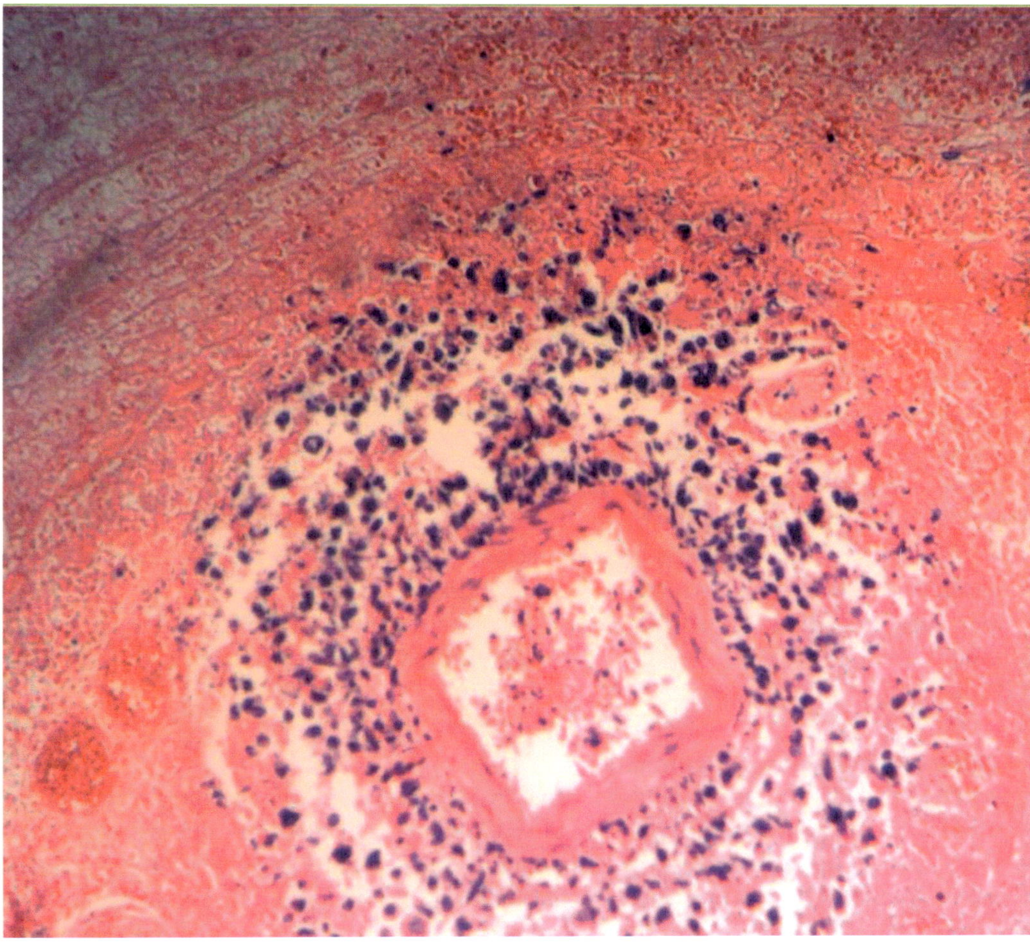

Fig. 8. Extranodal NK/T-cell lymphoma, nasal type. There is a lymphoid infiltrate, with angio-invasion and prominent coagulative necrosis (H-E 10X)

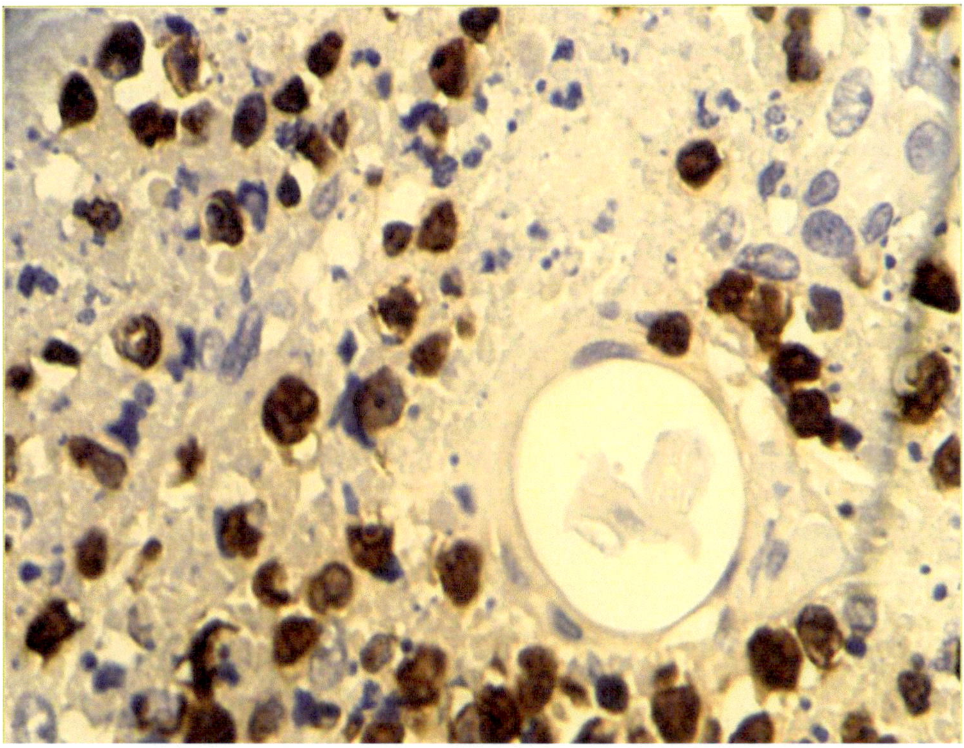

Fig. 9. *In situ* hybridization for EBV-encoded RNA (EBER), in this nasal tumor, practically all the neoplastic cells show nuclear labeling. (40X)

Relation between EBV infection and the origin of LH seems to be tighter in HIV infected patients than in the reamainder LH cases (Ree et al 1991). The combined use of in situ hybridation techniques, immunohistochemistry to determine the expression of LMP-1, indicative of latent EBV infection, and other molecular biology techniques have demonstrated that 78 to 100% of HIV+HL cases are associated to the EBV. On the other side, studies on the expression of bcl-6, generally expressed in centro-follicular lymphocytes, and of a proteglycan (CD138/Syndecan-1), characteristic of post-germinal differentiation have demonstrated the Reed-Sternberg cells of HL associated with HIV are post-germinal lymphocytes, in contrast to what occurs with the neoplastic cells of HL patients not HIV-infected (Carbone et al 1999). Incidence of HL in HIV patients has not increased (Seaberg et al 2010).

4.6 Other malignancies (Carcinoma)

Squamous cells carcinoma of different sites in HIV patients. Despite the association of infection with the human papiloma virus in HIV patients and cancer at different sites, such as anal, cervix, lip, conjunctiva, penis, vagina, and vulva, has increased the role of immunodepression in this type of epithelial cells is still unknown, nor do we know their incidence after antiretroviral drugs use. In a recently performed study by (Chaturvedi et al 2009), these authors found statistical significance between the number of CD4 lymphocytes and anal, vaginal, and vulva cancer, but not when dealing with cervical cancer.

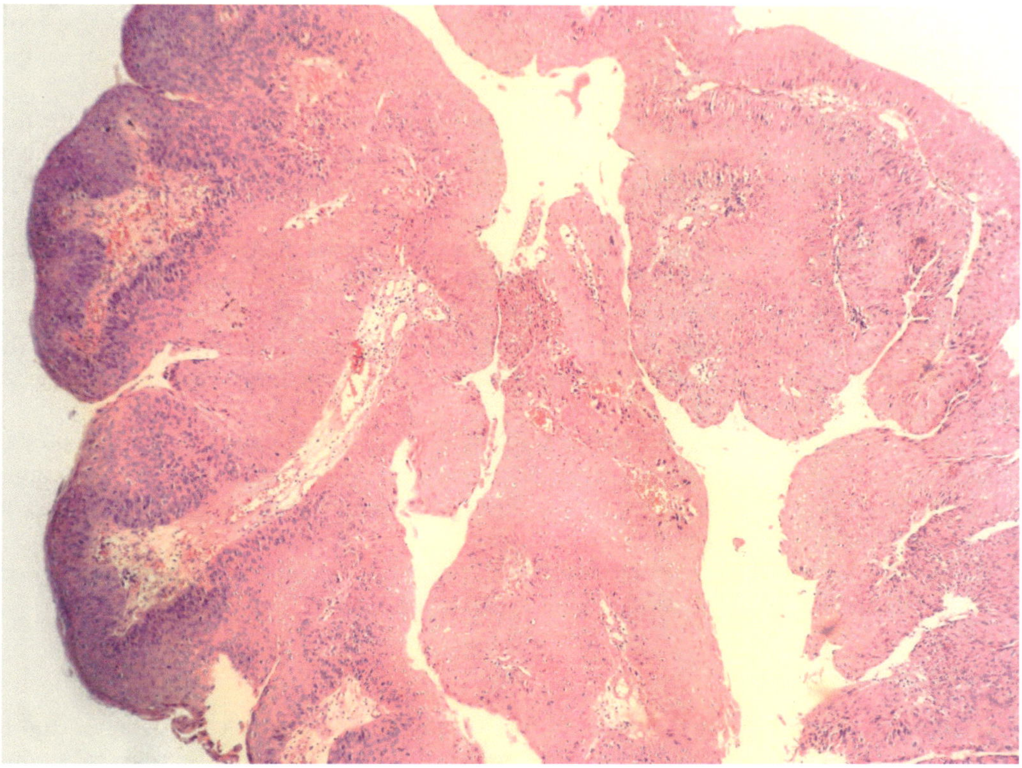

Fig. 10. Anal squamous cell carcinoma. (H-E 10X)

Anal cancer is a rare disease, it corresponds to only 4% of the malignant tumors of the gastrointestinal tract (Clark et al 2004).

Squamous cell carcinoma is by far the most common type of anal malignancy (Ryan and Mayer 2000). The incidence of anal carcinoma is higher in those who practise ano-receptive intercourse, those who are HIV-positive and in transplant recipients. Anal intraepithelial neoplasia is a premalignant lesion associated with human papilloma virus, thought to develop into invasive squamous cell carcinoma in a manner analogous to the progression of cervical intraepithelial neoplasia to cervical squamous cell carcinoma. Bleeding and pain are common in anal carcinoma. Anal carcinomas are divided into keratinized and non keratinized tumors with subtypes of the non keratinized tumors referred to as clacogenic or basaloid. The behavior of these subtypes is similar. Irrespective of the anatomic and histologic classification, anal squamous cell carcinoma can be thought of as a tumor that may show squamous, basaloid, ductal or a mixed morphology. The type 16 is the most frequently isolated type with 40-75% of all HPV positive samples. Verrucous carcinoma is a low-grade well-differentiated squamous cell carcinoma characterized by papillomatosis, acnathosis and boroad down growths with keratin clefts. The incidence of this disease is increasing in the United States, Europe and South America, especially in the male population.

In Mexico, cervical-uterine cancer remains a public health problem and patients infected with HIV, are at high risk of being infected with HPV, particularly with high risk subtypes, and develop invasive cervical carcinoma (Volkow et al 2001), that occurs in young women between the third and fourth decade of life and is clinically more aggressive. The most common morphological type is squamous cell carcinoma and there are no unique characteristics among carcinomas from patients without HIV.

Vulvar cancer is likely to be a multifactorial tumor in which recognized risk factors include advanced age, HPV infection, smoking habits, HIV infection, previous VIN (vulvar intraepithelial neoplasm) lesions, lichen sclerosus in the vulva and immunessupression. The expected proportion of vulvar cancers attributable to HPV lies within a range of 15-40% with a summary point estimate of 14%. Nevertheless, distinct subtypes of squamous cell carcinomas (SCCs) are recognized with different prevalence of HPV infection, but in HIV infection most patients are HPV positive. The warty and basaloid subtypes which account for 10-25% of all vulvar cancers have a range of HPV positivity of 59-90%, and the prevalence in the most common conventional squamous cell carcinoma the HPV prevalence is a low as 10-15% (Kurman et al 1993)

Recognized risk factor for vaginal cancer are HPV infection, exposure during pregnancy to diethylstilbestrol, previous history of cervical cancer and previous history or VAIN lesions. The most frequently isolated HPV types identified in cancers of the vagina are 16 and 18 (Srodon et al. 2006).

Other types of tumors have been reported in HIV patients, such as smooth muscle tumors (leiomyomas and leiomyosarcomas) related to EBV in children (Chadwick et al 1990)

5. Conclusions

In conclusion, despite the low morbidity and mortality of HIV infected patients due to opportunistic infections, such as atypical mycobacteral and some fungal infections, particularly in developed countries and thanks to the antiretroviral therapy, there is still much to learn, especially because of the resistant HIV strains and the resistance to antibiotic therapy of some opportunistic pathogens frequently occurring in this type of patients. It must also be taken into account that there are other infectious agents that may arise and it is necessary to know their clinical and diagnostic characteristics to be able to provide specific treatment. Neoplasms in HIV patients are well identified, however, with time and from future research, new types can up particularly in geographical regions were some oncogenic viruses are prevalent.

6. References

AIDS epidemic update: December 2005. Geneva: UNAIDS WHO, 2005.

Alcaide F, Telenti A. Molecular techniques in the diagnosis of drug-resistant tuberculosis. Ann Acad Med Singapore 1997, 26:647-650.

AK Chaturvedi, Madeleine MM, Biggar RJ, Engels EA. Risk of Human Papillomavirus-Associatted Cancers among Persons with AIDS. J Natl Cancer Inst 2009; 101:1120-1130

Anagnastopoulos Y, Hummel M. Epstein-Barr virus in Tumours. Histopathology 1999, 29:297-235.

Arthur RR, Dagostino S, Shah KV, Detection of BKV and JCV in urine and brain tissue by the polymerase chain reaction. J Clin Microbiol 1989, 27:1174-1179.

Arzoo KK, Bu X, Espina BM, Seneviratne L, Nathwani B and levin AM. T-cell lymphoma in HIV-infected Patients. J Acquir Immune Defic Syndr 2004, 36:1020-1027.

Ashley RL, Corey L. Herpes simplex viruses. In: Schmidt NJ, Emmons RW (eds). Diagnostic Procedures for Viral, Ricketsial and Chlamydial Infections. 6th ed. Washington, American Public Health Association, 1989.

Baiocchi RA, Caliguri MA, Cytokines in the evolution and Treatment of AIDS-lymphoma. Curr Opin Oncol 1999, 11:516-521.

Bellas C, Santon A, Manzanal A, Campo E, Martin C, Acevedo A, et al. Pathological Immunological, and molecular features of Hodgkn's disease associated with HIV Infection. Comparison with ordinary Hodgkin's disease. Am J Surg Pathol 1996, 20:1520-1524.

Carbone A, Gloghini A, Larocca LM, Antinori A, Falini B, Tirelli U, et al. Human immunodeficiency virus-associated Hodgkin's disease, derives from post-germinated center B cells. Blood 1999:93:2319-2326.

CDC. Public Health Service Task Force. Sexually Transmitted Diseases Treatment Guidelines. Moral Morbid Wkly Rep, 2002.

Cesarman E, Chang Y, Moore PS, Said JW, Knowles DM. Kaposi's sarcoma associated herpes-virus-like DNA sequences in AIDS-related body cavity lymphoma case. N Engl J Med 1995, 332:1186-1191.

Clark MA, Hartley A, Geh JI. Cancer of the anal canal. Lancet Oncol 2004, 5:149-157.

Chadwick EG, Connor EJ, Hanson IC, et al. Tumors of smooth-muscle origin in HIV-infected Children. JAMA 1990, 263:3182-3184.

Engels EA, Biggar RJ Marshall VA et al. Detection and Quantification of Kaposi's sarcoma-associated herpesvirus to predict AIDS-associated Kaposi's sarcoma. AIDS 2003, 17:1847-1851.

Euro HIV. HIV / AIDS Surveillance in Europe. End-year report 2004. Saint-Maurice: Institut de veille sanitaire, 2005. No 71.

Eisenman HC et al.New Insights on the pathogenesis of invasive Cryptococcus neoformans infection. Curr Infect Dis Rep 2007;9:457

Fischl MA, Richman DD, Grieco MH. Efficacy of azidothymdine (AZT) in the Treatment of Patients with AIDS and AIDS-related complex: A double-blind, placebo-controlled trial. N. Engl J Med 1987, 317:185-191.

Gaidano G, Pastore, C, Gloghin A, Canzoniery V, Capello D. Franceschi S, et al. Genetic heterogeneity of AIDS-related small non-cleaved cell lymphoma. Br J Haematol 1997, 98:726-732.

Gaidano G, Ghia P Fassone L, Cilia AM, Gloghini A et al. Patterns of cytokine expression in AIDS-related non-Hodgkin's lymphoma. Br J Haematol 1998, 103:143-149.

Ganem D. KSHV Infection and the pathogenesis of Kaposi's sarcoma. Annu Rev Pathol Mech Dis 2006, 1:273

Gern G, Perea M, Percival E et al. Human Cytomegalovirus viremia in HIV-1 seropositive Patients at Various Stages of Infection. AIDS 1990, 4:1027-1031

Gershon AA, Steinberg SP, Schmidt NJ. Varicella-Zoster virus. In: Ballows A, Hausler WJ, Hermann KL, Isenberg HD, Shadomy HJ (eds). Manual of Clinical Microbiology 5 th ed. Washington, American Society for Microbiology, 1991.

Gleaves CA, Smith TF, Shuster EA, Pearson GR. Rapid detection of cytomegalovirus in MCR-5 cells Inoculated with urine specimens by using low speed centrifugation and monoclonal antibody to an early antigen. J Clin Microbiol 1984, 19:917-919.

Goedert JJ, Coté TR, Virgo P, et al Spectrum of AIDS-associated Malignant disorders. Lancet 1998, 351:1833-1839.

González C, Ribera JM, Campo E, Bosch X, Montserrat E, Grau JM. Ki-1 anaplastic T-cell lymphoma of origin in an HIV infected patient. AIDS 1991, 5:751-755.

Hans CP, Weisenburger DD, Greiner TC, et al. Confirmation of the molecular classifcation of diffuse large B-cell lymphoma by using microarray mmunohistochemestry. Blood 2003, 103:275-282.

Ho-Yen C, Chung Fuju, Van der Walt J and Lucas S. Gastrointestinal Malignancies in HIV-infected or Immunosuppressed Patients. Adv Anat Pathol 2007, 14:431-443.

http: / / www.aids-sida.org/estadist05.htlm

Hue S, Pillay D, Clewley J et al. Genetic Analysis Reveals the complex structure of HIV transmission within Risk Groups defined. Proc Natl Acad Sci 2005.102: 4425-4429.

Isenberg HD. Clinical Microbiology Procedures Handbook. 2nd ed. ASM Press Washington, 2004

Kaplan JE et al: Epidemiology of human immunodeficiency virus-associated opportunistic infections in the United States in the era of Highly Active Antiretroviral therapy. Clin Infect Dis 2000, 30 (Suppl 1): S5.

Knowles DM. Immunodeficiency associated lymphoproliferative disorders. Mod Pathol 1999; 12: 200-217.

Knowles D, Chamulak GA, Subar M, Burke JS, Dugan M, Wernz J, et al. Lymphoid neoplasia associated with the Acquired immunodeficiency syndrome (AIDS). The New York University Medical Center experience with 105 Patients (1981-1986). Ann Intern Med 1988, 108:744-753

Kurman RJ, Toki T, Schffman MH. Basal and warty carcinomas of the vulva. Distinctive types of squamous cell carcinoma frequently associated with human papillomavruses. Am J Surg Pathol. 1993, 17:133-145.

Lalezari J, Eron J, Carlson M, Arduino R, Goodgame J, Chen C et al. Safety, pharmacokinetics and antiretroviral activity of T-20 as single agent in Heavily Pre-treated Patients. 6th Conference Retroviruses Opportunistic Infeccions. Chicago, 1999.

Lehloenya R. Menitjes G. Dermatologic Manifestations of the immune reconstitution inflammatory syndrome. Dermatol Clin 2006, 24:549-570

Luppi M Barozzi P, Malorama A, Tavato R, Z Masarea, Martelli F, et al. Expression of cell homologous genes of human herpesvirus 8 in human immunodefciency lymphoproliferatve negative virus diseases. Blood 1999, 94:2931-2933.

Lyons SF, Liebowitz DN. The roles of human viruses in the pathogenesis of lymphoma. Semin. Oncol 1998, 25:461-475.

Mellors JW, Rinaldo CR, Gupta P et al. Prognosis in HIV Infection Predicted by the quantity of virus in plasma. Science 1996, 272:1167-1169.

Mesri EA. Angiogenicity inflamatory and reactivation of Kaposi's sarcoma-associated herpesvirus HHV-8. A missing link in the pathogenesis of Acquired immunodeficiency syndrome associated Kaposi sarcoma. Blood 1999, 93:4031-4033.

Mitsuyasu RT. Clinical Aspects of AIDS-related Kaposi's sarcoma. Curr Opin Oncol 1993, 5:835-844.

Mudroch DM, Venter WDF Feldman C, VanR Rie A. Incidenci and Risk Factors for the immune reconstitution inflammatory syndorme in HIV Patients in South Africa: a prospective study. AIDS 2008, 22:601-610

Musher DM, Hamill RJ, Baughn RE. Effect of human immunodeficiency virus Infection on the course of syphilis and on the response to Treatment. Ann Intern Med 1990, 113: 872-880.

Ometto L, Menin C, Masieno S, Bonaldi L, Del Mistra A, Cattelan AM, et al. Molecular profile of Epstein-Barr virus in human immunodeficiency virus type 1 Virut related lymphadenopathies and Lymphoma. Blood 1997, 90:313-322.

Pfyffer GE, Brown Elliott BA, Wallace RJ Jr. Mycobacterium: General Characteristics, isolation, and staining procedures. In: Murray PR, Baron EJ, Jorgensen JH, Pfaller MA, Yolken RH (eds). Manual of Clinical Microbiology. The 8th ed. Washington DC: American Society for Microbiology 2003:532-559.

Pierson TC, Zhou Y, Kiefler T et al. Molecular characterization of pre-integration latency in HIV Infection. J Virol 2002, 76:8518-8531.

Ree HJ, Strauch JA, Khan AA, Gold JE, Crowley JP, Kahn H, et al. Human immunodeficiency virus-associated Hodgkin's disease. Clinicopathologic studies of 24 married and preponderance of mixed cellularity type Characterized by the Occurrence of fibrohistiocytoid stroma cells. Cancer 1991, 67:1614-1621.

Rickinson AB, Epstein Barr virus action in vivo. N Engl J Med 1998, 338:1461-1463.

Rodwell GEJ, CL Bayles, Towersey L, Aly R. The Prevalence of dermatophyte Infection in Patients infected with human immunodeficiency virus. Int J Dermatol 2008, 47:339-343.

Romani I. Immunity to fungal infections. Nat Rev Immunol 2004: 1-4

Romero-Guadarrama MB, Lazos M Ochoa, Cruz Ortiz H, Vázquez-Hernández P, Cruz Arroyo, Al et al. Non-Hodgkin lymphomas of nose, palate and oropharynx in patients from General Hospital of Mexico OD. Gen Hosp Med Rev 2008, 71:119-125.

Seaberg EC, Martinez Maza O, Chmiel JS, Kgsley L, Tang Y et al. Cancer incidence, AIDS in the Multicenter, Cohort Study Before and During The HAART era: 1984 to 2007. Cancer 2010, 116:5507-5516.

Secretary of the National AIDS Plan. Epidemiological Monitoring of AIDS in Spain. Madrid: Ministry of Health, Instituto de Salud Carlos III, 2005. Semi-annual report. 1.

Simonelli C, Spina M, Cinelli R et al. Clinical features and outcome of primary effusion lymphoma in HIV Infected Patients: a single-institution study. J Clin Oncol 2003, 21:3498-3954

Skies DJ, Crosby C. Survival is Prolonged by higly active antretrovial therapy in AIDS Patients with primary central nervous system lymphoma. AIDS 2003, 17:1787-1793.

Srodon M, Stoler MH, Baber GB, Kurman RJ. The distributon of low and high-risk HPV types in vulvar and vaginal intraepithelial neoplasia (VIN and VaIN). Am J Surg Pathol. 2006, 30:1513-1518.

Stremlau M, O Wens CM, Perron MJ et al. The cytoplasmic body component restricts HIV-1infection TRIM5alpha in Old World monkeys. Nature 2004, 427:484-853.

Swerdlow SH, Campo E, Harris NL, Jaffe ES, Pileri SA et als. WHO classification of Tumours of haematopaoietic and lymphoid tissues. International Agency for Research on Cancer Lyon 2008 4th edition 233-257.

Tirrelli U, Errante D, Dolcetti R, Gloghini A, Serraino D, Vacche E et al. Hodgkin's disease and human immunodeficiency virologic VRUs Infection and clinicopathologic features of 114 Patients from the Italian Cooperative Group on AIDS and Tumors. J Clin Oncol 1995, 13:1758-1767

Tirelli U, Vacche E, Zagonel V, Talamini R, Bernardi D, Tavio M, et al. CD 30 (Ki-1) anaplastic large cell lymphoma in 13 Patients with and 27 Patients Without Infection human immunodeficiency virus: the first comparative clinicopathologic study from a single institution That Also includes 80 Other Patients with human immunodeficiency virus-related systemic lymphoma. J Clin Oncol 1995, 13: 373-380.

Volkow P, Rubi S, Lizano M, Carrillo A, Vilar-Compte D, Garcia Carrancá A, et al. High Prevalence of oncogenic Papillomavirus in the Genital Tract of Women with Human Inmunodeficiency Virus. Gynecol Oncol 2001, 82:27-31.

Whiteway M, Oberholzer U. Candida morhogenesis and host-pathogen interactions. Curr Opin Microbiol 2004;7:350

Ziegler JL, Beckstead JA, Volkberding PA, et al. Non-Hodgkin's lymphoma in 90 homosexual men. Relation to generalized lymphadenopathy and the acquired immunodeficiency syndrome. N Engl J Med 1984, 311:565-570.

Part 5

Antiretroviral Therapy

12

Simplification of Antiretroviral Therapy (ART)

Maria Paloma Geijo Martinez
Internal Medicine, Infectious Disease Department. General Hospital. Cuenca
Angel Jesus García Imbroda. Cuenca-1 Health Center. Cuenca
Spain

1. Introduction

Simplification is the change of a therapeutic regimen that has achieved suppression of viral replication by a simpler one that continues this deletion. Its objectives are to improve the quality of life, facilitate adherence and prevent or reverse some adverse effects.
The simplification is achieved by reducing the number of tablets or frequency of shots, to change at the co-formulations, eliminate food, improve side effects and reduce or eliminate interactions.
This strategy was used, with the appearance of the NN. Most initial simplification studies carried out on standards with enhanced PI. RTV boosting with the IP was the first step to develop treatment regimens that do not present problems of complexity and tolerance of the initial PI. The second generation PI and new formulations of old, as well as co-formulations and new classes of drugs have also helped to build simple treatments.
At present the majority of patients starting treatment with simple combinations and subsequently, when they fail, become more complex treatments. Simplification has been a widely used strategy for a long period of time, but now with simple treatment guidelines from the beginning, are standard practice, leaving few for simplicity. ART can be simplified by reducing the number of drugs, the number of tablets or the number of shots.

2. Reducing the number of drugs

The first simplification of ART studies were aimed at reducing the number of drugs in what is called induction-maintenance strategy consisting of an initial induction phase with three or four-followed by maintenance with less than three drugs. This strategy was questioned by the failure of some initial trials. Some subsequent studies found no difference in the proportion of patients with < 50 copies / mL (79% vs. 77%) at 48 weeks between the branch of simplification and maintenance of initial antiretroviral therapy, adverse reactions were less frequent in the group simplification (15% vs. 6%) and improved lipid profile and adherencia[1].
He has explored the strategy of simplifying to monotherapy with LPV/r, after a period of induction with triple therapy involving this drug. In a pilot Spanish study comparing, open randomized, that included 42 patients, 21 were simplified to monotherapy with LPV/r. At 72 weeks the proportion of undetectable VL in the monotherapy group was the same (81%) and had declined to 90.5% in the triple therapy group ($p = 0.38$)[2]. In patients who failed were not observed genotypic resistance mutations and re-induced viral suppression NA

reintroducing the previously recalled. The data at 96 weeks confirmed the durability and safety of this estrategia[3].

After this study, is performed OK04 study including 205 patients with undetectable VL for at least 6 months (median 28), who were taking HAART including LPV/r associated with two NA. Is a randomized, open, non-inferiority comparing the strategy of continuation of triple therapy compared to monotherapy with LPV/r, followed by reinduction with 2 NA if viral rebound appeared. At 48 weeks the percentage of patients without virologic failure was 90 and 94% respectively (difference, -4%, upper limit 95% CI for difference 3.4%, meeting the criteria for noninferiority). The percentage of patients with VL <;50 copies/mL at 48 weeks (ITT), considering as failures reinduction was 85% in the monotherapy group and 90% in the continuation (p = 0.31). Episodes of low-level viremia between 50 and 500 copies / mL were more frequent in patients treated with monotherapy (4 vs. none) [4].

With patients in these two studies performed a multivariate analysis of predictors of loss of virologic response in the group treated with LPV/r monotherapy. Virologic failure was associated with lack of grip, low haemoglobin levels and nadir CD4 <100 cells/µL[5].

In another study of simplification to monotherapy with LPV/r was somewhat different strategy. We included 155 previously untreated patients who were randomized 2:1 to treatment with ZDV/3TC start with LPV / r (n = 104) or EFV (n = 51). Within 24 weeks of treatment and after at least 3 controls with VL < 50 copies / mL, patients taking LPV maintenance came to LPV/r monotherapy. Whereas failure to any positive viremia at 96 weeks of follow up, 48% of patients treated with LPV / r and 61% with EFV had CVP < 50 copies / mL (p = 0.17, 95% of the difference, -29% to 4%). In a new analysis that included patients as responders to reintroduce them after getting back NA CVP < 50 copies / mL, 60% of patients on LPV/r and EFV 63% responded to treatment (p = 0.73, CI 95% -19% 13%). Have been observed low viral loads in patients on monotherapy. As for security, lipoatrophy was observed in 5% of the monotherapy arm, compared to 34% of the EFV group. There were no differences in lipohypertrophy. Grade 3-4 lipid abnormalities were more frequent in the group of LPV/r. In these two studies highlights the importance of the period during which the CVP remains undetectable prior to the step alone.

This same strategy is being explored and DRV/r[6,7] ATV/r [8,10].

They have published the results at 48 weeks of a pilot study, single-arm open-simplification to ATV / r, the ACTG 5201. Were included in the same 34 patients who started treatment with 2 NA and IP, who were with undetectable viral load (<50 copies / mL) for at least 48 weeks, had not been treated with NN or prior virologic failure were HBsAg negative. Upon entering the study were switched to IP they were taking on ATV / r and 6 weeks after suspending the AN. The primary endpoint was time to virologic failure. At 48 weeks, 30 patients (88%) remained with undetectable viral load. In those with virologic failure were not detected resistance mutations. In addition, analysis of the residual viremia was observed that was not modified in patients in whom there was no virologic failure, but increased progressively in those who were detected from 4-12 weeks before they confirm the failure.

More recently, the study reported data OREY. This is a pilot, open, multicenter single-arm and 96 weeks follow-up evaluation of monotherapy with ATV / r. We included 61 patients who were receiving ART, which had had no previous failure (VL < 50 copies / mL at least 24 weeks) and treated with ATV / r 2 NA at least 8 weeks before inclusion. The analysis at 48 weeks, most patients maintained virologic suppression (79% <400 copies / mL) after switching to monotherapy, the reintroduction of triple therapy was generally satisfactory (7 of 9 patients). The development of primary mutations to PIs was rare[8].

As for the DRV / r have been reported in two clinical trials that explore two different scenarios in which explore the efficacy and safety of administration of DRV/r alone. MONET study[9] included 256 patients on antiretroviral therapy with 2 NAs and a NN or a PI / r with no previous experience with DRV / r and no history of virologic failure, with undetectable viral load (<50 copies / mL) for at least 6 months. They were randomized to either DRV / r (800/100 QD) (n = 129) alone or 2 AN optimized (n = 127). This is a non-inferiority study in which the primary objective is the time to loss of virologic response (TLOVR). Although the scheduled follow-up is 96 weeks, reported data are for 48 weeks; them confirming the no inferiority of the branch of DRV / r alone. In the ITT analysis, considering a change of treatment failure, 85.3% of patients receiving DRV / r compared to 84.3% of those taking 2 NA also had undetectable VL (-1; limit 95% CI: -9.9). As for the emergence of resistance, a patient is detected by branch genotypic evidence of resistance, but phenotypic DRV.

The study design MONOI [10] is different. This is an open randomized clinical trial which included patients who had received antiretroviral treatment for at least 18 months, who had VL of <400 copies / mL during the 18 months before and VL <50 copies / mL at the time of inclusion, who had not had virological failure to IP and had never received DRV / r. It consists of two phases, first introduced in the treatment DRV/r and 8 weeks later (second phase) were randomized 1:1 to DRV / r (600/100 mg BID) or DRV / r (600/100 BID) + 2 AN. It is a non-inferiority study of the pattern of monotherapy versus triple therapy with the primary goal is the percentage of patients who maintained virological response at week 48, although the scheduled follow-up is longer. In the initial phase included 242 patients, 226 were randomized. Data have been reported at 48 weeks (110 patients on triple therapy and 109 with DRV / r). In the per protocol results DRV / r alone shows non-inferiority versus triple therapy (94.1% vs. 99.0% of CVP < 50 copies / mL). In the ITT analysis similar results (87.5% vs. 92%).

Three virological failures were observed (> 400 copies / mL) in patients with DRV/r alone, undetected for DRV resistance mutations and subsequent viral resupresion after the reintroduction of NA. They review that two patients in the monotherapy group had clinical failure related to suppression of HIV in the central nervous system[11].

Also presented data from several studies that explore the possibility of another type of induction-maintenance is to initiate treatment with ATV / r and then suspend the RTV. This strategy has been raised given the amount of problems caused by even low-dose ritonavir. The most significant studies are INDUMA and ARIES. The INDUMA is a randomized, open, multicenter, non inferiority, which included 252 previously untreated patients who began treatment with induction 2AN + ATV / r in the week 26-30, which had PVL <50 copies / mL and continued treatment (172) are randomized 1:1 to continue the same treatment or take 2 NA + ATV 400 mg QD followed for 48 weeks [12,13].

The primary endpoint is the proportion of patients maintaining CVP <50 copies / mL at 48 weeks. Secondary objectives are the percentage of patients with PVL <400 copies / mL, CD4 count and data security. Half of the patients had been as a pair of NA ABC/3TC. At week 48, the ATV industry shows no inferiority to the ATV/r (proportion of patients with VL of <50 copies / mL is 75% in the group of ATV/r (n = 85) and 78% in the field of ATV (n = 87), a difference of 2.9 and a 95% CI 69.8-15.5). Regarding the safety profile, there were fewer cases of hyperbilirubinemia and dyslipidemia in the ATV industry. The authors conclude that this is a fairly safe option in patients not taking tenofovir. No resistance was detected over PI in either arm among patients with virological failure. The study is a study ARIES-similar. This is an open clinical trial, multicenter, non inferiority which includes patients without prior treatment regimen to which ABC/3TC + ATV / r and then at week 36 were randomized (1:1) to continue the same treatment or discontinue ritonavir for 48 weeks, if your PVL <50 copies / mL and have not submitted prior virologic failure. 419 patients were randomized and included in the analysis to the 379 (90%) who completed the 84 week follow up. The primary endpoint was the proportion of patients with VL <50 copies / mL at week 84 (TLOVR). The authors note that the effectiveness of both treatments is similar, sustained regardless of the CVP at baseline, virological failure is uncommon (2%).

3. Reducing the number of tablets and / or dose

Reducing the number of tablets and / or dose is achieved by replacing the IP by a drug from another group. In this strategy, widely studied, has been evaluated to replace the PI / r for EFV, NVP or ABC and the other PI / r can be administered in QD.

3.1 Simplification with EFV

There have been many studies about it, but few are comparative. In studies DMP-049 and -027 were randomized patients who were taking HAART with PI to continue with the same or substitute EFV. In both virologic failure was lower in the group EFV [14,15].

Another study compared the change of PI to EFV (n = 25), NVP (n = 26) or continue with the PI (n = 26), in patients on ART with PI, CD4> 300 cells / microL and CVP <80 copies / mL maintained over 9 months. At 48 weeks (ITT) there was no difference in the proportion of patients with undetectable VL with EFV (80%) or IP (77%) [16].

In a combined study design (case-control and randomized), we compared outcomes of 167 patients (who after discontinuation of IP were randomized to EFV or ABC), with another 167 patients who continued with IP (control). At 48 weeks (ITT) 70% of patients treated with EFV and 54% had CVP IP <500 copies / mL (p <0.05) [17].

3.2 NVP simplification

Several randomized studies and a study with case-control design that compares to continue with an PI switch to NVP.

In several randomized to continue with the same PI to simplify the treatment or therapeutic efficacy at 24-48 weeks was similar in both arms and showed improved lipid profile [18-20]. In one study there was a greater virological efficacy in the simplification group [20].In a case-control study of a cohort of patients receiving ART in the first IP and replaced by NVP (n = 125) or other IP (new formulation of SQV or PI / r, n = 321) was found at 48 weeks that the relative risk of failure due to change of treatment was 5 times higher with IP than with NVP and there were no differences in the risk of virologic failure [21].

With a different design, in another Spanish study (MULTINEKA) were randomized to 67 patients on stable and CVP <50 copies / mL for at least 6 months to receive LPV / r with NVP or two AN. At 48 weeks of treatment, virologic failure was not detected in any of the patients. He described a possible benefit in mitochondrial toxicity in patients with NVP[22].

NVP is contraindicated as initial treatment in women with CD4> 250 cells / uL and in men> 400 risk of severe hepatotoxicity. However, several independent studies agree that is not objectified increased hepatotoxicity or rash in patients with NVP is introduced as a strategy of simplification or substitution of toxicity regardless of the number of CD4. These results are very consistent about the number of patients[23].

3.3 ABC simplification

There have been multiple randomized trials and prospective case-control study to examine this strategy. The results are mixed. In one study, therapeutic efficacy was higher in the branch of ABC [24-26]. In the other, including the study COLA30305 TRIZAL[25], the efficacy was similar, but there was a higher incidence of failures in those patients who had come to take ABC and had previously taken sub-optim treatments. The study design and commented combined (case-control and randomized) comparing EFV or ABC to PI, 65% of patients treated with ABC and 54% of those who continued with PI had VL of <500 copies / mL (p <0.05) at 48 weeks.

In another study, 209 patients were randomized to receive ZDV/3TC/ABC in fixed combination with EFV or LPV / r, for 24-36 weeks. Patients who had PVL <50 copies / mL in both arms continued ZDV/3TC/ABC only. At 72 weeks 31 and 43% maintained undetectable VL (ITT), but 34% and 25% changed the standard by toxicidad[26].

Another pilot study included 17 patients after 12 months receiving a stable HAART containing a PI, went to take ZDV +3TC + ABC and TDF co-formulated. At 24 months, all continued with undetectable VL had an improvement in lipid profile and reduction of patients needed lipid-lowering drugs. It also aimed to a significant decrease in levels of DNA proviral[27].

Several studies have shown the existence of a high risk of treatment failure and development of mutations when used NA simplification patterns + 3TC + ABC and 3TC + ddI TDF + TDF so are not recommended as a strategy of simplification despite its simplicity.

3.4 Direct comparison of EFV, NVP and ABC simplifying ART

The NEFA is a prospective study in which 460 patients were randomized to treatment with 2 NA plus PI with PVL <200 copies / mL for ≥ 6 months [28, 29] It replaced the PI by NVP (n = 155), EFV (n = 156) or ABC (n = 149). 50%, 58% and 46% of patients respectively had received previous treatment with one or two suboptimal NA. The therapeutic efficacy (ITT) at 48 weeks (CVP <200 copies / mL) was similar in the three groups (77%, 72% and 77%, P = NS). Virologic failure was higher in the CBA group (6%, 4% and 12%, P <0.05) and occurred in patients who had received suboptimal treatment. These results were confirmed at 3 years. Genotypic analysis of strains from patients with virologic failure showed a higher number of resistance mutations in patients receiving NA ABC[29]. The numbers of patients who discontinued treatment because adverse events, was lower in the CBA group (17%, 17% and 6%, p<0,001). Simplification any NN, particularly NVP, produced benefits in lipid profile, reducing non-HDL cholesterol with ABC. Triglyceride levels were reduced in the three arms. Markers of insulin resistance showed a trend toward improvement. However, the alterations in the fat distribution improved.

A cohort study with data from the French Hospital Database on HIV is reproducing the data from the NEFA but in real life. We included 2462 patients followed for 12 months and the first treatment that included a PI; changed the IP for EFV, NVP or ABC. Predictors of regrowth of the CVP were female gender, younger age, previous suboptimal exposure to antiretrovirals, CPV high ddI/d4T use after the change and switch to NVP or ABC (if it had received suboptimal treatment). The differences from the NEFA are probably due to differences metodológicas[30]. Comparing the 3 NA simplification (ZDV+3TC+ABC co-formulated) vs. the combination of 2 NA (ZDV+3TC co-formulated) plus NVP. In the ITT analysis at 48 weeks there are no significant differences in CVP indetectable[31].

3.5 Simplification to Atazanavir

The ATV is a PI QD dosing, well tolerated, and with good metabolic profile and fewer tablets has a new simplification strategy in which a PI replaces another.

The SWAN is a phase IIIb open-label study in which 419 patients on stable treatment with PI (powered or not) with undetectable VL were randomized (2:1) to ATV 400 mg QD (if taking TDF was prescribed ATV/r 300/100 mg) (n = 278) or continue with the IP (n = 141). At week 48, virologic failure was lower in that simplified (7% vs. 16%, P <0.01). The virologic efficacy was higher in patients who switched from taking a PI unboosted ATV (22% vs. 5%, P <0.001) was not different between those continuing with a PI / r, which went from PI/r and ATV (11% vs. 8%, P = NS) 429. Regarding safety, the suspension of treatment was higher in patients in the control group (21% vs. 34%, p<0,01) and lipid profile was improved in the group simplified to ATV. SIMPATAZ and ATAZIP studies confirm the safety and efficacy of this strategy of simplification, in this case changing LPV/r by ATV/r [32,33].

The REAL study from which data were presented at 48 weeks, a clinical trial that includes patients in stable antiretroviral therapy for at least 12 weeks that contains a given BID PI, CVP undetectable and lipohypertrophy, which were randomized to continue the same treatment or change the PI to ATV / r 300/100 mg. Inmuno-virologic control was maintained, showed improved lipid profile in the field of ATC but no differences were observed in body composition. [34].

Another strategy is developed in the trial AI424-067-48 weeks [35]. This is a randomized, open, prospective study that included 246 patients treated with PI / r with hyperlipidemia and VL <50 copies / mL Patients were randomized to switch to ATV (400 MG) on day 1 (immediate change) or maintain their treatment and switching to ATV (400 MG) at 24 weeks (late switch). At 12 weeks both groups maintained a similar virologic control and those patients taking a significant improvement ATV figures for LDL-cholesterol (-15 and +1%, p <0.0001). The authors conclude that the change immediately or delayed, a boosted PI or unboosted ATV in patients with hyperlipemia is associated with improvement in lipid parameters without loss of virologic suppression.

4. Simplifying dosing regimens to once daily in

The change to a QD regimen simplification is another way in patients who are well controlled. Several trials have proven the validity of this strategy.

In a clinical trial, 355 patients were randomized to continue their ARV therapy or switching to a QD (ddI + FTC + EFV). At week 48 were still undetectable VL, 87% of the QD arm and 79% of those who had not changed (p <0.05)[36].

In another non-randomized study which included 169 patients, 84 continued their antiretroviral therapy and 85 switched to ddI + TDF + NVP QD; virologic efficacy was good (76 vs. 86%, ITT), but CD4 lymphocytes decreased in the branch QD with a half decrease of 95 cells / µL[37].

The combination ddI + TDF has demonstrated virological efficacy but poor recovery of CD4 lymphocytes or even declining in number while the CVP is suppressed. This decrease was more evident when given standard doses (full) of ddI [38]. The QD dosing regimens containing combination ddI + TDF should be avoided. Doing so should reduce the ddI dose to 250 mg / day in patients over 60 kg and 200 mg / day for patients below this weight.
With the advent of fixed-dose combinations of NA administered QD has simplified the situation. Clearly, their role in initial therapy and have begun trials to assess its use in simpler systems. The SWEET trial of 234 patients treated for at least 6 months with ZDV + 3TC (co-formulated) + EFV and CVP <50 copies / mL, were randomized to TDF + FTC (co-formulated) + EFV or to follow the same treatment. At 24 weeks there was improvement in haemoglobin levels and lipid profile in the TDF + FTC arm, maintaining the treatment response (VL <50 copies / mL, 93% versus 88%, P = 0.26). Recently results published 48 week[39], 206 patients. 5% of patients who continued the same treatment and 3% of patients who switched, discontinued due to adverse effects. No statistically significant differences were observed between the two arms by intention to treat (85% of patients who continued treatment versus 88% who had changed CVP <50 copies / mL). In the sub study of 100 patients has been performed DEXA fat tissue, it appears that the fat is maintained or increased in patients who switch treatment, but decreased in the group that continues (mean difference 448 g, 95% : 57-839 g, P = 0.025). As in other studies, the increase of fat is lower in patients with ZDV and those with less peripheral fat. No differences between groups in terms of renal toxicity. The researchers conclude that changing ZDV / 3TC by TDF / FTC in patients treated with EFV and virological sustained response is safe front the point of virologic view and is associated with an increase in haemoglobin and improvement in lipid parameters and distribution of body fat.
In another open randomized study[40], with 80 patients with VL <50 copies / mL and who are treated with ZDV/3TC (+PI or NN), who were randomized to ZDV/3TC / FTC continue or switch to TDF (RECOMB), at week 24 to 85% of patients treated with TDF / FTC, had PVL <50 copies / mL compared to 80% with ZDV/3TC (p = 0.77). It was also observed a significant increase in limb fat in patients with fat mass <7.2 kg at baseline, but also improve LDL cholesterol in the field of TDF / FTC. In 72 weeks data[41], there has been no virologic failure; (90% branch TDF / FTC vs. 83% branch AZT/3TC present CVP <50 copies / mL). (P = 0.52), with similar median increase of CD4. In addition, a significant improvement objective, with gradual increase in limb fat, especially if baseline BMI is> 25 kg/m2 and have over 5 years AZT/3TC treatment. The analysis was performed according to baseline BMI greater or not than 25 Kg/m^2, and the number of years AZT/3TC treatment and in all stages of peripheral fat improvement is statistically significant in the field of TDF / FTC. The authors conclude that it is a safe strategy from the point of immune-virologic and adverse effects view, which improves lipoatrophy and various biochemical parameters (haemoglobin, hematocrit and LDL cholesterol).
Another similar test is the totem of 91 patients with VL <400 copies / mL and dyslipidemia who were randomized to continue the same treatment or switch to TDF / FTC. In patients who switched showed a significant improvement in lipid profile at 12 semanas[42]. In BICOMBO study, randomized, open, with 335 patients receiving treatment regimen that included 3TC, and virologic suppression for ≥ 6 months were randomized to replace co-formulated with combinations AN ABC +3 TC (n = 167) or TDF + FTC (n= 168)[43]. The study was designed to assess non-inferiority of both combinations over, or virologic treatment

failure. In the TDF + FTC, treatment failure was 13.3% vs. 19.2% in the ABC +3 TC, did not demonstrate non-inferiority of ABC +3 TC compared to TDF + FTC (95% - 2% 14%). However ABC +3 TC demonstrate non-inferiority compared to TDF + FTC in order to virologic failure (2.4% vs. 0%, 95% CI 0.05% to 6%). Suspensions due to adverse events were 10% 0f ABC + 3TC group vs. 5% of TDF + FTC group (p = 0,004). Regarding the lipid profile, reductions in total cholesterol, HDL, LDL and triglycerides were higher in the TDF + FTC branch. The peripheral fat, the abnormal kidney functions or bone mineral density increase were similar. Liver toxicity was very low in both groups. By contrast, the immune response was better in the ABC +3TC. Prior determination of HLA B * 5701 might have changed these results.

He has recently published a prospective, randomized, controlled, open, multicenter trial[44], including patients treated with undetectable VL than those randomized to continue the same treatment or taking EFV + TDF + FTC co-formulated with a follow up to 48 weeks, showing the same efficiency in the two branches. It included 300 patients with PVL <200 copies / mL for> 3 months and no change in treatment. They were taking stratified as NN or PI and randomized 2:1 to simplify the treatment (taking single tablet) or continue with the same treatment (97 patients). The efficacy and safety was determined at baseline and weeks 4, 12, 24, 36 and 48. We also carried out an assessment of the quality of life and preferences for drugs. At 48 weeks, 89% of patients with TDF / FTC / EFV vs. 88% with the same treatment had PVL <200 copies / mL (TLOVR, 95%) with a difference between branches of 1.1% (- 6.7% to 8.8%), indicating non-inferiority of the branch of TDF / FTC / EFV. 87% of patients switched to TDF / FTC / EFV vs. 85% who did not change, CVP had <50 copies / mL: the difference between the two branches of 2.6% (95% CI -5.9% to 11.1 %. Discontinuation rates were similar, although the suspension due to adverse events was higher in the branch of TDF / FTC / EFV (5% VS 1%), mainly CNS-related symptoms. No differences regarding glomerular filtration rate, or adherence. There was an improvement in the number of triglycerides in the field of TDF / FTC / EFV (20 vs. 3 mg/dl, p = 0,035).

There is a new option to simplify a QD therapy since the publication of the study NODY, because it has demonstrated the efficacy and safety of Nevirapine simplifying administered twice daily to once a day. It is a study lasting 48 weeks, open, randomized, multicenter, which included 298 stable patients who were taking nevirapine twice daily for at least 12-18 weeks and had PVL <50 copies / mL. Were randomized to continue the same treatment or change to nevirapine QD. The primary study objective was to assess the hepatic safety of QD treatment, analyzing the proportion of patients with ALT/AST grade 3-4, and second endpoints were the development of clinical hepatitis and inmune-virological and clinical efficacy. The study demonstrated non-inferiority versus per protocol to maintain the initial pattern, with a no inferiority margin of 10% for hepatotoxicity, which was the primary objective.

A major unresolved issue is whether the impact of not taking a dose of medication due to forgetfulness or failure may be greater in a QD system in a regimen of multiple daily doses in the appearance of resistance mutations[45]. We currently have multiple drugs can be administered once a day, with a half life long enough to avoid this problem.

5. Other simplification

With the advent of new drugs with new families, it was possible to simplify the treatment given to patients multicoated. This simplification is not the number of pills but in the way of drug administration. This has already been presented studies that ENF is replaced by RAL, maintaining the treatment effectiveness [46-50]. Although most studies are observational, there has been a clinical trial [47] with included 170 patients with HIV resistant to three drug groups and VL <400 copies/mL for at least 3 months of treatment with ENF. They were randomized 1:1 to ENF continue or witch to RAL. The primary endpoint was the cumulative proportion of patients with virologic failure defined as CVP ≥ 400 copies / mL through week 24. Virologic failure was observed in 1patient per branch. The conclusion is that the change to RAL is effective and well tolerated at 24 weeks, which offers the advantage of simplicity, the same safety profile and you need a longer-term follow-up.

MVC could not be used in the context of simplification, in studies similar to those already made and in these circumstances cannot be performed tropism test.

But simplification cannot be performed if compromising treatment efficacy. As an example, include two clinical trials recently presented, SWITCHMRK 1 and 2 [51]. Two clinical trials are parallel, multicenter, double-blind, randomized studies encompassing virological controlled patients under treatment which included a Lopinavir/r stable, did not exclude patients who had failed other treatment regimens, provided that at the time of inclusion on CVP <50 copies / mL for at least 3 months. Patients were randomized 1:1 to maintain LPV / r switch to RAL, the same base analogs. Primary objectives were: percentage change in lipid levels at week 12, the proportion of patients with VL of <50 copies / mL at week 24 as well as safety and efficacy at 24 weeks. In SWITCHMRK 2, 355 patients were randomized at RAL and LPV/r. After the change, the RAL was confirmed to be well tolerated and produced significant improvements in lipid parameters, but did not demonstrate non-inferiority from the viewpoint virology at week 24: 154 of 175 patients (88%) vs. 167 of 178 (93.8%) had VL <50 copies / mL in groups of RAL and LPV / r respectively, the observed difference between the two treatments is -5.8% (95% CI: 12.2 to 0.22, ITT).

Probably these results are due to the inclusion criteria allowed entry into the study of patients with prior virologic failure, and lower genetic barrier of RAL. The teaching of this study is that it must choose well to patients whose treatment is simplified and the simplification strategy to follow.

6. Simplification of ART. Recommendations summary

- In patients with no history of prior failure to IP, with undetectable VL at least 6 months and signs or symptoms of toxicity of AN, is possible to simplify the DRV / r LPV / r monotherapy (A level).
- If you have not failed prior to NA, PI can be substituted for EFV, NVP. If the patient has received prior suboptimal treatment with NA, no one PI to simplify ABC, (A level).
- Simplification to ABC is contraindicated associated with 3TC and TDF or associated with TDF and ddI. (B level).
- In patients with high cardiovascular risk, the simplification to ATV or ATV/r or RAL can add metabolic advantages (A level).
- In patients at their first PI regimen with undetectable VL, can be simplified to a QD pattern as: EFV+ TDF+TCF (or 3TC), EFV+ ddI +3TC (or TDF), or ATV/r or (ATV) + TDF+TCF. (A level)
- ENF-substitution for virological suppressed patients to RAL has been shown effective and safe. (A level)

- It is important to select well the patients who should be simplified and strategy. The simplification is not possible at the expense of loss of virologic efficacy. You can only raise a simplification if there has been no previous failure of fully active drugs are used to maintain virologic success (A level)
- Other possible simplifications must be performed within clinical trials, in clinical practice (C level).

Strategy	**ART**	clinical trials
Reducing the number of drugs	monotherapy with LPV / r	OK04 study. Multivariate analysis
	monotherapy with DRV / r	MONET. MONOI
	monotherapy with ATV / r.	ACTG 5201. OREY
	ATV / r., Suspend the RTV	INDUMA. ARIES
Reducing the number of tablets and / or dose	Simplification with EFV	DMP-049 and -027
	Simplification with NVP	MULTINEKA.
	Simplification with ABC	COLA30305 TRIZAL
	Direct comparison of EFV, NVP and ABC simplifying ART	NEFA. French Hospital Database
	Simplification to ATV / r	SWAN. SIMPATAZ. ATAZIP. REAL
A QD regimen simplification	ddI + FTC + EFV	Molina, J Infect Dis 2005. Negredo, Antivir Ther 2004.
	ZDV +3 TC (co-formulated) + EFV	SWEET. RECOMB. BICOMBO
	TDF + FTC (co-formulated) + EFV	
	EFV + TDF + FTC co-formulated	Martin A, Clin Infect Dis 2009.
	QD regimen NVP	NODY
Other simplification	ENF is replaced by RAL	CHEER. ANRS 138
	maintain LPV/r vs switch to RAL	SWITCHMRK 1 and 2

Table 1. Simplification of antiretroviral therapy (ART)

Strategy	Significance level
- In patients with no history of prior failure to IP, with undetectable VL at least 6 months and signs or symptoms of toxicity of AN, is possible to simplify the DRV / r LPV / r monotherapy	(A level)
- If you have not failed prior to NA, PI can be substituted for EFV, NVP. If the patient has received prior suboptimal treatment with NA, no one PI to simplify ABC.	(A level)
- Simplification to ABC is contraindicated associated with 3TC and TDF or associated with TDF and ddI.	(B level)
- In patients with high cardiovascular risk, the simplification to ATV or ATV/r or RAL can add metabolic advantages.	(A level)
- In patients at their first PI regimen with undetectable VL, can be simplified to a QD pattern as: EFV+ TDF+TCF (or 3TC), EFV+ ddI +3TC (or TDF), or ATV/r or (ATV) + TDF+TCF.	(A level)
- ENF-substitution for virologically suppressed patients to RAL has been shown effective and safe.	(A level)
- It is important to select well the patients who should be simplified and strategy. The simplification is not possible at the expense of loss of virologic efficacy. You can only raise a simplification if there has been no previous failure of fully active drugs are used to maintain virologic success.	(A level)
-Other possible simplifications must be performed within clinical trials, in clinical practice.	(C level)

Table 2. Simplification of antiretroviral 1 therapy (ART). Recommendations summary.

7. References

[1] Castagna A, Danise A, Menzo S, Galli L, Gianotti N, Carini E et al. Lamivudine monotherapy in HIV 1 infected patients harbouring a lamivudine-resistant virus: a randomized pilot study (E184V study). AIDS 2006; 20(6):795-803

[2] Pulido F, Arribas J, González-García J, López Aldeguer J, Domingo P, Estrada V, et al. Risk factors for lossof virological suppression at 48 weeks in patients receiving Lopinavir/ritonavir monotherapy in 2 clinical trials comparing LPV/r monotherapy vs. triple therapy with LPV/r (OK and OK04 trials). 14th Conference on Retroviruses and Opportunistic Infections, Los Angeles, February 25-28 2007. Abstract 513.

[3] Cameron DW, da Silva BA, Arribas JR, Myers RA, Bellos NC, Gilmore N et al. A 96 week comparison of Lopinavir-ritonavir combination therapy followed by lopinavir-ritonavir monotherapy versus efavirenz combination therapy. J Infect Dis 2008; 198(2):234-240

[4] Nunes EP, Santini de OM, Mercon M, Zajdenverg R, Faulhaber JC, Pilotto JH et al. Monotherapy with Lopinavir/Ritonavir as maintenance after HIV-1 viral suppression: results of a 96 week randomized, controlled, open-label, pilot trial (KalMo study). HIV Clin Trials 2009; 10(6):368-374

[5] Gutmann C, Cusini A, Gunthard HF, Fux C, Hirschel B, Decosterd LA et al. Randomized controlled study demonstrating failure of LPV/r monotherapy in HIV: the role of compartment and CD4-nadir. AIDS 2010; 24(15):2347-2354

[6] Arribas JR, Horban A, Gerstoft J, Fatkenheuer G, Nelson M, Clumeck N et al. The MONET trial: darunavir/ritonavir with or without nucleoside analogues, for patients with HIV RNA below 50 copies/ml. AIDS 2010; 24(2):223-230

[7] Valentin MA, Flandre P, Kolta S, Duvivier C, Algarte-Genin M, Ponscarme D, Slama L, Cuzin L, et al. Fat tissue distribution changes in HIV-infected patients with viral suppression treated with DRV/r Monotherapy vs 2 NRTI+DRV/r in the MONOI-ANRS 136 randomized trial: results at 48 weeks. 17th Conference on Retroviruses and Opportunistic Infections, San Francisco, February 27-March 2 2010. Abstract 721.

[8] Wilkin TJ, McKinnon JE, DiRienzo AG, Mollan K, Fletcher CV, Margolis DM et al. Regimen simplification to atazanavir-ritonavir alone as maintenance antiretroviral therapy: final 48-week clinical and virologic outcomes. J Infect Dis 2009; 199(6):866-871

[9] Rieger A, Banhegyi D, Schmidt W, Arribas JR, Hill A, van Delft, Y, Moecklinghoff C. The MONET trial 96 week analysis: darunavir/r monotherapy versus darunavir/r + 2NRTIs, for patients with HIV RNA < 50 copies/mL at baseline. 18th International AIDS Conference, Vienna, July 18-23 2010. Abstract TBLBB209.

[10] Valentin MA, Flandre P, Kolta S, Duvivier C, Algarte-Genin M, Ponscarme D, Slama L, Cuzin L, et al. Fat tissue distribution changes in HIV-infected patients with viral suppression treated with DRV/r Monotherapy vs 2 NRTI+DRV/r in the MONOI-ANRS 136 randomized trial: results at 48 weeks. 17th Conference on Retroviruses and Opportunistic Infections, San Francisco, February 27-March 2 2010. Abstract 721.

[11] Curran A, Gutirerrez M, Deig E, Mateo G, Lopez RM, Imaz A et al. Efficacy, safety and pharmacokinetics of 900/100 mg of darunavir/ritonavir once daily in treatment-experienced patients. J Antimicrob Chemother 2010; 65(10):2195-2203

[12] Pulido F, Serrano O, Rivero A, Montes ML, Rubio R, López Bernaldo de Quirós JC, et al. Atazanavir/ritonavir en monoterapia como mantenimiento en pacientes con supresión virológica: Análisis primario a las 48 semanas del estudio OREY. 1er Congreso Nacional de Gesida, Madrid, 21-24 octubre 2009. PO-70.

[13] Ghosn J, Carosi G, Moreno S, Pokrovsky V, Lazzarin A, Pialoux G et al. Unboosted atazanavir-based therapy maintains control of HIV type-1 replication as effectively as a ritonavir-boosted regimen. Antivir Ther 2010; 15(7):993-1002

[14] Becker S, Rachlis A, Gill J, DeJesus E, Pierone G, Kirkland L, Koosian S, Farina D, Labriola D, Ruiz N,Bessen L, Villano S. Successful substitution of protease inhibitors with efavirenz in patients with undetectable viral loads: A prospective,

randomized, multicenter, open-label study (DMP 049). 8th Conference on Retroviruses and Opportunistic Infections, Chicago, February 4-8 2001. Abstract 20.

[15] Katlama C, Stazewsky S, Clumeck N, Arasteh K, Dellamonica P, Molina JM, et al. Successful substitution of protease inhibitors with Sustiva (efavirenz) in patients with undetectable plasma HIV-1 RNA: results of a prospective, randomized, multicenter, open-label study (DMP 006-027). XIII International AIDS Conference, Durban, South Africa, 2000 (Abstract LbPeB7044).

[16] Negredo E, Cruz L, Paredes R, Ruiz L, Fumaz CR, Bonjoch A et al. Virological, immunological, and clinical impact of switching from protease inhibitors to nevirapine or to efavirenz in patients with human immunodeficiency virus infection and long-lasting viral suppression. Clin Infect Dis 2002; 34(4):504-10

[17] Campo RE, Cohen C, Grimm K, Shangguan T, Maa J, Seekins D. Switch from protease inhibitor- to efavirenz-based antiretroviral therapy improves quality of life, treatment satisfaction and adherence with low rates of virological failure in virologically suppressed patients. Int J STD AIDS 2010; 21(3):166- 171.

[18] Maggiolo F, Ripamonti D, Ravasio L, Gregis G, Quinzan G, Callegaro A et al. Outcome of 2 simplification strategies for the treatment of human immunodeficiency virus type 1 infection. Clin Infect Dis 2003; 37(1):41-49

[19] Negredo E, Ribalta J, Paredes R, Ferre R, Sirera G, Ruiz L et al. Reversal of atherogenic lipoprotein profile in HIV-1 infected patients with lipodystrophy after replacing protease inhibitors by nevirapine. AIDS 2002; 16(10):1383-1389

[20] Arranz Caso JA, Lopez JC, Santos I, Estrada V, Castilla V, Sanz J et al. A randomized controlled trial investigating the efficacy and safety of switching from a protease inhibitor to nevirapine in patients with undetectable viral load. HIV Med 2005; 6(5):353-359

[21] Barreiro P, Soriano V, Blanco F, Casimiro C, de la Cruz JJ, Gonzalez-Lahoz J. Risks and benefits of replacing protease inhibitors by nevirapine in HIV-infected subjects under long-term successful triple combination therapy. AIDS 2000; 14(7):807-12

[22] Negredo E, Miro O, Rodriguez-Santiago B, Garrabou G, Estany C, Masabeu A et al. Improvement of mitochondrial toxicity in patients receiving a nucleoside reverse-transcriptase inhibitor-sparing strategy: results from the Multicenter Study with Nevirapine and Kaletra (MULTINEKA). Clin Infect Dis 2009; 49(6):892-900

[23] de Lazzari E, Leon A, Arnaiz JA, Martinez E, Knobel H, Negredo E et al. Hepatotoxicity of nevirapine in virologically suppressed patients according to gender and CD4 cell counts. HIV Med 2008; 9(4):221-226

[24] Katlama C, Fenske S, Gazzard B, Lazzarin A, Clumeck N, Mallolas J et al. TRIZAL study: switching from successful HAART to Trizivir (abacavir-lamivudine-zidovudine combination tablet): 48 weeks efficacy, safety and adherence results. HIV Med 2003; 4(2):79-86

[25] Pulvirenti J, Goodwin D, Slater L. Simplification of protease inhibitor- containing HAART regimens with abacavir maintains viral suppression and favourable adherence in HIV-1 infected adults (COLA30305). 39th Annual Meeting of the Infectious Disease Society of America, San Francisco, october 25-28 2001.Abstract 620.

[26] Mallolas J, Pich J, Penaranda M, Domingo P, Knobel H, Pedrol E et al. Induction therapy with trizivir plus efavirenz or lopinavir/ritonavir followed by trizivir alone in naive HIV-1-infected adults. AIDS 2008; 22(3):377-384

[27] d'Ettorre G, Zaffiri L, Ceccarelli G, Andreotti M, Massetti AP, Vella S et al. Simplified maintenance therapy with abacavir/lamivudine/zidovudine plus tenofovir after sustained HIV load suppression: four years of follow-up. HIV Clin Trials 2007; 8(3):182-188

[28] Martinez E, Arnaiz JA, Podzamczer D, Dalmau D, Ribera E, Domingo P et al. Substitution of nevirapine, efavirenz, or abacavir for protease inhibitors in patients with human immunodeficiency virus infection. N Engl J Med 2003; 349(11):1036-1046

[29] Ochoa de EA, Arnedo M, Xercavins M, Martinez E, Roson B, Ribera E et al. Genotypic and phenotypic resistance patterns at virological failure in a simplification trial with nevirapine, efavirenz or abacavir. AIDS 2005; 19(13):1385-1391

[30] Fisac C, Fumero E, Crespo M, Roson B, Ferrer E, Virgili N et al. Metabolic benefits 24 months after replacing a protease inhibitor with abacavir, efavirenz or nevirapine. AIDS 2005; 19(9):917-925

[31] Martinez E, Gatell JM. Considerations on the effectiveness of nevirapine in protease inhibitor-based regimen simplification. AIDS 2007; 21(13):1829-1830

[32] Mallolas J, Podzamczer D, Milinkovic A, Domingo P, Clotet B, Ribera E et al. Efficacy and safety of switching from boosted lopinavir to boosted atazanavir in patients with virological suppression receiving a LPV/r-containing HAART: the ATAZIP study. J Acquir Immune Defic Syndr 2009; 51(1):29-36

[33] Rubio R, Serrano O, Carmena J, Asensi V, Echevarria S, Flores J et al. Effect of simplification from protease inhibitors to boosted atazanavir-based regimens in real-life conditions. HIV Med 2010; 11(9):545-553

[34] Moyle G, Girard JM, Andrade J, Salvato P, Bogner JR, Hay P, et al. Continuation of BID boosted PI vs switch to once-daily ATV/RTV for the management of lipodystrophy: 48 week primary analysis of the 96 week multicenter, open-label, randomized, prospective ReAL study. 17th International AIDS Conference, Mexico DF, 3-8 August 2008. Abstract MOPDB103.

[35] Sension M, ndrade Neto JL, Grinsztejn B, Molina JM, Zavala I, Gonzalez-Garcia J et al. Improvement in lipid profiles in antiretroviral-experienced HIV-positive patients with hyperlipidemia after a switch to unboosted atazanavir. J Acquir Immune Defic Syndr 2009; 51(2):153-162

[36] Molina JM, Journot V, Morand-Joubert L, Yeni P, Rozenbaum W, Rancinan C et al. Simplification therapy with once-daily emtricitabine, didanosine, and efavirenz in HIV-1-infected adults with viral suppression receiving a protease inhibitor-based regimen: a randomized trial. J Infect Dis 2005; 191(6):830-839

[37] Negredo E, Molto J, Munoz-Moreno JA, Pedrol E, Ribera E, Viciana P et al. Safety and efficacy of oncedaily didanosine, tenofovir and nevirapine as a simplification antiretroviral approach. Antivir Ther 2004; 9(3):335-342.

[38] Barrios A, Rendon A, Negredo E, Barreiro P, Garcia-Benayas T, Labarga P et al. Paradoxical CD4+ T-cell decline in HIV-infected patients with complete virus suppression taking tenofovir and didanosine. AIDS 2005; 19(6):569-575

[39] Fisher M, Moyle GJ, Shahmanesh M, Orkin C, Kingston M, Wilkins E et al. A randomized comparative trial of continued zidovudine/lamivudine or replacement with tenofovir disoproxil fumarate/emtricitabine in favirenz-treated HIV-1-infected individuals. J Acquir Immune Defic Syndr 2009; 51(5):562-568.

[40] Martínez E, Ribera E, Pulido F, Rubio R, Negredo E, Sanz J et al. Early improvement of limb fat content in patients switching from AZT/3TC to FTC/TDF (TVD): a 24 week interim analysis of the RECOMB Trial. 17th International AIDS Conference, Mexico DF, 3-8 August 2008. Abstract MOPDB102.

[41] Ribera E, Martinez E, Clotet B, Estrada V, Sanz J, Berenguer J, et al. 72 week outcomes following switch from AZT/3TC to FTC/TDF (TVD) vs continuing on AZT/3TC. Final results of the RECOMB trial. 5th IAS Conference on HIV Pathogenesis, Treatment and Prevention, Cape Town, July 19-22 2009. Abstract CDB091.

[42] Valantin MA, Bittar R, de TP, Bollens D, Slama L, Giral P et al. Switching the nucleoside reverse transcriptase inhibitor backbone to tenofovir disoproxil fumarate + emtricitabine promptly improves triglycerides and low-density lipoprotein cholesterol in dyslipidaemic patients. J Antimicrob Chemother 2010; 65(3):556-561

[43] Martinez E, Arranz JA, Podzamczer D, Lonca M, Sanz J, Barragan P et al. A simplification trial switching from nucleoside reverse transcriptase inhibitors to once-daily fixed-dose abacavir/lamivudine or tenofovir/emtricitabine in HIV-1-infected patients with virological suppression. J Acquir Immune Defic Syndr 2009; 51(3):290-297

[44] Martin A, Bloch M, Amin J, Baker D, Cooper DA, Emery S et al. Simplification of antiretroviral therapy with tenofovir-emtricitabine or abacavir-Lamivudine: a randomized, 96-week trial. Clin Infect Dis 2009; 49(10):1591-1601

[45] Airoldi M, Zaccarelli M, Bisi L, Bini T, Antinori A, Mussini C et al. One-pill once-a-day HAART: a simplification strategy that improves adherence and quality of life of HIV-infected subjects. Patient Prefer Adherence 2010; 4:115-125.

[46] Towner W, Klein D, Kerrigan HL, Follansbee S, Yu K, Horberg M. Virologic outcomes of changing enfuvirtide to raltegravir in HIV-1 patients well controlled on an enfuvirtide based regimen: 24-week results of the CHEER study. J Acquir Immune Defic Syndr 2009; 51(4):367-373

[47] De Castro N, Braun J, Charreau I, Pialoux G, Cotte L, Katlama C, et al. Switch from Enfuvirtide to Raltegravir in highly treatment-experienced patients: a randomized open label non-inferiority trial, Easier-ANRS 138. 16th Conference on Retroviruses and Opportunistic Infections, Montreal, February 8- 11 2009. Abstract 572.

[48] Gatti F, Matti A, Nasta P, Cologni G, Costarelli S, Carosi G. Switch from enfuvirtide to raltegravir: a simplification option for heavily pretreated patients. 9th International Congess on Drug Therapy in HIV Infection, Glasgow, November 9-13 2008. Abstract P52.

[49] Talbot A, Machouf N, Thomas R, Marcotte S, Therrien R, Lessard B et al. Switch from enfuvirtide to raltegravir in patients with undetectable viral load: efficacy and

safety at 24 weeks in a Montreal cohort. J Acquir Immune Defic Syndr 2009; 51(3):362-364

[50] Santos JR, Llibre JM, Ferrer E, Domingo P, Imaz A, Molto J et al. Efficacy and safety of switching from enfuvirtide to raltegravir in patients with virological suppression. HIV Clin Trials 2009; 10(6):432-438

[51] Eron JJ, Young B, Cooper DA, Youle M, DeJesus E, ndrade-Villanueva J et al. Switch to a raltegravir-based regimen versus continuation of a lopinavir-ritonavir-based regimen in stable HIV-infected patients with suppressed viraemia (SWITCHMRK 1 and 2): two multicentre, double-blind, randomised controlled trials. Lancet 2010; 375(9712):396-407

13

Highly Active Antiretroviral Therapy (HAART) and Metabolic Complications

Beth S. Zha[1], Elaine J. Studer[1], Weibin Zha[1], Philip B. Hylemon[1,2], William Pandak[1,2] and Huiping Zhou[1,2]
[1]*Virginia Commonwealth University – School of Medicine*
[2]*McGuire Veterans Affairs Medical Center, Richmond, Virginia*
United States of America

1. Introduction

The overwhelming impact the Human Immunodeficiency Virus (HIV) has on the world is undeniable - by the end of 2009 there were 33.3 million people living with HIV in the world, with 1.8 million deaths in that year alone (WHO 2010). In addition, the high rate of deaths can be directly attributed to the lack of available medications - only 36% of the infected population received adequate antiretroviral therapy (WHO 2009). Besides the known political and monetary issues at hand, the multiple number of HIV virus subtypes and sub-subtypes that have been described are overwhelming pharmaceutical availability. In fact, most research completed on HIV therapies has occurred, and continues to occur, in Europe and America, targeting the HIV-1 strain, although much of the world population is also afflicted by HIV-2.

To combat viral strain mutations, Highly Active Antiretroviral Therapy (HAART) has increased in complexity and effectively decreased deaths from opportunistic infections in those that are candidates for this treatment. However, these advances are tainted with metabolic long-term side effects, some of which are directly attributed to HIV Protease Inhibitors (PIs).

HAART has been linked to cardiovascular complications in HIV-1 patients, and recent studies have shown that HIV PIs play critical roles in insulin resistance, dysregulation of lipid metabolism, and inflammation, which are all cornerstones of cardiovascular complications. In addition, HIV PI-induced atherosclerotic cardiovascular disease is becoming the leading cause of mortality in HIV-1 infected persons in developed countries. During the last decade, an extensive effort has been put forth to study HAART-induced side effects. Both *in vitro* and *in vivo* animal studies from our laboratory and others' have linked HIV PIs with the activation of endoplasmic reticulum (ER) stress and oxidative stress as well as an increase in inflammatory cytokine production from several cell types including macrophages, hepatocytes, intestinal epithelial cells and adipocytes. However, the underlying cellular and molecular mechanisms remain to be fully identified and therapeutic strategies are currently unavailable. Understanding the root causes of HAART-associated metabolic syndrome and its potential implications for HIV-infected patients will be critical to the design of effective interventions to combat the metabolic and cardiovascular diseases in a population chronically exposed to HAART. This chapter will discuss the current findings of HAART-associated metabolic complications and therapeutic challenges in the clinic.

2. FDA approved antiretrovirals in sequence of viral cycle

The first essential step in HIV infection of immune cells is fusion of the viral and cellular membranes. After an initial interaction, viral proteins utilize secondary receptors, especially CXCR4 (T cells) or CCR5 (macrophages), to gain entrance into the host cell. **Maraviroc** is a recently approved antiretroviral agent that inhibits fusion via binding and therefore prevents interactions with CCR5. Another, less commonly prescribed agent is **Fuzeon** (enfuvirtide), which binds to viral gp41. Due to the recent FDA approval of these two therapies, they will not be discussed in this chapter as there is little information on the long term clinical side effects of their usage. However, there is some positive evidence that there are minimal adverse metabolic effects.

After entry into the cellular cytoplasm, the viral genome (two copies of a single-stranded RNA) is reverse-transcribed into DNA by the viral enzyme, reverse transcriptase (RT). The first anti-HIV drugs to come on the market inhibited this enzyme. There are currently three classes of RT inhibitors **(RTI)**, **nucleotide and nucleoside analogues (NRTI)**, as well as **non-analogues (NNRTI)**. NRTIs are analogues to deoxynucleotides which are incorporated into the growing DNA chain, but lack one significant motif, a 3'-hydroxyl group, which is essential in linking each deoxyribose in the chain. Without this hydroxyl group, NRTIs cause a halt in synthesis, terminating chain growth. NNRTIs, on the other hand, bind directly to the RT itself, inhibiting the function of this essential enzyme.

The next step is integration of the newly synthesized DNA strand into the host genome by viral integrase. In 2007, the FDA approved **Raltegravir**, which directly inhibits this enzyme, and therefore does not allow latency of the virus in host cells. There has been some exciting evidence that Raltegravir has minimal side effects and may even reduce the side effects of some HIV PIs, as discussed later.

Upon host cell activation, often in times of stress such as infection and inflammation, the integrated virus cuts itself from the host genome and begins the viral replication cycle. Here, the virus utilizes the host RNA polymerase to produce multiple copies of package-able RNA strands from the DNA sequence. At the same time, the host cell machinery is recruited to translate RNA into viral proteins that are necessary for virion production and release. After protein production, the viral protease cleaves long HIV proteins into functional segments. Viral protease is unique in that it recognizes substrates with multi-folded domains and cleaves between a tyrosine/proline or phenylalanine/proline, something which human host cell enzymes cannot accomplish. This allowed for the specific design of HIV **protease inhibitors (PI)**.

2.1 Trails to current recommendations

Zidovudine, an NRTI, was the first drug approved in 1987, followed by approvals of zalcitabine, stavudine, and didanosine. The NRTIs seemed effective, yet the development of resistant strains caused a rebound of opportunistic infections in patients. In 1995, a major turning point occurred with the approval of HIV PIs ritonavir, saquinavir, and indinavir. Not only did these drugs work independently to help reduce viral load, but combination therapy with NRTIs drastically decreased opportunistic infections. This regimen is now known as Highly Active Antiretroviral Therapy (HAART), although the combinations have increased in variety. The classic HAART regimen includes two NRTIs with one PI, though 2 NRTIs with 1 NNRTI, or 3 NRTIs are also used. With the constant battle against resistant strains in the current HIV-infected population, addition of integrase or fusion inhibitors increases efficacy of these regimens, thus widening the arsenal of HIV drugs available to physicians.

In addition to different classes of drugs, each class has also increased in variety. For instance, within HIV PIs, there are now two generations of drugs, peptidic and non-peptidic, all of which have a hydroxyl group that mimics the transition state structure of hydrolysis (Mastrolorenzo et al. 2007). The peptidomimetic class is large in itself, and inherently diverse in structure. For example, some (i.e. ritonavir) are less peptidic in nature, but enhance stability of PI binding to the enzyme. In contrast, others are more effective but the viral protease may easily mutate with their use. As PIs are discussed extensively in this chapter due to their correlation with metabolic side effects, we will quickly mention them here.

Saquinavir (SQV) was the first PI approved by the FDA in 1995. Indinavir (IDV) reached the market in 1996 and, due to its efficacy with NRTIs, set the bar for HAART. Ritonavir (RITV) was marketed that same year, but currently is only given as a booster with other PIs as it inhibits cytochrome P450 (enzymes that metabolize most PIs and subsequently decrease their bioavailability). Nelfinavir (NFV) was marketed in 1997, and subsequently became the first PI to be recommended for pediatric patients. In 1999, Amprenavir (AMPV - now prescribed as prodrug fosamprenavir) was introduced. Atazanavir (ATZV) was approved in 2003, and was the first PI approved for once-daily dosing, raising the bar for development of more convenient PIs.

Lopinavir (LOPV) entered the prescription option in 2000. It was structurally designed for viral protease variants, but is similar to RITV. Due to low bioavailability, LOPV is prescribed only with a RITV combination. Now, the only form of LOPV available on the market is as a co-formulation pill, Kaletra (the first drug not available in single formulation). Kaletra was so successful in both drug-naïve and drug-experienced patients that it became first-line therapy in 2006, and now has only been surpassed by the newer non-peptidic PI, darunavir (DRV). Tipranavir (TRV) is the most recent PI, coming onto the market in 2006, but is only used in patients with resistant strains due to a high side effect profile.

2.2 Side effects of antiretrovirals

As the list of FDA approved antiretrovirals is long, so is the inventory of side effects. Even though the life expectancy of HIV-infected patients under HAART has been extended, the various HAART-induced side effects significantly affect quality of life. Therefore, treatment of HIV infection requires the balance between the beneficial effects of viral suppression and the drug-induced toxic effects.

The most common side effects of HAART are attributable to the NRTI/NNRTIs. These include general side effects such as rash, anemia, nausea, vomiting, diarrhea, and sleep disturbances. More severely, it is not uncommon to observe liver toxicities, pancreatitis and neuropathy in certain patients, often with underlying risk factors. Furthermore, in the past decade there has been increasing concern over long-term HAART patients experiencing early-onset cardiovascular risk factors such as hypertension and insulin resistance. With parallel observations in the American population, some attributed these to environmental factors not due to the drugs. However, numerous large clinical trials have determined that

HAART can induce such drastic metabolic changes, the most common of which are components of the clinically defined Metabolic Syndrome.

Metabolic Syndrome is a diagnosable syndrome that leaves patients at a high risk for heart attacks and strokes. To be diagnosed, according to the National Heart Lung and Blood Institute criteria (Grundy et al. 2006), a patient must have 3 out of the 5 diagnoses:

1. 35" central circumference in women, or 40" in men.
2. A triglyceride level >150mg/dL.
3. An HDL <50mg/dL in women or <40 in men.
4. A blood pressure >130/85.
5. High fasting blood glucose level or insulin resistance.

Importantly, each component is an individual risk factor for atherosclerosis.

In addition, some long term side effects have been given discrete labels, such as HIV-associated lipodystrophy (Caron-Debarle et al. 2010). This has pathophysiologically been defined as selective damage of adipose tissue with subcutaneous fat loss and/or central fat accumulation. A large clinical trial, the Data Collection on Adverse Events of Anti-HIV Drugs (DAD), has provided more insight on this and other phenomena, giving the base for other investigators to continue examining the details. Specifically, lipodystrophy and dyslipidemia are now better explained. Contrary to the belief at the start of HAART, peripheral wasting is no longer attributed to viral wasting, but to NRTIs (stavudine and zidovudine) (Barbaro 2007; Carr et al. 2000; Martinez et al. 2001; Lee, Hanes, and Johnson 2003); and fat accumulation is not a physiological phenomenon, but due to PI treatment (Mallon 2007; Mallon et al. 2003). Additional specific PI-induced side effects include glucose alterations and insulin resistance, which can lead to diabetes (DMII), hypertension, and cardiovascular (CV) dysfunctions (Calza, Manfredi, and Chiodo 2004; Friis-Moller et al. 2003; Group et al. 2007). The bottom line from these investigations is that myocardial infarction is directly correlated with PIs, and not other components of HAART (Friis-Moller et al. 2003; Kaplan et al. 2007).

3. HAART-induced dyslipidemia

Alterations in serum lipids of the HIV infected population have been noted since the beginning of the '90s. Before treatments began, patients often had a decrease in LDL and HDL plasma concentrations. NRTI treatment alone seemed to increase LDL to presumable baseline levels, without any effect on HDL, yet multi-drug treatments tended to increase serum triglycerides. In the late '90s, effort was carried out to tease apart the effect of infection versus particular therapies.

In the past decade, there has been an increase in average serum lipid levels in the general population due to poor diet and increasing age, and the HIV-HAART cohort is no different. In addition, the initial rise in serum lipid levels of HIV patients observed by clinicians was hypothesized to be immune reconstitution phenomena (Floris-Moore et al. 2006), which is a robust inflammatory response when HIV viral load decreases a few months to a year after treatment initiation. However, it has been found in numerous long-term and short-term studies, as well as in healthy versus HIV-infected persons, that HAART regimen, specifically PIs, induces dyslipidemia (Pere et al. 2008; Periard et al. 1999; Tsiodras et al. 2000; Friis-Moller et al. 2003; Calza et al. 2003; Carr et al. 1999; Purnell et al. 2000; Group et al. 2007). Often, clinicians combat this phenomenon with lipid-lowering drugs. At the same time, research has been attempting to determine which anti-HIV drugs induce the most change in lipid composition, and the mechanism underlying these changes.

Lipid homeostasis is centrally controlled by the liver. When fats are consumed in the diet, lipids are packaged into chylomicrons in the intestines whose final fate is the liver through an apoE endocytosis pathway. In order to effectively transport these to peripheral tissues, the liver packages triglycerides (TGs) and cholesterol into very low density lipoproteins (VLDL). VLDLs circulate and the TGs inside are taken up by muscle and adipose tissue after hydrolysis by lipase. The remnants are called intermediate density lipoproteins (IDL) which can be endocytosed by cells or further converted to low density lipoproteins (LDL) by lipases on the surface of cells. LDLs are cholesterol rich particles endocytosed through apoB-100, mostly in the liver or adipose tissue, and pathologically by macrophages. Another type of lipoprotein is high density (HDL), which is a way peripheral tissues 'send back' lipids, cholesterols, and proteins to the liver in an attempt not to be overloaded with these potentially toxic substances, as well as signal to the liver to stop synthesizing VLDLs.

HAART-induced dyslipidemia appears to affect many aspects of this pathway. Some studies have found that NNRTIs may even be able to increase HDL (Garcia-Benayas et al. 2001), a clinical advantage for dyslipidemic patients leading some to want to alter regimens to decrease PIs and increase NNRTIs (Barragan, Fisac, and Podzamczer 2006; Walli et al. 2001). In fact, there were successful studies in switching from PI-based treatments to NNRTI or NRTI-only regimes with success in attenuating dyslipidemia (Walli et al. 2001; Ruiz et al. 2001; Martinez et al. 2003). However, the effectiveness of PIs against HIV cannot be disputed. When PIs were added to the regimen in the mid-90s, there was a drastic decrease in patients who succumbed to opportunistic infections. The benefits of PIs far outweigh the side effects, but determining the mechanism behind these side effects may lead to alternative therapies in conjunction with PI use, or better-designed PIs.

4. HAART impact on liver lipid metabolism

The liver is a key organ in multiple processes, as well as the first organ to come into contact with ingested HAART medications. Hepatocytes are critical cells involved in lipid homeostasis, bile acid synthesis, gluconeogenesis, and metabolism of drugs. Therefore, alterations of normal cellular function can lead to global physiological consequences.

In regard to hepatic lipid metabolism, the endoplasmic reticulum (ER) is a central player. The ER is a critical organelle in cellular function as it is responsible for proper protein folding, cellular calcium level, lipid synthesis, and the secretory pathway. Inducing ER stress is thus relatively simple via depletion of ER calcium stores, changes in ER lipid membrane composition, reactive oxygen species (ROS), or accumulation of misfolded proteins. When triggered, the ER signals to the cell through the unfolded protein response (UPR) to cope with the increased accumulation of unfolded or misfolded proteins by downregulating protein synthesis and upregulating the degradation pathway. However, the extended activation of UPR will result in apoptosis.

UPR components identified in mammalian cells include three transducers [ER transmembrane kinase/endoribonuclease (IRE1), doubled-stranded RNA-activated protein kinase-like ER kinase (PERK), and activating transcription factor 6 (ATF-6)], as well as one master regulator [an ER chaperone protein (BiP/GRP78)]. In response to increased proteins in the ER lumen or calcium depletion, BiP/GRP78 releases the transducers, which induce differential control of gene transcription through transcription factors ATF-4 and spliced

XBP-1. Further activation of the downstream transcription factor GADD 153/CHOP will trigger apoptosis.

In addition, sterol regulatory element-binding proteins (SREBPs) are transcription factors that also reside in the ER membrane. There are three isoforms derived from two genes: SREBP-1a, SREBP-1c, and SREBP-2. SREBP-1c and SREBP2 are the predominant isoforms in the liver and play a major role in regulating the expression of key genes involved in lipid and lipoprotein metabolism such as 3-hydroxy-3-methylgutaryl-CoA (HMG-CoA) synthase, HMG-CoA reductase, squalene synthase, acetyl-CoA carboxylase (ACC), fatty acid synthase (FAS), and nuclear receptors. Therefore, ER stress induction not only alters protein production, but also lipid metabolism.

4.1 HIV PIs activate ER stress in hepatocytes

In HAART-induced metabolic dysfunctions, many features are similar to those observed in nonalcoholic fatty liver disease (NAFLD). NAFLD is a clinical term to describe a phenomenon in which patients have a fatty liver similar in all aspects to an equivalent alcoholic subject. Induction of NAFLD has been described in a range of conditions, such as obesity and diabetes, as well as by a variety of drugs. In addition, NAFLD is strongly associated with hepatic insulin resistance, yet it is hard to distinguish which comes first – fatty liver or the insulin resistance. To complicate the issue further, the exact cause of lipid accumulation in the liver can range from increased non-esterified fatty acids (NEFA) coming mostly from adipose tissue, excess lipids from the diet in the form of chylomicrons, impaired lipid processing in hepatocytes (*de novo* lipogenesis or DNL), or decreased release of VLDLs. However, Donnelly and colleagues were able to demonstrate that the majority of hepatic lipids in patients with NAFLD came from peripheral NEFA and DNL, not the diet (Donnelly et al. 2005).

This result is in agreement with HAART-induced NAFLD, as metabolic complications in these patients do not always seem to be correlated with diet. Importantly, although HAART-related NAFLD is not an entity of its own, many patients taking HIV PIs may have NAFLD with no symptoms, as does the majority of the overweight population. However, other patients progress to nonalcoholic steatohepatitis (NASH), which occurs with excess inflammation and scarring, potentially causing severe damage to the liver. Indeed, many studies have found NASH in greater than 50% of HAART-treated patients undergoing liver histopathological assessments (Ingiliz et al. 2009; Lemoine et al. 2006; Akhtar et al. 2008). HAART has been clearly shown to alter lipid and carbohydrate metabolism pathways, the underlying mechanism of NAFLD (Rector et al. 2008). Above all, NAFLD/NASH is most likely part of HAART-induced metabolic syndrome due to the strong correlations of hyperglycemia, insulin resistance, inflammation, and dyslipidemia.

Not all HAART components are associated with inducing constituents of NAFLD. RTIs can induce liver enzyme dysfunctions, but most studies are inconclusive. The two drugs with the strongest correlation are two NNRTIs, nevirapine and EFV (Waters, John, and Nelson 2007). Nevirapine-based HAART induces a faster liver fibrosis in those co-infected with hepatitis C (Macias et al. 2004), most likely due to a hypersensitivity reaction. In addition, some RTIs can have deleterious effects in the liver due to mitochondrial toxicities, which will not be discussed here due to a lack of correlation with metabolic side effects [reviewed in (Nunez 2010)]. However, HIV PIs are known to induce components of the metabolic syndrome, and hepatic alterations have been subsequently found to be at the core. Indeed, a connection has been found between western diet-induced NAFLD and HIV PIs - the induction of ER stress (Erickson 2009).

ER stress activation has been linked to various human diseases including NAFLD/NASH. Recent studies have shown that HIV PIs induce ER stress in many cell types including hepatocytes, macrophages and intestinal epithelial cells (Zhou et al. 2006; Zhou, Pandak, and Hylemon 2006; Zhou, Pandak et al. 2005; Zhou, Lhotak et al. 2005; Wu et al. 2010; Djedaini et al. 2009; Cho et al. 2009; Pyrko et al. 2007). We also have identified that HIV PI-induced ER stress is partially due to depletion of ER calcium stores. In addition, activation of ER stress has been linked to the upregulation of SREBPs and dysregulation of lipid metabolism in hepatocytes.

4.2 Autophagy in HIV PI-induced ER stress

Autophagy is similar to the UPR as its main purpose is to protect the cell from deleterious stimuli, but has the ability to increase cellular damage or death when over-stimulated. It can be triggered in a number of ways, but the best described is that of perceived starvation. In a nutrient-rich environment, growth factors stimulate the eukaryotic cell and activate phosphoinositide 3-kinase (PI3K) Class I proteins. In turn, protein Akt-1 becomes activated through phosphorylation, leading to inhibition of autophagosome formation. Consequently, lack of nutrients leads to autophagy, resulting in engulfment of cellular particles or organelles for energy through lysosomal degradation.

In addition to aiding cells during a starvation period, autophagy also helps regulate lipid stores. The exact mechanism behind autophagy-regulated lipid metabolism is not clearly defined, although it is known to be essential. When autophagy is inhibited in hepatocytes, lipids accumulate in droplets (Singh, Kaushik et al. 2009), and this is not due to increased triglyceride synthesis nor decreased VLDL secretions (Singh 2010). In addition, mice lacking autophagy in the liver have enlarged lipid-laden livers with increased triglyceride and cholesterol levels (Singh, Kaushik et al. 2009). Singh and colleagues have coined this process as lipophagy, in which lipid droplets are degraded through autophagy instead of lipolysis. Even further, components of the autophagosome may be necessary for lipid droplet formation, suggesting a flux of lipid metabolism in the cell dependent on this pathway (Shibata et al. 2009).

In recent years, different laboratories focusing on dissimilar topics have independently come upon an autophagy and ER stress link. For one, autophagy offers another pathway other than proteasomes to degrade unfolded proteins (Kawakami et al. 2009; Yorimitsu and Klionsky 2007; Ding and Yin 2008). However, prolonged UPR activation has now been shown to lead to autophagy-induced cell death (Yorimitsu and Klionsky 2007) and inhibition of autophagy increases cell viability with prolonged ER stress (Price et al. 2010; Qin et al. 2010). The exact mechanism of how ER stress induces autophagy is still being investigated. Recently, it was found that ER stress activation can inhibit Akt phosphorylation, which is a dose-dependent response caused by some HIV PIs (Gupta et al. 2007). However, the responsible protein(s) are still not known, and may be cell-type specific [reviewed in (Schleicher et al. 2010)].

A recent study has found a strong link between activation of ER stress, increased autophagy induction, and increased SREBP activation leading to lipid overload in hepatocytes (Nishina et al. 2010), although the exact pathway linking these three was not experimentally addressed. Our laboratory has recently found that HIV PIs induce ER stress in hepatocytes, leading to an increase in SREBP translocation to the nucleus, as well as induction of autophagy. However, the contribution of autophagy to HIV PI-induced metabolic syndrome remains to be determined and is the focus of our current studies [Figure 1].

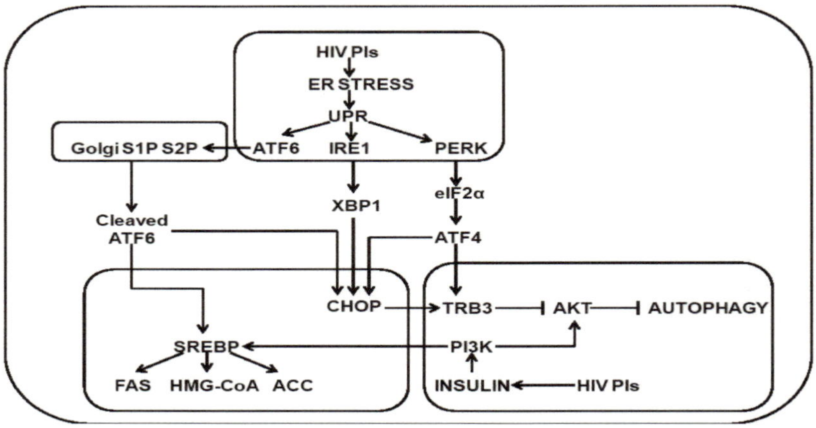

Fig. 1. Potential mechanisms of HIV PI-induced dysregulation of hepatic lipid metabolism.

4.3 HIV PI-induced hepatic insulin resistance

As discussed in the second section, HIV PIs have been directly linked to induction of HAART-metabolic syndromes, including lipodystrophy, glucose intolerance, and insulin resistance. These metabolic changes significantly increase the risk of DMII. There does not appear to be any one instigator in the spiral towards disease, but rather a mixture of increased lipolysis in the periphery, increased fat deposition in the liver and muscle, and peripheral and hepatic insulin resistance. In an attempt to tease these apart, a few clinical trials have found that HIV PIs first target a decrease in peripheral glucose uptake, although chronic treatment alters hepatic glucose production (Lee, Rao, and Grunfeld 2005; Woerle et al. 2003). Of specific note was an increase of fasting glucose - explained by endogenous liver production and decreased uptake in the periphery.

DNL occurs in the absence of insulin, when the body is in a presumably fasting state. This pathway may be directly activated without absence of insulin as the instigator, such as through growth hormones activating Akt (potentially linking the findings of ER stress above) or simply through cellular insulin insensitivity. In particular, diabetic mice demonstrated an increase of Tribbles 3 (TRB3). Du and colleagues have found that TRB3 complexes with Akt, causing an inhibition of its activity (Du et al. 2003). As Akt mediates insulin signaling, the inhibition of its action results in inducing cellular insulin resistance. Importantly, ER stress can activate TRB3 directly through transcription factors ATF-4 and CHOP. Again, TRB3 activation would also lead to autophagy through inhibition of Akt activity.

In addition to activating TRB3, ER stress also activates c-Jun N-terminal Kinase (JNK). JNK phosphorylates insulin receptor substrate (IRS-1), inhibiting its action of insulin-stimulated cell signaling (Ozcan et al. 2004). However, no current studies have been able to definitively show that HIV PI-induced ER stress leads to JNK activation, giving more support to the activation of TRB3 leading to both insulin insensitivity as well as autophagy.

The link between insulin insensitivity in the hepatocyte and that of metabolic consequences seen in HAART patients is now coming together. It is understood that insulin suppresses

VLDL secretion, most likely through inhibition of ApoB100 from packaging TGs. Therefore, loss of insulin stimulation will invariably lead to increased VLDL secretions, contributing to dyslipidemia. In addition, insulin actively stimulates SREBP-1c, but it cannot be assumed that loss of the insulin activation will lead to a decrease in SREBP-1c and thus a decrease in lipogenesis. In contrast, HIV PIs may be continually stimulating the UPR, leading to a continuation of SREBP-1c activation and lipogenesis. Therefore, HIV PI effects in the liver may, in fact, contribute directly to dyslipidemia and insulin insensitivity.

5. Impact of HAART on lipid metabolism in adipocytes

Although the average individual despises adipose tissue due to the displeasing aesthetics, there is no denying its importance in overall health. Adipose tissue is a much more complex and important endocrine organ than originally thought, composed of adipocytes, macrophages, and endothelial cells communicating in a matrix of complex extracellular proteins and proteoglycans. To make issues more complex, there is a constant turnover of cells in tissue (10% of adipocytes renew each year (Spalding et al. 2008)) and an influx of macrophages from the periphery at times of adipocyte hypertrophy or stress (Sell and Eckel 2010).

Different depots in the body have differing physiology (Hocking et al. 2010; Ray et al. 2009), most likely due to inconsistent derivations of tissue (Laharrague and Casteilla 2010; Billon et al. 2007). The differences between depots are seen both chemically and physiologically. It was found in the late '90s that preadipocytes isolated from different depots have different adipogenic induction responses (Adams et al. 1997) and gene expressions (Lefebvre et al. 1998), but these differences are still not well understood. Physiologically, it has been long known that those with increased visceral adipose mass have a higher risk of cardiovascular disease, although those with the same BMI, but more subcutaneous mass do not have the same risk. In HIV treatment, different drugs have differential effects on fat tissue - the RTIs seem to decrease subcutaneous depots while the HIV PIs increase visceral adipose mass (Mallewa et al. 2008). The result is a substantial increased risk of CV disease in HAART-treated patients, patients, which can be directly attributed to PIs can be attributed directly to PIs (Group et al. 2007).

However, the differences that lead to detrimental risks are still not understood. Basic researchers have probed the physiology of visceral versus subcutaneous depots for a decade now with no concrete results. Nevertheless, these studies have provided more information on the metabolism of adipocytes and adipose tissue than ever before, allowing more understanding not only of HAART side effects, but also those of diabetes.

5.1 Reverse transcriptase inhibitors

Most persons that are not treated for HIV infection experience wasting syndrome, or the involuntary loss of a significant amount of weight with associated weakness. With the advent of RTIs, physicians were able to combat this uncomfortable aspect of the disease, but soon realized another phenomenon - that of a patient gaining weight only centrally or even directly loosing fat mass from the legs, arms, and face. In the mid '90s when clinicians first began observing this occurrence, they attributed it to the PI component of HAART. This explanation was in good logic as the observance came soon after PIs were added to the regimen. After further clinical studies, they were able to tease apart this phenomenon termed HAART-induced lipodystrophy, finding that RTIs induce peripheral fat loss while

PIs increased central obesity. The next phase of studies determined which drugs were most likely to induce these aesthetic mishaps. It is now known that thymidine analogue-NRTIs in particular are most strongly associated with lipo-atrophy of the extremities (Mallon 2007; Stankov and Behrens 2007; Mallal et al. 2000). Even more so, the mechanism behind this attribution seems to stem from mitochondrial toxicity leading to adipose cell death.

Thymidine analogues are not initially active when they enter host cells as they must be phosphorylated before they can inhibit RT. This occurs in three steps, and generates two pharmacokinetic NRTIs in patients - active phosphate in cells and inactive drug in the plasma. Within the cells, intermediates occur that can have added effects, but the triphosphorylated NRTI is of most concern here, as it has been shown to directly inhibit mitochondrial DNA polymerase in many organs, including adipose (Kakuda 2000; Collins et al. 2004; Cote 2005). In fact, mitochondrial DNA was found to be depleted in HAART patient adipose biopsies (Nolan et al. 2003; Shikuma et al. 2001). However, this hypothesis seems insufficient to explain the total sum of physiological peripheral lipo-atrophy in patients. Therefore others have proposed supplementary mechanisms that may play a part in inhibition of the DNA polymerase for an additive effect on cells (Anderson, Kakuda, and Lichtenstein 2004; Lund and Wallace 2004). Most of these mechanisms are related to mitochondrial dysfunction, and may be partially due to the intermediate NRTIs. In addition, the balance of endogenous substrate with triphsophorylated NRTI may play a role, and help explain why only a certain proportion of patients experience lipo-atrophy (Anderson, Kakuda, and Lichtenstein 2004).

Another component to this story includes inhibition of adipogenesis. Peroxisome proliferator-activated receptor-γ (PPARγ) is an essential transcription factor required for maturation from a pre-adipocyte to a mature adipocyte. It has been shown that thymidine analogues can downregulate this nuclear receptor, inhibiting adipogenesis. Later, it was found that mitochondrial toxicity is related to this inhibition, and may be directly linked. In other words, the thymidine analogues are perhaps not inhibiting PPARγ directly, but inducing mitochondrial toxicity that results in crosstalk to the nucleus to stop differentiation of cells (Viengchareun et al. 2007; Stankov et al. 2007).

Importantly, the atrophy induced by RTIs may in fact contribute to HIV PI-induced NAFLD discussed previously. With the increase of cell death or inhibition of differentiation, there is a decrease in uptake of fats plus an increased release during cell death, increasing NEFA and contributing about 60% of the fats depositing in hepatocytes. Therefore, inhibition of RTI-induced cell death would not only aid a patient in an aesthetic discomfort, but also decrease the risk of NAFLD.

5.2 HIV protease inhibitors

As stated above, PIs appear to increase central adiposity, which is a major risk factor for CV disease. In addition, there are direct links of PIs and insulin resistance. The clinical significance of this has led to more research into PI-induced effects in adipose tissue than RTIs. Unfortunately, in the past decade we have only come a few steps closer to elucidating the exact mechanism of PI-induced adipose pathology.

At the start of investigating these drugs, many researchers focused on the possibility that HIV PIs can inhibit adipogenesis and induce apoptosis, which may help explain lipo-atrophy. However, depot-specific differences could not be explained and the conclusion that it was the NRTIs inducing the atrophy and not the PIs altered the focus of the field. In addition, the findings from these early investigations are still not conclusive. This is

explained by inherent difficulties in handling and processing adipose tissue, diversity in cell lines, and different subjective techniques used between laboratories. For example, some investigators found that RITV does not inhibit differentiation of adipocytes, while others stated that it significantly inhibits this pathway. Importantly, most laboratories focused on inhibition of differentiation, not the mechanism of this phenomenon nor how this effect in cell culture could be well correlated in the clinic.
An important turning point in this field came through parallel research conducted in obesity, diabetes, and endocrinology. Major conclusions demonstrated that adipose tissue was a significant player in the inflammatory state and insulin resistance. HIV PI-investigators began to turn from focusing on which drugs inhibited differentiation to the mechanism of HIV PI-induced lipid metabolism dysregulation, cytokine secretions, and connections to the metabolic syndromes seen in this patient population. Ensuing hypotheses included induction of ER stress, mitochondrial toxicity, inhibition of GLUT4, and autophagy induction.

5.2.1 HIV PI-induced ER stress, inflammation, and insulin resistance in adipocytes

As discussed in the previous section, ER stress activation is directly linked to dysregulation of hepatic lipid metabolism. In adipocytes, this is no different, and may be even more complex as cell maturation relies on lipids. In the preadipocyte state, the cell has more characteristics of a fibroblast than an adipocyte, in which it is elongated and located close to the blood vessel. At this stage, it releases minimal cytokines, and is relatively lipid droplet (LD) free. Upon induction of differentiation, the cell rearranges, begins to round when next to other adipocytes, and forms LDs. Although the complete understanding of LD formation is yet to be elucidated, it is known that they originate in some manner from the ER. It is also hypothesized that the two organelles stay connected in a manner that allows free exchange of lipids, but this hypothesis is not completely supported by evidence at this time.
Either way, the close proximity of the ER to LDs, as well as the dependence of the ER on the production of neutral lipids, demonstrates how much the UPR can affect an adipocyte. In addition, adipocytes need constitutive activation of the UPR as the IRE1-XBP-1 pathway is essential in adipogenesis (Sha et al. 2009; Basseri et al. 2009), while overstimulation of the UPR can inhibit differentiation altogether (Shimada et al. 2007). This dependence on the UPR has not been demonstrated in hepatocytes and, in addition, another difference is observed with SREBP-1c. In adipocytes, SREBP-1c is actually downregulated in times of ER stress (Gregor and Hotamisligil 2007), as it is also a major player in adipogenesis.
However, in addition to these differences, both cell types respond with some degree of insulin resistance upon UPR activation (Djedaini et al. 2009). In the fields of obesity and diabetes, we have come to realize that DMII is directly related to the inflammation and malfunction of overloaded adipose tissue. With increasing overload, adipocytes begin to hypertrophy, becoming stressed and signaling this with a release of proinflammatory cytokines. These cytokines cause an infiltration of circulating macrophages, which engulf over-stressed or dying cells, forming characteristic crown-like structures. Interestingly, HIV patients on HAART therapy appear to be in the same state as an obese individual in terms of inflammatory and dysfunctional adipose tissue. Patients often have a decrease in insulin sensitivity, as well as having dyslipidemia and liver disease as previously discussed. These factors can also be teased apart from over-nutrition, as shown in the D.A.D. studies, among other clinical investigations.

HIV PIs have been repeatedly shown to induce ER stress, and the results in our laboratory support others' work. This activation has been shown to be directly linked to alterations in SREBP-1c processing in adipocytes, as well as suggested to be the cause of inhibition of differentiation observed with these drugs. In addition, the inflammatory cascade is induced in adipocytes treated with HIV PIs (Jones et al. 2005; Kim et al. 2006; Leroyer et al. 2011). The inflammatory state is highly predictive of onset of insulin resistance, and once again this induction is also directly linked to ER stress. In fact, activation of the UPR can induce inflammatory activation through the JNK pathway as stated previously. Additionally, cytokine release from neighboring cells can induce ER stress in the host cell, causing a vicious cycle.

A key study in this field was done by Djedaini and colleagues, in which they treated human adipocyte cells with LOPV. They noted both increased activation of ER stress and decreased IRS1 phosphorylation, as well as reduced glucose uptake (Djedaini et al. 2009). What linked these phenomena was eIF2-α phosphorylation - a key protein activated during the UPR. When these investigators inhibited this phosphorylation with a specific molecule, salubrinal, they were able to decrease IRS1 phosphorylation slightly. However, when done in conjunction with minimal concentrations of LOPV, there was a significant decrease of IRS1 phosphorylation, demonstrating a synergistic effect of the two drugs.

Activation of the UPR leading to a decrease in insulin signaling may only be part of the story. Others have shown that PIs can actually inhibit the glucose transporter directly (Hertel et al. 2004). It has been proposed that this inhibition induces a starvation-like state in the cell with the decrease of intracellular glucose, causing activation of ER stress. This would lead to a decrease in insulin signaling, propagating insulin resistance further. At this point, adipocytes would rely heavily on lipids, hydrolyzing triglyceride stores and thus increasing NEFA release, causing lipotoxicity and insulin resistance at the physiological level. Despite these findings, more research is obviously needed to determine which pathway or proteins HIV PIs induce/inhibit when they first come into contact with an adipocyte. Only then can we be certain of the consequences of a given structure on the drugs currently on the market.

5.2.2 Adiponectin and autophagy

Adipocytes release not only pro-inflammatory cytokines, but also the anti-inflammatory cytokine adiponectin. Adiponectin is unique in a number of ways. It is exclusively secreted by adipose tissue and is negatively correlated with diseases such as atherosclerosis and insulin resistance. In overexpanded or stressed tissue, there is a decrease of adiponectin secretion (Kern et al. 2003), and an increase of macrophage-inducing TNF-α, IL-6, and MCP-1, implicating inflammatory diseases such as atherosclerosis and insulin resistance.

HIV PIs have been repeatedly reported to decrease adiponectin, from the RNA level to secretion. Our laboratory has also noted this phenomenon, as well as found a substantial increase in IL-6 secretion in mouse adipocytes treated with HIV PIs for 48 hours, in a dose-dependent manner. MCP-1 and TNF-α mRNA levels also increase. This is just one more piece of evidence that HIV PIs induce a pro-inflammatory state in adipose.

Interestingly, adiponectin can alleviate ER stress (Zhou et al. 2010). Zhou and colleagues found in their cellular studies that ER stress initiation is sufficient to decrease adiponectin release. In animal models, they reported stabilization of adiponectin further decreased obesity-induced ER stress in adipose tissue. Moreover, induction of autophagy could alleviate ER stress responses in the cell, stabilizing adiponectin secretions.

As discussed previously, increasing evidence points to autophagic dysregulation as a component of altered lipid metabolism in cells. In adipocytes, there is a constitutive base of autophagy aiding in the recycling of lipid stores. Indeed, with a decrease in autophagy in pre-adipocytes, there is a resulting inhibition of adipogenesis (Singh, Xiang et al. 2009). *In vivo* animal studies from the same group found a complete reduction of adipose mass when they induced a decrease in the autophagy pathway, resulting in smaller adipocytes and altered LD morphology. This is in seeming opposition to what occurs in the liver with a decrease in autophagy and may be best explained best by Singh and colleagues. They detail the need for autophagy to control adipose mass so lipids can be continually stored in adipose tissue, while in the liver, autophagy attempts to decrease TG accumulations (Singh 2010).

5.3 Other HIV PI effects in adipocytes

Although ER stress activation represents an important cellular mechanism underlying HIV PI-induced side effects in adiopocytes, HIV PIs may also influence cellular lipid metabolism through other mechanisms, such as mitochondrial toxicity. In this realm, most investigators who are proponents of this mechanism found concurrent inhibition of adipocyte differentiation with increased markers of mitochondrial dysfunction (Viengchareun et al. 2007). When considering this hypothesis, however, the close tie of ER and mitochondrial homeostasis must be contemplated, especially in the case of the apoptosis cascade. Indeed, some have shown the same close connection when mitochondrial dysfunction leads to the UPR (Burkart et al. 2011), and likewise the UPR has been shown to induce mitochondrial dysfunction (Lee et al. 2010). This tight interplay often makes it difficult to discern where the initial damage occurs, but it is irrefutable that ER stress activation plays a major role.

Another mechanism proposed is inhibition of PPARγ activity that leads to inhibition of differentiation. As stated before, many investigators discovered that RTIs and PIs were able to decrease the capability of adipogenesis. In these studies, it was found that PIs could inhibit PPARγ activity, and this was not through direct interaction[reviewed in (Caron et al. 2009)]. Affecting PPARγ will alter the cell physiology, such as a decrease of adiponectin secretion and alteration of lipid metabolism. However, without demonstrating a direct pathway of HIV PI-induced PPARγ downregulation, it is difficult to pursue this mechanism when there are also other promising pathways in the works.

6. HIV PIs increase inflammation at the vasculature and alter macrophage lipid metabolism

Macrophages are key cells involved in atherosclerotic plaques. Initiation of a plaque can occur very early, when the endothelial lining becomes damaged or inflamed, inducing leukocyte infiltration. The damage is often attributed to oxidized lipoproteins in the bloodstream, occurring with high LDL levels and decreased anti-oxidants. After initial damage, macrophages localize to the area. In addition to their innate role to induce inflammation in the process of healing, macrophages will also take up circulating lipids that are not being properly processed by peripheral tissues. Macrophages will keep accumulating lipids, expanding and releasing pro-inflammatory cytokines that call in more macrophages, all the while not 'fixing' the initial problem of damaged endothelium. As the plaque builds, more lipids tend to accumulate in the given area and stability decreases, having the potential of completely restricting flow or dislodging.

Patients taking HIV PIs have been found to have accelerated atherosclerotic lesions. An important causative factor is most likely the dyslipidemia discussed previously, potentially inducing initial damage, although direct influence on the endothelial layer could also be at fault. In fact, numerous clinical studies have noted decreased endothelial function in HAART-treated patients. This decrease has been directly attributed to the PI component (Teixeira et al. 2009). In cell culture investigations, it has been found that PIs can directly induce apoptosis of vascular smooth muscle cells, which could contribute to both endothelium dysfunction as well as plaque instability, maybe through increased reactive oxygen species (Rudich et al. 2005).

Once the initial damage ensues at the endothelium, macrophages can migrate through the endothelial layer into the intima and begin secreting inflammatory cytokines as well as developing scavenger receptors. These receptors are directly responsible for LDL uptake in macrophages, leading to foam cell formation. In regard to macrophages, HIV PIs actually have multiple affects. One of the more important of these was discovered by Dressman et al. who found that PIs actively induce CD36 (Dressman et al. 2003). CD36 is a fatty acid transporter in metabolically active tissues and, in macrophages, it binds and endocytoses oxidized LDLs. This directly leads to the formation of foam cells, which are at the core of plaques.

In addition to inducing CD36, HIV PIs can increase foam cell formation via other pathways. HIV PIs have been shown by several investigators to increase active SREBPs in macrophages. Our laboratory has demonstrated that HIV PI-induced upregulation of SREBPs occurs through the activation of ER stress (Zhou, Pandak et al. 2005). In addition, PIs were found to decrease cholesterol efflux in foam cells by inhibiting scavenger receptor B1 and caveolins (Wang et al. 2007). Thus, PIs can both induce the intake and inhibit the export of the ingredients of a foam cell.

Previous findings in our laboratory demonstrate that inner-membranes are overloaded with cholesterol in HIV PI-treated macrophages, and ER calcium stores depleted. Taking the above together, we hypothesize that HIV PIs induce cholesterol overload in macrophages, leading to an alteration in cholesterol composition of the ER membrane. As stated before, a slight alteration in membrane composition can induce the UPR, which would lead to an increase of SREBP-1 in macrophages, causing lipid overload and increasing foam cell formation of these cells. In addition, a proportion of these cells would die through the apoptotic pathway, inducing an unstable plaque, and a basis for the drastic side effects seen with these drugs.

7. Metabolic disease, cardiovascular dysfunction, and concluding remarks

As demonstrated throughout this chapter, PIs have drastic effects in multiple cell types and tissues. In addition to those listed above, PIs have also been shown to increase pro-insulin secretions from β-cells, demonstrating their altered functions (Behrens et al. 1999). It is postulated that PIs fist induce a transition from normal to impaired glucose tolerance due to insulin resistance induction in the liver and adipose tissues. With worsening glucose resistance, more insulin must be secreted, and over time this leads to β-cell dysfunction, which can be demonstrated by the release of inactive pro-insulin. However, as some investigators have shown direct effects of HIV PIs on the β-cell, it is possible these mechanisms are occurring simultaneously, accounting for the more rapid induction of insulin resistance seen in this patient population (Schutt et al. 2004).

In any case, there is no doubt that HAART has decreased total mortality in HIV-infected persons, but determining the mechanism behind life-altering side effects could help improve therapies. Also, not all HIV PIs have the same degree of metabolic disease-inductions; such as AMPV, which has the least effect on lipid metabolism and does not need a RITV booster. As mentioned previously, some have actually proposed to switch to NNRTIs and leave out the PIs for favorable lipid profiles in patients. Even more, we have recently shown that Raltegravir can actually mitigate HIV PI-induced ER stress, relieving lipid metabolism dysregulation in hepatocytes (Cao et al. 2010).

This leaves the question of cost versus benefit. HIV-specialists are sure to argue that some of the PIs that are controversial are keeping their patients' morbidity drastically down. Without these particular drugs, the chance of increased viremia and viral mutations is too large. Switching to AMPV, for instance, is not always feasible. In addition, although we have shown the potential of Raltegravir against the cellular side effects, this might not feasibly translate into the clinic due to pill-burden and expense. Therefore, physicians continue to push exercise and lipid-lowering drugs. Development of better therapeutic strategies for HIV infection and HAART-induced metabolic syndrome requires more extensive studies and efforts.

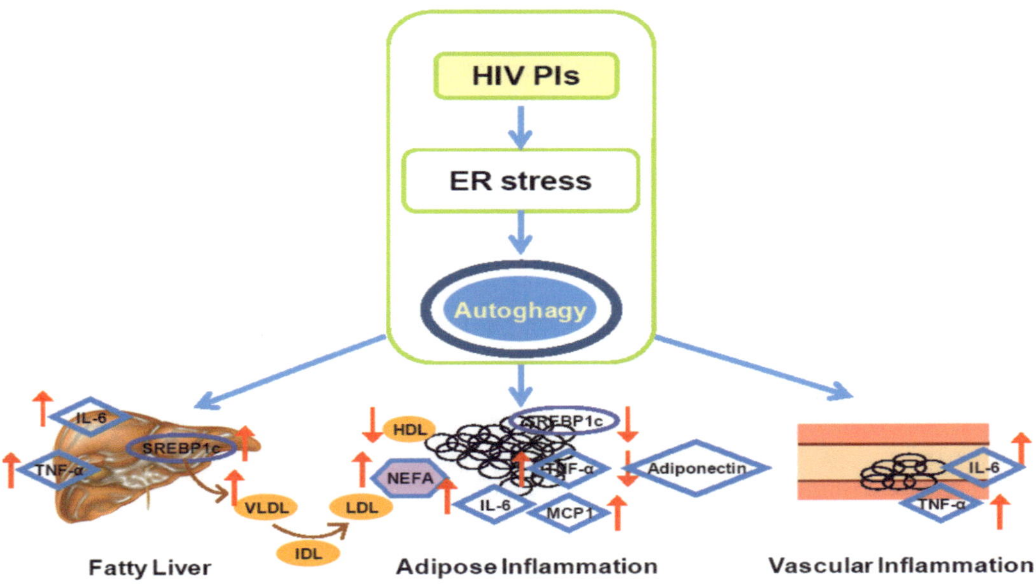

Fig. 2. Summary of HIV PI-induced pathological effects.

8. Acknowledgements

This work was supported by grants from the National Institutes of Health (R21AI068432, R01AT004148, R01AI057189, and 1F30DK085856-02) and A.D. Williams fund.

***Address request for reprints to**: Huiping Zhou, Ph.D, Department of Microbiology and Immunology, School of Medicine, Virginia Commonwealth University, PO Box 908678, Richmond, VA 23298-0678; Tel. (804)828-6817; Fax. (804) 828-0676; E-mail: hzhou@vcu.edu.

9. References

Adams, M., C. T. Montague, J. B. Prins, J. C. Holder, S. A. Smith, L. Sanders, J. E. Digby, C. P. Sewter, M. A. Lazar, V. K. Chatterjee, and S. O'Rahilly. 1997. Activators of peroxisome proliferator-activated receptor gamma have depot-specific effects on human preadipocyte differentiation. *J Clin Invest* 100 (12):3149-53.

Akhtar, M. A., K. Mathieson, B. Arey, J. Post, R. Prevette, A. Hillier, P. Patel, L. J. Ram, D. H. Van Thiel, and A. Nadir. 2008. Hepatic histopathology and clinical characteristics associated with antiretroviral therapy in HIV patients without viral hepatitis. *Eur J Gastroenterol Hepatol* 20 (12):1194-204.

Anderson, P. L., T. N. Kakuda, and K. A. Lichtenstein. 2004. The cellular pharmacology of nucleoside- and nucleotide-analogue reverse-transcriptase inhibitors and its relationship to clinical toxicities. *Clin Infect Dis* 38 (5):743-53.

Barbaro, G. 2007. Visceral fat as target of highly active antiretroviral therapy-associated metabolic syndrome. *Current pharmaceutical design* 13 (21):2208-2213.

Barragan, P., C. Fisac, and D. Podzamczer. 2006. Switching strategies to improve lipid profile and morphologic changes. *AIDS Rev* 8 (4):191-203.

Basseri, S., S. Lhotak, A. M. Sharma, and R. C. Austin. 2009. The chemical chaperone 4-phenylbutyrate inhibits adipogenesis by modulating the unfolded protein response. *J Lipid Res* 50 (12):2486-501.

Behrens, G., A. Dejam, H. Schmidt, H. J. Balks, G. Brabant, T. Korner, M. Stoll, and R. E. Schmidt. 1999. Impaired glucose tolerance, beta cell function and lipid metabolism in HIV patients under treatment with protease inhibitors. *Aids* 13 (10):F63-70.

Billon, N., P. Iannarelli, M. C. Monteiro, C. Glavieux-Pardanaud, W. D. Richardson, N. Kessaris, C. Dani, and E. Dupin. 2007. The generation of adipocytes by the neural crest. *Development* 134 (12):2283-92.

Burkart, A., X. Shi, M. Chouinard, and S. Corvera. 2011. Adenylate kinase 2 links mitochondrial energy metabolism to the induction of the unfolded protein response. *J Biol Chem* 286 (6):4081-9.

Calza, L., R. Manfredi, and F. Chiodo. 2004. Dyslipidaemia associated with antiretroviral therapy in HIV-infected patients. *The Journal of antimicrobial chemotherapy* 53 (1):10-14.

Calza, L., R. Manfredi, B. Farneti, and F. Chiodo. 2003. Incidence of hyperlipidaemia in a cohort of 212 HIV-infected patients receiving a protease inhibitor-based antiretroviral therapy. *Int J Antimicrob Agents* 22 (1):54-9.

Cao, R., Y. Hu, Y. Wang, E. C. Gurley, E. J. Studer, X. Wang, P. B. Hylemon, W. M. Pandak, A. J. Sanyal, L. Zhang, and H. Zhou. 2010. Prevention of HIV protease inhibitor-induced dysregulation of hepatic lipid metabolism by raltegravir via endoplasmic reticulum stress signaling pathways. *The Journal of pharmacology and experimental therapeutics* 334 (2):530-539.

Caron-Debarle, M., F. Boccara, C. Lagathu, B. Antoine, P. Cervera, J. P. Bastard, C. Vigouroux, and J. Capeau. 2010. Adipose Tissue as a Target of HIV-1 Antiretroviral Drugs. Potential Consequences on Metabolic Regulations. *Current pharmaceutical design*.

Caron, M., C. Vigouroux, J. P. Bastard, and J. Capeau. 2009. Antiretroviral-Related Adipocyte Dysfunction and Lipodystrophy in HIV-Infected Patients: Alteration of the PPARgamma-Dependent Pathways. *PPAR Res* 2009:507141.

Carr, A., J. Miller, M. Law, and D. A. Cooper. 2000. A syndrome of lipoatrophy, lactic acidaemia and liver dysfunction associated with HIV nucleoside analogue therapy: contribution to protease inhibitor-related lipodystrophy syndrome. *AIDS (London, England)* 14 (3):F25-32.

Carr, A., K. Samaras, A. Thorisdottir, G. R. Kaufmann, D. J. Chisholm, and D. A. Cooper. 1999. Diagnosis, prediction, and natural course of HIV-1 protease-inhibitor-associated lipodystrophy, hyperlipidaemia, and diabetes mellitus: a cohort study. *Lancet* 353 (9170):2093-2099.

Cho, H. Y., S. Thomas, E. B. Golden, K. J. Gaffney, F. M. Hofman, T. C. Chen, S. G. Louie, N. A. Petasis, and A. H. Schonthal. 2009. Enhanced killing of chemo-resistant breast cancer cells via controlled aggravation of ER stress. *Cancer Lett* 282 (1):87-97.

Collins, M. L., N. Sondel, D. Cesar, and M. K. Hellerstein. 2004. Effect of nucleoside reverse transcriptase inhibitors on mitochondrial DNA synthesis in rats and humans. *J Acquir Immune Defic Syndr* 37 (1):1132-9.

Cote, H. C. 2005. Possible ways nucleoside analogues can affect mitochondrial DNA content and gene expression during HIV therapy. *Antivir Ther* 10 Suppl 2:M3-11.

Ding, W. X., and X. M. Yin. 2008. Sorting, recognition and activation of the misfolded protein degradation pathways through macroautophagy and the proteasome. *Autophagy* 4 (2):141-150.

Djedaini, M., P. Peraldi, M. D. Drici, C. Darini, P. Saint-Marc, C. Dani, and A. Ladoux. 2009. Lopinavir co-induces insulin resistance and ER stress in human adipocytes. *Biochemical and biophysical research communications* 386 (1):96-100.

Donnelly, K. L., C. I. Smith, S. J. Schwarzenberg, J. Jessurun, M. D. Boldt, and E. J. Parks. 2005. Sources of fatty acids stored in liver and secreted via lipoproteins in patients with nonalcoholic fatty liver disease. *J Clin Invest* 115 (5):1343-51.

Dressman, J., J. Kincer, S. V. Matveev, L. Guo, R. N. Greenberg, T. Guerin, D. Meade, X. A. Li, W. Zhu, A. Uittenbogaard, M. E. Wilson, and E. J. Smart. 2003. HIV protease inhibitors promote atherosclerotic lesion formation independent of dyslipidemia by increasing CD36-dependent cholesteryl ester accumulation in macrophages. *J Clin Invest* 111 (3):389-97.

Du, K., S. Herzig, R. N. Kulkarni, and M. Montminy. 2003. TRB3: a tribbles homolog that inhibits Akt/PKB activation by insulin in liver. *Science* 300 (5625):1574-7.

Erickson, S. K. 2009. Nonalcoholic fatty liver disease. *J Lipid Res* 50 Suppl:S412-6.

Floris-Moore, M., A. A. Howard, Y. Lo, J. H. Arnsten, N. Santoro, and E. E. Schoenbaum. 2006. Increased serum lipids are associated with higher CD4 lymphocyte count in HIV-infected women. *HIV Med* 7 (7):421-30.

Friis-Moller, N., R. Weber, P. Reiss, R. Thiebaut, O. Kirk, A. d'Arminio Monforte, C. Pradier, L. Morfeldt, S. Mateu, M. Law, W. El-Sadr, S. De Wit, C. A. Sabin, A. N. Phillips, J. D. Lundgren, and D. A. D. study group. 2003. Cardiovascular disease risk factors in HIV patients--association with antiretroviral therapy. Results from the DAD study. *AIDS (London, England)* 17 (8):1179-1193.

Garcia-Benayas, T., F. Blanco, J. J. de la Cruz, M. J. Senchordi, J. M. Gomez-Viera, V. Soriano, and J. Gonzalez-Lahoz. 2001. Role of nonnucleosides in the development of HAART-related lipid disturbances. *J Acquir Immune Defic Syndr* 28 (5):496-8.

Gregor, M. G., and G. S. Hotamisligil. 2007. Adipocyte stress: The endoplasmic reticulum and metabolic disease. *J Lipid Res.*

Group, D. A. D. Study, N. Friis-Moller, P. Reiss, C. A. Sabin, R. Weber, A. Monforte, W. El-Sadr, R. Thiebaut, S. De Wit, O. Kirk, E. Fontas, M. G. Law, A. Phillips, and J. D. Lundgren. 2007. Class of antiretroviral drugs and the risk of myocardial infarction. *The New England journal of medicine* 356 (17):1723-1735.

Grundy, S. M., J. I. Cleeman, S. R. Daniels, K. A. Donato, R. H. Eckel, B. A. Franklin, D. J. Gordon, R. M. Krauss, P. J. Savage, S. C. Smith, Jr., J. A. Spertus, and F. Costa. 2006. Diagnosis and management of the metabolic syndrome: an American Heart Association/National Heart, Lung, and Blood Institute scientific statement. *Current opinion in cardiology* 21 (1):1-6.

Gupta, A. K., B. Li, G. J. Cerniglia, M. S. Ahmed, S. M. Hahn, and A. Maity. 2007. The HIV protease inhibitor nelfinavir downregulates Akt phosphorylation by inhibiting proteasomal activity and inducing the unfolded protein response. *Neoplasia* 9 (4):271-8.

Hertel, J., H. Struthers, C. B. Horj, and P. W. Hruz. 2004. A structural basis for the acute effects of HIV protease inhibitors on GLUT4 intrinsic activity. *J Biol Chem* 279 (53):55147-52.

Hocking, S. L., L. E. Wu, M. Guilhaus, D. J. Chisholm, and D. E. James. 2010. Intrinsic depot-specific differences in the secretome of adipose tissue, preadipocytes, and adipose tissue-derived microvascular endothelial cells. *Diabetes* 59 (12):3008-16.

Ingiliz, P., M. A. Valantin, C. Duvivier, F. Medja, S. Dominguez, F. Charlotte, R. Tubiana, T. Poynard, C. Katlama, A. Lombes, and Y. Benhamou. 2009. Liver damage underlying unexplained transaminase elevation in human immunodeficiency virus-1 mono-infected patients on antiretroviral therapy. *Hepatology* 49 (2):436-42.

Jones, S. P., O. Janneh, D. J. Back, and M. Pirmohamed. 2005. Altered adipokine response in murine 3T3-F442A adipocytes treated with protease inhibitors and nucleoside reverse transcriptase inhibitors. *Antiviral Therapy* 10 (2):207-213.

Kakuda, T. N. 2000. Pharmacology of nucleoside and nucleotide reverse transcriptase inhibitor-induced mitochondrial toxicity. *Clin Ther* 22 (6):685-708.

Kaplan, R. C., L. A. Kingsley, A. R. Sharrett, X. Li, J. Lazar, P. C. Tien, W. J. Mack, M. H. Cohen, L. Jacobson, and S. J. Gange. 2007. Ten-year predicted coronary heart disease risk in HIV-infected men and women. *Clinical infectious diseases : an official publication of the Infectious Diseases Society of America* 45 (8):1074-1081.

Kawakami, T., R. Inagi, H. Takano, S. Sato, J. R. Ingelfinger, T. Fujita, and M. Nangaku. 2009. Endoplasmic reticulum stress induces autophagy in renal proximal tubular cells. *Nephrology, dialysis, transplantation : official publication of the European Dialysis and Transplant Association - European Renal Association* 24 (9):2665-2672.

Kern, P. A., G. B. Di Gregorio, T. Lu, N. Rassouli, and G. Ranganathan. 2003. Adiponectin expression from human adipose tissue: relation to obesity, insulin resistance, and tumor necrosis factor-alpha expression. *Diabetes* 52 (7):1779-85.

Kim, R. J., C. G. Wilson, M. Wabitsch, M. A. Lazar, and C. M. Steppan. 2006. HIV protease inhibitor-specific alterations in human adipocyte differentiation and metabolism. *Obesity (Silver Spring, Md.)* 14 (6):994-1002.

Laharrague, P., and L. Casteilla. 2010. The emergence of adipocytes. *Endocr Dev* 19:21-30.

Lee, G. A., M. N. Rao, and C. Grunfeld. 2005. The effects of HIV protease inhibitors on carbohydrate and lipid metabolism. *Curr HIV/AIDS Rep* 2 (1):39-50.

Lee, H., J. Hanes, and K. A. Johnson. 2003. Toxicity of nucleoside analogues used to treat AIDS and the selectivity of the mitochondrial DNA polymerase. *Biochemistry* 42 (50):14711-14719.

Lee, J. W., W. H. Kim, J. Yeo, and M. H. Jung. 2010. ER stress is implicated in mitochondrial dysfunction-induced apoptosis of pancreatic beta cells. *Mol Cells* 30 (6):545-9.

Lefebvre, A. M., M. Laville, N. Vega, J. P. Riou, L. van Gaal, J. Auwerx, and H. Vidal. 1998. Depot-specific differences in adipose tissue gene expression in lean and obese subjects. *Diabetes* 47 (1):98-103.

Lemoine, M., V. Barbu, P. M. Girard, M. Kim, J. P. Bastard, D. Wendum, F. Paye, C. Housset, J. Capeau, and L. Serfaty. 2006. Altered hepatic expression of SREBP-1 and PPARgamma is associated with liver injury in insulin-resistant lipodystrophic HIV-infected patients. *Aids* 20 (3):387-95.

Leroyer, S., C. Vatier, S. Kadiri, J. Quette, C. Chapron, J. Capeau, and B. Antoine. 2011. Glyceroneogenesis is inhibited through HIV protease inhibitor-induced inflammation in human subcutaneous but not visceral adipose tissue. *J Lipid Res* 52 (2):207-20.

Lund, K. C., and K. B. Wallace. 2004. Direct, DNA pol-gamma-independent effects of nucleoside reverse transcriptase inhibitors on mitochondrial bioenergetics. *Cardiovasc Toxicol* 4 (3):217-28.

Macias, J., V. Castellano, N. Merchante, R. B. Palacios, J. A. Mira, C. Saez, J. A. Garcia-Garcia, F. Lozano, J. M. Gomez-Mateos, and J. A. Pineda. 2004. Effect of antiretroviral drugs on liver fibrosis in HIV-infected patients with chronic hepatitis C: harmful impact of nevirapine. *Aids* 18 (5):767-74.

Mallal, S. A., M. John, C. B. Moore, I. R. James, and E. J. McKinnon. 2000. Contribution of nucleoside analogue reverse transcriptase inhibitors to subcutaneous fat wasting in patients with HIV infection. *Aids* 14 (10):1309-16.

Mallewa, J. E., E. Wilkins, J. Vilar, M. Mallewa, D. Doran, D. Back, and M. Pirmohamed. 2008. HIV-associated lipodystrophy: a review of underlying mechanisms and therapeutic options. *J Antimicrob Chemother* 62 (4):648-60.

Mallon, P. W. 2007. Pathogenesis of lipodystrophy and lipid abnormalities in patients taking antiretroviral therapy. *AIDS reviews* 9 (1):3-15.

Mallon, P. W., J. Miller, D. A. Cooper, and A. Carr. 2003. Prospective evaluation of the effects of antiretroviral therapy on body composition in HIV-1-infected men starting therapy. *AIDS (London, England)* 17 (7):971-979.

Martinez, E., J. A. Arnaiz, D. Podzamczer, D. Dalmau, E. Ribera, P. Domingo, H. Knobel, M. Riera, E. Pedrol, L. Force, J. M. Llibre, F. Segura, C. Richart, C. Cortes, M. Javaloyas, M. Aranda, A. Cruceta, E. de Lazzari, and J. M. Gatell. 2003. Substitution of nevirapine, efavirenz, or abacavir for protease inhibitors in patients with human immunodeficiency virus infection. *N Engl J Med* 349 (11):1036-46.

Martinez, E., A. Mocroft, M. A. Garcia-Viejo, J. B. Perez-Cuevas, J. L. Blanco, J. Mallolas, L. Bianchi, I. Conget, J. Blanch, A. Phillips, and J. M. Gatell. 2001. Risk of lipodystrophy in HIV-1-infected patients treated with protease inhibitors: a prospective cohort study. *Lancet* 357 (9256):592-598.

Mastrolorenzo, A., S. Rusconi, A. Scozzafava, G. Barbaro, and C. T. Supuran. 2007. Inhibitors of HIV-1 protease: current state of the art 10 years after their introduction. From antiretroviral drugs to antifungal, antibacterial and antitumor agents based on aspartic protease inhibitors. *Curr Med Chem* 14 (26):2734-2748.

Nishina, S., M. Korenaga, I. Hidaka, A. Shinozaki, A. Sakai, T. Gondo, M. Tabuchi, F. Kishi, and K. Hino. 2010. Hepatitis C virus protein and iron overload induce hepatic steatosis through the unfolded protein response in mice. *Liver Int* 30 (5):683-92.

Nolan, D., E. Hammond, A. Martin, L. Taylor, S. Herrmann, E. McKinnon, C. Metcalf, B. Latham, and S. Mallal. 2003. Mitochondrial DNA depletion and morphologic changes in adipocytes associated with nucleoside reverse transcriptase inhibitor therapy. *Aids* 17 (9):1329-38.

Nunez, M. 2010. Clinical syndromes and consequences of antiretroviral-related hepatotoxicity. *Hepatology* 52 (3):1143-55.

Ozcan, U., Q. Cao, E. Yilmaz, A. H. Lee, N. N. Iwakoshi, E. Ozdelen, G. Tuncman, C. Gorgun, L. H. Glimcher, and G. S. Hotamisligil. 2004. Endoplasmic reticulum stress links obesity, insulin action, and type 2 diabetes. *Science* 306 (5695):457-61.

Pere, D., S. L. Ignacio, T. Ramon, L. Fernando, T. Alberto, V. Pompeyo, G. Juan, M. Jose G, G. Paloma, V. Antonio, C. Jaime, R. Esteban, R. Bernardino, M. Luisa GA, S. Trinitario, T. Ferran, L. Juan Ramon, and G. Myriam. 2008. Dyslipidemia and cardiovascular disease risk factor management in HIV-1-infected subjects treated with HAART in the Spanish VACH cohort. *Open AIDS J* 2:26-38.

Periard, D., A. Telenti, P. Sudre, J. J. Cheseaux, P. Halfon, M. J. Reymond, S. M. Marcovina, M. P. Glauser, P. Nicod, R. Darioli, and V. Mooser. 1999. Atherogenic dyslipidemia in HIV-infected individuals treated with protease inhibitors. The Swiss HIV Cohort Study. *Circulation* 100 (7):700-5.

Price, J., A. K. Zaidi, J. Bohensky, V. Srinivas, I. M. Shapiro, and H. Ali. 2010. Akt-1 mediates survival of chondrocytes from endoplasmic reticulum-induced stress. *Journal of cellular physiology* 222 (3):502-508.

Purnell, J. Q., A. Zambon, R. H. Knopp, D. J. Pizzuti, R. Achari, J. M. Leonard, C. Locke, and J. D. Brunzell. 2000. Effect of ritonavir on lipids and post-heparin lipase activities in normal subjects. *Aids* 14 (1):51-7.

Pyrko, P., A. Kardosh, W. Wang, W. Xiong, A. H. Schonthal, and T. C. Chen. 2007. HIV-1 protease inhibitors nelfinavir and atazanavir induce malignant glioma death by triggering endoplasmic reticulum stress. *Cancer Res* 67 (22):10920-8.

Qin, L., Z. Wang, L. Tao, and Y. Wang. 2010. ER stress negatively regulates AKT/TSC/mTOR pathway to enhance autophagy. *Autophagy* 6 (2):239-247.

Ray, H., C. Pinteur, V. Frering, M. Beylot, and V. Large. 2009. Depot-specific differences in perilipin and hormone-sensitive lipase expression in lean and obese. *Lipids Health Dis* 8:58.

Rector, R. S., J. P. Thyfault, Y. Wei, and J. A. Ibdah. 2008. Non-alcoholic fatty liver disease and the metabolic syndrome: an update. *World J Gastroenterol* 14 (2):185-92.

Rudich, A., R. Ben-Romano, S. Etzion, and N. Bashan. 2005. Cellular mechanisms of insulin resistance, lipodystrophy and atherosclerosis induced by HIV protease inhibitors. *Acta Physiol Scand* 183 (1):75-88.

Ruiz, L., E. Negredo, P. Domingo, R. Paredes, E. Francia, M. Balague, S. Gel, A. Bonjoch, C. R. Fumaz, S. Johnston, J. Romeu, J. Lange, and B. Clotet. 2001. Antiretroviral treatment simplification with nevirapine in protease inhibitor-experienced patients

with hiv-associated lipodystrophy: 1-year prospective follow-up of a multicenter, randomized, controlled study. *J Acquir Immune Defic Syndr* 27 (3):229-36.
Schleicher, S. M., L. Moretti, V. Varki, and B. Lu. 2010. Progress in the unraveling of the endoplasmic reticulum stress/autophagy pathway and cancer: implications for future therapeutic approaches. *Drug Resist Updat* 13 (3):79-86.
Schutt, M., J. Zhou, M. Meier, and H. H. Klein. 2004. Long-term effects of HIV-1 protease inhibitors on insulin secretion and insulin signaling in INS-1 beta cells. *J Endocrinol* 183 (3):445-54.
Sell, H., and J. Eckel. 2010. Adipose tissue inflammation: novel insight into the role of macrophages and lymphocytes. *Curr Opin Clin Nutr Metab Care* 13 (4):366-70.
Sha, H., Y. He, H. Chen, C. Wang, A. Zenno, H. Shi, X. Yang, X. Zhang, and L. Qi. 2009. The IRE1alpha-XBP1 pathway of the unfolded protein response is required for adipogenesis. *Cell Metab* 9 (6):556-64.
Shibata, M., K. Yoshimura, N. Furuya, M. Koike, T. Ueno, M. Komatsu, H. Arai, K. Tanaka, E. Kominami, and Y. Uchiyama. 2009. The MAP1-LC3 conjugation system is involved in lipid droplet formation. *Biochem Biophys Res Commun* 382 (2):419-23.
Shikuma, C. M., N. Hu, C. Milne, F. Yost, C. Waslien, S. Shimizu, and B. Shiramizu. 2001. Mitochondrial DNA decrease in subcutaneous adipose tissue of HIV-infected individuals with peripheral lipoatrophy. *Aids* 15 (14):1801-9.
Shimada, T., N. Hiramatsu, M. Okamura, K. Hayakawa, A. Kasai, J. Yao, and M. Kitamura. 2007. Unexpected blockade of adipocyte differentiation by K-7174: implication for endoplasmic reticulum stress. *Biochem Biophys Res Commun* 363 (2):355-60.
Singh, R. 2010. Autophagy and regulation of lipid metabolism. *Results and problems in cell differentiation* 52:35-46.
Singh, R., S. Kaushik, Y. Wang, Y. Xiang, I. Novak, M. Komatsu, K. Tanaka, A. M. Cuervo, and M. J. Czaja. 2009. Autophagy regulates lipid metabolism. *Nature* 458 (7242):1131-5.
Singh, R., Y. Xiang, Y. Wang, K. Baikati, A. M. Cuervo, Y. K. Luu, Y. Tang, J. E. Pessin, G. J. Schwartz, and M. J. Czaja. 2009. Autophagy regulates adipose mass and differentiation in mice. *J Clin Invest* 119 (11):3329-39.
Spalding, K. L., E. Arner, P. O. Westermark, S. Bernard, B. A. Buchholz, O. Bergmann, L. Blomqvist, J. Hoffstedt, E. Naslund, T. Britton, H. Concha, M. Hassan, M. Ryden, J. Frisen, and P. Arner. 2008. Dynamics of fat cell turnover in humans. *Nature* 453 (7196):783-7.
Stankov, M. V., and G. M. Behrens. 2007. HIV-therapy associated lipodystrophy: experimental and clinical evidence for the pathogenesis and treatment. *Endocr Metab Immune Disord Drug Targets* 7 (4):237-49.
Stankov, M. V., T. Lucke, A. M. Das, R. E. Schmidt, and G. M. Behrens. 2007. Relationship of mitochondrial DNA depletion and respiratory chain activity in preadipocytes treated with nucleoside reverse transcriptase inhibitors. *Antivir Ther* 12 (2):205-16.
Teixeira, H. N., E. T. Mesquita, M. L. Ribeiro, A. R. Bazin, C. T. Mesquita, M. P. Teixeira, C. Pellegrini Rda, and A. C. Nobrega. 2009. Study of vascular reactivity in HIV patients whether or not receiving protease inhibitor. *Arq Bras Cardiol* 93 (4):367-73, 360-6.

Tsiodras, S., C. Mantzoros, S. Hammer, and M. Samore. 2000. Effects of protease inhibitors on hyperglycemia, hyperlipidemia, and lipodystrophy: a 5-year cohort study. *Arch Intern Med* 160 (13):2050-6.

Viengchareun, S., M. Caron, M. Auclair, M. J. Kim, P. Frachon, J. Capeau, M. Lombes, and A. Lombes. 2007. Mitochondrial toxicity of indinavir, stavudine and zidovudine involves multiple cellular targets in white and brown adipocytes. *Antivir Ther* 12 (6):919-29.

Walli, R. K., G. M. Michl, J. R. Bogner, and F. D. Goebel. 2001. Improvement of HAART-associated insulin resistance and dyslipidemia after replacement of protease inhibitors with abacavir. *Eur J Med Res* 6 (10):413-21.

Wang, X., H. Mu, H. Chai, D. Liao, Q. Yao, and C. Chen. 2007. Human immunodeficiency virus protease inhibitor ritonavir inhibits cholesterol efflux from human macrophage-derived foam cells. *Am J Pathol* 171 (1):304-14.

Waters, L., L. John, and M. Nelson. 2007. Non-nucleoside reverse transcriptase inhibitors: a review. *Int J Clin Pract* 61 (1):105-18.

WHO, UNAIDS &. 2009. AIDS Epidemic Update.

———. 2010. Global Summary of the AIDS Epidemic.

Woerle, H. J., P. R. Mariuz, C. Meyer, R. C. Reichman, E. M. Popa, J. M. Dostou, S. L. Welle, and J. E. Gerich. 2003. Mechanisms for the deterioration in glucose tolerance associated with HIV protease inhibitor regimens. *Diabetes* 52 (4):918-25.

Wu, X., L. Sun, W. Zha, E. Studer, E. Gurley, L. Chen, X. Wang, P. B. Hylemon, W. M. Pandak, Jr., A. J. Sanyal, L. Zhang, G. Wang, J. Chen, J. Y. Wang, and H. Zhou. 2010. HIV protease inhibitors induce endoplasmic reticulum stress and disrupt barrier integrity in intestinal epithelial cells. *Gastroenterology* 138 (1):197-209.

Yorimitsu, T., and D. J. Klionsky. 2007. Eating the endoplasmic reticulum: quality control by autophagy. *Trends in cell biology* 17 (6):279-285.

Zhou, H., E. C. Gurley, S. Jarujaron, H. Ding, Y. Fang, Z. Xu, W. M. Pandak, Jr., and P. B. Hylemon. 2006. HIV protease inhibitors activate the unfolded protein response and disrupt lipid metabolism in primary hepatocytes. *American journal of physiology.Gastrointestinal and liver physiology* 291 (6):G1071-80.

Zhou, H., W. M. Pandak, Jr., and P. B. Hylemon. 2006. Cellular mechanisms of lipodystrophy induction by HIV protease inhibitors. *Future Lipidology* 1:163.

Zhou, H., W. M. Pandak, Jr., V. Lyall, R. Natarajan, and P. B. Hylemon. 2005. HIV protease inhibitors activate the unfolded protein response in macrophages: implication for atherosclerosis and cardiovascular disease. *Molecular pharmacology* 68 (3):690-700.

Zhou, J., S. Lhotak, B. A. Hilditch, and R. C. Austin. 2005. Activation of the unfolded protein response occurs at all stages of atherosclerotic lesion development in apolipoprotein E-deficient mice. *Circulation* 111 (14):1814-1821.

Zhou, L., M. Liu, J. Zhang, H. Chen, L. Q. Dong, and F. Liu. 2010. DsbA-L alleviates endoplasmic reticulum stress-induced adiponectin downregulation. *Diabetes* 59 (11):2809-16.

14

Future Perspectives in NNRTI-Based Therapy: Bases for Understanding Their Toxicity

Ana Blas-García[1,2], Nadezda Apostolova[1,3] and Juan V. Esplugues[1,2,3]
[1]*Departamento de Farmacología, Facultad de Medicina, Universidad de Valencia*
[2]*Fundación para la Investigación Hospital Universitario Dr. Peset*
[3]*Centro de Investigación Biomédica en Red-Enfermedades Hepáticas y Digestivas (CIBERehd), Valencia*
Spain

1. Introduction

Continuous administration of the drugs included under the term Highly Active Antiretroviral Therapy (HAART) has turned AIDS into a chronic disease, at least in developed countries (Panos et al., 2008). The initial development of these drugs was particularly rapid and focused on clinical efficacy before all other considerations. However, as the disease has come under control, there has been growing emphasis on the long-term adverse effects associated with this therapy.

The first drug for the treatment of HIV infection, zidovudine (AZT), was approved in 1987. The number of other antiretroviral drugs already approved for use or under development continues to grow, and the primary aim of researchers in the field is to improve their efficacy, safety and tolerability. Currently, there are 25 licensed antiretroviral drugs that belong to 6 different families: eight nucleoside (nucleotide) reverse transcriptase inhibitors (N[t]RTI) which inhibit competitively the viral reverse transcriptase, four non-nucleoside reverse transcriptase inhibitors (NNRTI), which produce a direct inhibition of the reverse transcriptase and a reduction in its catalytic activity, ten protease inhibitors (PI), which inactivate the HIV protease and prevent the generation of new viruses capable of infecting other cells, one fusion inhibitor, which prevents the fusion of the virus envelope with the host-cell membrane, one CCR5 inhibitor, which blocks the interaction of the virus with one of its receptors on the host cell, and, finally, one integrase inhibitor, whose function is to block viral DNA integration in the nuclear genome.

HAART aims to slow the rate of viral replication to the point of reducing the viral load and producing a significant immune system reconstitution that increases circulating levels of $CD4^+$ T cells. HAART usually combines the three major families of drugs: nucleoside reverse transcriptase inhibitors, non-nucleoside reverse transcriptase inhibitors and protease inhibitors. According to current guidelines, HAART regimens for initial treatment consist of two N(t)RTI plus either a NNRTI or a boosted PI (Hammer et al., 2008). NNRTI-based regimens have been in use for over a decade now, with the NNRTI of choice being Nevirapine (NVP) (for first line therapy in countries with limited resources) and Efavirenz (EFV) (for the treatment of naïve patients). Although considered to be safe and well-tolerated drugs, their low genetic barrier against the development of resistance and new and growing evidence of potential long-term toxicity associated with their use has generated a need for new improved drugs in this class. One new arrival is etravirine, which has already been approved by the Food and Drug Administration (FDA), and there are currently four other compounds in different stages of clinical development (rilpivirine, RDEA806, IDX899 and lersivirine).

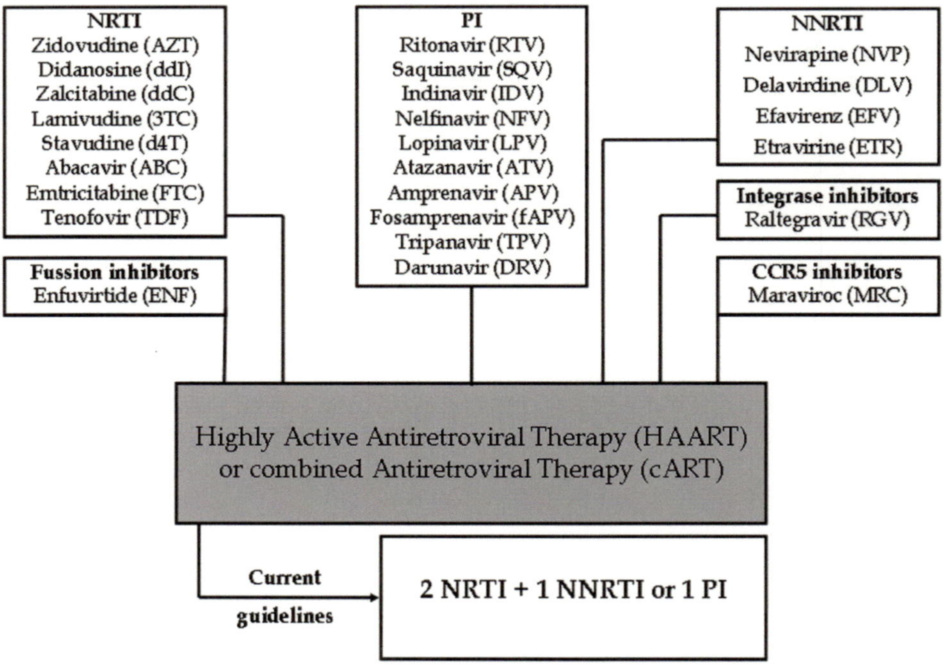

Fig. 1. Currently employed antiretroviral drugs and clinical guidelines in the treatment of HIV infection. The approved compounds are listed for each family.

2. NNRTI

This family is composed of highly specific inhibitors of HIV-1 characterized by a long-plasmatic half-life that allows once-daily dosing. Although all NNRTI have heterogenic chemical structures, they reduce HIV-1 replication through the same mechanism, which consists of non-competitive inhibition of the viral reverse transcriptase through binding to a hydrophobic pocket located close to the enzyme's catalytic site and inducing conformational changes that affect the catalytic activities of the enzyme (Sluis-Cremer, 2004). It is important to note that NNRTI are biotransformed in the liver via the cytochrome P450 pathway, which means there is potential for interactions with other drugs whose metabolism uses the same pathway.

The first member of this family to be approved by the FDA was NVP, in 1996, followed by Delavirdine (DLV) in 1997 and EFV in 1998. Nowadays, the NNRTIs of choice are NVP and EFV, which are still essential components of first-line HAART. On the other hand, DLV is no longer used due to its limited efficacy. First generation NNRTI exhibit a somewhat ineffective genetic barrier to the development of resistance, and have been shown to induce several moderate-to-severe side effects whose frequency and severity vary significantly with each compound, including hepatotoxicity, cutaneous reactions, central nervous system toxicity, metabolic alterations and gastrointestinal adverse events (van den Berg-Wolf, 2008; Jena, 2009). These disadvantages have fuelled the search of new NNRTI with an improved resistance profile and higher efficacy and tolerability, such as Etravirine (ETR), which was approved by the FDA in 2008 (Martínez, 2010). The chemical structures of the NNRTI currently available and in clinical development are shown in Figure 2.

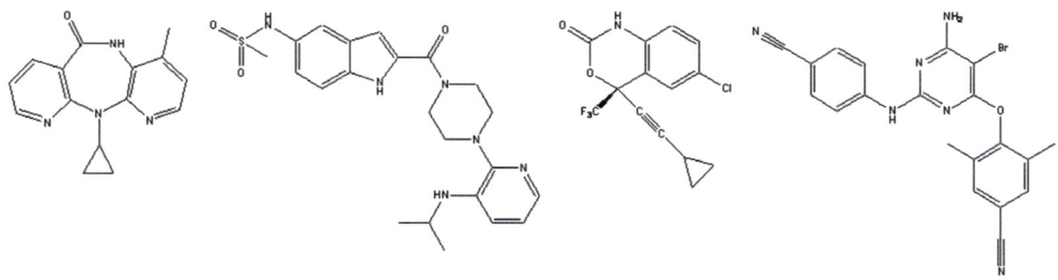

Nevirapine (Viramune®) **Delavirdine (Rescriptor®)** **Efavirenz (Sustiva™)** **Etravirine (Intelence™)**

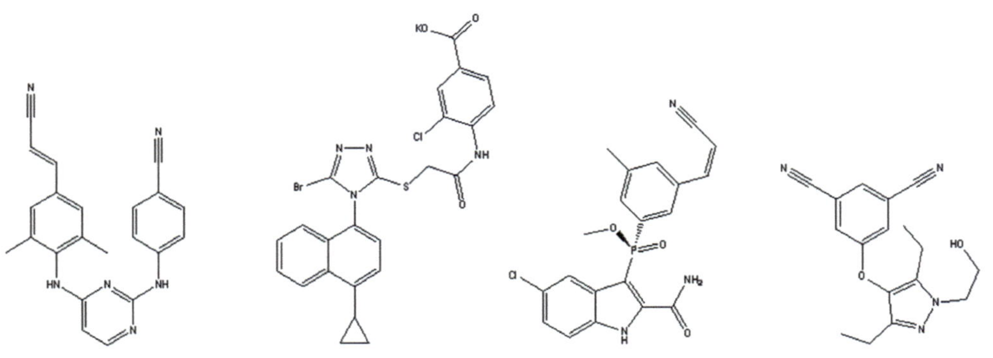

Rilpivirine **RDEA806** **IDX899** **Lersivirine**

Fig. 2. Chemical structures of approved NNRTI (nevirapine, delavirdine, efavirenz and etravirine) and NNRTI in clinical development (rilpivirine, RDEA806, IDX899 and lersivirine.

2.1 Nevirapine

This NNRTI is recommended for first line therapy in resource-limited countries, but, due to its low teratogenesis and paediatric toxicity, it is also widely employed in pregnant women and young children in the developed world. This dipyridodiazepinone is usually administered in twice-daily doses of 200mg, achieving peak plasma concentrations (2 ± 0.4μg/ml) at 4h. However, several clinical trials have also shown it to be safe and effective in a once-daily regimen of 400mg (Garcia, 2000; van Leth, 2004). Despite no major differences being reported between these two regimens, once-daily dosing has been shown to produce complications, including lower minimum concentration (C_{min}) and higher maximum concentration (C_{max}) levels and a high risk of rash, which can be minimized by generating tolerance through the administration of a twice-daily dose for a few weeks prior to treatment (Cooper, 2007). This compound is biotransformed via cytochrome P450 isoenzymes, mainly from the CYP3A family, into several hydroxylated metabolites, and its plasma half-life ranges from 45h (with a single dose) to 25 - 30h (with repetitive dosing) (Cooper, 2007). The most frequently described adverse effects of NVP are rash and hepatotoxicity.

2.2 Delavirdine

Regulatory agencies have advised against the use of DLV in initial therapy, and so current regimens rarely contain this bis(hetero-aryl)piperazine, as it is less effective than other NNRTI, is accompanied by complex drug interactions and requires a more inconvenient administration. It is characterized by a rapid absorption following oral administration, with peak plasma concentrations occurring approximately 1 hour after dosing. The recommended dosage of DLV is 400mg three times per day, which results in a C_{max} of $35 \pm 20\mu M$ and a C_{min} of $15 \pm 10\mu M$, and a mean half-life of 5.8h. CYP3A isoenzymes of the cytochrome P450 system are the main effectors of DLV conversion into several inactive metabolites, although *in vitro* data also suggest the involvement of CYP2D6. The major manifestation of its toxicity is rash (Rescriptor official FDA information, 2011).

2.3 Efavirenz

EFV, combined with two NRTI, is the recommended option for initial therapy and is the most widely used NNRTI. This benzoxazinone has a long half-life (at least 52h with single doses and 40 - 55h with multiple doses), which makes it suitable for once-daily dosing, with 600mg being the recommended dose for adults. Peak EFV plasma concentrations are reached 3 - 5h after a single oral dose and become steady at 6 - 7 days (Maggiolo, 2009). An important pharmacokinetic inter-individual variability has been reported in patients taking EFV: a daily dose of 600mg usually results in a C_{max} of $12.9 \pm 3.7\mu M$ and a C_{min} of $5.6 \pm 3.2\mu M$ (Starr, 1999; Staszewski, 1999), but higher levels (between 30 - 50μM) have been observed in as many as 20% of patients (Marzolini, 2001; Burguer, 2006).

This drug is extensively biotransformed into inactive hydroxylated metabolites via the cytochrome P450 system, and CYP2B6 is likely to be the corresponding isoenzyme. Moreover, *in vitro* studies suggest that the wide inter-individual variability in the expression and activity of CYP2B6, in addition to its genetic polymorphisms, could lie behind the variability in EFV pharmacokinetics (Ward, 2003). It is also important to note that EFV levels can vary if it is co-administered with other drugs that influence this isoenzyme. Despite its apparent safety, several adverse events of EFV-containing therapies have emerged, such as rash, neuropsychiatric disturbances, lipid and metabolic alterations, and hepatotoxicity (Maggiolo, 2009).

2.4 Etravirine

The most recent approved NNRTI is a di-aryl-pyrimidine. It has shown sustained clinical efficacy in HIV-1 strains that are resistant to other compounds of the same family and has a higher genetic barrier to the development of resistance than older NNRTI. ETR is less susceptible to drug-resistant mutations, probably due to the fact that it binds to the reverse transcriptase in multiple conformations (Dickinson, 2010; Martínez, 2010). Although several recent trials suggest that its long half-life (30 - 40h) makes it suitable for once-daily dosing

(400mg), the current recommended dosage for ETR is 200mg twice daily, which results in a C_{max} of 0.79 - 0.80μg/ml 4h after administration. As with other NNRTI, its metabolism depends on several isoforms of the cytochrome P450, primarily CYP3A4, CYP2C9 and CYP2C19. Thus, its use in combination with other drugs that also induce the cytochrome P450 is not recommended. Existing clinical evidence shows that ETR is well tolerated in patients, with low rates of discontinuation as a result of detrimental effects. In the PhaseIII trials DUET-1 and DUET-2, the primary adverse effect associated with ETR was mild-to-moderate rash, and no association was found with hepatic/lipid abnormalities or with a higher incidence of psychiatric disorders (Lazzarin, 2007; Madruga, 2007; Schiller, 2009). However, data about ETR are still limited due to its recent commercialisation, and further clinical and *in vitro* analyses are needed in order to determine the full side effects of this compound.

2.5 NNRTI in clinical development

New NNRTI are currently being developed as part of the quest to find efficient compounds with greater resistance and a lower frequency of adverse effects. The information available about the clinical relevance and pharmacokinetic and toxicological profiles of the four NNRTI currently under clinical development is limited, which makes it difficult to predict their potential as therapy for HIV infection. Nevertheless, several ongoing trials are investigating the efficacy, safety and tolerability of these drugs.

2.5.1 Rilpivirine (TMC278)

The pharmacokinetics of this di-aryl-pyrimidine compound allow once-daily dosing, usually with 25mg, and its good bioavailability makes it a potential candidate for co-formulation. In fact, studies are underway to develop a new once-daily fixed-dose antiretroviral regimen containing Emtricitabine, Tenofovir disoproxil fumarate and Rilpivirine hydrochloride (de Béthune, 2010). Rilpivirine has an *in vitro* resistance profile comparable to that of ETR (Azijn, 2010), and results from week 96 of a Phase IIB trial (TMC278-C204) in naïve patients have demonstrated a potent and sustained efficacy similar to that of EFV, while it seems to produce fewer adverse events. Indeed, rilpivirine is associated with fewer incidences of neuropsychiatric events and rash, and a smaller rise in lipid levels than EFV (Pozniak, 2010).

2.5.2 RDEA806

In vitro studies have reported that this triazole compound exerts a potent activity against both wild-type and NNRTI-resistant HIV-1 strains similar to that of ETR. Data from Phase IIA of a short-term monotherapy trial evaluating the antiviral activity, safety and pharmacokinetics of RDEA806 have demonstrated that this compound exerts a robust antiretroviral activity in HIV-1 positive, antiretroviral-naïve patients treated once daily for 7 days. All doses of RDEA806 tested were well tolerated and no patient's treatment was discontinued due to adverse effects (Moyle, 2010).

2.5.3 IDX899

This 3-phosphoindol compound also has a potent *in vitro* activity against wild-type and NNRTI-resistant strains of HIV-1, and possesses a high genetic barrier to resistance. Preliminary data from a Phase IIA trial of treatment-naïve patients undergoing 7 day monotherapy with IDX899 suggest a potent antiviral activity and tolerability with all the doses evaluated (Klibanov, 2010).

2.5.4 Lersivirine (UK-453061)

This compound belongs to the pyrazole family and exhibits a good resistance profile *in vitro*. Results from a phase IIA clinical trial in which asymptomatic HIV-1 infected adults were treated once or twice daily with lersivirine in a 7-day monotherapy regimen demonstrate its high antiviral activity and good safety and tolerability profile. Nevertheless, some minor adverse effects (headache, fatigue and nausea) have been reported (Corbau, 2010; Fätkenheurer, 2009).

3. NNRTI-associated adverse effects

NVP and EFV, the most widely employed NNRTI, share a similar efficacy and genetic barrier against the development of drug resistance, but differ in their toxicological profiles. Clinical trials have generally shown NNRTI, and especially EFV, to be safe and well-tolerated drugs. However, treatment discontinuation has been reported in patients receiving EFV- and NVP-based regimens, and is mainly attributed to the appearance of several moderate-to-severe side effects, some of which are drug-specific and unrelated to NNRTI as a pharmacological group. The most common adverse effects are cutaneous reactions, hepatotoxicity, neuro-psychiatric toxicity and metabolic alterations, but other toxicities have also been described to a lesser extent (Figure 3).

Discontinuation rates of up to 16% have been reported in patients receiving EFV and two NRTI, and similar or higher levels have been found following treatment with NVP. For example, in a study comparing EFV and NVP (each in combination with Lamivudine (3TC) and Stavudine (d4T)), discontinuation was necessary in 15.8% and 24.1% of treatments with EFV and NVP respectively (van Leth, 2004). It is important to note that the incidence of discontinuation of EFV-based therapy also depends on the NRTI co-administered, being more frequent when EFV is used with 3TC and Zidovudine (AZT) or with 3TC and Abacavir (Bartlett, 2007). In the FIRST study, severe (grade 4) adverse events were approximately half as common with EFV as with NVP (van der Berg-Wolf, 2008), especially in the case of rash and hepatotoxicity. Nevertheless, NVP can be considered an alternative therapy when there is a high risk of central nervous system (CNS) toxicity because of its lack of association with neuropsychiatric events (Hawkins, 2005; van Leth, 2004).

3.1 Cutaneous reactions

All NNRTI have been associated with skin reactions, but they differ in the frequency and severity of the adverse events, with being rash one of the most common manifestations. The majority of the cutaneous reactions associated NVP (including Stevens-Johnson syndrome, toxic epidermal necrolysis and hypersensitivity) appear within the first six weeks of treatment and can lead to therapy discontinuation if serious. Data from a metaanalysis revealed that 24% of NVP-treated patients suffered rash compared with 15% of controls, while 1.7% of patients showed severe grade 3 and 4 reactions vs 0.2% of controls [40]. One of the proposed mechanisms in NVP-mediated rash involves the 12-hydroxy metabolite of this drug, which can be converted to a reactive quinone methide in the skin, thus inducing an immune response and rash (Popovic, 2010).

NNRTI-induced adverse events

Cutaneous reactions

Grade 1: Erythema with/without pruritus

Grade 2: Diffuse erythematous macular or maculopapular eruption or dry desquamation with or without pruritus or typical target lesions, without blistering, vesicles or ulceration in the lesions; Urticaria

Grade 3: Diffuse erythematous macular or maculopapular eruption or moist desquamation with or without pruritus together with blistering and vesiculation. Angioedema, exfoliative dermatitis or diffuse rash and serum sickness or diffuse cutaneous eruption plus one of the following: cutaneos bullae with widespread sheet-like detachment of skin, Steven-Johnsons syndrome, two or more anatomically distinct sites of mucosal erosion or ulceration

Grade 4: Toxic epidermal necrolysis

CNS toxicity

Moderate: Dizziness, headache, confusion, depersonalization, drowsiness, euphoria, hallucinations, impaired concentration, amnesia, sleep abnormalities such as insomnia or vivid dreams, nerviousness, anxiety and/or depression.

Severe: Severe depression, delusions, suicidal ideation and paranoid reactions

Hepatotoxicity

Grade 1: Elevation of serum aminotransferases 1.25 to 2.5 times the upper normal limit

Grade 2: Elevation of serum aminotransferases 2.6 to 5 times the upper normal limit

Grade 3: Elevation of serum aminotransferases >5 times the upper normal limit

Grade 4: Elevation of serum aminotransferases >10 times the upper normal limit

Metabolic alterations

Lipodystrophy: reduction of lipogenesis and differentiation in adipocytes, decrease of adipokine release

Changes in metabolic profiles: hyperglycemia, hypertryglyceridemia, hypercholesterolemia

Other toxicities

Moderate gastrointestinal adverse events: nausea, diarrhoea, vomiting and abdominal pain; in some cases, anorexia, dyspepsia, and pancreatitis.

Cardiovascular complications: endothelial dysfunction, inflammatory processes, atherosclerotis lesions.

Vitamin D deficiency and bone toxicity.

Nephrotoxicity.

Hyperhidrosis.

Fig. 3. NNRTI-related adverse events

Mild-to-moderate rash has also been described in patients receiving EFV-based regimens, and is usually resolved as therapy continues, although approximately 2% of patients discontinue their treatment. These reactions usually appear as maculopapular skin eruptions within the first two weeks of treatment, but less than 1% patients develop severe rash, characterised by blistering, moist desquamation or ulceration, and only 0.1% suffer grade 4 rash, manifested as erythema multiforme or Stevens-Johnson syndrome. In controlled trials, the incidence of skin reactions was 26% in patients treated with 600mg per day of EFV compared to 18% in controls (AIDSinfo, 2010). In the 2NN trial, the frequency of moderate-to-severe rash was significantly greater with NVP than EFV when both were administered once daily, but there was no significant difference between NVP twice daily and EFV once daily (van Leth, 2004).

DLV and ETR have also been related to the onset of mild-to-moderate skin reactions. DLV-induced rash usually appears within 1 to 3 weeks of treatment and is resolved in 3 to 14 days. In the DUET studies, the only significant side effect observed in the ETR group was rash, which was usually maculopapular and of mild-to-moderate severity (1.3% grade 3), occurred a median of 14 days after initiation of therapy, and lasted approximately 15 days. Severe rash was not reported, and only 2.2% of patients discontinued treatment due to this side effect.

3.2 CNS toxicity

EFV is widely associated with CNS toxicity, which is responsible for the discontinuation of treatment in at least 4-10% of patients (Muñoz-Moreno, 2009). Between 25 and 70% of patients receiving EFV exhibit neuropsychiatric disturbances, including dizziness, headache, euphoria, hallucinations, impaired concentration, confusion, depersonalization, drowsiness, amnesia, sleep abnormalities (*e.g.* insomnia or vivid dreams), nervousness, anxiety and depression. More severe cases, consisting of depression, delusions, suicidal ideation and paranoid reactions, have been reported in 0.4 - 1.6% of EFV-treated patients (Staszewski, 1999; Hawkins, 2005; Fumaz, 2002). These side effects usually appear within the first few days of treatment and are resolved after 2-4 weeks, although there are cases in which they continue to manifest themselves for several months or even longer periods (Muñoz-Moreno, 2009; Arendt, 2007). The clinical evidence available, though extensive, is insufficient to clarify the mechanisms underlying EFV-induced CNS alterations, but recent data implicate neurotoxic events induced by HIV itself and cytokine production by EFV.

These adverse effects in the CNS seem to be dose-related (Marzolini, 2001). For instance, the higher incidence of such events in Afro-Americans than in European-Americans or Hispanic populations is attributed to the greater prevalence of the CYP2B6 T/T genotype in the former population, which results in a slower EFV metabolism and, consequently, higher plasma drug concentrations (Haas, 2004).

None of the remaining NNRTI has been associated with neuropsychiatric adverse effects. Moreover, switching from EFV to ETR produces an improvement in EFV-induced toxicity, with a significant reduction of CNS events such as insomnia, abnormal dreams and nervousness (Waters, 2011).

3.3 Metabolic alterations

Mounting evidence associates NNRTI with metabolic disorders involving lipid metabolism, such as alterations of body fat distribution (lipodystrophy) and dyslipidaemia (changes in plasma concentration of cholesterol, High Density Lipoprotein Cholesterol (HDL-c), Low Density Lipoprotein Cholesterol (LDL-c), triglycerides). Lipid alterations are sometimes accompanied by insulin resistance and can generate a metabolic syndrome-like condition. These effects seem to be drug-specific, but the mechanisms involved are still not fully understood. Increases in HDL-c have been reported in naïve patients treated with different NNRTI-based regimens (Negredo, 2004; van der Valk, 2001), but clinical studies have not clarified which drug(s) was/were responsible for these effects.

There is conflicting evidence as to whether HDL-c is significantly altered in patients switched from a PI- to a NNRTI-based regimen (Martínez, 2000; Negredo, 2002). The lipid profile of naïve patients receiving NVP or EFV plus d4T and 3TC was evaluated in a pre-planned study within the larger 2NN trial. NVP was associated with greater increases in HDL-c (42.5% with NVP vs 33.7% with EFV) and lower increases in total cholesterol (TC) levels (26.9% with NVP vs 31.1% with EFV), which led to a decrease in the TC:HDL-c ratio in patients receiving NVP (-4.1%). No significant differences were detected in LDL-c levels. Similarly, different dysmetabolic profiles were reported in a cross-sectional evaluation of EFV- and NVP-treated patients (Manfredi, 2005), with rates of hyperglycemia, hypertriglyceridemia and hypercholesterolemia being higher in the former group. The same report showed that, when patients were switched to NNRTI-containing therapies, dysmetabolism was ameliorated by NVP, whereas it was stabilised or worsened by EFV. In the case of DLV and ETR, neither has been significantly associated with lipid abnormalities.

The cellular and molecular mechanisms underlying NNRTI-induced metabolic alterations are still unclear, and many hypotheses have emerged to explain them. Some in vitro studies have suggested that EFV-induced lipodystrophy is a result of effects on adipocyte differentiation and function, whereas such effects are not observed with NVP. In particular, clinically relevant EFV concentrations have been shown to alter the lipogenic pathway of cell differentiation by preventing lipid storage in 3T3 or human preadipocytes and to deplete triacylglycerol accumulation in *3T3-F442A* mature adipocytes. These phenomena, which were attributed to the reduction in the expression of the lipogenic transcription factor SREBP-1c, may be involved in the atrophy of adipose tissue described in HAART-treated patients (Diaz-Delfin, 2008; El-Hadri, 2004). When the effects of EFV and a boosted IP, lopinavir/ritonavir (LPV/r; 4:1), were compared in human adipocytes during and after adipogenic differentiation, both compounds were found to impair adipogenesis and reduce transcript levels of adipogenic differentiation genes and master regulators of adipogenesis. In addition, they undermined the release of adipokine and enhanced the expression and release of inflammation-related cytokines. All these effects were more pronounced with EFV than with LPV/r (Gallego-Escuredo, 2010).

3.4 Hepatotoxicity

Hepatic adverse events are one of the main causes of mortality and morbidity in HIV-infected patients and are associated with the vast majority of antiretroviral drugs. Therefore, it is important to note that increased liver enzyme levels are a common feature of antiretroviral therapy (Palella, 2006; Weber, 2006). NNRTI , specially NVP and EFV, have been related to liver damage, but there is controversy regarding the level of toxicity of each compound and the relationship between NNRTI plasma levels and hepatotoxicity (Law, 2003). However, it is accepted that the risk of this adverse effect is increased in patients in whom liver enzymes levels were elevated prior to therapy and/or are co-infected with hepatitis B (HBV) and/or C (HCV) (Brück, 2008; Sulkowski, 2002).

Liver damage is particularly prevalent among NVP-treated patients, but most trials have not detected a positive correlation with the plasma concentration of this compound (Cooper, 2007; Kappelhoff, 2005). Liver enzyme levels normally increase within the first 18 weeks of therapy, but the risk continues thereafter, and so patients should be monitored at frequent intervals throughout their treatment. Severe life-threatening hepatotoxicity, including fatal fulminant hepatitis, has also been reported during therapy with NVP. In a recent study of NVP patients, 25.7% developed grade 1 hepatotoxicity and 2.8% displayed severe hepatotoxicity (Jena, 2009). There is also conflicting evidence about the involvement of NVP therapy in the progression of liver fibrosis in patients with a concomitant HCV infection, as some studies support this hypothesis (Macías, 2004) whereas others relate NVP to a reduction of fibrosis (Berenguer, 2008).

Up to 10% of EFV-treated patients exhibit increases of liver enzymes that may require discontinuation of therapy and which have been associated both with hypersensitivity to EFV and dose-dependent accumulative effects (Angel-Moreno-Maroto, 2006; Jena, 2009; Kappelhoff, 2005; Rivero, 2007). In fact, a substudy of the 2NN trial showed a correlation between the incidence of elevated levels of liver enzymes and plasma concentrations of EFV during the first 6 weeks of treatment. The risk of hepatotoxicity in EFV-treated patients increases considerably when HIV coexists with HBV and/or HCV infection (Ena, 2003; Sulkowski, 2002), and also when patients are treated with other potential hepatotoxic medicinal products. It has been claimed that hepatitis viral co-infection results in a higher exposure to EFV. In this context, there are studies that have failed to detect any differences

in plasma EFV concentrations between uninfected and HBV/HCV-infected patients (Katsounas, 2007; Pereira, 2008), while others report increased median plasma $C_{(min)}$ values leading to overdosing of NNRTI in HIV/HCV co-infected patients, especially in those at an advanced stage of liver fibrosis (Dominguez, 2010). Recent results from Phase III DUET trials have pointed to the good safety profile of ETR in patients co-infected with HIV and HBV and/or HCV, among whom the incidence and severity of hepatic adverse events were similar to those in the placebo group (Clotet, 2010). Finally, several cases of acute liver failure have been described with NVP and only a few with EFV, though this is a rarely reported hepatic event during antiretroviral therapy (Jao, 2010; Turkova, 2009).
The cellular and molecular mechanisms underlying NNRTI-induced hepatotoxicity remain elusive, and there is little and contradictory information about the *in vitro* toxic effects of EFV on hepatic cells.

3.5 Other toxicities

Less common side effects have also been associated with NNRTI-including therapies. Moderate gastrointestinal adverse effects have been reported with all NNRTI, but do not normally lead to the discontinuation of therapy. In general, NNRTI-related symptoms include nausea, diarrhoea, vomiting and abdominal pain, but EFV has also been associated with anorexia, dyspepsia and pancreatitis. These gastrointestinal EFV-associated adverse effects have been reported in up to 14% of patients, and increases in serum amylase concentration have been reported in 10% of patients receiving EFV compared to 6% of controls (AIDSinfo, 2010).
Several *in vitro* and clinical studies have raised the possibility that EFV contribute to HAART-associated cardiovascular complications in HIV-infected patients. Treatment of human coronary artery endothelial cells (HCAEC) with EFV leads to increased oxidative stress, evident in the induction of superoxide production and decrease of GSH levels, which significantly increases the *in vitro* monolayer permeability of these cells (Jamaluddin, 2009). In the study in question, antioxidant administration demonstrated that EFV-induced ROS also activated several cellular pathways mediated by JNK and NFκB and pointed to an involvement of this drug in inflammatory processes. Clinical evidence from a recent trial evaluating cardiovascular risk factors in patients treated for over 5 years with NVP- or EFV-based regimens associate the former drug with a better lipid and glucose profile and a lower tendency to develop subclinical atherosclerotic lesions than the latter drug (Maggi, 2011).
EFV therapy has recently been reported to induce vitamin D deficiency and elevated serum alkaline phosphatase levels, both of which are considered to be markers of bone toxicity and turnover (Welz, 2010). This compound has also been associated with significant decreases in 25-hydroxyvitamin D and an increased risk of hypovitaminosis D (Brown, 2010).
Preliminary studies in rats have suggested that high doses of EFV induce nephrotoxicity, expressed by necrosis of proximal tubular epithelial cells. Although humans are exposed to higher levels of EFV, this effect has not been corroborated in patients (Gerson, 1999; Mutlib, 2000). Species selectivity with respect to this toxic effect may result from differences in the production and/or processing of reactive metabolites. Some EFV-treated patients have reported hyperhidrosis, which is manifested as excessive nocturnal sweating and could be a consequence of alterations of the body's thermoregulation by high concentrations of this NNRTI in the cerebroespinal fluid. This adverse event can be controlled by dose reduction (Fuertes, 2009).

4. NNRTI-induced side effects: A potential role for mitochondria?

The mechanism of mitochondria-related toxicity most commonly associated with antiretroviral therapy is the inhibition of the enzyme responsible for mitochondrial DNA replication: DNA polymerase γ (Pol γ) (Walker, 2002). This toxicity is particularly related to NRTI treatment, and not to other antiretroviral drugs considered safer for mitochondrial function. However, recent evidence demonstrates that NNRTI act on various mitochondrial parameters without affecting Pol γ, which suggests a role for this organelle in NNRTI-induced toxicities (Pilon, 2002; Karamchand, 2008). Nevertheless, the identification of a specific clinical profile related to mitochondrial toxicity is challenged by the co-administration of these compounds with NRTI. Recent research has focused on the molecular and cellular mechanisms underlying NNRTI-associated adverse events, and on the potential role of mitochondria in such processes. Studies in endothelial cells have confirmed that EFV treatment induces ROS production and decreases GSH levels, contributing to endothelial dysfunction, an early stage of atherosclerosis (Jamaluddin, 2010). Additionally, EFV has been shown to induce mitochondrial apoptosis in Jurkat T cells and human peripheral blood mononuclear cells (Pilon, 2002). In this regard, we have recently characterized specific features of both EFV- and NVP-associated toxicity that are related to the induction of hepatic damage (Apostolova, 2010; Blas-García, 2010). In particular, we have reported evidence of a new mechanism of mitochondrial interference induced by EFV in human hepatic cells and which does not involve an effect on mitochondrial DNA replication. EFV decreased mitochondrial oxygen consumption by a direct inhibition of Complex I at the electron transport chain, and induced a reduction of mitochondrial membrane potential and an increase in reactive oxygen species (ROS) generation. The impairment of oxidative phosphorylation led to a reduction in cellular ATP levels and a subsequent activation of AMP-activated protein kinase (AMPK), which is the cellular master switch of energetic stress (Hardie, 2007). Indeed, the mitochondrial dysfunction observed produced alterations in lipid metabolism, increasing the lipid content in the cytoplasm in an AMPK-related fashion. These changes were accompanied by a relative increase in mitochondrial mass, without an increase in the mtDNA/nuclear DNA copy number ratio, which points to a lack of authentic mitochondrial biogenesis. EFV also compromised cellular viability and proliferation in both Hep3B and HeLa cells. Specifically, EFV led to cell cycle arrest and induced apoptotic cell death through the intrinsic (mitochondrial) pathway, which was evident in the translocation of mitochondrial apoptogenic proteins (cytochrome *c* and AIF), activation of caspase-3 and -9 and apoptotic changes in the nuclear morphology, such as chromatin condensation. EFV-induced toxic effects on cellular viability and proliferation were attenuated by an antioxidant treatment with the hydrosoluble analog of vitamin E, Trolox, thus implicating oxidative stress in these processes (Figure 4). Interestingly, NVP had no effect on the mitochondrial parameters analysed, but did produce a toxic effect on cellular viability and proliferation. In light of these findings, it is plausible that the deleterious mitochondrial effect induced by EFV is relevant to the development not only of hepatotoxicity but also to some of the more systemic metabolic side effects associated with this drug. These results are a strong endorsement of clinical evidence that the mechanisms of hepatotoxicity induced by NVP and EFV are drug-specific and unrelated to NNRTI as a drug family.

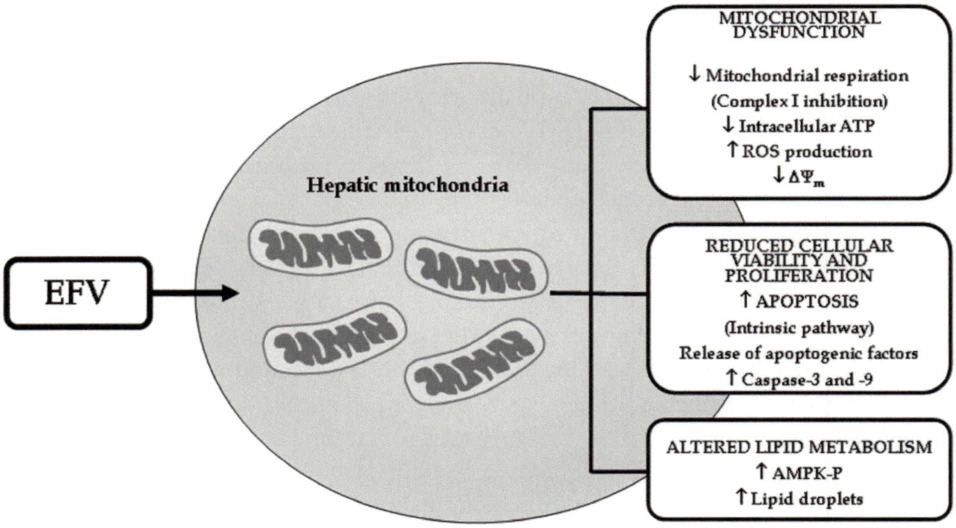

Fig. 4. Schematic representation of the direct mitotoxic effect induced by efavirenz (EFV) in hepatic cells *in vitro*.

5. Conclusions

Twenty years after the identification of NNRTI as a new class of antiretroviral drugs for the treatment of HIV-1 infection, recent advances in the characterization of the causes of their toxicity and the development of new compounds have put NNRTI in the spotlight. Given that these compounds are essential elements of antiretroviral therapy, the characterization of their toxic effects and the mechanisms that underlie them may help to improve HIV therapy. The real impact of newly developed compounds on HAART remains to be seen, but they are likely to play an important role in future antiretroviral regimens. Finally, the fact that HIV is now a chronic illness means that therapy must be administered for life; therefore, the choice of drugs to be taken should be based not only on their clinical efficacy but also on their toxicological profile, bearing in mind their profound influence on other concomitant infections and age-related diseases.

6. Acknowledgement

The authors thank Brian Normanly for his English language editing of the manuscript. This work was supported by grants PI081325 from "Fondo de Investigacion Sanitaria", and ACOMP2010/207 y PROMETEO/2010/060 from Generalitat Valenciana, Spain.

7. References

AIDSinfo. A service of the U.S. Department of Health and Human Services. Guidelines for the use of antiretroviral agents in HIV-1-infected adults and adolescents, http://aidsinfo.nih.gov/Guidelines/Default.aspx?MenuItem=Guidelines. (Accessed March 15, 2011).

Angel-Moreno-Maroto, A.; Suárez-Castellano, L.; Hernández-Cabrera, M. & Pérez-Arellano, J,L. (2006). Severe efavirenz-induced hypersensitivity syndrome (not-DRESS) with acute renal failure. *Journal of Infection*, Vol.52, No.2, pp.e39-40, ISSN 0163-4453.

Apostolova, N.; Gomez-Sucerquia, L.J.; Moran, A.; Alvarez, A.; Blas-Garcia, A. & Esplugues, J.V. (2010). Enhanced oxidative stress and increased mitochondrial mass during Efavirenz-induced apoptosis in human hepatic cells. *British Journal of Pharmacology*, Vol.160, No.8, pp.2069-84, ISSN 0007-1188.

Arendt, G.; de Nocker, D.; von Giesen, H.J. & Nolting, T. (2007). Neuropsychiatric side effects of efavirenz therapy. *Expert Opinion on Drug Safety*, Vol.6, No.2, pp.147-54, ISSN 1474-0338.

Azijn, H.; Tirry, I.; Vingerhoets, J.; de Béthune, M-P.; Kraus, G.; Boven, K.; Jochmans, D.; Van Craenenbroeck, E.; Picchio, G. & Rimsky, L.T. (2010). TMC278, a next-generation nonnucleoside reverse transcriptase inhibitor (NNRTI), active against wild-type and NNRTI-resistant HIV-1. *Antimicrobial Agents and Chemotherapy*, Vol.54, No.2, pp.718-727, ISSN 0066-4804.

Bartlett, J.A.; Chen, S.S. & Quinn, J.B. (2007). Comparative efficacy of nucleoside/nucleotide reverse transcriptase inhibitors in combination with efavirenz: results of a systematic overview. *HIV Clinical Trials*, Vol.8, No.4, pp.221-6, ISSN 1528-4336.

Berenguer, J.; Bellón, J.M.; Miralles, P.; Álvarez, E.; Castillo, I.; Cosín, J.; López, J.C.; Sánchez Conde, M.; Padilla, B. & Resino, S. (2008). Association between exposure to nevirapine and reduced liver fibrosis progression in patients with HIV and hepatitis C virus coinfection. *Clinical Infectious Diseases*, Vol.46, No.1, pp.137-43, ISSN 1058-4838.

Blas-García, A.; Apostolova, N.; Ballesteros, D.; Monleón, D.; Morales, J.M.; Rocha, M.; Victor, V.M. & Esplugues, J.V. (2010). Inhibition of mitochondrial function by efavirenz increases lipid content in hepatic cells. *Hepatology*, Vol.52, No.1, pp.115-25, ISSN 1665-2681.

Brown, T.T. & McComsey, G.A. Association between initiation of antiretroviral therapy with efavirenz and decreases in 25-hydroxyvitamin D. *Antiviral Therapy*, Vol.15, No.3, pp.425-9, ISSN 1359-6535.

Brück, S.; Witte, S.; Brust, J.; Schuster, D.; Mosthaf, F.; Procaccianti, M.; Rump, J.A.; Klinker, H.; Petzold, D. & Hartmann, M. (2008). Hepatotoxicity in patients prescribed efavirenz or nevirapine. *European Journal of Medical Research*, Vol.13, No.7, pp.343-8, ISSN 0949-2321.

Burger, D.; van der Heiden, I.; la Porte, C.; van der Ende, M.; Groeneveld, P.; Richter, C.; Koopmans, P.; Kroon, F.; Sprenger, H.; Lindemans, J.; Schenk, P. & van Schaik, R. (2006). Interpatient variability in the pharmacokinetics of tha HIV non-nucleoside reverse transcriptase inhibitor efavirenz: the effect of gender, race, and CYP2B6 polymorphism. *British Journal of Clinical Pharmacology*, Vol.61, pp.148-154, ISSN 0306-5251.

Clotet, B.; Clumeck, N.; Katlama, C.; Nijs, S. & Witek, J. (2010). Safety of etravirine in HIV-1/hepatitis B and/or C virus co-infected patients: pooled 96 week results from the Phase III DUET trials. *Journal of Antimicrobial Chemotherapy*, Vol.65, No.11, pp.2450-2454, ISSN 1460-2091.

Cooper, C.L. & van Heeswijk, R.P. (2007). Once-daily nevirapine dosing: a pharmacokinetics, efficacy and safety review. *HIV Medicine*, Vol.8, No.1, pp.1-7 ISSN 1468-1293.

Corbau, R.; Mori, J.; Phillips, C.; Fishburn, L.; Martin, A.; Mowbray, C.; Panton, W.; Smith-Burchnell, C.; Thornberry, A.; Ringrose, H.; Knöchel, T.; Irving, S.; Westby, M.; Wood, A. & Perros, M. (2010). Lersivirine, a nonnucleoside reverse transcriptase inhibitor with activity against drug-resistant human immunodeficiency virus type 1. *Antimicrobial Agents and Chemotherapy*, Vol.54, No.10, pp.4451-4463, ISSN 0066-4804.

de Béthune, M.P. (2010). Non-nucleoside reverse transcriptase inhibitors (NNRTIs), their discovery, development, and use in the treatment of HIV-1 infection: A review of the last 20 years (1989-2009). *Antiviral Research*, Vol.85, pp.75-90, ISSN 0166-3542.

Diaz-Delfin, J.; Gallego-Escuredo, J.M.; Milanski, M.; Domingo, J.C.; Gutierrez, M.M.; Mateo, M.G.; Domingo, P.; Giralt, M. & Villarroya, F. (2008). Comparison of the effects of lopinavir/ritonavir and efavirenz on gene expression and differentiation of human adipocytes. *Antiviral Therapy*, Vol.13, Suppl.4, pp.A23, ISSN 1359-6535.

Dickinson, L.; Khoo, S. & Back, D. (2010). Pharmacokinetics and drug-drug interactions of antiretrovirals: An update. *Antiviral Research*, Vol.85, No.1, pp.176-189, ISSN 0166-3542.

Dominguez, S.; Ghosn, J.; Peytavin, G.; Guiquet, M.; Tubiana, R.; Valantin, M.A.; Murphy, R.; Bricaire, F.; Benhamou, Y. & Katlama C. (2011). Impact of hepatitis C and liver fibrosis on antiretroviral plasma drug concentrations in HIV-HCV co-infected patients: the HEPADOSE study. *Journal of Antimicrobial Chemotherapy*, Vol.65, No.11, pp.2445-2449, ISSN 1460-2091.

El Hadri, K.; Glorian, M.; Monsempes, C.; Dieudonné, M.N.; Pecquery, R.; Giudicelli, Y.; Andreani, M.; Dugail, I. & Fève, B. (2004). *In vitro* suppression of the lipogenic pathway by the nonnucleoside reverse transcriptase inhibitor efavirenz in 3T3 and human preadipocytes or adipocytes. *Journal of Biological Chemistry*, Vol.279, No.15, pp.15130-41, ISSN 0021-9258.

Ena, J.; Amador, C.; Benito, C.; Fenoll, V. & Pasquau, F. (2003). Risk and determinants of developing severe liver toxicity during therapy with nevirapine-and efavirenz-containing regimens in HIV-infected patients. *International Journal of STD & AIDS*, Vol.14, No.11, pp.776-81.

Fätkenheurer, G.; Staszewski, S.; Plettenburg, A.; Hackman, F.; Layton, G.; McFayden, L.; Davis, T. & Jenkins, J. (2009). Activity, pharmacokinetics and safety of lersivirine (UK-453,061), a next-generation nonnucleoside reverse transcriptase inhibitor, during 7-day monotherapy in HIV-1-infected patients. *AIDS*, Vol.23, No.16, pp.2115-2122, ISSN 0269-9370.

Fumaz, C.R.; Tuldrà, A.; Ferrer, M.J.; Paredes, R.; Bonjoch, A.; Jou, T.; Negredo, E.; Romeu, J.; Sirera, G.; Tural, C. & Clotet, B. (2002). Quality of life, emotional status, and adherence of HIV-1-infected patients treated with efavirenz versus protease inhibitor-containing regimens. *Journal of Acquired Immune Deficiency Syndromes*, Vol.29, No.3, pp.244-53, ISSN 1525-4135.

Fuertes, A.; Cabrera, S.; Valverde, Mde.L. & Domínguez-Gil, A. Hyperhidrosis in association with efavirenz. *AIDS Patient Care STDS*, Vol.23, No.3, pp.143-5, ISSN 1087-2914.

Gallego-Escuredo, J.M.; Del Mar Gutierrez, M.; Diaz-Delfin, J.; Domingo, J.C.; Mateo, M.G.; Domingo, P.; Giralt, M. & Villarroya, F. (2010). Differantial effects of efavirenz and lopinavir/ritonavir on human adipocyte differentiation, gene expression and release of adipokines and pro-inflammatory cytokines. *Current HIV Research*, Vol.8, No.7, pp.545-553, ISSN 1570-162X.

Garcia, F.; Knobel, H.; Sambeat, M.A.; Arrizabalaga, J.; Aranda, M.; Romeu, J.; Dalmau, D.; Segura, F.; Gomez-Sirvent, J.L., Ferrer, E.; Cruceta, A.; Gallart, T.; Pumarola, T.; Miró, J.M. & Gatell, J.M.; Spanish SCAN Study Group. (2000). Comparison of twice-daily stavudine plus once- or twice-daily didanosine and nevirapine in early stages of HIV infection: the scan study. *AIDS*, Vol.14, pp.2485-2494, ISSN 0269-9370.

Gerson, R.J., Mutlib, A.E., Meunier, P.C.; Haley, P.J.; Gan, L.S.; Chen, H.; Davies, M.H.; Gemzik, B.; Christ, D.D.; Krahn, D.F.; Markwalder, J.A.; Seitz, S.P.; Miwa, G.T. & Robertson R.T. (1999). Species-specific nephrotoxicity induced by glutathione conjugation of efavirenz in rats. *Toxicological Sciences*, Vol.48, Suppl.1, pp.1833, ISSN 1096-0929.

Haas, D.W.; Ribaudo, H.J.; Kim, R.B.; Tierney, C.; Wilkinson, G.R.; Gulick, R.M.; Clifford, D.B.; Hulgan, T.; Marzolini, C. & Acosta, E.P. (2004). Pharmacogenetics of efavirenz and central nervous system side effects: an Adult AIDS Clinical Trials Group study. *AIDS*, Vol.18, No.18, pp.2391-400, ISSN 0269-9370.

Hammer, S.M.; Eron, J.J.Jr; Reiss, P.; Schooley, R.T.; Thompson, M.A.; Walmsley, S.; Cahn, P.; Fischl, M.A.; Gatell, J.M.; Hirsch, M.S.; Jacobsen, D.M.; Montaner, J.S.; Richman, D.D.; Yeni, P.G. & Volberding, P.A. (2008). International AIDS Society-USA. Antiretroviral treatment of adult HIV infection: 2008 recommendations of the international AIDS Society-USA panel. *Journal of the American Medical Association*, Vol. 300, pp.555-570, ISSN 0098-7484.

Hardie, D.G. (2007). AMP-activated/SNF1 protein kinases: conserved guardians of cellular energy. *Nature Reviews Molecular Cell Biology*, Vol.8, pp.774-785, ISSN 1471-0072.

Hawkins, T.; Geist, C.; Young, B.; Giblin, A.; Mercier, R.C.; Thornton, K. & Haubrich, R. (2005). Comparison of neuropsychiatric side effects in an observational cohort of efavirenz- and protease inhibitor-treated patients. *HIV Clinical Trials*, Vol.6, No.4, pp.187-96, ISSN 1528-4336.

Jamaluddin, Md.S.; Lin, P.H.; Yao, Q. & Chen C. (2010). Non-nucleoside reverse transcriptase inhibitor efavirenz increases monolayer permeability in human coronary artery endothelial cells. *Atherosclerosis*, Vol.208, pp.104-111, ISSN 0021-9150.

Jao, J.; Sturdevant, M.; del Rio Martin, J.; Schiano, T.; Fiel, M.I: & Huprikar, S. (2010). Nevirapine-induced stevens johnson-syndrome and fulminant hepatic failure requiring liver transplantation. *American Journal of Transplantation*, Vol.10, No.7, pp.1713-1716, ISSN 1600-6135.

Jena, A.; Sachdeva, R.K.; Sharma, A. & Wanchu, A. (2009). Adverse drug reactions to nonnucleoside reverse transcriptase inhibiotr-based antirretroviral regimen: a 24-

week prospective study. *Journal of the International Association of Physicians in AIDS Care*, Vol.8, No.5, 318-322, ISSN 1545-1097.

Kappelhoff, B.S.; van Leth, F.; Robinson, P.A.; MacGregor, T.R.; Baraldi, E.; Montella, F.; Uip, D.E.; Thompson, M.A.; Russell, D.B.; Lange, J.M.; Beijnen, J.H. & Huitema, A.D.; 2NN Study Group. (2005). Are adverse events of nevirapine and efavirenz related to plasma concentrations? *Antiviral Therapy*, Vol.10, No.4, pp.489-98, ISSN 1359-6535.

Karamchand, L.; Dawood, H. & Chuturgoon, A.A. (2008). Lymphocite mitochondrial depolarization and apoptosis in HIV-1 infected HAART patients. *Journal of Acquired Immune Deficiency Syndromes*, Vol.48, pp.381-388, ISSN 1525-4135.

Katsounas, A.; Frank, A.; Klinker, H. & Langmann, P. (2007). Efavirenz-therapy in HIV-patients with underlying liver disease: importance of continuous TDM of EFV. *European Journal of Medical Research*, Vol.12, No.8, pp.331-6, ISSN 0949-2321.

Klibanov, O.M. & Kaczor, R.L. (2010). IDX899, an aryl phosphinate-indole non-nucleoside reverse transcriptase inhibitor for the potential treatment of HIV infection. *Current Opinion in Investigational Drugs*, Vol.11, No.2, pp.237-245, ISSN 1472-4472.

Law, W.P.; Dore, G.J.; Duncombe, C.J.; Mahanontharit, A.; Boyd, M.A.; Ruxrungtham, K.; Lange, J.M.; Phanuphak, P. & Cooper, D.A. (2003). Risk of severe hepatotoxicity associated with antiretroviral therapy in the HIV-NAT Cohort, Thailand, 1996-2001. *AIDS*, Vol.17, No.15, pp.2191-2199, ISSN 0269-9370.

Lazzarin, A.; Campbell, T., Clotet, B.; Johnson, M.; Katlama, C.; Moll, A.; Towner, W.; Trottier, B.; Peeters, M.; Vingerhoets, J.; de Smedt, G.; Baeten, B.; Beets, G.; Sinha, R. & Woodfall, B.; DUET-2 study group. (2007). Efficacy and safety of TMC125 (etravirine) in treatment-experienced HIV-1-infected patients in DUET-2: 24-week results from a randomized, double-blind, placebo-controlled trial. *The Lancet*, Vol.370, pp.39-48, ISSN 0140-6736.

Macías, J.; Castellano, V.; Merchante, N.; Palacios, R.B.; Mira, J.A.; Sáez, C.; García-García, J.A.; Lozano, F.; Gómez-Mateos, J.M. & Pineda, J.A. (2004). Effect of antiretroviral drugs on liver fibrosis in HIV-infected patients with chronic hepatitis C: harmful impact of nevirapine. *AIDS*, Vol.18, No.5, pp.767-74, ISSN 0269-9370.

Madruga, J.V.; Cahn, P.; Grinsztejn, B.; Haubrich, R.; Lalezari, J.; Mill,s A.; Pialoux, G.; Wilkin, T.; Peeters, M.; Vingerhoets, J.; de Smedt, G.; Leopold, L.; Trefiglio, R. & Woodfall, B.; DUET-1 Study Group. (2007). Efficacy and safety of TMC125 (etravirine) in treatment-experienced HIV-1-infected patients in DUET-1: 24-week results from a randomized, double-blind, placebo-controlled trial. *The Lancet*, Vol.370, pp.29-38, ISSN 0140-6736.

Maggi, P.; Bellacosa, C.; Carito, V.; Perilli, F.; Lillo, A.; Volpe, A.; Trillo, G.; Angiletta, D.; Regina, G.; Angarano G. (2011). Cardiovascular risk factors in patients on long-term treatment with nevirapine- or efavirenz- based regimens. *Journal of Antimicrobial Chemotherapy*, Vol.66, pp.896-900, ISSN 1460-2091.

Maggiolo, F. (2009). Efavirenz: a decade of clinical experience in the treatment of HIV. *Journal of Antimicrobial Chemotherapy*, Vol.64, pp.910-928, ISSN 1460-2091.

Manfredi, R.; Calza, L. & Chiodo, F. (2005). An extremely different dysmetabolic profile between the two available nonnucleoside reverse transcriptase inhibitors: efavirenz and nevirapine. *Journal of Acquired Immune Deficiency Syndromes*, Vol.38, No.2, pp.236-8, ISSN 1525-4135.

Martínez, E.; García-Viejo, M.A.; Blanco, J.L.; Bianchi, L.; Buira, E.; Conget, I.; Casamitjana, R.; Mallolas, J. & Gatell, J.M. (2000). Impact of switching from human immunodeficiency virus type 1 protease inhibitors to efavirenz in successfully treated adults with lipodystrophy. *Clinical Infectious Diseases*, Vol.31, No.5, pp.1266-1273, ISSN 1058-4838.

Martínez, E. & Nelson, M. (2010). Simplification of antiretroviral therapy with etravirine. *AIDS Reviews*, Vol.12, pp.52-59, ISSN 1139-6121.

Marzolini, C.; Telenti, A.; Decosterd, L.A.; Greub, G.; Biollaz, J. & Buclin, T. (2001). Efavirenz plasma levels can predict treatment failure and central nervous system side effects in HIV-1 infected patients. *AIDS*, Vol.15, pp.71-75, ISSN 0269-9370.

Moyle, G.; Boffito, M.; Stoehr, A.; Rieger, A.; Shen, Z.; Manhard, K.; Sheedy, B.; Hingorami, V.; Raney, A.; Nguyen, M.; Nguyen, T.; Ong, V.; Yehk L.T. & Quart, B. (2010). Phase 2a randomized controlled trial of short-term activity, safety, and pharmakinetics of a novel nonnucleoside reverse transcriptase inhibitor, RDEA806, in HIV-1-positive, antiretroviral-naïve subjects. *Antimicrobial Agents and Chemotherapy*, Vol.54, No.8, pp.3170-3178, ISSN 0066-4804.

Muñoz-Moreno, J.A.; Fumaz, C.R.; Ferrer, M.J.; González-García, M., Moltó, J., Negredo, E. & Clotet, B. (2009). Neuropsychiatric symptoms associated with efavirenz: prevalence, correlates, and management. A neurobehavioral review. *AIDS Reviews*, Vol.11, No.2, pp.103-9, ISSN ISSN 1139-6121.

Mutlib, A.E.; Gerson, R.J.; Meunier, P.C.; Haley, P.J.; Chen, H.; Gan, L.S.; Davies, M.H.; Gemzik, B.; Christ, D.D.; Krahn, D.F.; Markwalder, J.A.; Seitz, S.P.; Robertson, R.T. & Miwa, G.T. (2000). The species-dependent metabolism of efavirenz produces a nephrotoxic glutathione conjugate in rats. *Toxicology and Applied Pharmacolology*, Vol.169, No.1, pp.102-13, ISSN 0041-008X.

Negredo, E.; Cruz, L.; Paredes, R.; Ruiz, L.; Fumaz, C.R.; Bonjoch, A.; Gel, S.; Tuldrà, A.; Balagué, M.; Johnston, S.; Arnó, A.; Jou, A.; Tural, C.; Sirera, G.; Romeu, J. & Clotet, B. (2002). Virological, immunological, and clinical impact of switching from protease inhibitors to nevirapine or to efavirenz in patients with human immunodeficiency virus infection and long-lasting viral suppression. *Clinical Infectious Diseases*, Vol.34, No.4, pp.504-10, ISSN 1058-4838.

Negredo, E.; Ribalta, J.; Ferré, R.; Salazar, J.; Rey-Joly, C.; Sirera, G.; Masana, L. & Clotet, B. Efavirenz induces a striking and generalized increase of HDL-cholesterol in HIV-infected patients. *AIDS*, Vol.18, No.5, pp.819-21, ISSN 0269-9370.

Palella, F.J. Jr.; Baker, R.K.; Moorman, A.C.; Chmiel, J.S.; Wood, K.C.; Brooks, J.T. & Holmberg, S.D.; HIV Outpatient Study Investigators. (2006). Mortality in the highly active antiretroviral therapy era: changing causes of death and disease in the HIV outpatient study. *Journal of Acquired Immune Deficiency Syndromes*, Vol.43, No.1, pp.27-34, ISSN 1525-4135.

Panos, G.; Samonis, G.; Alexiou, V.G.; Kavarnou, G.A.; Charatsis, G. & Falagas, M.E. (2008). Mortality and morbidity of HIV infected patients receiving HAART: a cohort study. *Current HIV Research*, Vol.6, No.3, pp. 257-260, ISSN 1570-162X.

Pereira, S.A.; Caixas, U.; Branco, T.; Germano, I.; Lampreia, F.; Papoila, A.L. & Monteiro, E.C. (2008). Efavirenz concentrations in HIV-infected patients with and without viral hepatitis. *British Journal of Clinical Pharmacolology*, Vol.66, No.4, pp.551-5, ISSN 0306-5251.

Pilon, A.A.; Lum, J.J.; Sanchez-Dardon, J.; Phenix, B.N.; Douglas, R. & Badley, A.D. (2002). Induction of apoptosis by a nonnucleoside human immunodeficiency virus type 1 reverse transcriptase inhibitor. *Antimicrobial Agents and Chemotherapy*, Vol.46, pp.2687-2691, ISSN 0066-4804.

Popovic, M.; Shenton, J.M.; Chen, J.; Baban, A.; Tharmanathan, T.; Mannargudi, B.; Abdulla, D. & Uetrecht J.P. (2010). Nevirapine hypersensitivity. *Handbook of Experimental Pharmacology*, Vol.196, pp.437-451, ISSN 0171-2004.

Pozniak, A.L.; Morales-Ramirez, J.; Katabira, E.; Steyn, D.; Lupo, S.H.; Santoscoy, M.; Grinsztejn, B.; Ruxrungtham, K.; Rimsky, L.T.; Vanveggel, S. & Boven, K.; TMC278-C204 study group. (2010). Efficacy and safety of TMC278 in antiretroviral-naïve HIV-1 patients: week 96 results of a phase Iib randomized trial. *AIDS*, Vol.24, No.1, pp.55-65, ISSN 0269-9370.

Rescriptor official FDA information, side effects and uses, http://www.drugs.com/pro/rescriptor.html (Accesed March 15, 2011).

Rivero, A.; Mira, JA. & Pineda, JA. (2007). Liver toxicity induced by non-nucleoside reverse transcriptase inhibitors. *Journal of Antimicrobial Chemotherapy*, Vol.59, No.3, pp.342-6, ISSN 1460-2091.

Schiller, D.S. & Youssef-Bessler, M. (2009). Etravirine: a second generation nonnucleoside reverse transcriptase inhibitor (NNRTI) active against NNRTI-resistant strains of HIV. *Clinical Therapeutics*, Vol.31, No.4, pp.692-704, ISSN 0149-2918.

Starr, S.E.; Fletcher, C.V.; Spector, S.A.; Yong, F.H.; Fenton, T.; Brundage, R.C.; Manion, D. ; Ruiz, N.; Gersten, M.; Becker, M. ; McNamara, J.; Mofenson, L.M. ; Purdue, L. ; Siminski, S. ; Graham, B. ; Kornhauser, D.M. ; Fiske, W. ; Vincent, C. ; Lischner, H.W. ; Dankner, W.M. & Flynn, P.M. (1999). Combination therapy with efavirenz, nelfinavir, and nucleoside reverse-transcriptase inhibitors in children infected with human immunodeficiency virus type 1. Pediatric AIDS Clinical Trials Group 382 Team. *The New England Journal of Medicine*, Vol.341, pp.1874-1881, ISSN 0028-4793.

Staszewski, S.; Morales-Ramirez, J.; Tashima, K.T.; Rachlis, A.; Skiest, D.; Stanford, J.; Stryker, R.; Johnson, P.; Labriola, D.F.; Farina, D.; Manion, D.J. & Ruiz, N.M. (1999). Efavirenz plus zidovudine and lamivudine, efavirenz plus indinavir, and indinavir plus zidovudine and lamivudine in the treatment of HIV-1 infection in adults. Study 006 Team. *The New England Journal of Medicine*, Vol.341, No.25, pp.1865-73, ISSN 0028-4793.

Sluis-Cremer, N.; Temiz, N.A. & Bahar, I. (2004). Conformational changes in HIV-1 reverse transcriptase induced by nonnucleoside reverse transcriptase inhibitor binding. *Current HIV Research*, Vol.2, pp.323-332, ISSN 1570-162X.

Sulkowski, M.S.; Thomas, D.L.; Mehta, S.H.; Chaisson, R.E. & Moore, R.D. (2002) Hepatotoxicity associated with nevirapine or efavirenz-containing antiretroviral therapy: role of hepatitis C and B infections. *Hepatology*, Vol.35, No.1, pp.182-9, ISSN 1665-2681.

Turkova, A.; Ball, C.; Gilmour-White, S.; Rela, M. & Mieli-Vergani, G. (2009). A paediatric case of acute liver failure associated with efavirenz-based highly active antiretroviral therapy and effective use of raltegravir in combination antiretroviral treatment after liver transplantation. *Journal of Antimicrobial Chemotherapy*, Vol.63, No.3, pp.623-5, ISSN 1460-2091.

van den Berg-Wolf, M.; Hullsiek, K.H.; Peng, G.; Kozal, M.J.; Novak, R.M.; Chen, L.; Crane, L.R. & Macarthur, R.D.; CPCRA 058 Study Team, the Terry Beirn Community Programs for Clinical Research on AIDS (CPCRA), and The International Network for Strategic Initiative in Global HIV Trials (INSIGHT). (2008). Virologic, immunologic, clinical, safety, and resistance outcomes from a long-term comparison of efavirenz-based versus nevirapine-based antiretroviral regimens as initial therapy in HIV-1-infected persons. *HIV Clinical Trials*, Vol.9, No.5, pp.324-36, ISSN 1528-4336.

van der Valk, M.; Kastelein, J.J.; Murphy, R.L.; van Leth, F.; Katlama, C.; Horban, A.; Glesby, M.; Behrens, G.; Clotet, B.; Stellato, R.K.; Molhuizen, H.O. & Reiss, P.; Atlantic Study Team. (2001). Nevirapine-containing antiretroviral therapy in HIV-1 infected patients results in an anti-atherogenic lipid profile. *AIDS*, Vol.15, No.18, pp.2407-14, ISSN 0269-9370.

van Leth, F.; Phanuphak, P.; Ruxrungtham, K.; Baraldi, E.; Miller, S.; Gazzard, B.; Cahn, P.; Lalloo, U.G.; van der Westhuizen, I.P.; Malan, D.R.; Johnson, M.A.; Santos, B.R.; Mulcahy, F.; Wood, R.; Levi, G.C.; Reboredo, G.; Squires, K.; Cassetti, I.; Petit, D.; Raffi, F.; Katlama, C.; Murphy, R.L.; Horban, A.; Dam, J.P.; Hassink, E.; van Leeuwen, R.; Robinson, P.; Wit, F.W. & Lange, J.M.; 2NN Study team. (2004). Comparison of first-line antiretroviral therapy with regimens including nevirapine, efavirenz, or both drugs, plus stavudine and lamivudine: a randomised open-label trial, the 2NN Study. *The Lancet*, Vol.363, No.9417, pp.1253-63, ISSN 0140-6736.

Walker, U.A.; Setzer, B. & Venhoff, N. (2002). Increased long-term mitochondrial toxicity in combinations of nucleoside analogue reverse transcriptase inhibitors. *AIDS*, Vol.16, pp.2165-2173, ISSN 0269-9370.

Ward, B.A.; Gorski, J.C.; Jones, D.R.; Hall, S.D.; Flockhart, D.A. & Desta Z. (2003). The cytochrome P450 2B6 (CYP2B6) is the main catalyst of efavirenz primary and secondary metabolism: implication for HIV/AIDS therapy and utility of efavirenz as a substrate marker of CYP2B6 catalytic activity. *Journal of Pharmacology and Experimental Therapeutics*, Vol.306, No.1, pp.287-300, ISSN 0022-3565.

Waters, L.; John, L. & Nelson, M. (2007). Non-nucleoside reverse transcriptase inhibitors: a review. *International Journal of Clinical Practice*, Vol.61, pp.105-108, ISSN 1369-5031.

Waters, L.; Fisher, M.; Winston, A.; Higgs, C.; Hadley, W.; Garvey, L.; Mandalia, S.; Perry, N.; Nicola, M. & Nelson, M. (2011). A phase IV, double-blind, multicentre, randomized, placebo-controlled, pilot study to assess the feasibility of switching individuals receiving efavirenz with continuing central nervous system adverse effects to etravirine. *AIDS*, Vol.25, No.1, pp.65-71, ISSN 0269-9370.

Weber, R.; Sabin, C.A.; Friis-Møller, N.; Reiss, P.; El-Sadr, W.M.; Kirk, O.; Dabis, F.; Law, M.G.; Pradier, C.; De Wit, S.; Akerlund, B.; Calvo, G.; Monforte, A.; Rickenbach, M.; Ledergerber, B.; Phillips, A.N. & Lundgren, J.D. (2006). Liver-related deaths in persons infected with the human immunodeficiency virus: the D:A:D study. *Archives of Internal Medicine*, Vol.166, No.15, pp.1632-41, ISSN 0003-9926.

Welz, T.; Childs, K.; Ibrahim, F.; Poulton, M.; Taylor, C.B.; Moniz, C.F. & Post, F.A. (2010). Efavirenz is associated with severe vitamin D deficiency and increased alkaline phosphatase. *AIDS*, Vol.24, No.12, pp.1923-8, ISSN 0269-9370.

Zhou, X.J.; Pietropaolo, K.; Damphousse, D.; Belanger, B. ; Chen, J.; Sullivan-Bólyai, J. & Mayers, D. (2009). Single-dose escalation and multiple-dose safety, tolerability, and pharmacokinetics of IDX899, a candidate human immunodeficiency virus type 1 nonnucleoside reverse transcriptase inhibitor, in healthy subjects. *Antimicrobial Agents and Chemotherapy*, Vol.53, No.5, pp.1739-1746, ISSN0066-4804.

15

Antiretroviral Therapy and HIV-Associated Neurocognitive Disorders

Cagla Akay[1] and Kelly L. Jordan-Sciutto[2]
[1]*Department of Pathology, University of Pennsylvania*
[2]*Department of Pathology, University of Pennsylvania*
United States of America

1. Introduction

Human immunodeficiency virus (HIV)-Associated Neurocognitive Disorders (HAND) define a wide spectrum of behavioral, cognitive and motor dysfunctions(Heaton, Clifford et al. ; Neuenburg, Brodt et al. 2002; McArthur 2004; Lindl, Marks et al. 2010). The initial criteria put forth by the American Association of Neurology described two levels of neurocognitive impairment in HIV (+) patients: HIV-associated dementia (HAD) and minor motor cognitive disorder (MCMD)(1996). However, the emergence of more subtle forms of cognitive impairment after the implementation of combination antiretroviral therapy (cART) in 1996 necessitated a revised classification, which now includes, in addition to HAD, asymptomatic neurocognitive impairment (ANI), and mild neurocognitive disorder (MND), while MCMD is no longer included in the classification (Antinori, Arendt et al. 2007). While the incidence of HAD has declined in the cART era, from 10-15% to approximately 2%; ANI and MND have become more prevalent (Heaton, Clifford et al. 2010). Overall, HAND continues to persist, affecting approximately 50% of HIV (+) patients in the cART era (Power, Boisse et al. 2009; Heaton, Clifford et al. 2010). The underlying neuropathology suggests a change from overt dementia to a more insidious neurocognitive impairment (Kusdra, McGuire et al. 2002; Anthony and Bell 2008; Everall, Vaida et al. 2009). Various factors, such as age-related vascular and metabolic changes and substance and alcohol abuse, the emergence of resistant virus species, persistent viral DNA in the central nervous system (CNS) despite successful plasma viral control, limited access of cART into the CNS, poor adherence to drug regimen, and possible cART-related neurotoxicities are suggested to contribute to these changes observed in the clinical and neuropathological presentation in the HAND brain. With the increased life expectancy, the ever-expanding repertoire of antiretroviral drugs (ARVs) and the patient-tailored, dynamic combination ARV regimens, the contribution of cART to the persistence of HAND is an urgent question that needs to be addressed to more successfully predict and prevent CNS related morbidity and mortality among HIV-infected patients.

2. Clinical presentation of HAND

HAND was initially characterized as a combination of acquired deficits in cognition and motor function, in addition to behavioral and emotional changes (Navia, Cho et al. 1986;

Portegies, Enting et al. 1993). When it became apparent that viral replication could not be controlled by the use of one or two antiretroviral drugs, and that the CNS was shown to provide a sanctuary for HIV (Brew, Pemberton et al. 1997; Pialoux, Fournier et al. 1997), more aggressive treatment plans employing multiple ARVs were implemented. Successful viral suppression due to cART led to the observed initial improvement in cognitive function and an overall decrease in the incidence of the most severe form of HAND, HAD. However, as patients are maintained on cART long-term, subtler forms of neurocognitive impairment, ANI and MND have since emerged (Power, Boisse et al. 2009; Heaton, Clifford et al. 2010). ANI is defined as mild neurocognitive impairment in the absence of a decline in activities of daily living (ADL), whereas mild-to moderate neurocognitive decline that affects ADL is considered MND. The areas of cognition affected include concentration and/or attention, executive functioning, memory, and visuospatial skills (Antinori, Arendt et al. 2007). Depression, psychosis and anxiety at varying severity are also commonly observed in HIV-infected patients (Owe-Larsson, Sall et al. 2009). The complexity of cognitive and behavioral presentations in cART treated patients has served to obfuscate the underlying causes of these changes.

The clinical course of disease progression of HAND has changed dramatically since the introduction of cART in 1996. In the pre-cART era, HIV-associated neurocognitive impairment tended to worsen over time, and was more likely to follow a fulminant course. In fact, when other risk factors were controlled for, HAD was associated with increased mortality (Ellis, Deutsch et al. 1997). In contrast, the neurocognitive symptoms associated with HIV appear to follow a more unpredictable course during the life-time of the patient in the cART era. While some patients may recover from MND with effective cART, others can worsen steadily with progression from ANI to HAD. Further yet, some patients might experience a fluctuating course (Cole, Margolick et al. 2007; Woods, Moore et al. 2009). However, while progression to HAD is still observed in a subset of patients, even though at a slower pace in most cases, the mortality is now less likely to associate with HAND, and more likely with co-existing factors, such as co-infections, substance and alcohol use, and age-related illnesses.

3. Neuropathology of HAND

HIV targets and leads to a selective loss of CD4$^+$ T cells, which eventually causes the severe immunodeficiency that develops in cases of uncontrolled HIV infection. HIV also targets monocytes and macrophages early during infection, which enable HIV to establish viral reservoirs in the lymphoid tissue and the CNS (Gendelman, Lipton et al. 1994; Gonzalez-Scarano and Martin-Garcia 2005; Kaul, Zheng et al. 2005). In fact, extensive *in vitro* and *in vivo* studies support the "Trojan Horse" model of HIV infection in the CNS (Liu, Lossinsky et al. 2002). According to this model, HIV enters the brain via infected monocytes that cross the blood-brain barrier (BBB). Once in the CNS, infected monocytes differentiate into macrophages, which then constitute viral reservoirs in the brain. A small number of neurons and glia may also become infected; however, such infection is not productive (Gendelman, Lipton et al. 1994; Gonzalez-Scarano and Martin-Garcia 2005; Kaul, Zheng et al. 2005).

Two major mechanisms of neuronal damage have been proposed: 1) Direct neurotoxicity by viral proteins such as HIV envelope glycoprotein (gp120) and HIV transactivator of transcription (Tat) protein, and, 2) Indirect neurotoxicity induced by soluble factors released by infected and/or activated macrophages including, but not limited to, quinolinic acid,

TNF-α, reactive oxygen species (ROS), and cytokines such as CXCL12 (stromal cell-derived factor-1, SDF-1), CCL2 (monocyte chemotactic protein-1, MCP-1), and interleukin-6 (IL-6)(Price, Brew et al. 1988; Giulian, Yu et al. 1996; Soontornniyomkij, Nieto-Rodriguez et al. 1998; Lindl, Marks et al. 2010). Most of these factors not only directly affect neurons but also induce the secretion of more of these and other neurotoxic soluble factors, such as excitatory amino acids such as glutamate from neighboring macrophages/microglia, and astrocytes (Gorry, Ong et al. 2003; Gonzalez-Scarano and Martin-Garcia 2005). In the chronic course of HIV infection, inflammatory events and oxidative stress that ensue in this environment in the CNS precipitate neuronal dysfunction and death. Several *in vitro* and *in vivo* studies lend support to the indirect mechanism of neurotoxicity. Increases in neuroinflammatory factors (e.g. TNF-α, CCL2, and IL-6) have been detected in the cerebrospinal fluid (CSF) of HIV-infected patients (Sippy, Hofman et al. 1995; Achim, Masliah et al. 1996; Achim and Wiley 1996; Conant, Garzino-Demo et al. 1998; Gisolf, van Praag et al. 2000). Further, markers of oxidative stress, such as 4-hydroxynonenal (4-HNE), are well documented in HAND patients (Haughey, Cutler et al. 2004; Sacktor, Haughey et al. 2004). In addition, several studies have reported that neopterin and β2-microglobulin, regarded as indirect markers of macrophage activation, are elevated in the CSF of HIV infected patients (Yilmaz, Fuchs et al. 2006; Edén, Fuchs et al. 2010; Hagberg, Cinque et al. 2010). Finally, the neuropathological correlates of inflammation, including astrocytosis and increased perivascular macrophage infiltration are commonly observed in the brains of HIV-infected patients (Kolson 2002; Kusdra, McGuire et al. 2002; Lindl, Marks et al. 2010).

The precise mechanisms by which inflammation leads to neuronal death in response to these functionally diverse factors are not known; however, several mechanisms are likely candidates. Intracellular ROS accumulation can directly alter neuronal mitochondrial function, leading to neuronal damage and death (Reynolds, Laurie et al. 2007; Hu, Sheng et al. 2009). On the other hand, pro-inflammatory factors can impair glutamate reuptake by astrocytes (Gorry, Ong et al. 2003; Gonzalez-Scarano and Martin-Garcia 2005). Increased extracellular glutamate that is not buffered by astrocytes can activate *N*-methyl-D-aspartate glutamate (NMDA) receptors and lead to excess Ca^{2+} influx into the neurons (Giulian, Yu et al. 1996; O'Donnell, Agrawal et al. 2006). Much evidence indicates that increased intracellular Ca^{2+} concentrations are detrimental to neurons. Ca^{2+} can precipitate oxidative stress via free radical production, to which neurons are likely to become more susceptible in the absence of normal functioning astrocytes and macrophages. Further, excess intracellular Ca^{2+} activates the death-associated proteases, calpains and caspases (Moore, Rothwell et al. 2002; Danial and Korsmeyer 2004). The pathological indicators of neuronal damage and death, dendritic simplification, axonal damage and synaptic loss, correlate best with the presence of infected macrophages and microglia (Masliah, Heaton et al. 1997; Ellis 2010). Interestingly, viral load (VL) does not correlate with neurodegeneration, suggesting that the indirect mechanisms might play a more important role in neuronal injury than the direct mechanisms (Tozzi, Balestra et al. 2007; Yilmaz, Price et al. 2008).

Several CSF markers have been utilized in an attempt to predict, diagnose and monitor the progression of HAND. Among those, as markers of immune activation, TNF-α, and CCL2 levels were shown to correlate with neurological deficits in the pre-cART era (Gisolf, van Praag et al. 2000; Sevigny, Albert et al. 2004; Ragin, Wu et al. 2010); however, a more recent study did not show such a correlation for either of these markers among a cohort of patients on cART (McArthur, McDermott et al. 2004). Additionally, contrary to expectations, in patients on cART regimens with high predicted CSF concentrations, the markers of inflammation and oxidative stress appear to persist (Roc, Ances et al. 2007). Further, while cART has been shown to decrease neopterin levels in the CSF, these levels still appear to be above those measured in uninfected individuals (Yilmaz, Fuchs et al. 2006). A recent study shows that the changes in CSF neopterin levels are not affected by ARVs with predicted high CSF concentrations (Eden and Fuchs 2010). These findings imply that neuroinflammation might be ongoing despite the success of cART in controlling viral replication; thus supplementary therapies that would alleviate inflammation appear necessary for a better control of HAND.

4. HAND and Combination Antiretroviral Therapy

The development of more sensitive reverse transcriptase polymerized chain reaction (RT-PCR) methods for the detection of HIV RNA during the 1990s revealed that single ARV treatments were not able to completely suppress viral replication. It also became apparent that the development of ARV resistance was hampering the efforts to successfully suppress VL. These major concerns led to a revision in the treatment plan for HIV infection, which was initially called highly active antiretroviral therapy (HAART), and was later changed to combination antiretroviral therapy (cART). Currently recommended cART for ARV-naïve HIV-infected patients includes a cocktail of ARVs from three different classes, nucleoside/nucleotide reverse-transcriptase inhibitors (NRTIs/NtRTIs), non-nucleoside reverse-transcriptase inhibitors (nNRTIs), and protease inhibitors (PIs). Sustained viral suppression, improved immune function and better control of HIV-related co-morbidities have contributed to the reduction in HIV-associated morbidity and mortality in the era of cART.

In addition to its success in the periphery, cART led to striking changes in the clinical presentation and disease progression of HAND. The incidence of frank HAD has decreased dramatically and HAND in the cART era follows a more protracted course. However, neurocognitive impairment still persists, albeit as a general rule it is not as severe as in the pre-cART era. Importantly, HAD patients on cART still exhibit increased levels of macrophage infiltration similar to those seen in patients with HAD in the pre-cART era. Virus-related factors, such as persistent viral DNA in the CNS despite successful suppression of plasma and CSF VL and the emergence of resistant virus species due to failure of ARV to reach therapeutically relevant concentrations in the CSF, likely account at least partially for these observations.

Studies in animal models of HIV infection suggest that the seeding of HIV in the CNS can occur as early as 4 days after the initial exposure to the virus. In addition, HIV RNA can be detected in the human brain as early as 14 days after infection. These studies indicate that viral escape to the CNS during the initial phase of asymptomatic viremia is possible; thus early and sustained VL control is necessary to limit the establishment of an HIV reservoir in the CNS, which, as a consequence, would have an immediate impact on the development of HAND. However, the timing for cART initiation in ARV-naïve HIV-infected individuals is not straightforward due to serious systemic ARV-related side effects and potential non-adherence, which in itself carries increased risk for selection of drug-resistant virus strains. Based on data from large clinical trials revealing that the initial CD4 cell count is a major predictor of morbidity and mortality in HIV patients, The United States Panel on Antiretroviral Guidelines for Adults and Adolescents recommends that cART should be initiated in patients with CD4 cell counts lower than 350 cells/μl or in those with an AIDS-defining illness irrespective of

CD4 counts (Panel on Antiretroviral Guidelines for Adults and Adolescents. (Revised January 10, 2011) Guidelines for the use of antiretroviral agents in HIV-1-infected adults and adolescents, April 14, 2011, available from http://www.aidsinfo.nih.gov/ContentFiles/AdultandAdolescentGL.pdf). cART is also recommended for patients with CD4 counts between 350-500 cells/µl. The panel also states that cART should be considered irrespective of the CD4 counts in patients who have either HIV-associated nephropathy, or Hepatitis B infection that needs treatment. For those who have CD4 counts above 500, the panel was evenly divided, with 50% of the panel members voted in favor of starting cART, whereas the other 50% of members voted cART treatment as optional under these conditions. However, the panel has not reached consensus with regard to the time to start cART in the context of HAND risk reduction, an important factor in the persistence of HAND in the cART era. Unfortunately, even with early initiation of cART, failure of ARVs to reach effective CSF concentrations may hamper the suppression of VL in the CNS. Thus in an attempt to assess the efficacy with which ARVs reach effective CSF concentrations, a scoring system coined CNS penetrance effectiveness (CPE) scoring is being increasingly investigated in clinical studies (Letendre, Marquie-Beck et al. 2008; Marra, Zhao et al. 2009; Tozzi, Balestra et al. 2009; Edén, Fuchs et al. 2010; Letendre, Ellis et al. 2010; Garvey, Winston et al. 2011; Smurzynski, Wu et al. 2011). An ARV drug with relatively poor CNS penetration is assigned a CPE score of 0, while one with an intermediate CNS penetration would have a CPE score of 0.5, and one with high penetration would receive a CPE score of 1. Each combination ARV treatment regimen includes ARVs from at least three different classes with distinct physicochemical properties and thus the sum of CPE scores from several types of drugs will affect the functional capacity of the regimen within the CNS.

5. Antiretroviral drugs

While each ARV is unique in structure, each ARV class has certain common characteristics that aid in determining the overall CPE score of any given cART. However, the unique properties of each drug also make it harder to accurately predict the CPE score for that particular ARV, and by extension, CPE score for specific cART regimens as well. For a better understanding of an ideal cART regimen for the control of HAND, we need to examine each ARV class. ARVs target HIV at distinct steps in the life cycle of the virus, including (1) virus attachment to the host cell, both fusion with the cell membrane and entry, (2) reverse transcription, (3) integration, (4) processing of viral proteins, and (5) maturation. The major classes of antiretroviral drugs are entry inhibitors, nucleoside/nucleotide reverse transcriptase inhibitors (NRTIs), non-nucleoside reverse transcriptase inhibitors (nNRTIs), integrase inhibitors, and protease inhibitors (PIs). In this section, we will summarize the mechanisms of action, the general and CNS-specific side effects and the predictors of CPE scores for each class with the relevant *in vitro* and *in vivo* findings.

5.1 Entry inhibitors

HIV entry to the host cell begins with the binding of the HIV surface protein, gp120, to the T cell surface receptor CD4. This attachment exposes specific conserved regions of gp120, enabling its binding to one of the two chemokine receptors on the host cell surface, CXCR4 or CCR5. This, in turn, unmasks gp41, a process that leads to the fusion of the viral membrane with the host cell and the subsequent release of the virus capsid into the host cell cytoplasm. This highly conserved, stepwise process provides three access points which a relatively new class of ARVs, collectively termed entry inhibitors, targets. At this point, only two entry inhibitors are approved by the Food and Drug Administration (FDA) for clinical use: enfuvirtide (T-20), and maraviroc.

5.1.1 Enfuvirtide

Enfuvirtide is a 36 amino-acid synthetic peptide that mimics a specific region in gp41 and competitively inhibits the fusion step and does not depend on co-receptor use (Joly, Jidar et al. 2010). It is not a substrate for major drug metabolism enzymes, CYP3A4 or CYP2B6, a trait that limits possible interactions that might occur with other ARVs that are inhibitors or activators of these enzymes. Further, enfuvirtide acts in the extracellular area, and lacks cross-resistance. In addition, enfuvirtide-related side effects are minimal, and are usually limited to injection site reactions. Due to these characteristics, enfuvirtide is currently prescribed to ARV-experienced patients, especially those with multi-ARV resistance (Yeni, Mills et al. 2010). However, its potential benefits for patients with CNS involvement are not known. The only study where CNS penetrance of enfuvirtide was assessed in humans, has found CSF enfuvirtide levels to be below plasma EC_{50} (plasma concentration required for obtaining 50% of a maximum effect *in vivo)* values, which is most likely due to the high level of binding of enfuvirtide to plasma proteins (92%), mainly albumin (Patel, Zhang et al. 2005; Price, Parham et al. 2008). CSF concentration of a given pharmaceutical does not reflect its parenchymal concentration with certainty, as will be discussed in section 6; however, as extracellular enfuvirtide concentration determines its antiviral activity; its CSF levels most likely reflect its concentrations in the parenchyma. Based on these data, enfuvirtide is given a CPE score of zero (table 1 for proposed CPE scores of currently used ARVs) (Smurzynski, Wu et al. 2011). Importantly, a limited number of studies have found no association between the use of enfuvirtide and peripheral neuropathy, a side effect associated with certain ARVs. These findings, in addition to its low CPE score, likely preclude any potential neurotoxicity issues in the CNS related to enfuvirtide. In summary, the impact of enfuvirtide on HAND, whether beneficial or toxic, is most likely minimal; however, its efficacy in controlling systemic VL will certainly contribute to better control of disease progression in the CNS.

5.1.2 Maraviroc

The second clinically approved member of the entry inhibitor family is maraviroc. Maraviroc is a specific, non-competitive CCR5 antagonist and is effective in both ARV-naïve and ARV-experienced patients who harbor a CCR5-tropic virus, which is determined by genotypic and phenotypic tests before the initiation of maraviroc-including regimens (Lieberman-Blum, Fung et al. 2008; Kromdijk, Huitema et al. 2010). It is a substrate for drug efflux proteins ((p-glycoprotein (p-gp) and multidrug resistance protein-1 (MDR-1)) expressed by the BBB; however, its binding affinity to plasma proteins is not very high. Thus, CSF and brain distribution studies in rats suggest that approximately 10% of the plasma maraviroc levels are achieved in the CNS, which falls within a range of reported IC_{50} (half maximal inhibitory concentration) values (Walker, Bowers et al. 2008). These predictions are further supported by multiple studies conducted in humans, where maraviroc achieves therapeutically relevant concentrations in the CSF, and also effectively suppresses CSF VL (table 1) (Smurzynski, Wu et al. 2011). Currently no data exists on the possible toxic effects of maraviroc in the CNS; however, given that the only cell types that express CCR5 are macrophages and T cells, direct neurotoxicity due to maraviroc is not likely. Thus, cART regimens that include maraviroc are increasingly prescribed and future studies are warranted to examine its impact on HAND.

Antiretroviral Class		CPE Score	
	1	0.5	0
Entry Inhibitors			Enfuvirtide
	Maraviroc		
Nucleoside/nucleotide reverse transcriptase inhibitors	Zidovudine (AZT)	Stavudine (d4T)	Tenofovir (TDF) *
	Abacavir (ABC)	Lamivudine (3TC)	
		Emtricitabine (FTC) *	
nNRTIs	Nevirapine (NVP)	Efavirenz (EFV)	
Protease Inhibitors	Darunavir	Amprenavir	Nelfinavir
		Atazanavir	Ritonavir *
		Fosamprenavir	Saquinavir *
		Indinavir	
Integrase Inhibitors		Raltegravir	

Table 1. CNS penetrance effectiveness (CPE) scores of antiretroviral drugs currently in clinical use. Higher CPE scores indicate better penetrance. * In vivo data suggests better CPE score

5.2 Nucleoside/nucleotide reverse transcriptase inhibitors

5.2.1 Mechanism

The single-stranded HIV RNA, once in the host cell, is reverse transcribed by the viral reverse transcriptase (HIV-RT) into a double-stranded complementary viral DNA, which migrates to the host nucleus as part of the pre-integration complex. Nucleoside and nucleotide reverse transcriptase inhibitors (NRTIs/NtRTIs) are analogues of the naturally occurring deoxynucleotides that are needed for the reverse-transcription (Warnke, Barreto et al. 2007); however, NRTIs/NtRTIs lack a 3'-hydroxyl group on the deoxyribose moiety. Three steps of phosphorylation are needed for NRTIs to become activated, while only two phosphorylation steps are necessary in the case of NtRTIs (Piliero 2004). Following activation, NRTIs/NtRTIs are incorporated into the viral DNA, thereby preventing the next 5′-3′phosphodiester bond formation and consequently leading to the early termination of viral DNA synthesis, named chain termination (Warnke, Barreto et al. 2007).

5.2.2 Clinical use

NRTIs/NtRTIs quickly and effectively decrease VL and increase CD4 counts (Hill and Sawyer 2009). As they are not metabolized by drug metabolizing enzymes, the activities of which are altered by certain ARV drugs from other classes, dose adjustment is usually not necessary. Currently, five NRTIs (zidovudine (AZT), stavudine (d4T), lamivudine (3TC), emtricitabine (FTC), abacavir (ABC)) and one NtRTI (tenofovir disoproxil fumarate (TDF)) are used and form the backbone of most initial cART regimens. The current initial cART regimen typically includes two NRTIs/NtRTIs in addition to an nNRTI or a PI boosted with ritonavir, which is also a PI. The recently revised recommendations suggest that initial cART in ARV-naïve patients should include one of the following cocktails: efavirenz/tenofovir/emtricitabine (EFV/TDF/FTC), ritonavir-boosted atazanavir/tenofovir/emtricitabine (ATV+r/TDF/FTC), ritonavir-boosted darunavir/tenofovir/emtricitabine (DRV+r/TDF/FTC), or raltegravir + tenofovir/emtricitabine (RAL + TDF/FTC). A similar cART regimen is also recommended for post-exposure prophylaxis (Grant 2010). In addition, TDF/FTC cocktail is recommended as a pre-exposure prophylaxis regimen in high risk persons (Grant 2010). Further, combinations that include AZT, 3TC, and ABC are proven to be the most effective in prevention of intrauterine and postnatal transmission, with relatively few side effects to both mother and child, when compared with regimens that include nNRTIs or PIs (Sturt, Dokubo et al. 2010). However, specific NRTIs/NtRTIs are not considered part of a first line therapy in certain patient populations. For example, in pregnant women TDF is only considered when the infecting virus shows resistance to other NRTIs or in the presence of chronic hepatitis infection. This is due to concerns regarding possible toxicity of TDF for the fetus, specifically in bone mineralization (Duarte-Rojo and Heathcote 2010). Similarly, d4T can lead to sometimes fatal lactic acidosis and hepatic failure in pregnant women and is only used when no other viable options remain (Nolan and Mallal 2004).

5.2.3 Side effects

Due to the low fidelity of HIV-RT and to the high rate of HIV replication, NRTI/NtRTI-resistant viral strains have developed. The emergence of these strains along with the severe NRTI/NtRTI-associated side effects, including lactic acidosis, lipoatrophy, and peripheral neuropathy, usually necessitates changes in the regimen, which can include switching ARVs, adding more ARVs, and/or adjusting dosing (Kohler and Lewis 2007). Interestingly, individual NRTIs/NtRTIs are associated with specific side effects. For example, d4T, and to a lesser extent, AZT, are associated with lipoatrophy, while TDF does not appear to cause this particular side effect. Peripheral neuropathy, which manifests in approximately 40% patients on cART, is associated with regimens that include d4T (Kohler and Lewis 2007). On the other hand, TDF is associated with increased risk of nephropathy and loss of bone density (Duarte-Rojo and Heathcote 2010). FTC-associated side effects are usually milder than those observed with other NRTIs/NtRTIs and include skin discoloration, nausea, and elevated liver enzymes (Nelson and Schiavone 2004).

One major mechanism underlying NRTI/NtRTI-associated side effects is mitochondrial toxicity, which is a result of DNA polymerase γ inhibition, leading to mitochondrial DNA depletion, oxidative stress, loss of mitochondrial membrane potential ($\Delta\Psi m$), and loss of oxidative phosphorylation (Dalakas 2001; Dagan, Sable et al. 2002; William 2003; Nolan and Mallal 2004). The potency of NRTIs in inhibiting DNA polymerase γ differs among the members, with d4T and AZT showing higher potency compared with other NRTIs/NtRTIs. Further, the activities of the different kinases responsible for phosphorylation of each type of NRTI/NtRTI show variability among different cell types and may account for the cell-type specificity of the side effects (Bazzoli, Jullien et al. 2010).

5.2.4 Considerations for the CNS

Based on extensive data compiled from animal and human studies, AZT, d4T, and ABC appear to reach effective concentrations in the CNS, while the access of 3TC to the CNS is predicted to be minimal (Anderson and Rower 2010). There is limited information on TDF distribution in the CNS; the only functional study investigating TDF access to the CNS suggests that its concentrations in the CNS might be limited, with varying degrees of accumulation in different brain regions (Anthonypillai, Gibbs et al. 2006). Currently, there is no information on CSF levels of FTC in the CSF (table 1) (Smurzynski, Wu et al. 2011). However, several reports suggest that regimens containing TDF and FTC may lead to improvements in neurocognitive impairment when compared with regimens that include other NRTIs or nNRTI/PIs (Allavena, Le Moal et al. 2006; Winston, Duncombe et al. 2010). Overall, clinical data from extensive studies show that NRTIs/NtRTIs, as part of cART regimens contribute significantly to the sharp decreases observed in the incidence of HAND. However, with regard to NRTIs/NtRTIs, several factors should be considered as possible contributors to the persistence of HAND. First, the emergence of NRTI/NtRTI resistance and possible less-than effective CSF concentrations, especially of 3TC and TDF, may limit their effectiveness in the eradication of the viral reservoirs in the CNS. In addition, mitochondrial toxicity due to NRTIs/NtRTIs may play a role in neuronal damage and death, as there is preliminary evidence that NRTIs may induce mitochondrial damage in neurons *in vitro* (Nolan and Mallal 2004). In conclusion, neurotoxicity as a result of prolonged exposure to NRTIs/NtRTIs should be monitored as a possible contributing factor to neurological deficits, especially since TDF and FTC are emerging as viable pre-exposure and post-exposure prophylaxis options.

5.3 Non-nucleoside reverse transcriptase inhibitors

5.3.1 Mechanism

Like NRTIs/NtRTIs, nNRTIs block the conversion of the viral RNA genome to a double-stranded DNA; however, the mechanism of action differs. nNRTIs bind to the allosteric, hydrophobic site of HIV RT, inhibiting its catalytic activity (de Bethune 2010). In addition, nNRTIs are not excised by pyrophosphates, which is a mechanism by which NRTI resistance can develop (de Bethune 2010). Thus, nNRTIs can circumvent certain NRTI-associated resistance mechanisms employed by the virus. However, it is now apparent that viral resistance to nNRTI still occurs, and has become a concern, especially in patients who are either ARV-experienced with previous exposure to nNRTIs or in those who are considered for nNRTI monotherapy. Further, there is an increased risk of cross-resistance development to NRTIs which can be triggered by the presence of nNRTI-associated mutations (de Bethune 2010). Thus, at least two NRTIs/NtRTIs need to be administered with nNRTIs, to achieve complete viral suppression and prevent resistance development.

5.3.2 Clinical use

Nevirapine (NVP), efavirenz (EFV) and etravirine (ETR) are the three nNRTIs currently approved for use. Efavirenz (EFV) is the nNRTI of choice in developed countries, whereas nevirapine (NVP) is included in initial cART regimens in resource limited countries. Additionally, NVP is used in the prevention of mother to child transfer, as EFV in pregnant patients is not recommended in the first trimester, due to the increased risk of neural tube defects associated with EFV (De Santis, Carducci et al. 2002). ETR is increasingly incorporated into cART regimens in recent years for treatment-experienced patients, as it maintains viral suppression in the presence of nNRTI-related resistance mutations, and has high tolerability with fewer side effects (de Bethune 2010).

5.3.3 Side effects

The side effects due to NVP include mild-to-moderate rash and hypersensitivity-induced hepatotoxicity, which can resolve spontaneously even when the therapy is continued (de

Bethune 2010). One major presentation of nNRTI related toxicity is neuropsychiatric disturbances. While NVP-induced CNS side effects, including impaired consciousness and psychotic episodes, have been rare, 40-70% patients on an EFV-containing cART regimen present with a range of CNS-related symptoms, such as insomnia, mood changes, and impaired attention span and concentration (Arendt, de Nocker et al. 2007).

5.3.4 Considerations for the CNS

While the exact mechanisms involved in EFV- and NVP-associated CNS side effects are not known, data from two recent studies have shown that chronic NVP or EFV administration in mice inhibited mitochondrial respiratory chain and creatine kinase activity *in vivo* (Streck, Scaini et al. 2008; Streck, Ferreira et al. 2011). As NVP and EFV show the highest CPE among all ARVs for which data is available (table 1), the changes in the energy metabolism these ARVs cause may affect particularly vulnerable cell populations in the brain, such as neurons with their high energy demands. Interestingly, a recent large scale study has shown that switching from an EFV containing cART to an ETR-based cART improved severe CNS side effects in ARV-experienced patients (Waters, Fisher et al. 2011). As will be mentioned in subsection 6.3, NVP and EFV are inducers of drug metabolism enzyme, CYP3A4, more so than ETR (Kakuda, Schöller-Gyüre et al. 2011), and may partially account for the partial alleviation in CNS-related side effects observed.

5.4 Protease inhibitors

5.4.1 Mechanism

HIV protease inhibitors (PIs) are peptidomimetics, and inhibit viral proteases that are needed for virus maturation and assembly. Ten protease inhibitors are currently in use: indinavir, ritonavir, saquinavir, lopinavir, atazanavir, nelfinavir, amprenavir, fosamprenavir, tipranavir and darunavir. PIs have been shown to control plasma viral replication and improve immunological parameters as effectively as nNRTIs; thus they form an essential component of cART regimens across most patient populations (Warnke, Barreto et al. 2007). Several factors are taken into consideration when choosing a specific PI to be included in a cART regimen: prior use of ARVs, adherence and cost-effectiveness, pre-existing conditions, and side effects are a few among these, and will be discussed below.

5.4.2 Clinical use

PIs are recommended for use with the NRTI/NtRTI backbone in initial cART regimens, just like nNRTIs (MacArthur, Novak et al. 2006). The decision between an nNRTI- and a PI-based cART regimen depends on several factors, such as cardiovascular risks (insulin resistance, dyslipidemia), liver disease (hepatitis B and C included), pregnancy, neuropsychiatric disease risk/history, potential drug-drug interactions, and emergence of resistant virus. When PIs are included in the cART regimen, ritonavir is added to increase plasma concentrations of the first PI, as it is a potent inhibitor of CYP3A4, a major drug metabolizing enzyme (Xu and Desai 2009); the aim is better viral control and decreased resistance development. In order to decrease the pill burden and increase adherence, new drug formulations that include two PIs are used increasingly in clinical practice. The most commonly used PI combination is lopinavir/ritonavir, which is recommended for use during pregnancy as well as in pediatric HIV cases. On the other hand, all combinations other than saquinavir/ritonavir can be used in hepatitis B-and C-infected patients (Stephan,

Carlebach et al. 2007). It should be noted that the virological failure due to lopinavir/ritonavir containing regimens are less associated with the emergence of PI-resistance (Prosperi, Zazzi et al. 2010), whereas nelfinavir has a lower barrier for PI-resistant virus emergence (Theys, Deforche et al. 2010). Lastly, regimens that include atazanavir/ritonavir and darunavir/ritonavir have less detrimental cardiovascular side effects compared with lopinavir/ritonavir-containing regimens (Hill, Sawyer et al. 2009). Thus, recently revised recommendations suggest atazanavir/ritonavir and darunavir/ritonavir as part of the initial cART regimen.

5.4.3 Side effects

Adverse effects associated with PIs are dyslipidemia, insulin resistance, and lipohypertrophy (Hui 2003). Numerous studies have shown that PIs alter lipid metabolism, and lead to dysregulation of blood lipid levels, which in itself increases risk of cardiovascular complications. Further, PIs induce oxidative and endoplasmic reticulum stress in macrophages, inducing these cells to release cytokines (CCL2, CCL3 (macrophage inflammatory protein-1α, MIP-1α), TNF-α and IL-1β) and ROS (Touzet and Philips 2010). These effects of PIs on macrophages are readily observed as increased risk for atherosclerosis and are more commonly associated with lopinavir/ritonavir-including regimens (Hill, Sawyer et al. 2009).

5.4.4 Considerations for the CNS

Most PIs, including ritonavir and saquinavir, are highly lipophilic and strongly bind to plasma proteins; thus, they are predicted to have low CSF concentrations (table 1). These predictions are backed by various *in vitro* and *in vivo* studies (Lledo-Garcia, Nacher et al. 2007; Best, Letendre et al. 2009). However, a study conducted in an *in situ* guinea pig model suggests that ritonavir can achieve choroid plexus and parenchymal concentrations that are comparable to plasma levels, mainly by diffusion through the blood-choroid plexus barrier; interestingly CSF levels remain lower than those measured in the choroid plexus and the parenchymal compartments (Anthonypillai, Sanderson et al. 2004). Further, altered drug transport across the BBB due to viral proteins and neuroinflammation, in addition to a leaky BBB and blood-CSF barrier during the course of infection, can affect the actual CNS concentrations of ARVs. In the presence of a dysfunctioning BBB, PIs may induce indirect neuronal damage/death by triggering an inflammatory or oxidative stress response in macrophages in the CNS. Interestingly, one study has reported CNS-related side effects of PIs in an animal model where mice received ritonavir at doses comparable to those in cART regimens (Huisman, Smit et al. 2003). In that study, 2 out of 7 mice that received ritonavir co-administered with an inhibitor of the drug efflux protein p-gp developed the CNS-specific symptoms, ataxia and tremor, before death one hour following treatment. Thus, long-term effects of PIs on CNS-specific toxicities warrant further investigation.

5.5 Integrase inhibitors

5.5.1 Mechanism

Integrase inhibitors are a recently developed class of ARVs, which block the integrase enzyme that facilitates viral DNA integration into the host DNA. Currently, raltegravir is the only clinically approved drug of its class, and there are 3 more integrase inhibitors currently in different phases of clinical trials.

5.5.2 Clinical use and side effects

The first clinical studies examining the efficacy and safety of raltegravir have shown that it facilitates viral suppression when added to the optimized regimens, even in patients with poor prognostic factors (Burger 2010). Further studies have shown that raltegravir efficacy was comparable to that of EFV when either drug is added to standard cART regimens (Powderly 2010; Steigbigel, Cooper et al. 2010). In addition, raltegravir is associated with few resistance mutations so far (Varghese, Liu et al. 2010), and its side effects are usually limited (Burger 2010). In fact, studies in rat hepatocytes *in vitro* and in mouse liver *in vivo* have suggested that the addition of raltegravir may inhibit PI-induced hepatotoxicity by blocking endoplasmic reticulum stress and lipid accumulation (Cao, Hu et al. 2010). Further, raltegravir does not appear to have an effect on drug metabolizing enzymes, which limits its possible drug-drug interactions. Thus, the FDA has now expanded its recommendations for raltegravir use in both ARV-naïve and ARV-experienced patients.

5.5.3 Considerations for the CNS

Raltegravir is a potential substrate of p-gp (Zembruski, Buchel et al. 2011), which would limit the entrance of this drug into the CNS. However, there are currently two clinical studies that have reported that raltegravir can achieve therapeutically relevant CSF concentrations (Yilmaz, Gisslen et al. 2009; Croteau, Letendre et al. 2010). Thus, raltegravir is given a CPE score of 0.5. While future studies are needed to determine its access to the CNS over the long-term, raltegravir appears to be a safe drug to use in the prevention and treatment of HAND, considering its minimal toxic effects in the periphery and its favorable CPE score, and that fewer viral resistance mutations hamper its efficacy. However, its long term effects on CNS specific cell populations are not known and caution should be exercised due to its high CPE score.

6. Determinants of CNS drug penetrance

The anatomical barriers between the CNS and the periphery are critical for protection of the brain from a multitude of factors; however, HIV appears to be able to circumvent these barriers. Early CNS seeding with HIV continues as a major obstacle in the efforts to eliminate the viral reservoirs throughout the body with the use of cART. In addition to the considerations regarding how long to delay the start of cART following infection, tailored cART regimens with better CNS penetrance, higher CSF ARV concentrations, and better parenchymal distribution are being increasingly sought after in an attempt to prevent and manage HAND. As the methodologies to determine the actual drug concentrations in the CSF and parenchyma of patients are not feasible, CPE algorithms are increasingly considered in determining which ARV drugs to include in a regimen to achieve therapeutically relevant CNS concentrations. Currently, the CPE score of a given ARV is based on the chemical structure, pharmacodynamics, pharmacokinetics, and available clinical correlative data (Letendre, Marquie-Beck et al. 2008; Marra, Zhao et al. 2009; Smurzynski, Wu et al. 2011). In this section, we will summarize the factors that determine the CPE score of ARVs in the presence of HAND.

In general, for an ARV to have a high CPE score, it needs to be small in size (molecular mass below 400-500 kDa), with high lipid solubility and low protein binding, and it should not be a substrate for drug efflux or transport proteins, namely p-gp and multidrug resistance protein-1 (MRP-1). The integrity of the BBB, which HIV infection can compromise, should also be considered in predicting CSF concentrations of ARVs. Also, due to the chronic nature of HIV infection, co-morbidities such as cancer, infections, and drug and alcohol abuse can also alter BBB integrity and should be considered as confounding factors in establishing effective and safe CPE algorithms.

6.1 Blood-brain barrier

The brain microvascular endothelial cells (BMVEC) within the brain parenchyma are the main constituents of the BBB. The BMVECs form an elaborate tight junction network, which, acts with the underlying basal lamina, pericytes, astrocyte foot processes, and microglia, to compose the BBB and to contribute to its function. A multitude of transporters and membrane proteins expressed by BMVECs regulate the cellular and molecular exchange between the CNS and the periphery, including the delivery of pharmaceuticals across the BBB into the brain parenchyma (Wolburg, Noell et al. 2009).

The accumulation of serum proteins in the CSF and brain parenchyma of HAND patients indicates that BBB dysfunction occurs in these individuals (Roberts, Buckner et al. 2010). Both *in vitro* and *in vivo* studies have shown that the viral proteins, gp120 and Tat, can impair BBB integrity by induction of oxidative stress in BMVECs (Louboutin, Agrawal et al. 2010). In addition, the disruption of tight junctions, loss of membrane glycoproteins, and apoptosis of BMVECs, as well as pericytic and perivascular astrocytic injury, have been reported following HIV infection (Persidsky, Stins et al. 1997). Given that predictions indicate that HIV-infected monocyte transmigration across the BBB will occur multiple times during the course of infection even with the successful control of peripheral VL (HIV RNA < 50 copies/ml), the continued assault on the BBB integrity in the presence of neuroinflammation is expected to exacerbate BBB dysfunction. Other factors that can increase the permeability of BBB are concomitant use of other pharmaceuticals for coexisting infections, substance and alcohol abuse, and co-infections.

The basal ganglia, hippocampus, and frontal cortex are the regions that show the most striking evidence of neuroinflammation and neuronal damage in the HIV-infected brain. This regional preference of HAND correlates with the proximity of these structures to the BBB, the dysfunction of which has multiple implications in HAND pathogenesis, clinical course, and response to treatment. First, the breakdown of this natural barrier is likely to increase the recruitment of HIV-infected monocytes from the periphery, hampering the efforts to limit neuroinflammation. Further, the risk for secondary infections increases with compromised BBB integrity. Further, altered functions of drug efflux and transport proteins are likely to affect ARV penetrance into the CNS, and consequently increase the possibility of ARV-associated toxicities in this compartment. Thus, in situations where exacerbated BBB compromise is likely, such as substance use, cART regimens with the least CNS-specific toxicities should be considered.

6.2 Drug transport across BBB

Complex drug efflux and transport mechanisms, which are controlled by a number of proteins that are expressed mainly on the BMVEC membrane, ultimately determine the effectiveness of any given ARV in gaining access to the CNS. P-gp and MRP-1 are the two major and well-characterized members of this regulatory mechanism. P-gp is a membrane bound, ATP-dependant drug efflux pump and regulates concentration-time profiles of its substrates, which range from amphipathic lipid-soluble compounds and metabolites to certain classes of ARVs, including most PIs and raltegravir (Urquhart and Kim 2009). PIs are both substrates and inhibitors of p-gp, while raltegravir appears to be a substrate but not an inhibitor of p-gp (Huisman, Smit et al. 2000). Ritonavir and saquinavir are the most extensively evaluated PIs in this regard. Findings from *in vitro* and *in vivo* studies show that p-gp limits the permeability of both ritonavir and saquinavir across the BBB. Interestingly, these drugs increase the expression of p-gp as well (Huisman, Smit et al. 2000). Ritonavir is added to most cART regimens in both ARV-naïve and ARV-experienced patients in order to exploit its ability to boost plasma concentrations of other ARVs (Xu and Desai 2009). However, the ability of ritonavir to increase the expression of p-gp can limit CNS access of concomitantly administered ARVs that are also p-gp substrates. Further, HIV infection can increase p-gp expression in T cells and monocytic cell lines and this capacity may extend to other cell-types, further contributing to the limited penetrance of ARVs to the CNS (Zhong, Hennig et al. 2010).

MRP-1 provides an additional level of regulation of drug concentrations in the CNS. This BBB-resident protein mainly transports neutral drugs conjugated to glutathione, sulfate, or glucuronate, in addition to negatively charged anionic drugs and organic anionic drugs (Dallas, Miller et al. 2006). Numerous *in vitro* and *in vivo* studies show that PIs, as well as a number of NRTIs and nNRTIs, can inhibit MRP-1 function. A recent study reports that two NRTIs included in the recommended cART regimens, TDF and FTC, as well as the two most commonly used nNRTIs, EFV and NVP, can inhibit MRP-1 in a concentration-dependent manner *in vitro* (Weiss, Theile et al. 2007). Further, while TDF concentration in the CSF is limited, as measured in patient samples (Anthonypillai, Gibbs et al. 2006), clinical data show that TDF or FTC-including regimens are associated with better neurological outcomes (Winston, Duncombe et al. 2010), suggesting that the effect of cART on MRP-1 can influence the outcomes of antiretroviral therapy in the CNS.

6.3 Pharmacokinetics

In the liver, where the majority of drug metabolism occurs via the Cytochrome P450 (CYP) family of enzymes, Cytochrome P450 3A4 (CYP3A4) is the major enzyme that metabolizes the vast majority of drugs, including ARVs (Lakhman, Ma et al. 2009). Conversely, some drugs, including ARVs can enhance or inhibit the activity of CYP3A4 and can precipitate decreased drug efficacy or increased drug concentrations and toxicity, respectively, when added to the existing treatment plan (Fichtenbaum and Gerber 2002). For example, several non-ARV drugs prescribed concurrently with ARVs for co-existing conditions, such as macrolide antibiotics, cholesterol-lowering drugs, and calcium channel blockers, are CYP3A4 inhibitors, as is ritonavir. The addition of one of the aforementioned non-ARV drugs to a cART regimen that already includes ritonavir necessitates the lowering of ARV doses. EFV and NVP, on the other hand are strong inducers of CYP3A4, further complicating treatment strategies (Mugundu, Hariparsad et al. 2010). Data from a guinea pig model of drug diffusion showed that NVP limited CSF distribution of ritonavir (Anthonypillai, Sanderson et al. 2004). This example further highlights the importance of drug-drug interactions in determining the CPE score of a cART regimen.

Intriguingly, CYP2B6, another member of the CYP family, is also induced by EFV and NVP (Ngaimisi, Mugusi et al. 2010). CYP2B6 is expressed in a number of extrahepatic tissues in addition to the liver, including the neurons and astrocytes of the different brain regions (Wang and Tompkins 2008). Thus, the predicted concentrations of drugs that are CYP2B6 substrates in the CNS can be compounded by the concurrent use of EFV or NVP. On the other hand, the activity of CYP2B6 varies widely among individuals due to the common occurrence of SNPs (Elens, Vandercam et al. 2010), as well as its transcriptional regulation (Wang and Tompkins 2008), and pharmacogenomic profiling may be necessary for successful dosing for regimens that include EFV and NVP.

In summary, the factors discussed in this section contribute to the CPE scoring and provide a starting point for clinicians for devising the most effective cART regimen to control HAND. However, dose adjustments and drug replacements have become a necessary part of the treatment plans while trying to find a balance between maximum efficiency and minimum side effects. At the present, the implications of these changes during the long course of HIV infection are not known; however, several clinical studies suggest that insufficient suppression of CSF VL, which can arise from fluctuations in the CSF ARV concentrations, is associated with treatment failure, i.e. emergence of resistant virus, worsening of neurological symptoms. Thus, utmost effort should be made to minimize such fluctuations in order to decrease the prevalence of HAND.

7. The impact of CPE scores on HAND

To date, six studies have investigated the effectiveness of CPE scoring in the prevention and management of HAND (Letendre, Marquie-Beck et al. 2008; Cysique, Vaida et al. 2009; Marra, Zhao et al. 2009; Garvey, Winston et al. 2011; Lanoy, Guiguet et al. 2011; Smurzynski, Wu et al. 2011). The most important conclusion these studies suggest is that the use of ARVs with high CPE scores is beneficial for suppressing CSF HIV RNA levels and for improving neurocognitive deficits. Further, this correlation between CPE scores and neurological improvements is independent of the success of the given regimen at suppressing peripheral VL. Interestingly, data suggest that ARV-naive patients show better improvement in neurocognitive deficits than ARV-experienced patients, likely due to the existence of drug-resistant virus harbored by the latter group.

While the majority of these studies have found a positive correlation between CPE scores and neurological outcomes, a study by Marra *et al.* reported that cART regimens with higher CPE scores were associated with worse neurocognitive performance (Marra, Zhao et al. 2009). The authors argued that this result was most likely due to the small size of the cohort and a possible bias towards prescription of more CPE penetrant regimens to patients with worse baseline neurocognitive impairment. However, cART regimens with higher CPE scores carry a risk of neurotoxicity in the already compromised brains of patients.

There are surprisingly few animal studies that investigated CNS-specific side effects of ARVs; however, findings suggest that NVP and EFV can induce cognitive deficits and anxiety when administered at doses that are reflective of doses used in humans over a short term (Streck, Scaini et al. 2008; Streck, Ferreira et al. 2011). The underlying mechanisms of NVP or EFV-induced CNS side effects are not known but given that these ARVs can achieve therapeutically relevant concentrations in the CNS, the long-term exposure to these ARVs may contribute to the persistence of HAND despite successful control of VL and further investigation is warranted.

Interestingly, one study has reported that ritonavir can induce acute signs of CNS-related toxicity, including ataxia and tremor in mice followed by death within an hour, when it is administered in the presence of a p-gp inhibitor (Huisman, Smit et al. 2003). These data suggests that acute exposure to high doses of ritonavir might be neurotoxic. In addition, mice that were administered lopinavir/ritonavir for 3 weeks at clinically relevant doses showed significant cognitive impairment, as determined by a multi-unit T-maze (Pistell, Gupta et al. 2010). Further, PIs cause increases in inflammatory markers via oxidative and endoplasmic reticulum stress response of macrophages (Touzet and Philips 2010). Thus, some of the CNS-related toxicities observed in animal models might be a result of activated macrophages by these ARVs. In the presence of a neuroinflammatory environment, the recruitment ARV-activated macrophages from the periphery in the presence of a compromised BBB can potentiate indirect neurotoxicity due to these ARVs. In addition, as mentioned in section 5.4, ritonavir concentrations in the brain parenchyma might be higher than predicted by the classical determinants of CPE (Anthonypillai, Sanderson et al. 2004), and direct neurotoxicity via oxidative stress can further precipitate neuronal damage and death.

In summary, in a setting where long-term administration of cART is inevitable to control infection and as a prophylactic measure, animal studies which better represent the inflammatory conditions observed in HIV-infected brain are needed to more successfully predict the CPE scores of ARVs and determine the most efficient combinations with minimal CNS related toxicities. Further, large-scale, longitudinal studies will be instrumental to tease out the contribution of ARV-related neurotoxicities to the persistence of HAND.

8. CNS-specific co-morbidities and cART effectiveness

Since its inception, cART has changed the landscape of HIV infection. However, it has also introduced unique challenges in the management of HIV. Due to longer life expectancy, co-morbidities such as substance abuse, chronic co-infections, and aging have become major contributors to HAND development and persistence. These co-morbidities need to be taken into consideration when cART regimens are determined on a patient-by-patient base.

8.1 Drugs of abuse

Perhaps the most important HIV associated co-morbidity is illicit drug use. For example, HIV-infected patients using methamphetamine (METH) show more neurocognitive deficits, compared to those not using METH (Nath 2010). These findings are not surprising, as illicit drugs, such as morphine and methamphetamine, alter the BBB permeability through direct damage to the BMVECs (Ramirez, Potula et al. 2009). In addition, these drugs exert neurotoxic effects in the CNS through oxidative stress and mitochondrial dysfunction (Yamamoto, Moszczynska et al. 2010). As mentioned in previous sections, BBB dysfunction and neurotoxicity are observed during the course of HIV infection as well as in response to ARV exposure and include similar mechanisms. Considering that the prevalence of HIV infection is 12-17% among illicit drug users (Cadet and Krasnova 2007), animal and clinical studies are essential to tailor cART regimens that reach sufficient CSF concentrations and yet do not augment neurotoxicity that might already be occuring in response to drug abuse.

8.2 Chronic alcohol use

A second co-morbidity that needs to be considered in the era of cART is chronic alcohol use. Chronic alcohol consumption has been established as a major confounding factor in the development of HAND (Durazzo, Rothlind et al. 2007; Miguez-Burbano, Lewis et al. 2008; Miguez-Burbano, Nair et al. 2009). Extensive studies have shown that chronic ethanol exposure causes neuronal damage and death (Brust 2010). Further, ethanol directly damages the BBB structure, and elicits a pro-inflammatory response in the parenchyma, as detected by increases in CCL2 and IL1-β, and increased ROS accumulation in the hippocampus(Shiu, Barbier et al. 2007; Qin, He et al. 2008). These effects are expected to be augmented in the presence of HIV infection. Further, ARV-induced neurotoxicity due to loss of BBB integrity in the setting of neuroinflammation is a possibility over the long term. Finally, chronic alcohol use will impair adherence to cART regimens. Thus, chronic alcohol use remains an important obstacle in the eradication of HAND.

8.3 Co-infections

The possible CNS-related effects of co-infections also need to be considered in HIV-infected population. Hepatitis B and C (HBV and HCV) were major co-morbidity and mortality factors in the pre-cART era. cART not only improved immunological functions, altering the detrimental effects of these viruses on the immune system, but also helped control the hepatitis virus replication to a certain extent. However, mortality due to liver disease remains the second most common following AIDS-related deaths. Recent data from Anti-HIV study group (D:A:D) revealed that, of all the deaths that are due to liver disease, 66% were a result of HCV, while 17% was due to HBV, and 3% was related to cART-related hepatotoxicity (Turner, Bansi et al. 2010). While these viruses do not target the cells of the CNS and there is no direct evidence of hepatitis as a contributing factor for the persistence of HAND; there is evidence that viral suppression and CD4 cell recovery is not as successful in the presence of HCV or HBV. These findings might partially explain the sporadic data suggesting that worse neurocognitive impairment is observed in HIV-HCV co-infected patients (Winston, Duncombe et al. 2010).

8.4 Aging

The contribution of cART to the increased life span of HIV-infected individuals cannot be overstated. However, longer life expectancy has brought new complications to the management of disease, one of which is the age-related metabolic and functional changes in the CNS. The neuroinflammation is still observed in the hippocampus of patients with suppressed CNS and peripheral VL, in addition to the accumulation of phosphorylated Tau, and intracellular and extracellular β-amyloid (Aβ) in the frontal cortex and the hippocampus(Brew, Pemberton et al. 2005; Green, Masliah et al. 2005; Anthony, Ramage et al. 2006; Achim, Adame et al. 2009). Interestingly, while increased accumulation of amyloid precursor protein (APP) was observed in the brains of HIV-infected individuals, the presence of phospho-Tau and Aβ were not demonstrated before the implementation of cART. Among the factors that may contribute to this shift are increased life span and prolonged neuroinflammation. It is established that risk of developing Alzheimer Disease (AD) increases with age. In addition, prolonged and/or uncontrolled neuroinflammation due to the emergence of new co-morbidities, adjustments in the cART regimens, and direct and indirect cART-related neurotoxicity can further exacerbate the neuropathological changes that classically occur in the aging brain.

Both HAND and AD brains show increases in markers of neuroinflammation, oxidative stress, and endoplasmic reticulum stress (Lindl, Akay et al. 2007). Interestingly, several *in vitro* and *in vivo* studies have shown that ARVs can lead to cellular toxicity via oxidative stress and endoplasmic reticulum stress (Zhou, Gurley et al. 2006; Gavilan, Pintado et al. 2009; Salminen, Kauppinen et al. 2009). Interestingly, these aforementioned stress pathways have been shown to increase Aβ secretion both *in vitro* and *in vivo* (Velliquette, O'Connor et al. 2005; O'Connor, Sadleir et al. 2008). Thus, age-related changes might be partially due to cART-related amyloidogenic processes, and the possible contributions of cART to these age-related changes need to be studied while establishing regimens with high CNS concentrations.

9. Adjunctive therapies

In addition to the utilization of the CPE scoring system, alternative delivery methods such as nanoparticle delivery are being explored. Further, adjunctive therapies are currently being studied for their efficiency in alleviating neuroinflammation, and decreasing neuronal damage and death. While the initial data obtained from these studies suggest limited success, the results are encouraging and constitute a newly expending field in the management of HAND.

9.1 Anti-excitotoxicity agents

The excitotoxins, such as glutamate and quinolinic acid that accumulate as a result of activated and/or infected macrophages and astrocytes cause direct neuronal dysfunction via activation of the NMDA receptor, as mentioned previously(O'Donnell, Agrawal et al. 2006; Lindl, Marks et al. 2010). Thus, memantine, an NMDA receptor antagonist that is approved for use in AD (Lipton and Chen 2004) is explored for its neuroprotective effects in HAND (Schifitto, Navia et al. 2007). Clinical trials so far report that memantine appears to be associated with few side effects, with favorable tolerance. Further, patients that received memantine showed improved neurocognitive functions. Given that memantine has shown benefits in patients with AD, it emerges as an attractive treatment option in a patient population that increasingly consists of aging patients.

9.2 Anti-oxidants

Oxidative stress, as mentioned before, is a major component of HIV-induced neuroinflammation. The increases in 4-HNE, protein carbonyls, long-chain sphingomyelins and ceramides are still observed in the presence of cART (Haughey, Cutler et al. 2004; Sacktor, Haughey et al. 2004). Use of illicit drugs and ethanol can induce oxidative stress, exacerbating the accumulation of oxidative products, and ARVs might contribute to this process. Thus, antioxidants were among the first to be tested as adjuncts to ARVs. Selegiline is one such antioxidant that was tested in several small clinical trials (Sacktor, Schifitto et al. 2000; Schifitto, Zhang et al. 2007). While initial studies conducted in patients receiving selegiline and NRTIs showed slight improvement in cognitive functions, a more comprehensive study that enrolled patients who received cART reported that neither the CSF and neuroimaging markers of oxidative stress nor cognitive and functional deficits improved with selegiline over a 24 week period (Schifitto, Yiannoutsos et al. 2009). One caveat of this study is its small number of patients, while a second caveat is the lack of stratification of patients according to the CPE scores. Thus, future studies that will take CPE scores of the cART regimens into account are necessary to better assess the efficacy of selegiline. This approach of utilizing antioxidants will be beneficial at multiple levels, such as virus-related direct and indirect neurotoxicity, ARV-related oxidative changes in the CNS, and alcohol and illicit drug-induced oxidative responses.

9.3 Anti-inflammatory agents

The neuroinflammation in the brains of HIV-infected patients are partially due to the activation of macrophages in response to HIV, or co-morbid conditions such as chronic alcohol and illicit drug use. In an attempt to resolve the persistent neuroinflammation, adjunctive agents to alleviate the inflammatory component of HAND are currently sought. One such agent is minocycline, a tetracycline antibiotic with both neuroprotective and anti-inflammatory effects. Its efficacy has been shown in models of traumatic and ischemic brain injury, and other neurodegenerative diseases such as AD and multiple sclerosis (Chen, Ona et al. 2000; Du, Ma et al. 2001; Van Den Bosch, Tilkin et al. 2002; Metz, Zhang et al. 2004). Further, it has been shown to be effective in limiting HIV replication *in vitro* and its close relative simian immunodeficiency virus (SIV) *in vivo* (Zink, Uhrlaub et al. 2005). Further, neuroinflammation markers in the CNS in the animal model of SIV encephalitis were decreased with minocycline administration. Currently, clinical trials are being conducted to assess its potential. In summary, its favorable safety profile, ease of administration and efficient BBB permeability makes it a viable adjunctive agent.

10. Conclusion

One of the paradoxical outcomes of cART is the persistence of HAND despite successful CNS viral control. Moreover, there seems to be a shift from overt dementia to more subtle presentations of neurocognitive impairment. Probable cART-related neuronal perturbations might contribute, and even precipitate, some of these changes in the chronic course of HAND, considering that cART regimens with higher CPE scores are prescribed in cases of higher or uncontrollable viral burden. However, the data regarding the impact of co-morbidities and possible cART-related side effects on CPE scores and the success of cART on HAND need to be expanded, given the ever-expending repertoire of ARVs and the patient-tailored, dynamic cART regimens in a multiple-system therapy management to ensure more successful outcomes of cART. The information gained from such studies will help physicians to determine the most efficient cART regimens with minimal CNS side effects, and further help design and determine adjunctive therapeuticals in the management of CNS perturbations in HIV-infected patients on long-term cART.

11. References

(1996). "Clinical confirmation of the American Academy of Neurology algorithm for HIV-1-associated cognitive/motor disorder. The Dana Consortium on Therapy for HIV Dementia and Related Cognitive Disorders." Neurology 47(5): 1247-1253.

Achim, C. L., A. Adame, et al. (2009). "Increased accumulation of intraneuronal amyloid beta in HIV-infected patients." J Neuroimmune Pharmacol 4(2): 190-199.

Achim, C. L., E. Masliah, et al. (1996). "Macrophage Activation Factors
in the Brains of AIDS Patients." J NeuroAIDS 1(2): 1-16.

Achim, C. L. and C. A. Wiley (1996). "Inflammation in AIDS and the role of the macrophage in brain pathology." Current Opinion in Neurology 9(3): 221-225.

Allavena, C., G. Le Moal, et al. (2006). "Neuropsychiatric adverse events after switching from an antiretroviral regimen containing efavirenz without tenofovir to an efavirenz regimen containing tenofovir: a report of nine cases." Antivir Ther 11(2): 263-265.

Anderson, P. L. and J. E. Rower (2010). "Zidovudine and Lamivudine for HIV Infection." Clin Med Rev Ther 2: a2004.

Anthony, I. C. and J. E. Bell (2008). "The Neuropathology of HIV/AIDS." Int Rev Psychiatry 20(1): 15-24.

Anthony, I. C., S. N. Ramage, et al. (2006). "Accelerated Tau deposition in the brains of individuals infected with human immunodeficiency virus-1 before and after the advent of highly active anti-retroviral therapy." Acta Neuropathol 111(6): 529-538.

Anthonypillai, C., J. Gibbs, et al. (2006). "The distribution of the anti-HIV drug, tenofovir (PMPA), into the brain, CSF and choroid plexuses." Cerebrospinal Fluid Research 3(1): 1.

Anthonypillai, C., R. N. Sanderson, et al. (2004). "The Distribution of the HIV Protease Inhibitor, Ritonavir, to the Brain, Cerebrospinal Fluid, and Choroid Plexuses of the Guinea Pig." Journal of Pharmacology and Experimental Therapeutics 308(3): 912-920.

Antinori, A., G. Arendt, et al. (2007). "Updated research nosology for HIV-associated neurocognitive disorders." Neurology 69(18): 1789-1799.

Arendt, G., D. de Nocker, et al. (2007). "Neuropsychiatric side effects of efavirenz therapy." Expert Opin Drug Saf 6(2): 147-154.

Bazzoli, C., V. Jullien, et al. (2010). "Intracellular Pharmacokinetics of Antiretroviral Drugs in HIV-Infected Patients, and their Correlation with Drug Action." Clinical Pharmacokinetics 49(1): 17-45 10.2165/11318110-000000000-000000000.

Best, B. M., S. L. Letendre, et al. (2009). "Low atazanavir concentrations in cerebrospinal fluid." Aids 23(1): 83-87.

Brew, B. J., L. Pemberton, et al. (2005). "CSF amyloid beta42 and tau levels correlate with AIDS dementia complex." Neurology 65(9): 1490-1492.

Brew, B. J., L. Pemberton, et al. (1997). "Levels of human immunodeficiency virus type 1 RNA in cerebrospinal fluid correlate with AIDS dementia stage." J Infect Dis 175(4): 963-966.

Brust, J. C. (2010). "Ethanol and cognition: indirect effects, neurotoxicity and neuroprotection: a review." Int J Environ Res Public Health 7(4): 1540-1557.

Burger, D. M. (2010). "Raltegravir: a review of its pharmacokinetics, pharmacology and clinical studies." Expert Opin Drug Metab Toxicol 6(9): 1151-1160.

Cadet, J. and I. Krasnova (2007). "Interactions of HIV and methamphetamine: Cellular and molecular mechanisms of toxicity potentiation." Neurotoxicity Research 12(3): 181-204.

Cao, R., Y. Hu, et al. (2010). "Prevention of HIV protease inhibitor-induced dysregulation of hepatic lipid metabolism by raltegravir via endoplasmic reticulum stress signaling pathways." J Pharmacol Exp Ther 334(2): 530-539.

Chen, M., V. O. Ona, et al. (2000). "Minocycline inhibits caspase-1 and caspase-3 expression and delays mortality in a transgenic mouse model of Huntington disease." Nat Med 6(7): 797-801.

Cole, M. A., J. B. Margolick, et al. (2007). "Longitudinally preserved psychomotor performance in long-term asymptomatic HIV-infected individuals." Neurology 69(24): 2213-2220.

Conant, K., A. Garzino-Demo, et al. (1998). "Induction of monocyte chemoattractant protein-1 in HIV-1 Tat-stimulated astrocytes and elevation in AIDS dementia." Proc Natl Acad Sci U S A 95(6): 3117-3121.

Croteau, D., S. Letendre, et al. (2010). "Total raltegravir concentrations in cerebrospinal fluid exceed the 50-percent inhibitory concentration for wild-type HIV-1." Antimicrob Agents Chemother 54(12): 5156-5160.

Cysique, L. A., F. Vaida, et al. (2009). "Dynamics of cognitive change in impaired HIV-positive patients initiating antiretroviral therapy." Neurology 73(5): 342-348.

Dagan, T., C. Sable, et al. (2002). "Mitochondrial dysfunction and antiretroviral nucleoside analog toxicities: what is the evidence?" Mitochondrion 1(5): 397-412.

Dalakas, M. C. (2001). "Peripheral neuropathy and antiretroviral drugs." J Peripher Nerv Syst 6(1): 14-20.

Dallas, S., D. S. Miller, et al. (2006). "Multidrug resistance-associated proteins: expression and function in the central nervous system." Pharmacol Rev 58(2): 140-161.

Danial, N. N. and S. J. Korsmeyer (2004). "Cell death: critical control points." Cell 116(2): 205-219.

de Bethune, M. P. (2010). "Non-nucleoside reverse transcriptase inhibitors (NNRTIs), their discovery, development, and use in the treatment of HIV-1 infection: a review of the last 20 years (1989-2009)." Antiviral Res 85(1): 75-90.

De Santis, M., B. Carducci, et al. (2002). "Periconceptional exposure to efavirenz and neural tube defects." Arch Intern Med 162(3): 355.

Du, Y., Z. Ma, et al. (2001). "Minocycline prevents nigrostriatal dopaminergic neurodegeneration in the MPTP model of Parkinson's disease." Proc Natl Acad Sci U S A 98(25): 14669-14674.

Duarte-Rojo, A. and E. J. Heathcote (2010). "Efficacy and safety of tenofovir disoproxil fumarate in patients with chronic hepatitis B." Therap Adv Gastroenterol 3(2): 107-119.

Durazzo, T. C., J. C. Rothlind, et al. (2007). "Chronic cigarette smoking and heavy drinking in human immunodeficiency virus: consequences for neurocognition and brain morphology." Alcohol 41(7): 489-501.

Edén, A., D. Fuchs, et al. (2010). "HIV-1 Viral Escape in Cerebrospinal Fluid of Subjects on Suppressive Antiretroviral Treatment." Journal of Infectious Diseases 202(12): 1819-1825.

Elens, L., B. Vandercam, et al. (2010). "Influence of host genetic factors on efavirenz plasma and intracellular pharmacokinetics in HIV-1-infected patients." Pharmacogenomics 11(9): 1223-1234.

Ellis, R. (2010). "HIV and antiretroviral therapy: impact on the central nervous system." Prog Neurobiol 91(2): 185-187.

Ellis, R. J., R. Deutsch, et al. (1997). "Neurocognitive impairment is an independent risk factor for death in HIV infection. San Diego HIV Neurobehavioral Research Center Group." Arch Neurol 54(4): 416-424.

Everall, I., F. Vaida, et al. (2009). "Cliniconeuropathologic correlates of human immunodeficiency virus in the era of antiretroviral therapy." J Neurovirol 15(5-6): 360-370.

Fichtenbaum, C. J. and J. G. Gerber (2002). "Interactions between antiretroviral drugs and drugs used for the therapy of the metabolic complications encountered during HIV infection." Clin Pharmacokinet 41(14): 1195-1211.

Garvey, L., A. Winston, et al. (2011). "Antiretroviral therapy CNS penetration and HIV-1-associated CNS disease." Neurology 76(8): 693-700.

Gavilan, M. P., C. Pintado, et al. (2009). "Dysfunction of the unfolded protein response increases neurodegeneration in aged rat hippocampus following proteasome inhibition." Aging Cell 8(6): 654-665.

Gendelman, H. E., S. A. Lipton, et al. (1994). "The neuropathogenesis of HIV-1 infection.[see comment]. [Review] [107 refs]."

Gisolf, E. H., R. M. van Praag, et al. (2000). "Increasing cerebrospinal fluid chemokine concentrations despite undetectable cerebrospinal fluid HIV RNA in HIV-1-infected patients receiving antiretroviral therapy." J Acquir Immune Defic Syndr 25(5): 426-433.

Gisolf, E. H., R. M. E. van Praag, et al. (2000). "Increasing Cerebrospinal Fluid Chemokine Concentrations Despite Undetectable Cerebrospinal Fluid HIV RNA in HIV-1-Infected Patients Receiving Antiretroviral Therapy." JAIDS Journal of Acquired Immune Deficiency Syndromes 25(5): 426-433.

Giulian, D., J. Yu, et al. (1996). "Study of receptor-mediated neurotoxins released by HIV-1-infected mononuclear phagocytes found in human brain." J Neurosci 16(10): 3139-3153.

Gonzalez-Scarano, F. and J. Martin-Garcia (2005). "The neuropathogenesis of AIDS." Nat Rev Immunol 5(1): 69-81.

Gonzalez-Scarano, F. and J. Martin-Garcia (2005). "The neuropathogenesis of AIDS. [Review] [173 refs]."

Gorry, P. R., C. Ong, et al. (2003). "Astrocyte infection by HIV-1: mechanisms of restricted virus replication, and role in the pathogenesis of HIV-1-associated dementia." Curr HIV Res 1(4): 463-473.

Grant, R. M. (2010). "Antiretroviral agents used by HIV-uninfected persons for prevention: pre- and postexposure prophylaxis." Clin Infect Dis 50 Suppl 3: S96-101.

Green, D. A., E. Masliah, et al. (2005). "Brain deposition of beta-amyloid is a common pathologic feature in HIV positive patients." Aids 19(4): 407-411.

Hagberg, L., P. Cinque, et al. (2010). "Cerebrospinal fluid neopterin: an informative biomarker of central nervous system immune activation in HIV-1 infection." AIDS Research and Therapy 7(1): 15.

Haughey, N. J., R. G. Cutler, et al. (2004). "Perturbation of sphingolipid metabolism and ceramide production in HIV-dementia." Ann Neurol 55(2): 257-267.

Heaton, R. K., D. B. Clifford, et al. "HIV-associated neurocognitive disorders persist in the era of potent antiretroviral therapy: CHARTER Study." Neurology 75(23): 2087-2096.

Heaton, R. K., D. B. Clifford, et al. (2010). "HIV-associated neurocognitive disorders persist in the era of potent antiretroviral therapy: CHARTER Study." Neurology 75(23): 2087-2096.

Hill, A. and W. Sawyer (2009). "Effects of nucleoside reverse transcriptase inhibitor backbone on the efficacy of first-line boosted highly active antiretroviral therapy based on protease inhibitors: meta-regression analysis of 12 clinical trials in 5168 patients." HIV Med 10(9): 527-535.

Hill, A., W. Sawyer, et al. (2009). "Effects of first-line use of nucleoside analogues, efavirenz, and ritonavir-boosted protease inhibitors on lipid levels." HIV Clin Trials 10(1): 1-12.

Hu, S., W. S. Sheng, et al. (2009). "Preferential sensitivity of human dopaminergic neurons to gp120-induced oxidative damage." J Neurovirol 15(5-6): 401-410.

Hui, D. Y. (2003). "Effects of HIV protease inhibitor therapy on lipid metabolism." Progress in Lipid Research 42(2): 81-92.

Huisman, M. T., J. W. Smit, et al. (2000). "Significance of P-glycoprotein for the pharmacology and clinical use of HIV protease inhibitors." Aids 14(3): 237-242.

Huisman, M. T., J. W. Smit, et al. (2003). "Assessing safety and efficacy of directed P-glycoprotein inhibition to improve the pharmacokinetic properties of saquinavir coadministered with ritonavir." J Pharmacol Exp Ther 304(2): 596-602.

Joly, V., K. Jidar, et al. (2010). "Enfuvirtide: from basic investigations to current clinical use." Expert Opin Pharmacother 11(16): 2701-2713.

Kakuda, T. N., M. Schöller-Gyüre, et al. (2011). "Pharmacokinetic Interactions between Etravirine and Non-Antiretroviral Drugs." Clinical Pharmacokinetics 50(1): 25-39 10.2165/11534740-000000000-000000000.

Kaul, M., J. Zheng, et al. (2005). "HIV-1 infection and AIDS: consequences for the central nervous system. [Review] [199 refs]."

Kohler, J. J. and W. Lewis (2007). "A brief overview of mechanisms of mitochondrial toxicity from NRTIs." Environmental and Molecular Mutagenesis 48(3-4): 166-172.

Kolson, D. L. (2002). "Neuropathogenesis of central nervous system HIV-1 infection." Clin Lab Med 22(3): 703-717.

Kromdijk, W., A. D. Huitema, et al. (2010). "Treatment of HIV infection with the CCR5 antagonist maraviroc." Expert Opin Pharmacother 11(7): 1215-1223.

Kusdra, L., D. McGuire, et al. (2002). "Changes in monocyte/macrophage neurotoxicity in the era of HAART: implications for HIV-associated dementia." Aids 16(1): 31-38.

Lakhman, S. S., Q. Ma, et al. (2009). "Pharmacogenomics of CYP3A: considerations for HIV treatment." Pharmacogenomics 10(8): 1323-1339.

Lanoy, E., M. Guiguet, et al. (2011). "Survival after neuroAIDS." Neurology 76(7): 644-651.

Letendre, S., J. Marquie-Beck, et al. (2008). "Validation of the CNS Penetration-Effectiveness rank for quantifying antiretroviral penetration into the central nervous system." Arch Neurol 65(1): 65-70.

Letendre, S. L., R. J. Ellis, et al. (2010). "Neurologic complications of HIV disease and their treatment." Top HIV Med 18(2): 45-55.

Lieberman-Blum, S. S., H. B. Fung, et al. (2008). "Maraviroc: a CCR5-receptor antagonist for the treatment of HIV-1 infection." Clin Ther 30(7): 1228-1250.

Lindl, K. A., C. Akay, et al. (2007). "Expression of the endoplasmic reticulum stress response marker, BiP, in the central nervous system of HIV-positive individuals." Neuropathol Appl Neurobiol 33(6): 658-669.

Lindl, K. A., D. R. Marks, et al. (2010). "HIV-associated neurocognitive disorder: pathogenesis and therapeutic opportunities." J Neuroimmune Pharmacol 5(3): 294-309.

Lipton, S. A. and H. S. Chen (2004). "Paradigm shift in neuroprotective drug development: clinically tolerated NMDA receptor inhibition by memantine." Cell Death Differ 11(1): 18-20.

Liu, N. Q., A. S. Lossinsky, et al. (2002). "Human immunodeficiency virus type 1 enters brain microvascular endothelia by macropinocytosis dependent on lipid rafts and the mitogen-activated protein kinase signaling pathway." J Virol 76(13): 6689-6700.

Lledo-Garcia, R., A. Nacher, et al. (2007). "Bioavailability and pharmacokinetic model for ritonavir in the rat." J Pharm Sci 96(3): 633-643.

Louboutin, J. P., L. Agrawal, et al. (2010). "HIV-1 gp120-induced injury to the blood-brain barrier: role of metalloproteinases 2 and 9 and relationship to oxidative stress." J Neuropathol Exp Neurol 69(8): 801-816.

MacArthur, R. D., R. M. Novak, et al. (2006). "A comparison of three highly active antiretroviral treatment strategies consisting of non-nucleoside reverse transcriptase inhibitors, protease inhibitors, or both in the presence of nucleoside reverse transcriptase inhibitors as initial therapy (CPCRA 058 FIRST Study): a long-term randomised trial." Lancet 368(9553): 2125-2135.

Marra, C. M., Y. Zhao, et al. (2009). "Impact of combination antiretroviral therapy on cerebrospinal fluid HIV RNA and neurocognitive performance." Aids 23(11): 1359-1366.

Masliah, E., R. K. Heaton, et al. (1997). "Dendritic injury is a pathological substrate for human immunodeficiency virus-related cognitive disorders. HNRC Group. The HIV Neurobehavioral Research Center." Ann Neurol 42(6): 963-972.

McArthur, J. C. (2004). "HIV dementia: an evolving disease." J Neuroimmunol 157(1-2): 3-10.

McArthur, J. C., M. P. McDermott, et al. (2004). "Attenuated Central Nervous System Infection in Advanced HIV/AIDS With Combination Antiretroviral Therapy." Arch Neurol 61(11): 1687-1696.

Metz, L. M., Y. Zhang, et al. (2004). "Minocycline reduces gadolinium-enhancing magnetic resonance imaging lesions in multiple sclerosis." Ann Neurol 55(5): 756.

Miguez-Burbano, M. J., J. E. Lewis, et al. (2008). "Cognitive performance and the thymus among HIV-infected subjects receiving HAART." Biologics 2(2): 321-327.

Miguez-Burbano, M. J., M. Nair, et al. (2009). "The role of alcohol on platelets, thymus and cognitive performance among HIV-infected subjects: are they related?" Platelets 20(4): 260-267.

Moore, J. D., N. J. Rothwell, et al. (2002). "Involvement of caspases and calpains in cerebrocortical neuronal cell death is stimulus-dependent." Br J Pharmacol 135(4): 1069-1077.

Mugundu, G. M., N. Hariparsad, et al. (2010). "Impact of ritonavir, atazanavir and their combination on the CYP3A4 induction potential of efavirenz in primary human hepatocytes." Drug Metab Lett 4(1): 45-50.

Nath, A. (2010). "Human immunodeficiency virus-associated neurocognitive disorder: pathophysiology in relation to drug addiction." Ann N Y Acad Sci 1187: 122-128.

Navia, B. A., E. S. Cho, et al. (1986). "The AIDS dementia complex: II. Neuropathology." Annals of Neurology 19(6): 525-535.

Nelson, M. and M. Schiavone (2004). "Emtricitabine (FTC) for the treatment of HIV infection." Int J Clin Pract 58(5): 504-510.

Neuenburg, J. K., H. R. Brodt, et al. (2002). "HIV-related neuropathology, 1985 to 1999: rising prevalence of HIV encephalopathy in the era of highly active antiretroviral therapy." J Acquir Immune Defic Syndr 31(2): 171-177.

Ngaimisi, E., S. Mugusi, et al. (2010). "Long-term efavirenz autoinduction and its effect on plasma exposure in HIV patients." Clin Pharmacol Ther 88(5): 676-684.

Nolan, D. and S. Mallal (2004). "Complications associated with NRTI therapy: update on clinical features and possible pathogenic mechanisms." Antivir Ther 9(6): 849-863.

O'Connor, T., K. R. Sadleir, et al. (2008). "Phosphorylation of the translation initiation factor eIF2alpha increases BACE1 levels and promotes amyloidogenesis." Neuron 60(6): 988-1009.

O'Donnell, L. A., A. Agrawal, et al. (2006). "Human immunodeficiency virus (HIV)-induced neurotoxicity: roles for the NMDA receptor subtypes." J Neurosci 26(3): 981-990.

O'Donnell, L. A., A. Agrawal, et al. (2006). "Human immunodeficiency virus (HIV)-induced neurotoxicity: roles for the NMDA receptor subtypes." Journal Of Neuroscience.

Owe-Larsson, B., L. Sall, et al. (2009). "HIV infection and psychiatric illness." Afr J Psychiatry (Johannesbg) 12(2): 115-128.

Patel, I. H., X. Zhang, et al. (2005). "Pharmacokinetics, pharmacodynamics and drug interaction potential of enfuvirtide." Clin Pharmacokinet 44(2): 175-186.

Persidsky, Y., M. Stins, et al. (1997). "A model for monocyte migration through the blood-brain barrier during HIV-1 encephalitis." J Immunol 158(7): 3499-3510.

Pialoux, G., S. Fournier, et al. (1997). "Central nervous system as a sanctuary for HIV-1 infection despite treatment with zidovudine, lamivudine and indinavir." Aids 11(10): 1302-1303.

Piliero, P. J. (2004). "Pharmacokinetic properties of nucleoside/nucleotide reverse transcriptase inhibitors." J Acquir Immune Defic Syndr 37 Suppl 1: S2-S12.

Pistell, P. J., S. Gupta, et al. (2010). "Metabolic and neurologic consequences of chronic lopinavir/ritonavir administration to C57BL/6 mice." Antiviral Res 88(3): 334-342.

Portegies, P., R. H. Enting, et al. (1993). "Presentation and course of AIDS dementia complex: 10 years of follow-up in Amsterdam, The Netherlands." AIDS 7(5): 669-675.

Powderly, W. G. (2010). "Integrase inhibitors in the treatment of HIV-1 infection." Journal of Antimicrobial Chemotherapy 65(12): 2485-2488.

Power, C., L. Boisse, et al. (2009). "NeuroAIDS: an evolving epidemic." Can J Neurol Sci 36(3): 285-295.

Price, R. W., B. Brew, et al. (1988). "The brain in AIDS: central nervous system HIV-1 infection and AIDS dementia complex." Science 239: 586-592.

Price, R. W., R. Parham, et al. (2008). "Enfuvirtide cerebrospinal fluid (CSF) pharmacokinetics and potential use in defining CSF HIV-1 origin." Antivir Ther 13(3): 369-374.

Prosperi, M. C., M. Zazzi, et al. (2010). "Low rate of virological failure and maintenance of susceptibility to HIV-1 protease inhibitors with first-line lopinavir/ritonavir-based antiretroviral treatment in clinical practice." J Med Virol 82(12): 1996-2003.

Qin, L., J. He, et al. (2008). "Increased systemic and brain cytokine production and neuroinflammation by endotoxin following ethanol treatment." J Neuroinflammation 5: 10.

Ragin, A. B., Y. Wu, et al. (2010). "Biomarkers of neurological status in HIV infection: a 3-year study." Proteomics Clin Appl 4(3): 295-303.

Ramirez, S. H., R. Potula, et al. (2009). "Methamphetamine disrupts blood-brain barrier function by induction of oxidative stress in brain endothelial cells." J Cereb Blood Flow Metab 29(12): 1933-1945.
Reynolds, A., C. Laurie, et al. (2007). "Oxidative stress and the pathogenesis of neurodegenerative disorders." Int Rev Neurobiol 82: 297-325.
Roberts, T. K., C. M. Buckner, et al. (2010). "Leukocyte transmigration across the blood-brain barrier: perspectives on neuroAIDS." Front Biosci 15: 478-536.
Roc, A. C., B. M. Ances, et al. (2007). Detection of Human Immunodeficiency Virus Induced Inflammation and Oxidative Stress in Lenticular Nuclei With Magnetic Resonance Spectroscopy Despite Antiretroviral Therapy. 64: 1249-1257.
Sacktor, N., N. Haughey, et al. (2004). "Novel markers of oxidative stress in actively progressive HIV dementia." J Neuroimmunol 157(1-2): 176-184.
Sacktor, N., G. Schifitto, et al. (2000). "Transdermal selegiline in HIV-associated cognitive impairment: pilot, placebo-controlled study." Neurology 54(1): 233-235.
Salminen, A., A. Kauppinen, et al. (2009). "ER stress in Alzheimer's disease: a novel neuronal trigger for inflammation and Alzheimer's pathology." J Neuroinflammation 6: 41.
Schifitto, G., B. A. Navia, et al. (2007). "Memantine and HIV-associated cognitive impairment: a neuropsychological and proton magnetic resonance spectroscopy study." Aids 21(14): 1877-1886.
Schifitto, G., C. T. Yiannoutsos, et al. (2009). "Selegiline and oxidative stress in HIV-associated cognitive impairment." Neurology 73(23): 1975-1981.
Schifitto, G., J. Zhang, et al. (2007). "A multicenter trial of selegiline transdermal system for HIV-associated cognitive impairment." Neurology 69(13): 1314-1321.
Sevigny, J. J., S. M. Albert, et al. (2004). "Evaluation of HIV RNA and markers of immune activation as predictors of HIV-associated dementia." Neurology 63(11): 2084-2090.
Shiu, C., E. Barbier, et al. (2007). "HIV-1 gp120 as well as alcohol affect blood-brain barrier permeability and stress fiber formation: involvement of reactive oxygen species." Alcohol Clin Exp Res 31(1): 130-137.
Sippy, B. D., F. M. Hofman, et al. (1995). "Increased expression of tumor necrosis factor-alpha receptors in the brains of patients with AIDS." J Acquir Immune Defic Syndr Hum Retrovirol 10(5): 511-521.
Smurzynski, M., K. Wu, et al. (2011). "Effects of central nervous system antiretroviral penetration on cognitive functioning in the ALLRT cohort." Aids 25(3): 357-365 310.1097/QAD.1090b1013e32834171f32834178.
Smurzynski, M., K. Wu, et al. (2011). "Effects of central nervous system antiretroviral penetration on cognitive functioning in the ALLRT cohort." Aids 25(3): 357-365.
Soontornniyomkij, V., J. A. Nieto-Rodriguez, et al. (1998). "Brain HIV burden and length of survival after AIDS diagnosis." Clin Neuropathol 17(2): 95-99.
Steigbigel, R. T., D. A. Cooper, et al. (2010). "Long-term efficacy and safety of Raltegravir combined with optimized background therapy in treatment-experienced patients with drug-resistant HIV infection: week 96 results of the BENCHMRK 1 and 2 Phase III trials." Clin Infect Dis 50(4): 605-612.
Stephan, C., A. Carlebach, et al. (2007). "Dose reduction effective in alleviating symptoms of saquinavir toxicity." Int J STD AIDS 18(2): 81-84.

Streck, E. L., G. K. Ferreira, et al. (2011). "Non-Nucleoside Reverse Transcriptase Inhibitors Efavirenz and Nevirapine Inhibit Cytochrome C Oxidase in Mouse Brain Regions." Neurochem Res.

Streck, E. L., G. Scaini, et al. (2008). "Effects of the HIV treatment drugs nevirapine and efavirenz on brain creatine kinase activity." Metab Brain Dis 23(4): 485-492.

Sturt, A. S., E. K. Dokubo, et al. (2010). "Antiretroviral therapy (ART) for treating HIV infection in ART-eligible pregnant women." Cochrane Database Syst Rev(3): CD008440.

Theys, K., K. Deforche, et al. (2010). "Estimating the individualized HIV-1 genetic barrier to resistance using a nelfinavir fitness landscape." BMC Bioinformatics 11: 409.

Touzet, O. and A. Philips (2010). "Resveratrol protects against protease inhibitor-induced reactive oxygen species production, reticulum stress and lipid raft perturbation." Aids 24(10): 1437-1447.

Tozzi, V., P. Balestra, et al. (2007). "Persistence of neuropsychologic deficits despite long-term highly active antiretroviral therapy in patients with HIV-related neurocognitive impairment: prevalence and risk factors." J Acquir Immune Defic Syndr 45(2): 174-182.

Tozzi, V., P. Balestra, et al. (2009). "Changes in Cognition During Antiretroviral Therapy: Comparison of 2 Different Ranking Systems to Measure Antiretroviral Drug Efficacy on HIV-Associated Neurocognitive Disorders." JAIDS Journal of Acquired Immune Deficiency Syndromes 52(1): 56-63 10.1097/QAI.1090b1013e3181af1083d1096.

Turner, J., L. Bansi, et al. (2010). "The prevalence of hepatitis C virus (HCV) infection in HIV-positive individuals in the UK - trends in HCV testing and the impact of HCV on HIV treatment outcomes." J Viral Hepat 17(8): 569-577.

Urquhart, B. L. and R. B. Kim (2009). "Blood-brain barrier transporters and response to CNS-active drugs." Eur J Clin Pharmacol 65(11): 1063-1070.

Van Den Bosch, L., P. Tilkin, et al. (2002). "Minocycline delays disease onset and mortality in a transgenic model of ALS." Neuroreport 13(8): 1067-1070.

Varghese, V., T. F. Liu, et al. (2010). "HIV-1 integrase sequence variability in antiretroviral naive patients and in triple-class experienced patients subsequently treated with raltegravir." AIDS Res Hum Retroviruses 26(12): 1323-1326.

Velliquette, R. A., T. O'Connor, et al. (2005). "Energy inhibition elevates beta-secretase levels and activity and is potentially amyloidogenic in APP transgenic mice: possible early events in Alzheimer's disease pathogenesis." J Neurosci 25(47): 10874-10883.

Walker, D. K., S. J. Bowers, et al. (2008). "Preclinical assessment of the distribution of maraviroc to potential human immunodeficiency virus (HIV) sanctuary sites in the central nervous system (CNS) and gut-associated lymphoid tissue (GALT)." Xenobiotica 38(10): 1330-1339.

Wang, H. and L. M. Tompkins (2008). "CYP2B6: new insights into a historically overlooked cytochrome P450 isozyme." Curr Drug Metab 9(7): 598-610.

Warnke, D., J. Barreto, et al. (2007). "Antiretroviral drugs." J Clin Pharmacol 47(12): 1570-1579.

Waters, L., M. Fisher, et al. (2011). "A phase IV, double-blind, multicentre, randomized, placebo-controlled, pilot study to assess the feasibility of switching individuals

receiving efavirenz with continuing central nervous system adverse events to etravirine." Aids 25(1): 65-71.
Weiss, J., D. Theile, et al. (2007). "Inhibition of MRP1/ABCC1, MRP2/ABCC2, and MRP3/ABCC3 by nucleoside, nucleotide, and non-nucleoside reverse transcriptase inhibitors." Drug Metab Dispos 35(3): 340-344.
William, L. (2003). "Mitochondrial DNA replication, nucleoside reverse-transcriptase inhibitors, and AIDS cardiomyopathy." Progress in cardiovascular diseases 45(4): 305-318.
Winston, A., C. Duncombe, et al. (2010). "Does choice of combination antiretroviral therapy (cART) alter changes in cerebral function testing after 48 weeks in treatment-naive, HIV-1-infected individuals commencing cART? A randomized, controlled study." Clin Infect Dis 50(6): 920-929.
Winston, A., C. Duncombe, et al. (2010). "Does Choice of Combination Antiretroviral Therapy (cART) Alter Changes in Cerebral Function Testing after 48 Weeks in Treatment-Naive, HIV-1–Infected Individuals Commencing cART? A Randomized, Controlled Study." Clinical Infectious Diseases 50(6): 920-929.
Wolburg, H., S. Noell, et al. (2009). "Brain endothelial cells and the glio-vascular complex." Cell Tissue Res 335(1): 75-96.
Woods, S., D. Moore, et al. (2009). "Cognitive Neuropsychology of HIV-Associated Neurocognitive Disorders." Neuropsychology Review 19(2): 152-168.
Xu, L. and M. C. Desai (2009). "Pharmacokinetic enhancers for HIV drugs." Curr Opin Investig Drugs 10(8): 775-786.
Yamamoto, B. K., A. Moszczynska, et al. (2010). "Amphetamine toxicities: classical and emerging mechanisms." Ann N Y Acad Sci 1187: 101-121.
Yeni, P., A. Mills, et al. (2010). "Etravirine in the treatment of HIV-1: a clinical overview for healthcare professionals." Curr HIV Res 8(7): 564-576.
Yilmaz, A., D. Fuchs, et al. (2006). "Cerebrospinal fluid HIV-1 RNA, intrathecal immunoactivation, and drug concentrations after treatment with a combination of saquinavir, nelfinavir, and two nucleoside analogues: the M61022 study." BMC Infectious Diseases 6(1): 63.
Yilmaz, A., M. Gisslen, et al. (2009). "Raltegravir cerebrospinal fluid concentrations in HIV-1 infection." PLoS One 4(9): e6877.
Yilmaz, A., R. W. Price, et al. (2008). "Persistent intrathecal immune activation in HIV-1-infected individuals on antiretroviral therapy." J Acquir Immune Defic Syndr 47(2): 168-173.
Zembruski, N. C., G. Buchel, et al. (2011). "Potential of novel antiretrovirals to modulate expression and function of drug transporters in vitro." J Antimicrob Chemother 66(4): 802-812.
Zhong, Y., B. Hennig, et al. (2010). "Intact lipid rafts regulate HIV-1 Tat protein-induced activation of the Rho signaling and upregulation of P-glycoprotein in brain endothelial cells." J Cereb Blood Flow Metab 30(3): 522-533.
Zhou, H., E. C. Gurley, et al. (2006). "HIV protease inhibitors activate the unfolded protein response and disrupt lipid metabolism in primary hepatocytes." Am J Physiol Gastrointest Liver Physiol 291(6): G1071-1080.
Zink, M. C., J. Uhrlaub, et al. (2005). "Neuroprotective and anti-human immunodeficiency virus activity of minocycline." JAMA 293(16): 2003-2011.

Part 6

Special Clinical Cares

16

Special Considerations in the Management of HIV Infection in Pregnancy

Chi Dola, Sean Kim and Juliet Tran
Department of Obstetrics and Gynecology, Tulane University School of Medicine
New Orleans, Louisiana
USA

1. Introduction

In the industrialized world, significant development and interventions were made since the HIV epidemic and they contributed to improved maternal health and low perinatal transmission rates. However, not all questions about this infection in pregnancy were answered. At times, obstetric health care providers for HIV-infected pregnant women were faced with certain clinical situations where there was limited available data to help direct treatment planning. This chapter will discuss recent data on various special considerations encountered in the management of HIV infection in pregnancy.

2. Apparent lack of prenatal care and the lack of knowledge of available treatment to decrease perinatal transmission among HIV-infected women

Vertical transmission of HIV infection was significantly reduced by offering HIV testing to pregnant women and implementing the Pediatrics AIDS Clinical Trials Group (PACTG) protocol 076 (Connor et al., 1994). The success of this protocol was dependent on women seeking prenatal care, where they were offered HIV screening and appropriate treatment for affected pregnancies and their newborns. However, HIV-infected women often do not obtain prenatal care. As a whole, 5–10% of women in the United States receive inadequate or no prenatal care (Kogan et al., 1998). HIV-infected women are even less likely to seek prenatal care. According to a study by Minkoff et al., 50% of HIV-infected women who gave birth at a municipal hospital in New York City did not have prenatal care (Minkoff et al., 1990). In a survey of HIV-infected women in Philadelphia, only a third of these pregnant women reported adequate prenatal care and 20% had no prenatal care (Turner et al., 1996).

Additionally, these women often failed to disclose their HIV infectious status when they presented for labor and delivery. Fifty percent of the women with inadequate prenatal care were actually aware of their HIV infection but did not choose to disclose to their caretaker when they presented for delivery at the Medical Center of LA in New Orleans (Centers for Disease Control and Prevention [CDC], 2004). This troubling data implies that many HIV-infected women unknowingly, as a consequence of a lack of knowledge, infect their unborn children despite the availability of treatments to reduce vertical transmission (Dola et al., 2010). These findings stress the importance of educating the public on the currently available interventions to reduce vertical transmission of HIV infection.

One of the barriers to decreasing perinatal transmission is that HIV-infected women do not obtain early prenatal care and thus exclude themselves from available interventions. Heath care providers must understand why HIV infected women are less likely to utilize prenatal services. Lancioni et al. reported that issues normally encountered in women without prenatal care - such as transportation, lack of child care, lack of insurance, and scheduling of appointments - were not found to be the reason why HIV infected women do not seek prenatal care. Rather, these women opted out of prenatal services because they feared the risk of disclosure and the anticipated anger from health care providers because they chose to continue their pregnancy (Lancioni et al., 1999). Eliminating the social stigma about HIV infection and educating health care providers about these women's fears and concerns could help reduce the barriers in seeking prenatal care (Dola et al., 2010).

3. Limitations of benefits of rapid HIV testing in labor and delivery

In the United States, approximately 144 - 226 infants are infected annually with HIV (CDC, 2007). Many of these infants were born of mothers who were not tested early in pregnancy or did not receive the appropriate prophylaxis treatment (CDC, 2007). Approximately a quarter of all people currently infected with HIV are not aware of their infectious status (Marks et al, 2006). Therefore, HIV screening during prenatal care is a necessity for the success of PACTG protocol 076. In addition, there is a high rate of HIV infection amongst women without prenatal care (Lindsay et al., 1991). Thus, those who most need it are excluded from the benefits of the PACTG protocol 076 and other obstetrical interventions to decrease perinatal transmission.

Rapid HIV testing is now available to allow undiagnosed HIV-infected women one last vital opportunity to be tested for the infection and to decrease the risk of transmitting the disease to their newborns. By virtue of the fast availability of the rapid HIV test result, it is hoped that interventions can be instituted to decrease perinatal transmission. If a woman tested reactive on the rapid HIV test, she will be counseled appropriately and if agreed, she will be administered zidovudine prophylaxis during labor along with obstetrical interventions, and her neonate will receive prophylactic zidovudine after birth. This abbreviated regimen of zidovudine has been shown to be cost-effective (Stringer et al., 1999) and can decrease vertical transmission (Wade et al., 1998). Studies by Wade et al. show a reduction of vertical HIV transmission to 10% when zidovudine prophylaxis begins intrapartum compared to 27% in those without any treatment (Wade et al., 1998).

Rapid HIV testing is an excellent concept to allow undiagnosed HIV-infected women one last chance to decrease the risk of infecting their newborn, however, the benefits of rapid HIV tests may not be fully appreciated due to a large percentage of these women presenting in advanced labor, after rupture of membranes, or when they deliver shortly after arrival to the labor unit. Dola et al. retrospectively analyzed 350 parturients without prior prenatal care at their institution who presented to the labor unit with unknown HIV serostatus (Dola et al., 2010). These women often presented in active labor with cervical dilation of $\geq$ 5 cm (48.6%); another 15.2% presented at complete cervical dilation of 10 centimeters, and 43% presented after ruptured membranes. The benefit of early detection of HIV infection via rapid testing may be less obvious in these women as perinatal transmission might already have occurred. Another 5.5% of these women even missed the benefits of rapid HIV testing by delivering their baby prior to their arrival to the hospital. It could be postulated that no benefit can be gained from a rapid HIV test result to direct effective management of these patients during their labor and delivery (Dola et al., 2010). However, early oral zidovudine treatment for the newborn can be facilitated by early detection of the infection by rapid HIV testing on admission. Even so, recent studies reported conflicting data regarding the effectiveness of administering only zidovudine prophylaxis to neonates after delivery (Wade et al., 1998; Fiscus et al., 1999).

Although results from rapid HIV testing is readily available - the median turn-around time is 66 minutes based on the CDC-sponsored MIRIAD Study (Bulterys et al.,2004), or 45 minutes with the OraQuick Rapid HIV-1 Antibody Test at point-of-care hospitals (Cohen et al., 2003), Dola et al. reported that 22% of their study patients delivered within one hour after arrival to the labor and delivery unit, 31.6% within 2 hours, 38.4% within 3 hours, and 47.2% within 4 hours. Therefore, in order for any rapid HIV test to be of use, the test result turnaround time, the time for counseling, and the time to availability of the zidovudine treatment must be constricted to within a few hours after admission (Dola et al., 2010).

As a consequence, the full benefit of the rapid HIV tests may not be realized in patients who typically present without prenatal care - mostly in advanced labor and with rupture membranes (Dola et al., 2010). Due to the high prevalence of HIV infection in women without prenatal care (Lindsay et al., 1991), and until the rapid HIV testing results become available, obstetricians should consider these unregistered parturients as infected with HIV when they present for labor and delivery - refraining from certain common obstetrics practices (i.e. artificial rupture of membranes and the placement of an invasive fetal scalp electrode) to avoid inadvertly increasing the risk of perinatal transmission (Dola et al., 2010).

4. HIV rescreening in late pregnancy – should all women be rescreened?

A case report from Steele (Steele, 2010) describes three cases of infants whose mothers were screened negative for HIV infection in their first trimester of pregnancy. Since their mothers were not considered at high risk for HIV infection, they were not retested in the later stage of pregnancy according to the revised Centers for Disease Control and Prevention (CDC) guidelines (CDC, 2006; Branson et al., 2006). These mothers must have been infected with HIV later in their pregnancy as they were diagnosed with HIV infection shortly after delivery. Of these 3 infants, 2 developed an HIV infection (Steele, 2010).

The revised CDC guidelines (Branson et al., 2006) recommended repeat testing for HIV infection in late pregnancy but before 36 weeks of gestation for women at high risk for acquiring the infection. Women requiring repeat testing would include: those with high risk behaviors, those living in 20 states with high incidence of HIV infection, those receiving care at facilities with incidence of HIV infection of at least 1 per 1,000 women screened, and those with signs and symptoms consistent with acute HIV infection (Branson et al., 2006). These guidelines were placed as beneficial interventions to reduce mother-to-child transmission (MTCT) of HIV could have been implemented in mothers not identified as HIV infected until late in pregnancy or until the onset of labor (Wade et al., 1998).

Sansom et al, further supports the necessity of rescreening for HIV in the third trimester as it could prove to be cost-effective in preventing MTCT in a community with an HIV incidence of 1 per 1,000 person-years or higher. They argue that primary HIV infection may go undetected in women who continue to practice high-risk behaviors during pregnancy and in those with initial tests performed before HIV antibody development (Sansom et al., 2003). According to one study of 407 HIV-positive mothers, eight seroconversions happened after a negative test result during or just before pregnancy. Three of the 8 seroconversions resulted in perinatal HIV transmissions (Fiscus et al., 1999).

In an effort to further reduce perinatal transmission, Patterson et al. recommended that repeat HIV testing should be done in late pregnancy and again at time of labor and delivery along with the use of reflex RNA testing for women with negative antibody to detect acute HIV infection (Patterson et al, 2007). Furthermore, Gray et al reported that the risk of acquisition of HIV infection increased by 2-fold in pregnancy after adjustment for behaviors risk factors (Gray et al., 2005). Although the evidence is inconclusive, this increased risk could be due to the hormonal changes in pregnancy, which could affect genital tract mucosa (Jacobson et al., 2000; Michael et al., 1997) or immune responses (Brahin, 2002; Beagley & Gockel, 2003), resulting in susceptibility to HIV infectivity.

This above case report presented by Steele and the above arguments on cost-effectiveness of rescreening in late pregnancy support a recommendation for late pregnancy HIV screening - possibly including RNA reflex testing for those with negative antibody to the virus- of all women instead of only women known to have risk factors. However, a barrier to putting this into practice is that not all insurance companies will cover the cost of a repeat HIV screening in late pregnancy for all pregnant women unless the CDC revises its guidelines (Steele, 2010).

5. Cesarean section in HIV-infected women – Are there any maternal or neonatal morbidities?

Scheduled cesarean section prior to labor is recommended at 38 weeks gestation for women with a viral load above 1,000 copies/ml to further prevent vertical transmission of HIV infection (American College of Obstetricians and Gynecologists [ACOG], 2004). The combination of cesarean delivery and antiretroviral medications have been demonstrated to effectively reduce mother-to-child transmission of HIV disease (The International Perinatal HIV Group, 1999; The European Mode of Delivery Collaboration, 1999;Mofenson, 2002; Burdge et al., 2003; Mandelbrot et al., 1998; Kind et al., 1998). Cesarean deliveries are not without significant complications even for HIV-negative women (Allen et al., 2003; Makoha et al., 2004). Therefore, HIV-positive women could theoretically be at greater risk for post-operative complications due to a relatively weakened immune system or immunodeficient status. However, there are conflicting reports from the currently available data with regard to post-cesarean morbidities incurred by HIV-infected women (The European Mode of Delivery Collaboration, 1999; Maiques-Montesinos et al., 1999; Grubert et al., 2002; Rodriguez et al., 2001; Marcollet et al., 2002; Watts et al., 2000). Most studies report an increased risk of post-operative morbidity, mostly infectious, in HIV-positive women compared with HIV-negative control subjects (Coll et al., 2002; Grubert el al., 1999; Vimercati et al., 2000). Additionally, the risk of complications is correlated with the degree of immunosuppression (Jamieson et al., 2007). Thus, those who most benefit from scheduled cesarean delivery to decrease vertical transmission would sustain the highest risk of complication from the procedure.

A Cochrane review (Read & Newell; 2005) summarizes six studies (European Mode of Delivery Collaboration, 1999; Marcollet et al., 2002; Watts et al., 2000; Read et al., 2001; Faucher et al., 2001; Fior et al., 2004) which compare the complication rates in women receiving scheduled cesarean delivery, non-elective cesarean delivery, and vaginal delivery. Post-operative morbidity was highest in women who underwent a non-elective cesarean delivery.

Vaginal delivery resulted in the lowest post-partum morbidity. Of note, most of these morbidities were post-operative fever, anemia, endometritis, and wound infection (Jamieson et al., 2007). Maternal deaths are rare, and these studies did not have adequate sample sizes to assess any potential differences in maternal mortality rate (Jamieson et al., 2007).

Given that these HIV-infected women are at high risk for post-operative infectious morbidities, prophylactic antibiotics should be given according to ACOG guidelines for all women who undergo cesarean delivery (American College of Obstetricians and Gynecologists [ACOG], 2003). However, most of these studies were performed prior to the recommendation to give prophylactic antibiotics at least 30 minutes prior to cesarean delivery instead of after cord clamping, which has been shown to decrease the risk of post-operative infection. It would be interesting to determine whether this newly recommended practice would reduce the risk of post-operative infection in these HIV-infected women.

Current ACOG guidelines recommends scheduled cesarean delivery in HIV infected women, emphasizing the importance of performing the surgery prior to the onset of labor or rupture of membranes to reduce the risk of vertical transmission (ACOG, 2004) and that cesarean delivery performed after the onset of labor or after rupture of membranes is of unclear benefit with regard to decreasing vertical transmission. Based on the previously mentioned data, these cesarean deliveries after onset of labor or after rupture of membrane could be associated with an increase in maternal infectious morbidity (Rodriguez et al., 2001; Marcollet et al., 2002; Read et al., 2001; Duarte et al., 2006). Therefore, when an HIV-infected woman attempts vaginal delivery, she should be counseled for the increased risk of post-operative morbidity should she require an emergent cesarean delivery (Cavasin et al., 2009). Marcollet et al. recommends that HIV-infected women with a low probability of having a successful vaginal delivery should consider a scheduled cesarean delivery (Marcollet et al., 2002).

Overall, as the cost for treating postpartum morbidity is relatively low in comparison to the cost incurred by pediatric HIV infection, it appears that scheduled cesarean delivery is cost-effective (Halpern et al., 2000; Mrus et al., 2000; Ratcliffe et al., 1998).

ACOG recommends that scheduled cesarean delivery in the absence of medical or obstetrical indications should not be performed at less than 39 weeks of gestation, due to increased risk of neonatal respiratory morbidity (ACOG, 2001). This risk of respiratory morbidity for neonates born via cesarean section would closely approximate that of neonates born via the vaginal route at 39 weeks of gestation (Tita et al., 2009). In HIV-infected women with viral load greater than 1,000 copies/ml, both ACOG and the U.S. Public Health Service recommend scheduled cesarean delivery at 38 weeks for prevention of vertical transmission of the HIV infection (ACOG, 2001; Public Health Service Task Force, 2010). The gestational age of 38 weeks instead of 39 weeks was chosen as the timing for scheduled cesarean delivery with the intent to avoid spontaneous labor and rupture of membranes. Recent data reaffirmed an increased risk of neonatal morbidity even for those neonates born just a few days before 39 weeks of gestation (Tita et al., 2011). To address this valid clinical concern of a potential increase in neonatal respiratory distress syndrome in deliveries at 38 weeks in an effort to prevent mother-to-child transmission of HIV disease, Livingston et al and the IMPACT Protocol 1025 Study group (Livingston et al., 2010) performed a prospective cohort study. They concluded that after adjustment for gestational age and birth weight, the mode of delivery was not significantly associated with respiratory distress syndrome (p=.10), although a trend toward an increased risk for respiratory distress syndrome was noted among neonates delivered by cesarean section (either elective and non-elective) when compared to those delivered via the vaginal route. The overall rate of neonatal respiratory distress syndrome among those born beyond 37 weeks by all modes of delivery is low: 3.4% for 37 weeks, 1.0% for 38 weeks, and 1.1% at 39 weeks. Among those neonates born via elective cesarean delivery at 38 weeks of gestation, there were only 2 out of 227 neonates who had respiratory distress syndrome. This is reassuring data and it appears that respiratory distress syndrome at this late gestational age could be readily managed, although, an admission to the intensive care nursery for treatment might invoke significant parental distress. In the counseling of patients on scheduled cesarean section at 38 weeks to prevent vertical transmission, one must include the small potential risk of neonatal respiratory distress syndrome. This small risk from iatrogenic premature delivery must then be balanced against the risk of less effective prevention of vertical transmission with the onset of labor or rupture of membranes if expectant management is continued until 39 weeks of gestation. The results from this study are the first available data and are reassuring with regard to the low rate of neonatal morbidity associated with current guidelines recommending scheduled cesarean delivery at 38 weeks, therefore further research in this area is needed to provide more robust data regarding this intervention for decreasing vertical transmission.

6. The challenge of prenatal diagnosis in HIV infected - women

The current standard of care offers prenatal diagnosis to the general obstetrics population. In pregnancies complicated by HIV infection, there is a suspicion of a higher rate of false-positive results when these women are screened with the maternal serum multiple marker test (Yudin et al., 2003). This may lead to a higher risk for HIV infected women to require definitive testing with genetic amniocentesis. Therefore it is important to review the current data on the usefulness of biochemical marker screening test in pregnant HIV-infected women.

Variations in beta-hCG and AFP levels have been shown in HIV-infected pregnancies (Yudin et al., 2003; Einstein et al., 2004). This may make calculating the risk for Down syndrome difficult and might result in further diagnostic procedures. Additionally, a patient's immune status (CD4+ count) and viral load may be associated with abnormal screening test results (Neale et al., 2001; Gross et al., 2003). However, the mechanism for these alterations of the tested biochemical markers is unclear. It has been postulated to be due to the altered maternal immune status or the impact of highly active antiretroviral therapy on feto-maternal transfer of these markers, their metabolism or their excretion by the mother (Yudin et al., 2003).

In contrast to the above findings, Brossard et al (Brossard et al., 2008) concluded that these tests were still useful in a HIV-infected population composed of 214 women for first trimester screening tests and 209 women for risk assessment for neural tube defects. Although, they also found a lower median of the MoM of beta-human chorionic gonadotrophin and pregnancy-associated plasma protein-A in HIV-infected women when compared to controls, they did not believe that such differences impacted the risk estimation for Down syndrome or neural tube defects (Brossard et al., 2008).

Similarly, Le Meaux et al. studied a cohort of HIV-infected women in France and noted that untreated HIV-infection was associated with lower maternal alpha fetoprotein levels but there was no increase in false-positive rates in their double marker screening test (which included serum AFP and total beta-hCG levels) (Le Meaux et al., 2008). Therefore, future research - with larger sample sizes - is needed to further investigate the plausible mechanisms for the alterations in these biochemical markers in HIV-infected women.

If indeed HIV-infected women had a higher rate of false-positive maternal serum multiple marker screening test results it may warrant that they are more likely to require definitive diagnostic testing, which includes invasive procedures such as amniocentesis. Caution is required for HIV infected pregnant women who need amniocentesis because there is a potentially iatrogenic risk for perinatal transmission which might be related to elevated maternal viral load (Bucceri et al., 2001). Such invasive procedures might result in infected maternal blood leaking into the amniotic cavity as the needle is traversing the uterine wall or an anterior placenta (Giorlandino et al., 1996).

Data regarding the safety of prenatal diagnostic procedures - in pregnancies complicated by HIV infection - are scant and based on a very small number of participants. Older studies conducted prior to the widespread use of zidovudine suggest an increased risk of infecting the unborn child through invasive diagnostic tests - such as amniocentesis, amnioscopies and other needle puncture procedures (Mandelbrot et al., 1996). With the use of zidovudine and HAART, the risk of perinatal transmission from invasive diagnostic tests may be greatly reduced (Shapiro et al., 1999; Maiques et al., 2003). Other studies with small numbers of study patients (ranging from 6-11 women) reported no perinatal transmission in newborns (Bucceri et al., 2001; Ekoukou et al., 2008; Coll et al., 2006). In total, of the data collected from published studies, amongst the women who underwent invasive procedures there were 28 infected newborns from 82 women who did not receive antiretroviral treatment, 2 infected newborns from 24 women who received zidovudine treatment only, and no infected newborns from 78 women who received HAART treatment, ($p = 0.0001$) (Ekoukou et al., 2008). Thus, it appears that the significant decline in the rate of perinatal transmission after invasive procedures performed during pregnancy could possibly reflect the beneficial impact of anti-retroviral therapy (Ekoukou et al., 2008). Additionally, the potential risk of perinatal transmission might not be as great as it was once thought to be with the implementation of HAART. However, we must consider that the above studies are limited by their small number of study participants.

A policy to guide physicians to provide adequate counseling to HIV-infected women regarding the potential risks of early invasive prenatal diagnostic tests, and the optimal approach to such procedures is much needed. We venture to offer the following conclusions regarding prenatal diagnosis in HIV-infected women based on the above limited data. HIV-infected pregnant women should be offered biochemical marker testing for prenatal diagnosis since it is unclear whether the variations in these marker levels are significant. If invasive sampling of the amniotic fluid is warranted, then careful judgment must be used to consider the patient's risk factors for vertical transmission. Patient should be counseled that based on studies with small sample sizes, the risk of iatrogenic transmission of the HIV virus to the fetus is much lower than previously thought in the setting of optimal viral suppression and HAART. Ideally, patients undergoing invasive testing should be on antiretroviral therapy and have undetectable viral loads (Watts, 2002). Additionally, care should be taken to avoid penetrating the placenta during the procedure as this could theoretically increase maternal and fetal blood mixing, or directly inoculate the fetal blood (Giorlandino et al., 1996). Prenatal diagnosis should not be performed in women whose HIV serology is unknown, given the above concern of iatrogenic risk and the need for appropriate therapy prior to the procedure. There is a great need for continued investigations on which to establish future policy and protocol on this topic.

7. Management of PPROM in women infected with HIV

The duration of rupture of membrane plays an important role in vertical transmission of HIV infection in term pregnancies. Minkoff et al. described a significantly increased rate of perinatal transmission of HIV infection in term women with low CD 4 count if they have ruptured their membranes for more than 4 hours (Minkoff et al., 1995). Other studies confirmed Minkoff's work and found an increase of perinatal transmission from 14% to 25% in the setting of rupture of membranes for greater than 4 hours (Landesman et al., 1996). Furthermore, there is a significant rise in transmission - from 8% to 31% - among women with AIDS if delivery is postponed past 24 hours after rupture of membranes (International Perinatal HIV Group, 2001).

These data reporting an increase in vertical transmission of the HIV infection after prolonged period of ruptured membranes pose a significant obstetrical dilemma for the management of women infected with HIV who had preterm premature rupture of the membranes (PPROM). The question is should all these HIV-infected women with PPROM be delivered at the time of first diagnosis with PPROM to avoid prolonged rupture of membranes, which potentially can lead to an increase in perinatal transmission of the disease? Does current data suggest that we should commit these HIV-infected pregnancies with PPROM to extreme prematurity with immediate delivery to avoid the risk of perinatal transmission of HIV? Available data on expectant management of PPROM in HIV infected women are limited. Currently available are two studies on PPROM in HIV infected women.

The first study by Aagaard-Tillery et al. (Aagaard-Tillery et al. 2006) in 2006 evaluated the management and outcomes of 7 HIV pregnancies complicated by PPROM. They were diagnosed with PPROM, were expectantly management, and subsequently delivered between 25 to 32 weeks gestation. The mean latency for these patients was 17.1 days with a median of 5 days; one woman had a latency of 92 days. Two of 6 infants became infected with HIV through vertical transmission. The mothers of these two HIV-infected infants either did not receive antepartum or intrapartum antiretroviral therapy or only received treatment in the antepartum period with zidovudine monotherapy. Based on their results, the authors questioned whether expectant management is possible in the setting of PPROM in HIV-infected women, provided that they receive prophylactic combination antiretroviral therapy.

A second study in 2007 by Alvarez et al. (Alvarez et al., 2007) reported data on 18 cases of HIV infected women with PPROM at ≤ 34 weeks of gestation from a single center, delivering at an average gestational age of 31 weeks. The latency period before delivery ranged from 4 to 336 hours. Of those cases, 10 patients had been managed with antenatal antiretroviral therapy and did not have mother-to-child-transmission of HIV regardless of the duration of ruptured membranes, viral load, or maternal CD4 count. The remaining 8 cases did not receive antenatal antiretroviral therapy and received only intrapartum nevirapine. Two of these eight neonates sustained perinatal transmission of HIV; their mothers did not have prenatal care and did not receive antenatal antiretroviral therapy. In this study, the perinatal transmission rate for HIV was 11.1% (2/18).

Although these two studies show encouraging outcomes and are very thought provoking, safety of expectant management of PPROM could not be ascertained based on the small number of study participants. From the above data, we concluded that for HIV-infected women with PPROM at a very young gestational age who has suppressed viral load and on antenatal HAART, expectant management to allow in-utero lung maturation might be considered. However, as risk of morbidity from preterm birth is decreased at tertiary care center beyond 30-32 weeks, there might be more advantageous for expedite delivery. The benefits of expectant management are still uncertain in patients not receiving antiretroviral treatment. Future studies on HIV infected women with PPROM prior to 34 weeks gestation are necessary to arrive at the optimal care plan.

8. Could viral load in genital tract secretions have a role in perinatal transmission?

Maternal viral load was determined to be the most important risk factor in perinatal transmission of HIV infection (The European Collaborative Study, 1999). Efforts in reduction of MTCT of HIV involve optimal suppression of viral load with the implementation of HAART. However, perinatal transmission was reported among women with undetectable maternal serum viral load (Cao et al., 1997; Sperling et al., 1996). Provocative data was gathered by the European Collaborative study. The investigators reported a 2% risk of vertical transmission among women with low viral load who delivered after 37 weeks by elective cesarean section and 11% among those delivered via the vaginal route (The European Collaborative Study, 1999). This might imply that other factors play an important role in the perinatal transmission besides maternal serum viral load. One explanation for the perinatal transmission in the setting of low plasma viral load and the protective effect from cesarean section could be that viral shedding in the female genital tract could have a role in perinatal transmission and that there might be a discordance between HIV-1 RNA levels in blood and cervicovaginal secretions (Garcia-Bujalance et al., 2004). HIV-1 RNA has been detected from the female cervicovaginal tract (Cu Uvin & Caliendoa, 1997) and treatment with HAART can suppress HIV-1 RNA to below detectable levels in both the genital tract and plasma of non-pregnant women (Cu Uvin et al., 2000).

Several studies noted a strong correlation between the level of HIV-1 viral load in the genital tract and the plasma (Hart et al., 1999; Kovacs et al., 1999). However, in non-pregnant women with undetectable plasma viral load, HIV-1 RNA load can be found in their genital tract (Debiaggi et al., 2001). Conversely, some studies reported no correlation between the viral load in the plasma and genital shedding of non-pregnant women (Rasheed et al., 1996). One study from Kovacs et al. (Kovacs et al., 2001) reports that although there was a positive correlation between RNA concentrations in the plasma and the genital tract, 4% (9 of 252 women) of their population had higher RNA concentrations in the genital secretions and two women had at least 10-fold higher RNA levels in genital tract secretions than in plasma. Different genotypic variants of HIV-1 were found in the blood and cervicovaginal lavage according to another study (Shaheen et al., 1999). Garcia-Bujalance et al. reported 2 cases in 38 HIV-1 infected pregnant women with a low plasma viral load of <50 copies/mL but with detectable viral load in their vaginal secretions (Garcia-Bujalance et al., 2004).

Another factor in reducing MTCT of HIV infection can perhaps be determined by viral shedding in the female genital tract. The lack of correlation between the viral load in blood plasma and genital tract secretions might suggest that there is still risk for perinatal transmission in women with undetectable viral load in the plasma (Iribarren et al., 2001). More studies are needed to investigate on the roles of genital tract viral shedding in perinatal transmission and the possible benefit of using both plasma and cervicovaginal secretion viral loads despite undetectable viral plasma load in choosing the vaginal route of delivery.

9. Should assisted reproductive technology be available for HIV-infected men and women?

Currently, about 80% of women infected with HIV are of reproductive age (CDC, 2001). With the current advent and widespread use of HAART in industrialized countries, HIV infection has become a chronic disease and those who are affected with the disease can now live longer and with a better quality of life (Kambin & Batzer, 2004). Furthermore, with current interventions, the risk of MTCT of HIV infection is now significantly declined to approximately 2% (The Ethics Committee of the American Society for Reproductive Medicine [ASRM], 2010). As a result, HIV-infected men and women may elect to have children. However, for discordant couple, reproduction may result in the risk of horizontal transmission to the uninfected partner.

The Ethics Committee of the American Society for Reproductive Medicine (ASRM) established guidelines in 1994 for patients infected with HIV who might request or require assisted reproductive technologies (Ethics Committee of the American Fertility Society, 1994). The committee made the following recommendations due to their concern about potential horizontal transmission to the uninfected partner and vertical transmission to the couple's child and the potential problem to the offspring as the infected parent might succumb to the disease. Their recommendations are as follows: couples seeking support are encouraged to test for HIV infection, development of written policies on infertility treatment for HIV-infected people by each institution, counseling of consequences of using infected sperm, and advising couples on the alternative options of donor sperm, adoption, or not having children (Ethics Committee of the American Fertility Society, 1994).

Since then, better understanding of the disease has been achieved, and the beneficial impact of HAART significantly improved survival and quality of life for HIV-infected persons, along with improved technique to provide virus-free sperm for reproductive assistance. Thus, in 2006, ASRM published its revision of the original guidelines. Obstetric health care providers should be aware of these revisions so that they can appropriately counsel their patients.

Approximately 1 in 500 – 1,000 episodes of unprotected intercourse is estimated to result in horizontal transmission of the HIV infection to an uninfected partner (Mandelbrot et al., 1997). Therefore, in discordant couples where the woman is infected with HIV and her partner is negative, ASRM discussed the use of homologous insemination with the uninfected male partner's sperm to achieve pregnancy and to avoid the risk of transmission (ASRM, 2010).

In discordant couples (with the male partner being infected), intercourse without condom use at the time of ovulation to attempt conception could reduce but does not eliminate the risk of infecting the partner. According to one study, the reported seroconversion rate was 4.3% for couples that employed timed intercourse to attempt conception (Sauer et al., 2009). Couples should be counseled against this unsafe method as they could still infect their partner. For these instances of male-infected sero-discordant couples, specific methods for sperm preparation and testing (density gradient and swim-up technique to obtain sperm and PCR virus detection assay) have been described (Kambin et al., 2004; Sauer et al., 2009; Semprini et al., 1998). The final sperm sample was used only if it tested negative on these assays (Semprini et al., 1998). These techniques resulted in less than 1% of the samples testing positive for the virus and thus was discarded (Semprini et al., 1998). These techniques can markedly reduce the chance of HIV transmission to the female partner and child. Specifically, Semprini et al. reported data on almost 1,600 inseminations of 513 HIV-uninfected women in which there were 228 pregnancies. At a follow-up rate of 97.5% at 3 months, and 92% at one year, all mothers and children were uninfected (Semprini et al., 1998). Similarly, there was no report of transmitted HIV infection to the mother or child with intrauterine insemination (Kambin et al., 2004) or intracytoplasmic sperm injection (Sauer et al., 2009) technique. For these male-positive discordant couples, extensive counseling should be performed regarding transmission risk-reduction techniques (ASRM, 2000). Health care providers should not overlook HIV-infected men and women's desire to have children. They should make every effort to encourage these men and women to obtain care at the institutions with most effective methods to provide appropriate treatment and to reduce the chance of infecting their partner and child.

10. Conclusion

Significant progress was made in understanding HIV virology and important interventions were developed to reduce mother-to-child-transmission of this disease since the epidemic of this disease. Most obstetricians caring for HIV-infected women are familiar with these commonly employed interventions. However, there are still many difficult clinical situations where only scant data is available to direct management, in part due to the fortunately low prevalence of the disease in industrialized countries. We hope readers of this chapter would continue to report their challenging clinical encounters and thus, would contribute to the better care of these pregnant HIV-infected women. The review of these special considerations, hopefully, will aid obstetricians in their plan of care, raise valid questions, and suggest areas of future research directions.

11. References

Aagaard-Tillery, K., Lin, M.G., Lupo, V., Buchbinder, A., & Ramsey, P.S. (2006). Clinical Study - Preterm Premature Rupture of Membranes in Human Immunodeficiency Virus Infected Women: A Novel Case Series. Infectious Diseases in Obstetrics and Gynecology; 2006:53234.

ACOG Committee on Obstetric Practice.(2004) Scheduled Cesarean Delivery and the Prevention of Vertical Transmission of HIV Infection. ACOG Committee Opinion No 234, May 2004.

Allen, V.M., O'Connell, C.M., Liston, R.M., & Baskett, T.F. (2003). Maternal morbidity Associated with cesarean delivery without labor compared with spontaneous onset of labor at term. Obstet Gynecol 2003; 102:477-82.

Alvarez, J.R., Bardeguez, A, Iffy, L., & Apuzzio, J.J.(2007). Preterm premature rupture of membranes in pregnancies complicated by human immunodeficiency virus infection: A single center's five-year experience. The Journal of Maternal-Fetal and Neonatal Medicine, 2007; 20(12):853-857.

American College of Obstetricians and Gynecologists. (2001). Scheduled cesarean delivery and the prevention of vertical transmission of HIV infection. ACOG Committee Opinion 234. Int J Gynaecol Obstet. 2001;73:279–81.

American College of Obstetricians and Gynecologists. (2003). Prophylactic antibiotics in labor and delivery: ACOG practice bulletin no. :47. Obstet Gynecol 2003;102:875-82.

Beagley, K.W., & Gockel, C.M. (2003). Regulation of innate and adaptive immunity by female sex hormones oestradiol and progesterone. FEMS Immunol Med Microbiol, 2003;39:13-22.

Brabin L. (2002). Interactions of the female hormonal environment, susceptibility to viral infections, and disease progression. AIDS Patient Care STDS 2002; 16: 211-21.

Branson, B.M., Handsfield, H.H., Lampe, M.A., Janssen, R.S., Taylor, A.W., Lyss, S.B., et al. (2006). Revised recommendations for HIV testing of adults, adolescents, and pregnant women in health-care settings. MMWR Recomm Rep 2006;55(RR-14): 1-17.

Brossard, P., Boulvain, M., Coll, O., Barlow, P., Aebi-Popp, K., Bischof, P., Martinez de Teja, B. (2008). Swiss HIV Cohort Study; Swiss HIV Mother and Child Cohort Study. Is screening for fetal anomalies reliable in HIV-infected pregnant women? A multicentre study. AIDS, 2008;22(15):2013-7.

Bucceri, A.M., Somigliana, E., Vignali, M. (2001). Early invasive diagnostic techniques During pregnancy in HIV-infected women. Acta Obstet Gynecol Scand, 2001;80(1):82-3.

Bulterys, M., Jamieson, D.J., O'Sullivan, M.J., & et al. (2004). Rapid HIV-1 Testing During Labor. A Multicenter Study. JAMA.2004;292:219-223.

Burdge, D.R., Money, D.M., Forbes, J.C., Walmsley, S.L., Smaill, F.M., Boucher, M., & et al. (2003). Canadian consensus guidelines for the management of pregnancy, labour and delivery and for postpartum care in HIV-positive pregnant women and their offspring. CMAJ 2003; 168.

Cao, Y., Krogstad, P., Korber, B.T., et al. (1997). Maternal HIV-1 viral load and vertical transmission of infection: the Ariel Project for the prevention of HIV transmission from mother to infant. Nat Med, 1997;3:549-552.

Cavasin, H., Dola, T., Uribe, O., & et al. (2009). Postoperative infectious morbidities of cesarean delivery in Human Immunodeficiency Virus-Infected Women. Infect Dis Obstet Gynecol. 2009;2009:827405. Epub 2009 May 25

Centers for Disease Control and Prevention (CDC). (2004). Rapid HIV Antibody Testing During Labor and Delivery for Women of Unknown HIV Status. A Practical Guide and Model Protocol. January 2004.

CDC. (2006). Sexually transmitted diseases treatment guidelines. Morb Mortal Wkly Rep, 2006;55(RR-11):14.

CDC. (2007). HIV/AIDS Fact sheet. Mother-to-Child (Perinatal) HIV transmission and prevention. October 2007.

CDC. (2001). HIV/ADIS Surveillance Report. 2001;13.

Cohen, M.H., Olszewski, Y., Brandon, B., & et al. (2003) Using point-of-care testing to make rapid HIV-1 tests in labor really rapid. AIDS. 2003;17:2121-2123.

Coll, O., Fiore, S., Floridia, M., & et al. (2002). Pregnancy and HIV infection: a European consensus on management. AIDS, 2002; 16(suppl):S1-18.

Coll, .O, Suy, A., Hernandez, S., Pisa, S., Lonca, M., Thorne, C., & Borrell, A. (2006). Prenatal diagnosis in human immunodeficiency virus-infected women: a new screening program for chromosomal anomalies. Am J Obstet Gynecol, 2006;194(1):192-8.

Connor, E.M., Sperling, R.S., Gelber, R., & et al. (1994). Reduction of maternal-infant transmission of human immunodeficiency virus type 1 with zidovudine treatment. N. Engl J Med. 1994;331:1173-1180.

Cu Uvin, S. & Caliendoa, A.M. (1997). Cervicovaginal human immunodeficiency virus secretion and plasma viral load in human immunodeficiency virus-seropositive women. Obstetrics & Gynecology, 1997;90(3): 739-743.

Cu Uvin, S., Caliendoa, A.M., Reinert, S., Chang, A., Juliano-Remollino, C., Flanigan, T.P., Mayer, K.H., & Carpenter, C.C.J. (2000). Effect of highly active antiretroviral therapy on cervicovaginal HIV-1 RNA. AIDS, 2000;14:415-421.

Debiaggi, M., Zara, F., Spinillo, A., De Santolo ,A., Maserati, R., Bruno, R., Sacchi, P., Achilli, G., Pistorio, A., Romero, E., & Filice, G. (2001). Viral excretion in cervicovaginal secretions of HIV-1 infected women receiving antiretroviral therapy. Eur J Clin, 2001; 20:91-96.

Dola, C.P., Tran, T., Duong, C., Federico, C., DeNicola, N., & Maupin, R. (2010). Rapid HIV testing and obstetrical characteristics of women with unkown HIV serostatus at time of labor and delivery. J Natl Med Assoc. 2010; 102(12):1158-64.

Duarte, G., Read, J., Gonin, R., & et al. (2006). Mode of delivery and postpartum morbidity in Latin American and Caribbean countries among women who are infected with human immunodeficiency virus-1: The NICHD International Site Development Initiative (NISDI) Perinatal Study. Am J Obstet Gynecol (2006) 195: 215-29.

Einstein, F.H., Wright, R.L., Trentacoste, S., Gross, S., Merkatz, I.R., & Bernstein, P.S. (2004). The impact of protease inhibitors on maternal serum screening analyte levels in pregnant women who are HIV positive. Am J Obstet Gynecol, 2004;191(3):1004-8.

Ekoukou, D., Khuong-Josses, M.A., Ghibaudo, N., Mechali, D., & Rotten, D. (2008). Amniocentesis in pregnant HIV-infected patients. Absence of mother-to-child viral transmission in a series of selected patients. Eur J Obstet Gynecol Reprod Biol, 2008;140(2):212-7. Epub 2008 Jun 27.

Ethics Committee of the American Fertility Society. (1994). Ethical considerations of assisted reproductive technologies. Fertil Steril 1994;62 (Suppl1):85s.

Ethics Committee of the American Society for Reproductive Medicine. (2010). Human immunodeficiency virus and infertility treatment. Fertility and Sterility, 2010;94(1): 11-15.

Faucher, P., Batallan, A., Bastian, H., & et al. (2001). Management of pregnant women infected with HIV at Bichat Hospital between 1990 and 1998: analysis of 202 pregnancies. Gynecol Obstet Fertil 2001;29:211-25.

Fiore S, Newell ML, Thorne C. Higher rates of post-partum complications in HIV-infected than in uninfected women irresptive of mode of delivery. AIDS 2004;18:933-8

Fiscus SA, Adimora AA, Schoenbach VJ, McKinney R, Lim W, Rupar D, et al. Trends in human immunodeficiency virus (HIV) counseling, testing, and antiretroviral treatment of HIV-positive women and perinatal transmission in North Carolina. J Infect Dis 1999;180:99–105.

Fiscus SA, Schoenbach VJ, Wilfert C. Short courses of zidovudine and perinatal transmission of HIV. N Engl J Med. 1999 Apr 1; 340 (13): 1040 – 1.

García-Bujalance S, Ruiz G, De Guevara CL, Peña JM, Bates I, Vázquez JJ, Gutiérrez A. Quantitation of human immunodeficiency virus type 1 RNA loads in cervicovaginal secretions in pregnant women and relationship between viral loads in the genital tract and blood. Eur J Clin Microbiol Infect Dis.,2004;23(2):111-5. Epub 2004 Jan 20.

Giorlandino C, Gambuzza G, D'Alessio P, Santoro ML, Gentili P, Vizzone A. Blood contamination of amniotic fluid after amniocentesis in relation to placental location. Prenat Diag, 1996;16:180-2

Gray R, Li X, Kigozi G, Serwadda D, Brahmbhatt H, Wabwire-Mangen F, et al. Increased risk of incident HIV during pregnancy in Rakai, Uganda: a prospective study. Lancet 2005; 366:1182–1188.

Gross S, Castillo W, Crane M, Espinosa B, Carter S, DeVeaux R, Salafia C. Maternal serum alpha-fetoprotein and human chorionic gonadotropin levels in women with human immunodeficiency virus. Am J Obstet Gynecol, 2003;188(4):1052-6.

Grubert TA, Reindell D, Belohradsky BH, Gurtler L, Stauber M, Dathe O. Rates of postoperative complication among human immunodeficiency virus-infected women who have undergone obstetric and gynecologic surgical procedures. CID 2002; 34:822-30.

Grubert TA, Reindell D, Kastner R, Lutz-Friedrich R, Belohradsky BH, Datha O. Complications after caesarean section in HIV-1 infected women not taking antiretroviral treatment. Lancet, 1999;354:1612-3.

Halpern MT, Read JS, Ganoczy DA, Harris Dr. Cost-effectiveness of cesarean section delivery to prevent mother-to-child transmission of HIV-1. AIDS 2000;14:691-700.

Hart CE, Lennox JL, Pratt-Palmore M, Wright TC, Schinazi RF, Evans-Strickfaden TE, Bush TJ, Schenell C, Conley LJ, Clancy KA, Ellerbrock TV. Correlation of human immunodeficiency virus type 1 RNA levels in blood and the female genital tract. J Infect Dis, 1999;179:871-882.

International Perinatal HIV Group. Duration of ruptured membranes and vertical transmission of HIV-1: A metaanalysis ßfrom 15 prospective cohort studies. AIDS 2001;15:357–368.

Iribarren JA, Ramos JR, Guerra L, Coll O, De Jose MI, Domingo P, Fortuny C, Miralles P, Parras F, Pena JM, Rodrigo C, Vidal R. Prevencion de la transmison vertical y tratamiento de la infeccion por el virus de la immunodeficiencia humana en la mujer embarazada. Enferm Infec Microbiol Clin, 2001;19:314-335.

Jacobson DL, Peralta L, Farmer M, Graham NMH, Gaydos C, Zenilman J. Relationship of hormonal contraception and cervical ectopy as measured by computerized planimetry to chlamydial infection in adolescents. Sex Transm Dis 2000; 27: 313–19.

Jamieson DJ, Read JS, Kourtis AP, Durant TM, Lampe MA, Dominguez KL. Cesarean delivery for HIV-infected women: recommendations and controversies. Am J Obstet Gynecol. 2007 Sep;197(3 Suppl):S96-100.

Kambin S, Batzer F. Assisted reproductive technology in HIV serodiscordant couples. Sex Reprod Menopause 2004;2:92–100.

Kind C, Rudin C, Siegrist C, Wyler C, Biedermann K, Lauper U. Prevention of vertical HIV transmission: additive protective effect of elective Cesarean section and zidovudine prophylaxis. AIDS 1998; 12:205–10.

Kogan, MD, Martin JA, Alexander GR, Kotelchuck M, Ventura SJ, Frigoletto FD. The changing pattern of prenatal care utilization in the US, 1981 - 1995, using different prenatal care indices. JAMA 1998; 279: 1623 - 8.

Kovacs, A., Chan, L.S., Chen, Z.C., Meyer, W., Muderspach, L., Young, M., Anastos, K., & Levine, A.M. (1999). HIV-1 RNA in plasma and genital tract secretions in women infected with HIV-1. J Acquir Immune Defic Syndr, 1999;22:124-131.

Kovacs, A., Wasserman, S., Burns, D., Wright, D., Cohn, J., Landay, A., Weber, K., Cohen, M., Levine, A., Minkoff, H., Miotti, P., Palefsky, J., Young, M., Reichelderfer, P., & the DATRI and WIHS Study Groups. (2001). Determinants of HIV-1 shedding in the genital tract of women. The Lancet, 2001;358(9293): 1593-1601.

Lancioni, C., Harwell, T., & Rutstein, R.M. (1999). Prenatal care and HIV infection. AIDS Patient Care STDS. 1999 Feb; 13 (2); 97 - 102.

Landesman, S.H., Kalisha, L.A., Burns, D.N,. Minkoff, H,. Fox, H.E., Zorrilla, C., Garcia, P., Fowler, M.G., Mofenson, L., & Tuomala, R. (1996). Obstetrical factors and the transmission of human immunodeficiency virus type 1 from mother to child. The Women and Infants Transmission Study. N Engl J Med, 1996;334:1617–1623.

Le Meaux, J.P., Tsatsaris, V., Schmitz, T., Fulla, Y., Launay, O., Goffinet, F., & Azria, E. (2008). Maternal biochemical serum screening for Down syndrome in pregnancy with human immunodeficiency virus infection. Obstet Gynecol, 2008;112(2 Pt 1):223-30.

Lindsay, M.K., Feng, T.I., Peterson, H.B., & et al. (1991). Routine human immunodeficiency infection screening in unregistered and registered inner-city parturients. Obstet Gynecol. 1991; 77: 599 - 603.

Livingston, E., Huo, Y., Patel, K., Brogly, S.B., Tuomala, R., Scott, G.B., Bardeguez, A., Stek, A., & Read, J.S. (2010). For the International Maternal Pediatric Adolescent AIDS Clinical Trials Group (IMPAACT) Protocol 1025 Study. Mode of Delivery and Infant Respiratory Morbidity Among Infants Born to HIV-1 infected Women. Obstet Gynecol, 2010; 116(2 Pt 1): 335–343.

Maiques, V., García-Tejedor, A., Perales, A., Córdoba, J., & Esteban, R.J. (2003). HIV detection in amniotic fluid samples. Amniocentesis can be performed in HIV pregnant women? Eur J Obstet Gynecol Reprod Biol, 2003;108(2):137-41.

Maiques-Montesinos, V., Cervera-Sanchez, J., Bellver-Pradas, J., Abad-Carrascosa, A., & Serra, V. (1999). Post-cesarean section morbidity in HIV-positive women. Acta Obstet Gynecol Scand 1999; 78:789-92.

Makoha, F.W., Felimban, H.M., Fathuddien, M.A., Roomi, F., & Ghabra, T. (2004). Multiple cesarean section morbidity. Int J Gynaecol Obstet 2004; 87:227-32.

Mandelbrot, L., Heard, I., Henrion-Geant, E., & Henrion, R. (1997). Natural conception in HIV-negative women with HIV-infected partners. Lancet 1997;349:850–1.

Mandelbrot, L., Le Chenadec, J., Berrebi, A., Bongain, A., Bénifla, J.L., Delfraissy, J.F., & et al. (1998). Perinatal HIV-1 transmission: interaction between zidovudine prophylaxis and mode of delivery in the French Perinatal Cohort. JAMA 1998; 280:55-60.

Mandelbrot, L., Mayaux, M.J., Bongain, A., Berrebi, A., Moudoub-Jeanpetit, Y., Bénifla, J.L., Ciraru Vigneron, N., Le Chenadec, J., Blanche, S., & Delfraissy, J.F. (1996). Obstetric factors and mother-to-child transmission of human immunodeficiency virus type 1: the French perinatal cohorts. SEROGEST French Pediatric HIV Infection Study Group. Am J Obstet Gynecol, 1996;175(3 Pt 1):661-7.

Marcollet, A., Goffinet, F., Firtion, G., Pannier, E., Le Bret, T., Brival, M., & et al. (2002). Differences in postpartum morbidity in women who are infected with the human immunodeficiency virus after elective cesarean delivery, emergency cesarean delivery, or vaginal delivery. Am J Obstet Gynecol 2002; 186:784-9.

Marks, G., Crepaz, N., & Janssen, R.S. (2006). Estimating sexual transmission of HIV from persons aware and unaware that they are infected with the virus in the USA. AIDS 2006;20(10):1447-1450.

Michael, C.W. & Esfahani, F.M. (1997). Pregnancy-related changes: a retrospective review of 278 cervical smears. Diagn Cytopathol 1997; 17: 99–107.

Minkoff, H., Burns, D.N., Landesman, S., Youchah, J., Goedert, J.J., Nugent, R.P., Muenz, L.R., & Willoughby, A.D. (1995). The relationship of the duration of ruptured membranes to vertical transmission of human immunodeficiency virus. American Journal of Obstetrics and Gynecology, 1995;173:585–589.

Minkoff, H., McCalla, S., & Feldman, J. (1990). The relationship of cocaine use to syphilis and HIV infection among inner city parturient women. Am J Obstet Gynecol. 1990;163:521-526.

Mofenson, L.M. (2002). U.S. Public Health Service Task Force Recommendations for use of antiretroviral drugs in pregnant HIV-1 –infected women for maternal health and interventions to reduce perinatal HIV-a transmission in the United States. MMWR Recomm Rep 2002; 51(RR-18):1-58.

Mrus, J.M., Goldi, S.J., Weinstein, M.C., & Tsevat, J. (2000). The cost-effectiveness of elective cesarean delivery for HIV-infected women with detectable HIV RNA during pregnancy. AIDS, 2000;14:2543-52.

Neale, D., Magriples, U., Simpson, J., & Copel, J. (2001). HIV and biochemical screening: Is there a higher false-positive rate in the HIV population? Am J Obstet Gynecol, 2001;185(suppl):S189.

Patterson, K.B., Leone, P.A., Fiscus, S.A., Kurue, J., McCoy, S.I., Wolf, L., Foust, E., Williams, D., Eron, J.J., & Pilcher, C.D. (2007). Frequent detection of acute HIV infection in pregnant women. AIDS, 2007;21(17): 2303-2308.

Public Health Service Task Force. (2010). Recommendations for use of antiretroviral drugs In pregnant HIV-1-infected women for maternal health and interventions to reduce perinatal HIV-1 transmission in the United States. 2010. Available at: http://aidsinfo.nih.gov/contentfiles/PerinatalGL.pdf Retrieved April 13, 2011.

Rasheed, S., Li, Z., Xu, D., & Kovacs, A. (1996). Presence of cell-free human immunodeficiency virus in cervicovaginal secretions is independent of viral load in the blood of human immunodeficiency virus-infected women. Am J Obstet Gynecol, 1996;175:122– 130.

Ratcliffe, J., Ades, A.E., Gibb, D., Sculpher, M.J., & Briggs, A.H. (1998). Prevention of mother-to-child transmission of HIV-1 infection: alternative strategies and their cost-effectiveness. AIDS 1998;12:1381-8.

Read, J.S. & Newell, M.K. (2005). Efficacy and safety of cesarean delivery for prevention of mother-to-child transmission of HIV-1. Cochrane Database Syste Rev 2005;4:CD005479.

Read, J.S., Tuomala, R., Kpamegan, E., & et al. (2001). Mode of Delivery and postpartum morbidity among HIV infected women: The Women and Infants Transmission Study. JAIDS March, 2001 26(3): 236-45.

Rodriguez, E.J., Spann, C., Jamieson, D., & Lindsay, M. (2001). Postoperative morbidity associated with cesarean delivery among human immunodeficiency virus-positive women. Am J Obstet Gynecol 2001; 184:1108-11.

Sansom, S., Jamieson, D., Farnham, P.G., Bulterys, M., & Fowler, M.G. (2003). Humman Immunodeficiency Virus Retesting During Pregnancy: Costs and Effectiveness in Preventing Perinatal Transmission. Obstetrics & Gynecology, 2003;102(4): 782-790.

Sauer, M.V., Wang, J.G., Douglas, N.C., Nakhuda, G.S., Vardhana, P., Jovanovic, V., & Guarnaccia, M.M. (2009). Providing fertility care to men seropositive for human immunodeficiency virus: reviewing 10 years of experience and 420 consecutive cycles of in vitro fertilization and intracytoplasmic sperminjection. Fertil Steril 2009;91:2455–60.

Semprini, A.E., Levi-Setti, P., Ravizza, M., & Pardi, G. (1998). Assisted conception to reduce the risk of male-to female sexual transfer of HIV in serodiscordant couples: an update [abstract]. Presented at the 1998 Symposium on AIDS in Women, Sao Paulo, Brazil, September 14–15, 1998.

Shaheen, F., Sison, A.V., McIntosh, L., Mukhart, M., & Pomerantz, R.J. (1999). Analysis of HIV-1 in the cervicovaginal secretions and blood of pregnant and nonpregnant women. J Hum Virol, 1999;2:154-166.

Shapiro, D.E., Sperling, R.S., Mandelbrot, L., Britto, P., & Cunningham, B.E. (1999). Risk factors for perinatal human immunodeficiency virus transmission in patients receiving zidovudine prophylaxis. Pediatric AIDS Clinical Trials Group protocol 076 Study Group. Obstet Gynecol, 1999;94(6):897-908.

Sperling, R.S., Shapiro, D.E., Cooms, R.W., & et al. (1996). Maternal viral load, zidovuidine treatment, and the risk of transmission of human immunodeficiency virus type 1 from mother to infant. N Engl J Med, 1996;355:1621-1629.

Steele, R.W. (2010). Late Pregnancy Screening for Human Immunodeficiency Virus. The Pediatric Infectious Disease Journal, 2010: 72-73. E-pub ahead of print.

Stringer, J.S. & Rouse, D.J. (1999). Rapid Testing and Zidovudine Treatment to Prevent Vertical Transmission of Human Immunodeficiency Virus in Unregistered Parturients: A Cost-Effectiveness Analysis. Obstetric & Gynecology. 1999; 94:34-40.

The European Collaborative study. (1999). Maternal viral load and vertical transmission of HIV-1: an important factor but not the only one. AIDS, 1999;13(11): 1377-1385).

The European Mode of Delivery Collaboration. (1999). Elective caesarean-section versus Vaginal delivery in prevention of vertical HIV-1 transmission: A randomized clinical trial. Lancet 1999; 353:1035-9.

The International Perinatal HIV Group. (1999). The mode of delivery and the risk of vertical transmission of human immunodeficiency virus type 1: a meta-analysis of 15 prospective cohort studies. N Engl J Med 1999; 340:977-87.

Tita, A.T., Lai, Y., Landon, M.B., Spong, C.Y., Leveno, K.J., Varner, M.W., Caritis, S.N., Meis, P.J., Wapner, R.J., Sorokin, Y., Peaceman, A.M., O'Sullivan, M.J., Sibai, B.M., Thorp, J.M., Ramin, S.M., & Mercer, B.M. (2011). Eunice Kennedy Shriver National Institute of Child Health and Human Development (NICHD) Maternal-Fetal Medicine Units Network (MFMU). Timing of elective repeat cesarean delivery at term and maternal perioperative outcomes. Obstet Gynecol, 2011;117(2 Pt 1):280-6

Tita, A.T., Landon, M.B., Spong, C.Y., Lai, Y., Leveno, K.J., Varner, M.W., Moawad, A.H., Caritis, S.N., Meis, P.J., Wapner, R.J., Sorokin, Y., Miodovnik, M., Carpenter, M., Peaceman, A.M., O'Sullivan, M.J., Sibai, B.M., Langer, O., Thorp, J.M., Ramin, S.M., Mercer, B.M.; Eunice Kennedy Shriver NICHD Maternal-Fetal Medicine Units

Network. Timing of elective repeat cesarean delivery at term and neonatal outcomes. N Engl J Med, 2009;360(2):111-20.

Turner, B.J., McKee, L.J., Siverman, N.S., &et al. (1996). Prenatal care and birth outcomes of a cohort of HIV-infected women. J Acquir Immune Defic Syndr 1996; 12:259 - 67.

Vimercati, A., Greco, P., Loverro, G., Lopalco, P.L., Pansini, V., & Selvaggi, L. (2000). Maternal complications after caesarean section in HIV infected women. Eur J Obstet Gynecol Reprod Biol, 2000;90:73-76.

Wade, N.A., Birkhead, G.S., Warren, B.L., & et al. (1998). Abbreviated regimens of zidovudine prophylaxis and perinatal transmission of the human immunodeficiency virus. N Engl J Med 1998; 339:1409-14.

Watts, D. (2002). Management of human immunodeficiency virus infection in pregnancy. N Engl J Med, 2002;346:1879-91.

Watts, D.H., Lambert, J.S., Stiehm, R., & et al. (2000). Complications according to mode of delivery among human immunodeficiency virus-infected women with CDS lymphocyte counts of ≤500/μL. Am J Obstet Gynecol July, 2000; 183 (1): 100-7.

Yudin, M.H., Prosen. T.L., & Landers. D.V. (2003). Multiple-marker screening in human Immunodeficiency virus-positive pregnant women: Screen positivity rates with the triple and quad screens. Am J Obstet Gynecol, 2003;189(4):973-6.

17

HIV-1 Treatment-Experienced Patients: Treatment Options and Management

Gail Reid and Richard M. Novak
University of Illinois, Chicago
U.S.A.

1. Introduction

Human immunodeficiency virus (HIV) and acquired immune deficiency syndrome (AIDS) are a global health crisis of unprecedented dimensions, causing over 25 million deaths worldwide since it was first recognized as a disease entity in the early 1980s.(Joint United Nations Program on HIV/AIDS 2008) In 2008 alone, there were approximately 2.7 million newly infected and over 33 million persons living with HIV globally, of whom between 1.8 and 2.3 million died.(Joint United Nations Program on HIV/AIDS 2011) In the 24 years since zidovudine was approved for the treatment of HIV infection, remarkable advances have been made in the understanding of disease pathogenesis and translating that knowledge into practical therapeutics. Most notably, the advent of highly active antiretroviral therapy (HAART) has transformed HIV from an inevitably fatal disease to one that, if managed appropriately, can be considered a chronic condition. As a result, the overall number of people living with HIV is increasing as these regimens extend life and as new infections outnumber AIDS deaths. (www.unaids.org; Joint United Nations Program on HIV/AIDS 2011)

The number of HIV treatment regimens has grown exponentially, particularly in the past decade. This, coupled with advances in the understanding of disease pathogenesis and progression, has made HIV disease management among the most dynamic fields in modern medicine. A number of guidelines have been developed to assist practitioners with often complex treatment decisions. These include the 2010 International AIDS Society (IAS/IAS-USA) guidelines and the 2011 US Department of Health and Human Services (DHHS) HIV treatment guidelines.(Thompson, et al., 2010; http//:www.aidsinfo.nih.gov; Thompson, et al., 2010; United States Department of Health and Human Services (US DHHS) Panel on Antiretroviral Guidelines for Adults and Adolescents 2011)

Close to 30 individual drugs and fixed-dose combinations are available to treat HIV. Despite the availability of a broad range of individual antiretroviral treatments and combinations, drug resistance remains a common phenomenon, and treatment failure is still frequently observed. Moreover, treatment advances—together with recent demographic shifts—have resulted in a dramatic expansion in the population of treatment-experienced patients. This group comprises an ever-increasing proportion of the patients whom HIV clinicians are called upon to treat. This review attempts to integrate guideline recommendations and evidence from recent clinical trials to identify best practices in the management of these patients.

2. The treatment-experienced patient

According to the IAS, the primary goal of antiretroviral therapy is to increase disease-free survival through the maximal suppression of viral replication and preservation of immunologic function.(Thompson, et al., 2010; Hammer, et al., 2008) Optimal therapy for patients with HIV depends on carefully balancing these benefits with the risks for drug toxicity, potential emergence of viral resistance, and the understanding that HIV infection is a chronic disease that requires continuous therapy—often for decades. These considerations are complicated in the treatment-experienced patient, as these patients often have accumulated resistance mutations to a number of drugs in existing antiretroviral drug classes. Modifications of treatment regimens may be forced by undue toxicity, drug-drug interactions, or outright virologic failure. While, theoretically, it is optimal for patients to remain on a single treatment until virologic failure, regimens may also be modified to improve convenience and/or ameliorate minor or cosmetic side effects, ultimately improving adherence and increasing time to virologic failure.(Thompson, et al., 2010; Hammer, et al. 2008)

3. Defining treatment failure

Treatment failure may be defined based on HIV RNA response to therapy (virologic failure), changes in CD4+ cell count (immunologic failure), and the occurrence or recurrence of HIV-related events after ≥ 3 months on an antiretroviral regimen (clinical progression). (US Department of Health and Human Services (DHHS) Panel on Antiretroviral treatment guidelines for adults and adolescents 2011, http://aidsinfor.nih.gov)

Virologic failure may be characterized as persistent HIV RNA viral load above 200 copies/mL. (US DHHS HIV treatment guidelines 2011) Occasional episodes of viral detection between 51 and 1000 copies/mL may occur due to laboratory variation or other transient viral illness. However, frequent and/or consistent viremia is a strong indicator of treatment failure and must be addressed to prevent selection of drug-resistant virus.

Immunologic failure is the failure to achieve and maintain an adequate CD4+ T-cell response despite virologic suppression. Although an absolute definition has not been agreed upon by experts, immunologic failure can generally be considered as failure to increase CD4+ cell counts above 350–500 cells/mm^3 over 4–7 years of treatment.(US DHHS HIV treatment guidelines 2011) Alternatively, it may be defined as failure to increase CD4+ cell count by 50–100 cells/mm^3 above baseline during the first year of a new therapy, or a decline in CD4+ cell count to below baseline while on therapy.(US DHHS HIV treatment guidelines 2011)

Clinical progression is the occurrence or recurrence of HIV-related conditions (a new AIDS defining illness or death) after ≥3 months of HAART, excluding immune reconstitution syndromes.(US DHHS HIV treatment guidelines 2011)

While virologic failure, immunologic failure, and clinical progression are closely related, all three may not occur simultaneously. In general, virologic failure precedes immunologic failure and clinical progression of disease; however, the period between overt virologic failure and detectable suppression of CD4+ cell count and/or HIV-related events can span from months to years.(US DHHS HIV treatment guidelines 2011; Deeks, et al., AIDS 2002)

4. Assessing treatment failure

In general, treatment failure cannot be attributed to any single cause. When assessing individual patients with treatment failure, it is important to recognize that multiple reasons for failure may occur in a single patient. These include:

1. patient-specific factors, such as earlier calendar year of starting therapy, high baseline HIV RNA level, lower nadir CD4+ cell count, prior AIDS diagnosis, the presence of comorbidities such as depression or active substance use, and infection with a drug-resistant virus;
2. medication noncompliance and/or missed clinic appointments;
3. medication side effects and toxicity, potentially leading to noncompliance;
4. suboptimal pharmacokinetics, including variable absorption, metabolism, penetration, food/fasting requirements, and drug and natural product interactions; and
5. suboptimal potency of the antiretroviral regimen.(http://aidsinfo.nih.gov)

Of these reasons, suboptimal adherence and toxicities account for the majority (26%–64%) of treatment failures and discontinuations.(d'Arminio Monforte, et al. AIDS 2000; Mocroft A, et al. AIDS 2001)

5. Addressing treatment failure

Careful assessment of the reasons for treatment failure is critical, as approaches to subsequent therapy differ based on the combination of risk factors in the individual patient. Of the potential reasons for failure summarized above, all except certain patient-specific risk factors can be addressed through appropriate attention to maintaining adherence (either to the current regimen or to a new regimen) and careful assessment of all of the patients' current medications, including but not limited to HAART, treatments for comorbid conditions, and natural health products.

5.1 Noncompliance

Unless the patient was infected with resistant virus, treatment failure implies inadequate adherence to antiretroviral therapy. The development of drug resistance requires concurrent antiretroviral drug exposure and ongoing viral replication. Thus, even intermediate adherence (e.g., 70%–90% compliance) is associated with considerable risk for the development of drug-resistant strains of HIV, as a result of ongoing low-level drug exposure and intermittent viral replication. (Lucas GM, et al., J Antimicrob Chemother 2005) For this reason, it is worthwhile to target 90%–100% compliance in patients with HIV.

The causes of nonadherence must be identified and addressed in cooperation with the patient to avoid future treatment failures and the accumulation of drug-resistance mutations. Numerous reasons for nonadherence to medication have been described in the literature. These include, but are not limited to, regimen complexity (a particular problem in HIV treatment), (Ammassari, et al., Neurology 2003) side effects, (Ammassari, et al., JAIDS 2001) failure to understand dosing directions, illiteracy,(Kalichman, et al., J Natl Med Assoc 1999) substance abuse, (Power , et al., AIDS Pt Care STDS 2003) psychological issues, (Gibbie, et al., Sex Health 2007) cost, missed appointments, and lack of social supports..

Routinely discussing adherence with patients at each visit may improve medication adherence. Pill boxes are helpful for patients who are busy or forgetful and have the additional benefit of being highly cost-effective. In one study, its use resulted in a significant

4% improvement in adherence that correlated with a significant reduction in viral load. (Petersen M, et al. CROI 2007)

5.2 Side effects and toxicities

When treatment fails, the patient should be carefully assessed for side effects and their duration and severity. In some cases, side effects are transiently associated with the initiation of a new regimen. However, ongoing side effects should first be managed, if possible, by using symptomatic treatment (e.g., antiemetics and antidiarrheals). Alternatively, substitution of one drug for another in the same therapeutic class may reduce symptoms. For example, tenofovir or abacavir may be used to replace zidovudine in patients with gastrointestinal symptoms or anemia.(US DHHS HIV treatment guidelines 2011) Changing drug classes altogether is also an option in patients who experience side effects with multiple alternative drugs within the same class.

5.3 Pharmacokinetic parameters

The risk for treatment failure is increased if the patient is not taking the medication correctly (e.g., with or without food and otherwise, as directed). Similarly, treatment may fail if the patient is taking other medications, prescription or over the counter, that may affect drug absorption or metabolism (e.g., proton pump inhibitors).

The effect of natural health products, such as herbs and vitamins, is underappreciated as a source of potentially detrimental interactions with antiretroviral treatment. Data suggest that more than two thirds of HIV patients take natural or alternative health products, (Rivera, et al., J Natl Med Assoc 2005) and that many physicians are not aware of their patients' use of "natural" or alternative health products. The complexities of accounting for interactions between these products and antiretroviral treatments are compounded by the fact that natural health products are not produced to a generally accepted standard, and there may be wide variability in potency between and within brands. Moreover, many natural health products are complex mixtures that may contain components that influence drug metabolizing enzymes and drug transporters.(Lee LS, et al. CID 2006) Table 1 presents some known interactions between antiretroviral drugs and natural health products.

5.4 Drug resistance

When noncompliance, side effects and toxicities, and potential pharmacokinetic interactions have been excluded, drug resistance should be considered. Resistance testing should be performed while the patient is still on the failing regimen or within 4 weeks of discontinuation, and before starting a new regimen. In general, changing therapy for virologic failure is warranted for detectable viremia >1000 copies/mL. Some authorities suggest a more aggressive approach, in which therapy is changed for any repeated, detectable viremia (e.g., two consecutive HIV RNA >50 copies/mL after suppression to <50 copies/mL in a patient receiving antiretroviral treatment), but this is not routine practice.(http://aidsinfo.nih.gov)

5.4.1 Drug resistance testing

Resistance testing may be accomplished through genotype or phenotype testing. Two types of resistance assays are available in clinical practice. Genotypic assays involve sequencing HIV-1 genes to detect mutations that confer HIV-1 drug resistance, whereas phenotypic assays use cell-culture based viral replication assays in the presence and absence of drugs.

	St. John's wort	*Echinacea*	*Milk thistle*	*Garlic*	*Vitamin E*
PIs	Should not be coadministered; may cause significant decrease in PI levels	Possible interaction; echinacea may interact with ARVs that are CYP 3A4 or CYP 2C9 substrates	Possible interaction, except for indinavir; milk thistle may inhibit CYP3A4	Possible interaction; garlic may inhibit CYP3A4 GI toxicity has been reported with coadministration of garlic and ritonavir	Should not be coadministered with tipranavir/ritonavir; may increase the risk of bleeding
NNRTIs	Should not be coadministered; may cause significant decrease in NNRTI levels (including etravirine)	Possible interaction; echinacea may interact with ARVs that are CYP 3A4 or CYP 2C9 substrates	Possible interaction; milk thistle may inhibit CYP 3A4	Possible interaction; garlic may inhibit CYP 3A4	Unknown
NRTIs	No evidence for interaction	No evidence for interaction	No evidence for interaction	No evidence for interaction	No evidence for interaction
Integrase inhibitor (raltegravir)	No evidence for interaction	No evidence for interaction	No evidence for interaction	No evidence for interaction	No evidence for interaction
CCR5 antagonist (maraviroc)	Coadministration not recommended; expected to decrease maraviroc concentrations	Possible interaction; echinacea may interact with ARVs that are CYP 3A4 and CYP 2C9 substrates	Possible interaction; milk thistle may inhibit CYP 3A4	Possible interaction; garlic may inhibit CYP 3A4	No evidence for interaction

Table 1. Known Interactions Between Antiretroviral (ARV) Therapies and Natural Health Products
CYP, cytochrome P; GI, gastrointestinal; NNRTI, non-nucleoside reverse transcriptase inhibitor; NRTI, nucleoside reverse transcriptase inhibitor; PI, protease inhibitor.
(Reyataz, Intelence, Aptivus, & Selzentry package inserts; Gorski, et al., 2004; Mills, et al., 2005; Venkataramanan, et al., 2000; Foster, et al., 2001; Laroche, et al., 1998; Lee, et al., 2006)

Both tests can accurately identify resistance only in the predominant virus in patients, so a substantial proportion of the circulating virus may be resistant even in patients with negative results.(Schuurman, et al., J Clin Microbiol 1999) Furthermore, drug resistance testing is limited, because it does not predict the activity of antiretroviral agents when used in combination and requires a viral load >1000. Also, it only reveals resistance based on drug pressure, so it is important to consider all prior genotype tests, as these mutations will remain, even if not currently detectable. In addition to these methods, "virtual phenotyping" utilizes

genotype data to evaluate *in vitro* drug susceptibility of the virus; for most antiretroviral agents, this test predicts actual phenotypic resistance.(Perez-Elias, et al., Antivir Ther 2003)
Despite limitations, the preponderance of evidence suggests an advantage for the use of genotypic testing over standard of care in the selection of regimens for patients with treatment failure.(Hirsch, et al., CID 2003) Compared with standard of care, the patients allocated to the genotyping arms of these studies had substantially greater decreases in plasma HIV RNA levels and were more likely to achieve undetectable HIV RNA levels. In contrast, trials of phenotypic testing versus standard of care have not produced such clear-cut results, with variable outcomes in different studies. (Hirsch, CID 2003; Melnick, et al., abstract #786 CROI 2000; Cohen, et al., AIDS 2002; Torti, et al., CID 2005; Dunn, et al., JAIDS, 2005; Vray, et al., 2003; Wegner, et al., CID 2004). A recent clinical study compared outcomes in patients randomly assigned to either genotypic testing or genotypic plus virtual phenotypic testing. (Hales, et al, PLoS Clin Trials 2006) After 48 weeks, no significant differences were observed between the two groups in terms of mean change from baseline plasma HIV RNA and mean change from baseline CD4+ cell count, suggesting that resistance testing with genotyping alone is sufficient for the management of HIV infection. Tables 2, 3, and 4 indicate resistance mutations for the three major classes of antiretrovirals.

6. 2011 Guidelines for the management of treatment-experienced patients

When selecting appropriate treatment, all resistance testing should be considered, as should the patient's treatment history, comorbidities, concomitant medications, and prior intolerance. Treatment should be individualized based on these factors.
In patients with limited prior treatment but with no resistance, the potential for nonadherence should be evaluated and strongly considered. Resumption of the same regimen or initiation of a new regimen should be considered, with genotypic testing within 4 - 6 weeks to determine whether a resistant viral strain emerges if viral suppression cannot be achieved. In patients with limited prior treatment who are receiving protease inhibitors (PIs), thought should be given to intensifying one drug or boosting. The primary goal of therapy is to resuppress HIV RNA levels to undetectable levels and to prevent further selection of resistance mutations. (http://aidsinfo.nih.gov)
In patients with limited prior treatment and recognized drug resistance, maximal HIV RNA suppression (e.g., to <50 copies/mL) is required to prevent the selection of additional resistance mutations. (Thompson, et al, 2010; http://aidsinfo.nih.gov) Changes in the treatment regimen should be considered to minimize selection of resistance mutations. New regimens should include ≥2 active agents. (Thompson, et al, 2010; http://aidsinfo.nih.gov)
Resistance mutations for nucleoside analog reverse transcriptase inhibitors (NRTIs), non-NRTIs (NNRTIs), and PIs are noted in Tables 2, 3, and 4, respectively. Effects of Protease mutations are noted in Table 5.
In patients with extensive prior treatment and drug resistance, maximal viral suppression is warranted to prevent the accumulation of additional resistance mutations. Antiretroviral drugs from newer classes should be considered. If viral suppression is impossible to achieve, the primary goal is to preserve immunologic function and prevent clinical progression. When a new regimen with two fully active agents cannot be identified, it is reasonable to observe the patient on the same regimen rather than changing the regimen, depending on the stage of HIV disease. (Thompson, et al, 2010; http://aidsinfo.nih.gov)
Patients with significant treatment experience and drug-resistant virus can often still achieve undetectable viral loads and the goal is still to reestablish suppression of the virus.

NRTI	*Resistance mutations* (IAS-USA)	*Mutations associated with reduced* RC
All currently approved NRTIs	69 insertion complex: M41L, A62V, 69 insert, K70R, L210W, T215Y/F, K219Q/E	
All currently approved NRTIs except tenofovir	151 complex: A62V, V75I, F77L, F116Y, Q151M	Q151M
All currently approved NRTIs	Thymidine analogue-associated mutations (TAMs): M41L, D67N, K70R, L210W, T215Y/F, K219Q/E	
Abacavir	K65R, L74V, Y115F, M184V	K65R, M184V
Didanosine	K65R, L74V	K65R
Emtricitabine	K65R, M184V/I	K65R, M184V
Lamivudine	K65R, M184V/I	K65R, M184V
Stavudine	M41L, D67N, K70R, L210W, T215Y/F, K219O/E	
Tenofovir	K65R, K70E	K65R
Zidovudine	M41L, D67N, K70R, L10W, T215Y/F, K219Q/E	

Table 2. NRTI resistance mutations
IAS, International Aids Society; NRTI, nucleoside reverse transcriptase inhibitor; RC, replicative capacity.
(Johnson, et al., 2009; Garcia-Perez, et al., 2005; Girardet, et al., 2007; White, et al., 2002)

NNRTI	*Resistance mutations* (IAS-USA)	*Mutations associated with reduced* RC
Delavirdine	K103N, V106M, Y181C, Y188L, P236L	V106A, G190C/S/E/Q/V/T, P225H, M230L, and P236L
Efavirenz	L100I, K103N, V106M, V108I, Y181C/I, Y188L, G190S/A, P225H	V106A, G190C/S/E/Q/V/T, P225H, M230L, and P236L
Nevirapine	L100I, K103N, V106A/M, V108I, Y181C/I, Y188C/L/H, G190A	V106A, G190C/S/E/Q/V/T, P225H, M230L, and P236L

Table 3. NNRTI Resistance Mutations
NNRTI, non-nucleoside reverse transcriptase inhibitor; RC, replicative capacity.
(Johnson, et al., 2009; Archer, et al., 2000; Huang, et al., 2003; Wirden, et al., 2003)

(US DHHS HIV management guidelines) NRTIs, in particular, have been shown to retain antiviral activity in patients with drug-resistant virus. Moreover, continued use of both NRTIs and PIs can select for drug-resistance mutations that reduce viral fitness. (Deeks, et al., 2005)
If complete viral suppression is not feasible, the goals of treatment should be maintenance or improvement of CD4+ cell count and preventing clinical progression. Discontinuation is not recommended unless the patient has a high CD4+ count. Data suggest that partial virologic suppression of >0.5 to 1.0 $\log_{10}$ copies/mL below baseline is associated with clinical benefit; larger and more sustained reductions in HIV RNA are directly correlated with lower risk for disease progression. (Murray, et al., 1999) In addition, a "holding regimen" will maintain poor viral fitness. For example, the M184V mutation, which increases resistance to lamivudine and emtricitabine, decreases viral fitness and increases

the antiviral activity of zidovudine, stavudine, and tenofovir. (Whitcomb, et al., 2003) Therefore, maintaining this resistance mutation by continuing lamivudine or emtricitabine can enhance the effect of zidovudine, stavudine, and/or tenofovir. (Wegner, et al., CID 2004)

Protease inhibitor	*Major resistance mutations* (IAS-USA)	*Mutations associated with reduced* RC
Atazanavir +/- ritonavir	I50L, I84V, N88S	I50L
Fosamprenavir/ritonavir	I50V, I84V	I50V, I84V
Darunavir/ritonavir	I47V, I50V, I54M/L, L76V, I84V	
Indinavir/ritonavir	M46I/L, V82A/F/T, I84V	
Lopinavir/ritonavir	V32I, I47V/A, L76V, V82A/F/T/S	
Nelfinavir	D30N, L90M	D30N, N88S, L90M
Saquinavir/ritonavir	G48V, L90M	
Tipranavir/ritonavir	I47V, Q58E, T74P, V82L/T, I84V	

Table 4. Major Protease Inhibitor Resistance Mutations
IAS, International Aids Society; RC, replicative capacity.
(Johnson, et al., 2009; Archer, et al., 2000; Martinez-Picado, et al., 1999; Prado, et al., 2002; Resch, et al., 2002; Wirden, et al., 2003; Reyataz prescribing information)

In some highly treatment-experienced patients, the addition of enfuvirtide should also be considered. In the T-20 versus Optimized Regimen Only (TORO) studies, adding enfuvirtide to an optimized background regimen was associated with significant antiretroviral and immunologic benefit in patients with >6 months of previous treatment with agents in three classes of antiretroviral drugs and/or resistance to drugs in these classes.(Lalezari, et al., 2003) Notably, enfuvirtide is most effective when given with other active drugs. As shown in the TORO study, enfuvirtide monotherapy is associated with a high rate of emerging resistance. (Lalezari, et al., 2003)
DHHS guidelines indicate no consensus on how to define or treat immunologic failure in the setting of a virologic response. (US DHHS HIV management guidelines) Patients with discordant responses (e.g., undetectable HIV RNA but low CD4+ cell counts) should continue to receive their current treatment, unless they are taking zidovudine or didanosine, which have been shown to be myelosuppressive. However, time to immune response is variable and may even take years. In these cases, changing these drugs, if possible, is recommended. Additionally, changing trimethoprim-sulfamethoxazole prophylaxis to dapsone or aerosolized pentamidine may be warranted in this group in order to enhance immunologic response further. This should be considered prior to changing an antiretroviral regimen that is successfully suppressing viral load.

7. Beyond the guidelines: Investigational therapeutic approaches

Numerous permutations of various treatment strategies have been attempted. Below are several of the more commonly investigated therapeutic approaches.

7.1 Structured treatment interruptions

The CPCRA 064 study found that there was an increased risk of death, a long-term negative effect on CD4+ cell count, and no virologic or clinical benefit associated with a structured treatment interruption.(Lawrence, et al., 2006) Based on these, it is advised to not discontinue an ARV regimen in an adherent patient except for in the presence of drug resistance and when awaiting genotype results.

7.2 Double-boosted PIs

Double-boosted PIs (two PIs plus ritonavir) may be clinically effective by increasing blood levels to the point where resistance is overcome.(Staszewski, et al., 2006) This approach raises major issues, however, in terms of drug interactions and may be suitable only for patients who have exhausted all other options. This is not strongly advised or recommended and the patient should be referred to an HIV specialist.

7.3 Mega-HAART

Multiple-drug rescue therapy (e.g., >5 antiretrovirals) has the complication of severe drug interactions. Thus, this is a last resort in highly selected patients and should be managed by an HIV specialist.(Montaner, et al., 2001)

8. New treatment options

Over the past 3 years, a number of new treatment options have been approved by the US Food and Drug Administration, including drugs from entirely new classes: maraviroc, a CCR5 antagonist, and raltegravir, an integrase inhibitor. Drug interactions of these newly approved agents are summarized in Table 6.

Effect	TPV	LPV	ATV	DRV
Decreased virologic response	no firm data	6 or more mutations	Increasing number of mutations	I47V, I54M, T74P, I84V
High level resistance	no firm data	7 - 8 mutations; I47A, V32I; L76V+3 mutations	I50L, I84V, N88S	3+of: V11I, V32I, L33F, I47V, I50V I54M/L, G73S, L76V, I84V, L89V
Possible increased virologic response	L24I, I50L/V, F53Y/L/W, I54L, L76V		M46I + L76V without other mutations	V82A

Table 5. Impact of Protease Inhibitor Resistance Mutations: Effects of different PI mutations on different PIs

*ATV, atazanavir; DRV, darunavir; LPV, lopinavir; TPV, tipranavir. PI, Protease Inhibitor (Norton, et al., 2008; DeMeyer, et al., 2009; Descamps, et al., 2009; Mo, et al., 2005; Friend, et al., 2004; Kagan, et al., 2005; Rhee, et al., 2010; Schapiro, et al., 2010, and Marcelin, et al., 2008; all as cited by Johnson, et al., 2010)

8.1 Newer protease inhibitors

In the RESIST-1 and RESIST-2 trials (Randomized Evaluation of Strategic Intervention in Multidrug Resistant Patients with Tipranavir), tipranavir-ritonavir plus optimized best regimen provided superior virologic and immunologic responses over 48 weeks compared with patients who received an investigator-selected ritonavir-boosted comparator PI plus optimized background regimen. (Hicks, et al., 2006) Gastrointestinal disorders, transaminitis, and hyperlipidemia were more frequent in patients who received tipranavir-ritonavir compared with the control group. Tipranavir carries black-box warnings regarding the risk for hepatitis and hepatic decompensation as well as fatal and non-fatal intracranial hemorrhage. (Aptivus package insert, Boehringer Ingelheim Pharmaceuticals 2008) Tipranavir's unique resistance profile makes it valuable in patients who have failed prior PI-containing regimens. (Marcelin, et al., 2008) Tipranavir is approved for highly treatment-experienced HIV patients or those with multiple PI resistance mutations.

Ritonavir-boosted darunavir has shown superiority to boosted comparator PIs in treatment-experienced patients, including those with PI mutations. (Clotet, et al., 2007) The POWER 1, POWER 2, and POWER 3 (Performance Of TMC114/r When evaluated in treatment-Experienced patients with PI Resistance) studies found 40%−44% attained viral suppression among treatment-experienced patients who had previously failed other PI-based regimens. Thus, darunavir is also valuable in patients with significant resistance. (Lefebvre, et al., Abstract H-1387, ICAAC 2006) Darunavir is approved for both treatment-experienced and treatment-naïve patients. Table 5 shows the impact of protease mutations on resistance to various PIs.

8.2 New non-NRTI

The DUET 1 and 2 (TMC125-0216: a phase 3 study to investigate the efficacy, tolerability, and safety of TMC125(etravirine) as part of an antiretroviral regimen, with optimized background regimen in HIV-1 infected patients with limited to no treatment options) trials examined the efficacy of etravirine, a second-generation NNRTI, in treatment-experienced adult patients with virological failure on stable antiretroviral therapy and documented genotypic evidence of NNRTI resistance, viral load >5000 copies/mL, and ≥3 primary PI mutations.(Lazzarin, et al., 2007; Madruga, et al., 2007) Etravirine was associated with superior virologic suppression compared with placebo, with up to 62% of patients in the etravirine group achieving undetectable viral loads, compared with 44% in the placebo group. (Lazzarin, et al., 2007; Madruga, et al., 2007) Etravirine exhibits retained activity despite multiple NNRTI mutations, with high rates of sustained efficacy at 48 weeks in heavily treatment-experienced patients. (Haubrich, et al, Abstract #790, CROI 2008; Johnson M, et al., Abstract #792, CROI, 2008) The tolerability profile is comparable to placebo, with the exception of a rash. It is associated with significant drug interactions and should not be used with unboosted PIs, boosted atazanavir, fosamprenavir, tipranavir, or other NNRTIs.[49](Intelence package insert, Tibotech Therapeutics 2008) The mutation Y181 decreases susceptibility to etravirine, but does not eliminate efficacy altogether. (Johnson, et al, 2010; http://aidsinfo.nih.gov)

8.3 New class: CCR5 antagonist

Maraviroc, the first drug in this class to be licensed, is active against chemokine receptor R5- but not X4-tropic viruses in vitro. In the MOTIVATE 1 and MOTIVATE 2 (Maraviroc versus Optimized Therapy in Viremic Antiretroviral Treatment-Experienced Patients) trials, patients who had R5-tropic virus and had been treated with or had resistance to three antiretroviral drug classes, and had HIV RNA >5000 copies/mL, demonstrated increased CD4+ counts and more sustained viral suppression at 48 weeks following treatment with maraviroc compared with placebo, and with comparable adverse event outcomes. (Gulick, et al., 2008) Maraviroc is not effective in patients with mixed-tropic virus infection; it is indicated for the treatment of patients infected with only CCR5-tropic HIV who are either treatment naïve, or who have evidence of viral replication and HIV strains resistant to multiple antiretroviral agents.(Selzentry package insert, Pfizer, Inc.) Patients that may benefit from having a regimen including maraviroc can be identified via any of several assays available to assess the presence of the CCR5 tropic virus and the minority CXCR4 (X4) strains. (Reeves, et al., Abstract H-1026, ICAAC, 2007)

8.4 New class: Integrase inhibitor

Raltegravir, the first-in-class integrase inhibitor, was examined in combination with optimized background regimen in two identical, placebo-controlled trials in patients infected with triple-class drug-resistant HIV-1 in whom antiretroviral therapy had failed. (Steigbigel, et al., 2008) At 48 weeks of therapy, 62.1% and 32.9% of raltegravir and placebo patients, respectively, had suppressed HIV RNA viral load. Raltegravir is approved in combination with other antiretroviral agents for the treatment of HIV infection in treatment-naïve or treatment-experienced adult patients who have evidence of viral replication and HIV-1 strains resistant to multiple antiretroviral agents. (Isentress package insert, Merck & Co)

9. Drugs under investigation

A new integrase inhibitor, Dolutegravir (Glaxo Smith Kline) is in phase 2 clinical trials and is active against raltegravir-resistant strains, revealing a higher genetic barrier to resistance (Seki, et al., abstract #555, CROI 2010; Eron, et al., abstract #151LB, CROI 2011).

GSK2248761 is a once daily NNRTI currently in phase 2b studies with activity against virus with many NNRTI mutations, including efavirenz resistant strains. (Kim, et al., abstract #628, CROI 2011; Kim, et al., abstract #631, CROI 2011) In addition, this drug appears to have an additive to synergistic antiviral effect when coadministered with other antiretrovirals. (Vavro, et al. abstract #520, CROI 2011)

BI-C is a non-cataytic site integrase inhibitor that may have activity against virus resistant to other integrase inhibitors. It has shown very good biological and pharmacological profiles and is now in Phase 1 clinical trials. (Fenwick, et al., abstract #523, CROI 2011)

9.1 New classes(future)

These are not currently approved and have yet to start Phase 3 clinical trials, however, they show promise as potential future new drug classes. Their possible addition to the current arsenal of antiretrovirals is particularly important for the treatment experienced patient.

9.1.1 Attachment inhibitors

Currently in very early trials, this class shows the possibility for potent antiretroviral activity against HIV-1 infection. (Nettles, et al., abstract #49, CROI 2011). New targets include the gp 120 glycoprotein, which allows attachment of virus to CD4+ cells. (Nowicka-Sans, et al., abstract #518, CROI 2011)

9.1.2 Gag inhibitors

Another potentially new class of antiviral drugs being investigated are gag inhibitors. This drug targets the HIV-1 capsid and exhibited inhibition of the early phase of its life cycle. (Urano, et al., abstract #525, CROI 2011)

	Interactions with other ARVs	*Selected interactions with non-ARV drugs*
Etravirine	Should not be coadministered with: • Tipranavir/ritonavir • Fosamprenavir/ritonavir • Atazanavir/ritonavir • Unboosted PIs • NNRTIs Dose adjustment not established with Saquinavir, consider Saquinavir 1000mg bid + Ritonavir 100mg bid If with Maraviroc: MVC 600mg bid MVC 150mg bid (if with Ritonavir boosted darunavir)	Drug concentration monitoring recommended when used with antiarrythmics INR monitoring recommended when used with warfarin; clopidogrel should not be coadministered Certain anticonvulsants, including carabamazepine, phenobarbital, and phenytoin, can cause significant decreases in etravirine plasma concentrations Dose adjustments may be necessary for coadministration with itraconazole, ketoconazole, voriconazole; coadminister with caution and follow drug levels Clarithromycin alternatives should be considered Rifampin, rifapentine, and rifabutin may cause significant decreases in etravirine plasma concentrations Etravirine may increase plasma concentrations of diazepam , dose adjustment may be necessary Dexamethasone should be used with caution, as etravirine levels may decrease. Interaction with certain statins has been detected Etravirine may be coadministered with methadone; however, clinical monitoring for withdrawal symptoms is recommended, as methadone maintenance therapy may need to be adjusted Administer with immunosuppressants with caution; levels of cyclosporine, tacrolimus, and sirolimus may be decreased
Raltegravir	No effect expected on the following drug classes: PIs, NNRTIs that would	No effect expected on methadone, opioid analgesics, statins, azole antifungals,

	require dose adjustments No clinically meaningful effect on lamivudine, tenofovir Recommended dose of raltegravir may be coadministered with efavirenz, nevirapine Recommended dose of raltegravir may be coadministered with boosted tipranavir or atazanavir	proton pump inhibitors, oral contraceptives, anti-erectile dysfunction agents Caution recommended when coadministering with rifampin; reduces plasma concentrations of raltegravir Recommended dose of raltegravir may be coadministered with rifabutin ; recommend 800 mg twice daily with coadministered rifampin
Maraviroc	Dose reduction to 150 mg twice daily with PIs (except tipranavir/ritonavir), delaviridine No dose adjustment (300 mg twice daily) with tipranavir/ritonavir, nevirapine, NRTIs Dose increase to 600 mg twice daily with CYP 3A inducers including efavirenz No effect on zidovudine, lamivudine	Dose reduction to 150 mg twice daily with ketoconazole, itraconazole, clarithromycin, other strong CYP 3A inhibitors (e.g., nefazadone, telithromycin) Dose increase to 600 mg twice daily with CYP 3A inducers including rifampin, carbamazepine, phenobarbital, phenytoin No clinically relevant effect on midazolam, oral contraceptives (ethinylestradiol and levonorgestrel)

Table 6. Drug Interactions of Newly Approved Antiretroviral Therapies
ARV, antiretroviral; INR, International Normalized Ratio; CYP, cytochrome; NNRTI, non-nucleoside reverse transcriptase inhibitor; NRTI, nucleoside reverse transcriptase inhibitor; PI, protease inhibitor.
(Aptivus, Invirase, Isentress, Kaletra, Lexiva, Prezista, Reyataz, Selzentry, Sustiva, Viracept, and Viramune prescribing information)

10. Conclusion

Managing treatment-experienced patients poses considerable challenges, not the least of which includes selecting appropriate therapy to maximize clinical benefit, minimize toxicities, and avoid drug-drug interactions. The best approach to these patients is preventative. As noted above, with appropriate attention to medication adherence and addressing the side effects and toxicities of antiretroviral medications proactively, many patients can remain on the first regimen for many years. In the real world, however, a substantial proportion of patients fail to adhere to their medication. Many suffer from overt toxicities and/or minor/cosmetic side effects that affect compliance with treatment and eventually necessitate a switch in regimen. Given the broad spectrum of available agents—including the recent advent of two entirely new classes of antiretroviral agents—the majority of patients have reasonably well-tolerated therapeutic options that, with appropriate attention to all aspects of the clinical and patient experience, can provide sufficient long-term efficacy which has transformed HIV from an inevitably fatal disease to one that can truly be considered a chronic condition.

11. Author disclosure statement

Gail Reid has no competing financial interests.
Richard Novak has been the Recipient of Research Grants from Merck, GlaxoSmithKline, and Abbott Laboratories.

12. References

Ammassari, A., R. Murri, et al. (2001). "Self-reported symptoms and medication side effects influence adherence to highly active antiretroviral therapy in persons with HIV infection." J Acquir Immune Defic Syndr 28(5): 445-9.

Ammassari, A. A., F. Starace, et al. (2003). "Medication adherence among HIV+ adults: effects of cognitive dysfunction and regimen complexity." Neurology 61(5): 723-4; author reply 724.

Boehringer Ingelheim Pharmaceuticals (2008). "Aptivus Prescribing Information."

Bristol-Meyers Squibb Inc (2008). "Reyataz Prescribing Information."

Clotet, B., N. Bellos, et al. (2007). "Efficacy and safety of darunavir-ritonavir at week 48 in treatment-experienced patients with HIV-1 infection in POWER 1 and 2: a pooled subgroup analysis of data from two randomised trials." Lancet 369(9568): 1169-78.

Cohen, C. J., S. Hunt, et al. (2002). "A randomized trial assessing the impact of phenotypic resistance testing on antiretroviral therapy." Aids 16(4): 579-88.

d'Arminio Monforte, A., A. C. Lepri, et al. (2000). "Insights into the reasons for discontinuation of the first highly active antiretroviral therapy (HAART) regimen in a cohort of antiretroviral naive patients. I.CO.N.A. Study Group. Italian Cohort of Antiretroviral-Naive Patients." Aids 14(5): 499-507.

Deeks, S. G., J. D. Barbour, et al. (2002). "Duration and predictors of CD4 T-cell gains in patients who continue combination therapy despite detectable plasma viremia." Aids 16(2): 201-7.

Deeks, S. G., R. Hoh, et al. (2005). "Interruption of treatment with individual therapeutic drug classes in adults with multidrug-resistant HIV-1 infection." J Infect Dis 192(9): 1537-44.

Archer RH, Dykes C, Gerondelis P, et al. Mutants of human immunodeficiency virus type 1 (HIV-1) reverse transcriptase resistant to nonnucleoside reverse transcriptase inhibitors demonstrate altered rates of RNase H cleavage that correlate with HIV-1 replication fitness in cell culture. J Virol. 2000 Sep;74(18):8390-401.

Dunn DT, Green H, et al. (2005). "A randomized controlled trial of the value of phenotypic testing in addition to genotypic testing for HIV drug resistance: evaluation of resistance assays (ERA) trial invetigators."Journal of Acquired Immune Deficiency Syndrome. 38:553-9.

Eron, J., Kumar, P., Lazzarin, A., Richmond, G., Soriano, V., Huang, J., Vavro., C., Ait-Khaled, M., Min, S., and Yeo., J. "DTG in Subjects with HIV Exhibiting RAL Resistance: Functional Monotherapy Results of VIKING Study Cohort II" Abstract #151LB, CROI 2011.

Fenwick, C, Bethel, R, Bonneau, P., et al., "Identification of BI-C, a Novel HIV-1 Non-catalytic Site Integrase Inhibitor." abstract #523, CROI 2011, Boston.

Foster, B. C., M. S. Foster, et al. (2001). "An in vitro evaluation of human cytochrome P450 3A4 and P-glycoprotein inhibition by garlic." J Pharm Pharm Sci 4(2): 176-84.

Garcia-Perez J, Sanchez-Palomino S, Perez-Olmeda M, Fernandez B, Alcami J. (2007). A new strategy based on recombinant viruses as a tool for assessing drug susceptibility of human immunodeficiency virus type 1.J Med Virol. 79:127-37.

Gibbie, T., M. Hay, et al. (2007). "Depression, social support and adherence to highly active antiretroviral therapy in people living with HIV/AIDS." Sex Health 4(4): 227-32.

Gorski, J. C., S. M. Huang, et al. (2004). "The effect of echinacea (Echinacea purpurea root) on cytochrome P450 activity in vivo." Clin Pharmacol Ther 75(1): 89-100.

Gulick, R. M., J. Lalezari, et al. (2008). "Maraviroc for previously treated patients with R5 HIV-1 infection." N Engl J Med 359(14): 1429-41.

Hales, G., C. Birch, et al. (2006). "A randomised trial comparing genotypic and virtual phenotypic interpretation of HIV drug resistance: the CREST study." PLoS Clin Trials 1(3): e18.

Hammer, S. M., J. J. Eron, Jr., et al. (2008). "Antiretroviral treatment of adult HIV infection: 2008 recommendations of the International AIDS Society-USA panel." JAMA 300(5): 555-70.

Haubrich, R, Cahn, P, Grinsztejn, B., et al., "DUET-1: Week 48 Results of a pase III Randomized double blind trial to evaluate the efficacy and safety of TMC125 vs placebo in 612 treatment experienced HIV-1 infected patients." abstract #790, CROI, 2008, Boston.

Hicks, CB, Cahn, P, cooper, DA, et al. (2006) "Durable efficacy of tipranavir-ritonavir in combination with an optimised background regimen of antiretroviral drugs for treatment-experienced HIV-1 infected patients at 48 weeks in the Randomized Evaluation of Strategic Intervention in multi-drug reSistant patients with Tipranavir (RESIST) studies: an analysis of combined data from two randomised open-label trials. Lancet 368:466-475.

Hirsch, M. S., F. Brun-Vezinet, et al. (2003). "Antiretroviral drug resistance testing in adults infected with human immunodeficiency virus type 1: 2003 recommendations of an International AIDS Society-USA Panel." Clin Infect Dis 37(1): 113-28.

Johnson, M, Campbell, T, Clotet, B., et al. "DUET-2: Week 48 Results of a Phase III Randomized double blind Trial to Evaluate the Efficacy and Safety of TMC125 vs Placebo in 591 Treatment experienced HIV-1 infected patients . Abstract #792. CROI, 2008, Boston.

Johnson VA, Brun-Vézinet F, Clotet B, et al. (2010) Update of the Drug Resistance Mutations in HIV-1: December 2010. Top HIV Med. 18;5: 156-163

Joint United Nations Program on HIV/AIDS (2008). "Report on the global AIDS epidemic. Available at: http://www.unaids.org/en/KnowledgeCentre/HIVData/GlobalReport/2008/2008_Global_report.asp. Accessed 6 December 2008."

Kalichman, S. C., S. Catz, et al. (1999). "Barriers to HIV/AIDS treatment and treatment adherence among African-American adults with disadvantaged education." J Natl Med Assoc 91(8): 439-46.

Kim, J, Wire, MB, Lovern, M.. "Dose seclection for Phase IIb studies of GSK2248761, a next generation NNRTI, using PK/PD/VD Model and Trial Simulation." abstract #628, CROI, 2011, Boston.

Kim, J, Gould, E, Lou, Y, Piscitelli, S. "Lack of drug-drug interaction between the NRRTI GSK2248761 and RAL." abstract #631, CROI, 2011, Boston.

Lalezari, J. P., K. Henry, et al. (2003). "Enfuvirtide, an HIV-1 fusion inhibitor, for drug-resistant HIV infection in North and South America." N Engl J Med 348(22): 2175-85.

Laroche, M. and S. Choudhri (1998). "Severe gastrointestinal toxicity with concomitant ingestion of ritonavir and garlic." Can J Infect Dis 9(Suppl A): 76A.

Lawrence, J., K. H. Hullsiek, et al. (2006). "Disadvantages of structured treatment interruption persist in patients with multidrug-resistant HIV-1: final results of the CPCRA 064 study." J Acquir Immune Defic Syndr 43(2): 169-78.

Lazzarin, A., T. Campbell, et al. (2007). "Efficacy and safety of TMC125 (etravirine) in treatment-experienced HIV-1-infected patients in DUET-2: 24-week results from a randomised, double-blind, placebo-controlled trial." Lancet 370(9581): 39-48.

Lee, L. S., A. S. Andrade, et al. (2006). "Interactions between natural health products and antiretroviral drugs: pharmacokinetic and pharmacodynamic effects." Clin Infect Dis 43(8): 1052-9.

Lefebvre, E., M. De Bethune, et al. (2006). "Impact of use of TPV, LPV & (f)APV at screening on TMC114/r virologic response in treatment-experienced patients in POWER 1,2, & 3. Interscience Conference on Antimicrobial Agents and Chemotherapy 2006. Abstract no. H-1387."

Lucas, G. M. (2005). "Antiretroviral adherence, drug resistance, viral fitness and HIV disease progression: a tangled web is woven." J Antimicrob Chemother 55(4): 413-6.

Madruga, J. V., P. Cahn, et al. (2007). "Efficacy and safety of TMC125 (etravirine) in treatment-experienced HIV-1-infected patients in DUET-1: 24-week results from a randomised, double-blind, placebo-controlled trial." Lancet 370(9581): 29-38.

Marcelin, A. G., B. Masquelier, et al. (2008). "Tipranavir-ritonavir genotypic resistance score in protease inhibitor-experienced patients." Antimicrob Agents Chemother 52(9): 3237-43.

Melnick, D. A., J. Rosenthal, et al. "Impact of phenotypic antiretroviral drug resistance testing on the response to salvage antiretroviral therapy (ART) in heavily experienced patients. In: Program and abstracts of the 7th Conference on Retroviruses and Opportunistic Infections (San Francisco). Alexandria, VA: Foundation for Retrovirology and Human Health, 2000:222. Abstract no. 786."

Merck & Co (2008). "Isentress prescribing information."

Mills, E., K. Wilson, et al. (2005). "Milk thistle and indinavir: a randomized controlled pharmacokinetics study and meta-analysis." Eur J Clin Pharmacol 61(1): 1-7.

Mocroft, A., M. Youle, et al. (2001). "Reasons for modification and discontinuation of antiretrovirals: results from a single treatment centre." Aids 15(2): 185-94.

Montaner, J. S., P. R. Harrigan, et al. (2001). "Multiple drug rescue therapy for HIV-infected individuals with prior virologic failure to multiple regimens." Aids 15(1): 61-9.

Murray, J. S., M. R. Elashoff, et al. (1999). "The use of plasma HIV RNA as a study endpoint in efficacy trials of antiretroviral drugs." Aids 13(7): 797-804.

Nettles, R, Schurmann, D, Zhu, L, et al. "Pharmacodynamics, Safety, and Pharmacokinetics of BMS-663068: A Potentially First-in-class oral HIV Attachment Inhibitor." Abstract #49, CROI, 2011, Boston.

Nowicka-Sans, B, Gong, Y-F, Ho, H-T, et al., "Antiviral Activity of a New SMall Molecule HIV-1 Attachment Inhibitor, BMS-626529, the Parent of BMS-663068." abstract #518, CROI 2011, Boston.

Perez-Elias, M. J., I. Garcia-Arata, et al. (2003). "Agreement degree between simultaneous real phenotype and virtual phenotype in patients from the REALVIRFEN study. Abstract no 808." Antivir Ther 8(Suppl 1).

Petersen, M., Y. Wang, et al. (2007). "Pill-box organizers are associated with improved ARV adherence, and viral suppression and are cost effective. Conference on Retroviruses and Opportunistic Infections CROI 2007. Abstract no. 524."

Pfizer Inc (2007). "Selzentry Prescribing Information."

Piliero, PJ, Parkin, N, Mayers, D. "Impact of protease (PR) mutations L33F/I, V82A, I84V, and L90M on ritonavir (RTV)-boosted protease inhibitor susceptibility. abstract H-998, ICAAC, 2006, San Francisco.

Power, R., C. Koopman, et al. (2003). "Social support, substance use, and denial in relationship to antiretroviral treatment adherence among HIV-infected persons." AIDS Patient Care STDS 17(5): 245-52.

Reeves, JD, Han, D, Liu, Y, et al. "Enhancements to the Trofile HIV Coreceptor Tropism Assay Enable Reliable Detection of CXCR4-using subpopulations at less than 1%. " abstract #H-1026, ICAAC, 2007, Chicago.

Resch W, Ziermann R, Parkin N, Gamarnik A, Swanstrom R. (2002) Nelfinavir-resistant, amprenavir-hypersusceptible strains of human immunodeficiency virus type 1 carrying an N88S mutation in protease have reduced infectivity, reduced replication capacity, and reduced fitness and process the Gag polyprotein precursor aberrantly. J Virol. Sep;76(17):8659-66.

Rivera, J. O., A. Gonzalez-Stuart, et al. (2005). "Herbal product use in non-HIV and HIV-positive Hispanic patients." J Natl Med Assoc 97(12): 1686-91.

Schuurman, R., L. Demeter, et al. (1999). "Worldwide evaluation of DNA sequencing approaches for identification of drug resistance mutations in the human immunodeficiency virus type 1 reverse transcriptase." J Clin Microbiol 37(7): 2291-6.

Seki, T, Kobayashi, M, Wakasa-Morimoto, C., et al. "S/GSK1349572 Is a Potent Next Generation HIV Integrase Inhibitor and Demonstrates a Superior Resistance Profile Substantiated with 60 Integrase Mutant Molecular Clones." abstract #555, CROI, 2010, San Francisco.

Staszewski, S., E. Babacan, et al. (2006). "The LOPSAQ study: 48 week analysis of a boosted double protease inhibitor regimen containing lopinavir/ritonavir plus saquinavir without additional antiretroviral therapy." J Antimicrob Chemother 58(5): 1024-30.

Steigbigel, R. T., D. A. Cooper, et al. (2008). "Raltegravir with optimized background therapy for resistant HIV-1 infection." N Engl J Med 359(4): 339-54.

Thompson MA, Aberg JA, Cahn P, et al; International AIDS Society-USA. (2010) "Antiretroviral treatment of adult HIV infection: 2010 recommendations of the International AIDS Society-USA panel." JAMA 304;3:321−333.

Tibotech Therapeutics (2008). "Intellence prescribing information."

Torti C, Quiros-Roldan E, Regazzi M, et al. (2005) "A randomized controlled trial to evaluate antiretroviral salvage therapy guided by rules-based or phenotype-driven HIV-1 genotypic drug-resistance interpretation with or without concentration-controlled intervention: the Resistance and Dosage Adapted Regimens (RADAR) Study." Clinical Infectious Disease, 40: 1828-36

United States Department of Health and Human Services (US DHHS) Panel on Antiretroviral Guidelines for Adults and Adolescents (2008). "Guidelines for the use of antiretroviral agents in HIV-1-infected adults and adolescents. Available at: http://aidsinfo.nih.gov/contentfiles/AdultandAdolescentGL.pdf. Accessed 13 December 2008."

Urano, Emiko, Kuramochi, N, et al., "A Novel HIV-1 Inhibitor Targeting Gag Screened by Yeast Membrane-associated 2-hybrid System." abstract #525, CROI 2011, Boston.

Vavro, Cindy, Ferris, R, Edelstein M, Standring D, and StClair M. "GSK2248761 Retains potency against many NNRTI resiance mutants and is additive to synergistc in combination with other ART." abstract #520, CROI 2011, Boston.

Venkataramanan, R., V. Ramachandran, et al. (2000). "Milk thistle, a herbal supplement, decreases the activity of CYP3A4 and uridine diphosphoglucuronosyl transferase in human hepatocyte cultures." Drug Metab Dispos 28(11): 1270-3.

Vray M, Meynard JL, Dalban C, et al. (2003) "Predictors of the virological response to a change in the antiretroviral treatment regimen in HIV-1 infected patients enrolled in a randomized trial comparing genotyping, phenotyping and standard of care (Narval trial)". Antiviral Therapy. 8:427-34.

Wegner, S, Wallace, MR, Aronson, NE, et al. (2004) "Long-term efficacy of routine access to antiretroviral-resistance testing in HIV type I infected patients: results of the clinical efficacy of resistance testing trial." CID, 38:723-30.

Whitcomb, J. M., N. T. Parkin, et al. (2003). "Broad nucleoside reverse-transcriptase inhibitor cross-resistance in human immunodeficiency virus type 1 clinical isolates." J Infect Dis 188(7): 992-1000.

White KL, Margot NA, Wrin T, Petropoulos CJ, Miller MD, Naeger LK. (2002) "Molecular mechanisms of resistance to human immunodeficiency virus type 1 with reverse transcriptase mutations K65R and K65R+M184V and their effects on enzyme function and viral replication capacity. Antimicrob Agents Chemother. Nov;46(11):3437-46.

Wirden M, Simon A, Schneider L, et al. (2003) "Interruption of nonnucleoside reverse transcriptase inhibitor (NNRTI) therapy for 2 months has no effect on levels of human immunodeficiency virus type 1 in plasma of patients harboring viruses with mutations associated with resistance to NNRTIs." J Clin Microbiol. Jun;41(6):2713-5.

InforMatrix Nucleoside/Nucleotide Reverse Transcriptase Inhibitors "Backbones"

Gerrit Schreij[1] and Rob Janknegt[2]
[1]*Maastricht University Medical Centre, Maastricht*
[2]*Orbis Medical Centre, Sittard-Geleen*
The Netherlands

1. Introduction

InforMatrix is an interactive matrix model, in which pharmacotherapeutic strategies are supported in a rational manner by means of a transparent selection methodology. This is achieved through the use of an independent reporting made by interactive workshops in the field, in which participants are facilitated in the determination of their own preference.
The treatment of AIDS is directed by guidelines and continually being modified as a result of ongoing research and the arrival of new treatment options. The goal of this InforMatrix program on backbones of nucleoside/nucleotide reverse transcriptase inhibitors is to make a rational selection of a first choice medication possible. It is important in this to describe the selection process and to make this process transparent. The InforMatrix methodology is a tool in this, in which selection criteria are described; tested against the available literature and the various therapeutic alternatives evaluated as to their clinical value.
Below follows a short description of the InforMatrix methodology, of the subject, and a description of the various selection criteria.

1.1 InforMatrix methodology

InforMatrix is a so-called decision matrix technique, with which a group of experts in the subject determine, on the basis of criteria, an order of merit within various treatment options which have similar objectives. In this order of merit, the criteria are weighed against each other. After all, they do not all carry the same weight. Next, the various options per criterion are compared to each other. Data is necessary for this, both from literature as well as from own practice experience. The literature is tested by an independent ethisor for clinical value and evaluated per criterion.
The InforMatrix technique has six set criteria. These criteria are:

- *Effectiveness* (the actualization of positive outcomes and treatment goas)
- *Safety* (the avoidance of negative outcomes, such as hazardous side effects)
- *Tolerance* (the interruption of the care process due to less hazardous, generally transitory, but disturbing side effects)
- *Users' ease* (ease for the patient, for example, dosing frequency)
- *Usability* (what is the scope of the treatment freedom (interactions and such) and the ease for the caregiver)
- *Costs* (price per month)

These criteria are specifically described per selection subject ("operationalized").
The InforMatrix technique takes place in the following steps:

- Operationalization of the six criteria
- Literature synthesis
- Relative weighing of the six criteria
- Evaluation of the various treatment options on the basis of the literature and own knowledge and experience
- Synthesis of the weightings and evaluations in the selection matrix: calculation of order of merit

A group of experts in the field are requested to test the operationalization of the above six selection criteria in the framework of the treatment of HIV/AIDS in the care process for relevance. Following on to these selection aspects, the authors execute a literature synthesis. This results in a report, in which these means are evaluated on the basis of these selection criteria by a group of experts in the field. In this, the report is tested as far as its applicability in making a rational consideration of the treatment options possible.
The choice of nucleoside/nuclotide reverse transcriptase inhibitors and the assessment criteria
After the introduction of nucleoside/nuclotide reverse transcriptase inhibitors (NRTIs), the first antiretroviral drugs approved for the treatment of HIV, patients were initially treated with one drug (monotherapy) and later with two NRTIs (duotherapy). After the introduction of protease inhibitors effective treatment of the HIV infection was possible. This so called HAART (highly active antiretroviral therapy) initially consisted of a combination of 2NRTIs with a proteaseinhibitor (PI).
New classes of antiretrovirals have been developed and nowadays many more combinations of antiretrovirals are possible. A backbone therapy consisting of 2NRTIs in combination with a third drugs like a PI, a non-nucleoside reverse transcriptase inhibitor (NNRTI) or an integrase inhibitor is still chosen as an initial combination antiretroviral therapy (cART).
The treatment goal of cART is to attain an undetectable plasma viral HIV-1 load (VL), after which a recovery of immunity usually follows.
In a meta-analysis covering 64 clinical trials with in total 10,559 naive patients HAART consisting of 2NRTI/PI/ritonavir or 2NRTI/NNRTI both produce significantly higher percentages of patients with undetectable VL and a significantly higher increase of CD4 positive T-lymphocytescount (CD4 cell count) than cART consisting of 2NRTI/PI or 3NRTI **(1).**
Although stavudine (d4T) is a effective anti-retroviral drug, especially in combination with didanosine, its use is no longer recommended because of the increased change for the development of lipoatrophy during treatment and high rates of mitochondrial toxicity **(2).**
Combining ddI with tenofovir leads to a specific renal interaction causing high drug levels of didanosine and ddI toxicity resulting in decrease of CD4 cell count **(3)**. Lowering of ddI dosing leads to an increased change of developing virological failure **(4)**.
The following combinations are compared in this InforMatrix because they are recommended in the three major guidelines, the American DHHS Panel (December, 2009) **(5),** the European AIDS Clinical Society (November, 2009) **(6)** and the International AIDS Society-USA Panel **(7)**

a. Abacavir/lamivudine (fixed dose combination Kivexa® or Epzicom®) abbreviated as ABC/3TC

b. Didanosine/lamivudine or emtricitabine abbreviated as ddI/3TC or FTC
c. Tenofovir/emtricitabine (fixed dose combination Truvada®) abbreviated as TDF/FTC
d. Zidovudine/eamivudine (fixed dose combination Combivir®) abbreviated as ZVD/3TC

The following criteria and subcriteria were used:

1. Efficacy of anti-retroviral backbones
   1.1 Parameters of efficacy of anti-retroviral backbones
   1.2 Compliance, quality of life and durability of anti-retroviral backbones
   1.3 Development of resistance during treatment with anti-retroviral backbones
2. Safety of anti-retroviral backbones
   1.4 Grade 3 and 4, serious adverse events
   1.5 Documentation
3. Tolerability of anti-retroviral backbones
   1.6 Grade 1 and 2, mild to moderate adverse events
4. Easy of use
   1.7 Dosage frequency, number of tablets per day
5. Applicability
   1.8 Available strengths
   1.9 Drug interactions
   1.10 Approved indications
   1.11 Contra-indications
   1.12 Use in children and elderly
   1.13 Use in renal and hepatic disease
   1.14 Use in pregancy and lactation
   1.15 Special precautions
6. Cost

2. Efficacy of anti-retroviral backbones

2.1 Parameters of efficacy of anti-retroviral backbones

The efficacy of a cART, usually consisting of 2NRTIs in combination with a PI or NNRTI is judged by the results of its anti-retroviral efficacy, increase of CD4 cell count and change of developing resistance.

The combination of 3 NRTIs as initial therapy is no longer used since the availability of the results of the ACTG 5095 study **(8)**. Limited data are available on combinations of one NRTI + NNRTI+PI the so called NUC-sparing regimen or other combinations. In has been shown in meta-analyses that HAART consisting of 2NRTIs + PI, not combined with ritonavir (as a booster) is virologically and immunologically less effective than 2NRTIs+NNRTI or 2NRTIs + PI combined with ritonavir **(1)**.

The anti-retroviral efficacy of cART must lead to undetectable VL, less than 50 copies/mL (VL<50 c/mL), in older studies a pVL < 400 c/mL is used as measure of undetectability.

If the VL does not become undetectable this almost always leads to the development of resistance and to antiviral inefficacy of a certain drug or a whole class of drugs resulting in a decrease of the CD4 cells. This ongoing decrease in the number of CD4 cells leads to HIV related diseases, AIDS and death. The antiviral efficacy is one of the most important parameter for the efficacy of a certain regimen. Te so called "regimen failure" which is a

broader measure effectivity of an antiretroviral regimen includes not only virological failure but all other reaons for stopping a regimen such as adverse effects or death and indicates its clinical efficacy.
Studies in patients who are not pretreated (naive patients) and harbouring no significant resistant mutations provide the best indication of the antiviral and clinical efficacy.
The percentage of naive patients in a certain study after 48 weeks, but preferably longer, in the intent to treat analysis (ITT) showing a VL<50 c/mL, is regarded as the best parameter for clinical efficacy. Often missing data on participants (M) are considered as virologic failures (F) (ITT analysis M=F) **(5).**
Increase of CD4 cell count is of less importance as a parameter of efficacy, because an undetectable VL almost always leads to recovery of CD4 cell count and the mean increase in CD4 cell count is probably similar in the different strata of CD4 cell count when starting cART. For instance in the Athena Dutch cohort study the average increase in CD4 cell count after initiation of therapy was around 70 cells/mm^3 per year during seven years of continuous cART with an undetectable VL. In the first six months after start of cART the increase was on average around 140 cells/mm^3 . Patients starting cART when the CD4 cell count was above 500 cells/mm^3 had on average a lower increase CD4 cell of around 40 cells/mm^3 per year **(9).**
There are seven major randomized studies **(10-17)** comparing backbones combined with a similar third drug. The results of these comparative studies are summarised in Table 1.
In the three above mentioned guidelines two **(3,5)** recommend to start with TDF/FTC and ABC/3TC as an alternative to start with.
-In the HEAT **(10)** and ACTG 5202 **(11,12)** these two fixed dose combinations were compared with each other. In the HEAT study the third drug was a PI, lopinavir/ritonavir and in the ACTG 5202 it was a NNRTI, efavirenz or a PI, atazanavir/ritonavir. The HEAT study is an industry sponsered study.
ABC is known for its hypersensitivity reaction usually appearing in the first six week after starting ABC therapy. This hypersensitivity can lead to serious complications and death if not recognized. The presence of HLA-B5701 antigen is highly predictive for the chance of developing this hypersensitivity reaction **(18).**
In boths studies no determination for the presence of HLA-B5701 antigen was done.
In the HEAT study **(10)** the effectivity and CD4 cell count increase of both regimens after 48 weeks of treatment and safety after 96 weeks of treatmet was similar. In both treatment arms 2% of the participants had a grade 3-4 **(19)** decrease in renal function.
Of importance in this study is the fact that there was no difference in anti-vial efficacy between both treatment arms for participants with a high screening VL greater than 100,000 copies/ml (high VL). In the ACTG 5202 the anti-viral efficacy of the regimens were similar for participants with a screening VL less than 100,000 copies/ml **(12)** but not for those participants with a high screening VL. In the ACTG 5202, 43% of the participants had a high screening VL **(11).** At a median follow-up of 60 weeks, among the 797 patients with high VL, the time to virologic failure was significantly shorter in the ABC/3TC group than in the TDF/FTC group. There were 57 virologic failures (14%) in the ABC/3TC group versus 26 (7%) in the TDF/FTC group. The time to the first adverse event was also significantly shorter in the ABC/3TC arm. The increase in CD4 cells from baseline at week 48 was similar.
In an analysis of five pharmaceutical company sponsored trials with 872 paticipants with high sreening VL treated with ABC/3TC and using the same criteria for virological

failure as in the ACTG 5202 study there was no inceased chance for virological failure in this group **(20).**

But in a meta-analysis of 12 trials with 4896 participants and also using the same criteria for virological failure as in the ACTG 5202 study TDF/FTC showed to be virological more effective than ABC/3TC **(21).**

-In a number of trials **(13-17)** (see table 1) combination regimens with ZVD or combination regimens with d4T are less effective or result in a lower increase of CD4 cell count than in the comparative study arm.

For instance in two trials comparing ABC/3TC with ZVD/3TC **(14)** and TDF/FTC with ZVD/3TC **(13)** a significant lower increase in CD4 count is seen in both ZVD/3TC study arms than in the comparative study arms. In the 934 study **(13)** significant differences were seen in the proportion of patients with VL less than 50 copies/ml (80% versus 70%). Significant more patients in de ZVD/3TC arm had virologic failure, 4% versus <1% in the TDF arm.

More patients in theZVD/3TC group than in the TDF/FTC group had adverse events resulting in discontinuation of the study drugs **(13)**. These adverse events were mainly anemia, nausea, vomiting and fatigue. The authors concluded that through week 48, TDF/FTC proved to be superior in terms of virologic suppression, CD4 response and adverse events resulting in discontinuation of the study drugs.

Also in other studies, serious adverse events like anemia and leukopenia are seen in patients taking ZVD and are often a reason for stopping ZVD **(14, 15).**

2.2 Compliance, quality of life and durability of anti-retroviral backbones

Good compliance is the cornerstone for succes of anti-retroviral therapy. Stress reduction, a good sociaal network and adequate information play an important role **(22).** Irregular intake of medication by inadequate compliance leads to suboptimal plasma levels of the medication, thereby increasing development of resistance **(23, 24)** Compliance which leads to actual intake of > 95% of the prescribed medication is a predictor of efficacy of a regimen **(23,24).**

Adverse events, the number of pills and dosage frequency determine compliance.

In different meta-analyses of 64 **(25)** and 20 **(26)** clinical trials it was shown that the number of tablets per day, dosage fequency and diet restrictions (with food or on an empty stomach) are important determinants of success of antiretroviral therapy. In the meta-analysis of 64 clinical trials **(25)** the number of tablets per day was the most important factor for success of cART.

A meta-analysis of 11 randomized trials revealed that the adherence rate was better with once-daily regimens than twice-daily regimens and this effect was more pronounced at the time of treatment initiation **(27).**

No studies on quality of life (QoL) and compliance have been done linked to the seven major randomized studies mentioned above.

In a meta analysis, initial ART regimens, regimens containing TDF are equivalent to those containing AZT concerning serious adverse events. However, TDF showed to be superior to AZT in terms of immunologic response and adherence and less frequent emergence of resistance **(28).**

In a review of twenty-two randomized controlled trials including all above mentioned backbones, including 8,184 HIV-treatment-naïve patients, the combination ddI/3TC was anti-virologic more effective and less toxic for discontinuation due to adverse events and more tolerable than its comparators. The combination TDF/3TC or FTC was more effective and less toxic only in the 144-week follow-up data (two trials, 1,119 patients). ABC/3TC had similar efficacy to its comparators, but more AIDS-defining events **(29)**. In the Swiss cohort study, including 1318 naïve patients, between 2005 and 2008 drug toxicity remained a frequent reason for treatment modification. Initial treatment with ZVD/3TC was associated with a high rate of drug toxicity. **(30)** In general QoL is beter with a higher CD4 cell count and QoL is decreased in patients with a high VL. The effects of adverse events on QoL are independent of CD4 cell count and VL **(31).**

Acronime of study	Set up of study	Treatment arms Number of patients in each treatment arm ()	Third drug	ITT analysis: % patients with VL< 50 cop/mL	% patients with screening VL >100.000 copies/mL with VL< 50 copies/mL	CD4 increase cells/mm³	% patients stopping study drugs due to adverse events
HEAT Sudy #(10)	randomised dubble blind placebo controlled	ABC/3TC (343) versus TDF/FTC (345)	lopinavir/r	68% vs 67%	63% vs 65%	214 vs 193	up to week 96: 6% vs 6%
ACTG 5202# (11,12)	randomised blinded for backbone	ABC/3TC (388) versus TDF/FTC (393)	atazanavir/r or efavirenz	similar	75% vs 80%	194 vs 199	up to week 112: 5% vs 4%
Gilead 934 Study (13)	randomised open label	TDF/FTC(258) versus ZVD/3TC (259)	efavirenz	77% vs 68%**	not available	190 vs 158*	up to week 48: 5% vs 19%* up to week 144: 13% vs 34%*
CNA30024# (14)	randomised dubble blind	ABC/3TC (327) versus ZVD/3TC (327)	efavirenz	70% vs 69%	67% vs 67%	209 vs 155**	up to week 48: 14% vs 18%
GESIDA (15)	randomised open label	ddI/3TC (189) versus ZVD/3TC (187)	efavirenz	67% vs 63%	67% vs 63%	158 vs 163	up to week 48: 14% vs 26%
FTC 301 (16)	randomised dubble blind	ddI/FTC (286) versus d4T/ddI (285)	efavirenz	78% vs 59%***	67% vs 50%***	168 vs 134	up to week 60: 7% vs 15%
Gilead 903 Study(17)	randomised dubble blind placebo controlled	TDF/FTC (299) versus d4T/3TC (303)	efavirenz	82% vs 81%	not available	169 vs 167	up to week 48: 9% vs 9% up to week 96: 14% vs 15%

Table 1. Major characteristics and parameters of effectiviness of the seven important clinical trials comparing different backbones of during 48 to 96 weeks of treatment
HLA-B57 screening test not done at inclusion
Degree of significance between treatment arms * $p< 0{,}05$ ** $p<0{,}005$ *** $p<0.001$

2.3 Resistance development during treatment with anti-retroviral backbones

Inadequate compliance is the most important cause of virologic failure and resistance development **(23,24)**. Repeated virologic failure with cumulation of resistances will lead to a decrease of the number of CD4 cells (immunologic failure), leading to HIV-related diseases, AIDS and death (clinical failure).

Development of resistance varies per class of anti-retroviral drugs and also within a class of antiretrovirals. For NRTIs, the development of resistance after initiation of cART is stongly associated with adherence. Resistance to antiretrovirals from the start of cART will develop first and during follow-up in highest frequency to lamivudine, followed by development of resistance to NNRTIs, NRTIs and PIs **(32).**

A distinction between the different mutations to NRTI's is made between thymidine analoge mutations (TAMs), TAMs-associated mutations, evolving mainly during virologic failure when on therapy with thymidine analogues ZVD and d4T and the discriminatory mutations and the Q151M pathway mutations conferring for multiresistance. Mutations, an acumulation of mutations or the occurrence of multi-resistant mutations limit the number of effective combinations of NRTIs in the backbone for a second or third regimen.

For instance the K65R mutation (discriminatory mutation) can develop during failing therapy with TDF and will make ABC and ddI ineffective.

These drug-resistant viruses can be tranmitted and may limit the treatment options in treatment naïve patients.

The prevalence of transmitted drug resistance viruses since 2004 is similar in different Eropean countries and the Netherlands. In the Netherlands the prevalence of NRTI drug resistance in recent infection (naïve patients) is found to be around 5-6% and for intermediate or high level of resistance is around 2% **(33)**

Since2003 treatment guidelines recommend onbtaining a genotypic sequence at the start of cART.

3. Safety of anti-retroviral backbones

3.1 Grade 3 and 4, serious adverse events

The prevalence and incidence of grade 3 (severe adverse event) and grade 4 (potentially life threatening adverse event) adverse events (table according to NIAID, Division of AIDS) (19) provide information on the safety of anti-retrovirals. It is not always possible to determine which adverse events are caused by an individual drug or by the combination of drugs in a regimen. Grade 3-4 adverse events have major consequences for the patient and may lead to significant morbidity, hospitalisation and mortality. The medication must almost always be stopped, leading to an increased risk of resistant mutations, decrease in CD4 cell count and resulting impairment of physical condition and a lower quality of life **(22,23,24,31).**

Adverse events in the studies with mainly naive patients show highly variable incidences of grade 3 and 4 adverse events, ranging from 0-57%. On the basis of these studies, it is not possible to determine a certain pattern of side-effects. It is not clear which side-effects can be linked to the individual NRTI, to the backbone or other drugs. In some studies all grade 2-4 side-effects are summarised without full details **(10,14,16).** In other studies report only a selection of grade 3 and 4 clinical and or only laboratory adverse events are reported **(11,12).** The percentage of patients stopping study drugs because of adverse events ranged up to 34% (see table1). Several adverse events with changing severity have been associated with NRTIs **(34).**

Anemia, neutropenia and thrombocytopenia

Anemia and neutropenia (granulocytopenia) occur are 1.1-9.7% of the patients treated with ZVD. Higher percentages is seen in patients with AIDS, 15-61% **(35).** Serious grade 3 of 4 anemia and neutropenia are relatively rare with earlier initiation of treatment. Hematologic toxicity is more often seen with ZVD and rarely to never in treatment with other NRTIs. Combinations of NRTIs with other hemato-toxic medication may increase the incidence of serious anemia and neutropenia **(35).** Serious grade 3 of 4 thrombocytopenia due to cART, necessitating thrombocytes transfusions have been reported **(35).**

Pancreatitis:

In the older studies pancreatitis was seen in 4-7% of patients treated with ddI and d4T. In 6% of these patients pancreatis was fatal **(35).** Combinations of ddI/d4T double the risk and ddI/TDF also increase the risk of development of pancreatitis **(36)**.

In the ACTG studies from October 1989 through July 1999 the overall pancreatitis rates were 0.61 per 100 person-years clinical and 2.23 per 100 person-years clinical/laboratory **(36).** The incidence of pancreatitis in the EuroSida cohort decreased over the years with earlier start of therapy and with higher CD4 cell counts. The incidence was 0.127 per 100 person-years over the years 2001-2006 **(38).**

Lactate acidosis (mitochondrial toxicity):

Lactate acidosis is a serious complication of the treatment with NRTIs, which occurs in around 0.9 times per 1000 years of treatment and often leads to serious morbidity and mortality **(35).**

In vitro studies have shown that inhibition of DNA polymerase gamma and other mitochondrial enzymes by NRTIs may lead to mitochondrial disfunction and cellular toxicity.

The clinical symptomatology of NRTI-induced mitochondrial toxicity consists of steatosis, hepatitis, lactate acidosis, myopathy, nephrotoxicity, peripheral neuropathy and pancreatitis. Studies with NRTIs in enzym assays and in cell cultures have shown that the following NRTIs are responsible for this mitochondrial toxicity, to a decreasing extent: ddI > d4T > ZVD **(39)**. DNA polymerase gamma inhibition is not found in normal concentrations of ABC, 3TC and TDF **(39).**

Lipodystrophy:

Three forms of lipodystrophy are distinguished: lipoatrophy caused by loss of subcutaneous fat, fat accumulation or lipohypertrophy and mixed forms. It was described with cART in 1997 and may occur in all combinations of cART medication with a prevalence between 2-84%. Lipo-accumumulation like buffelo-hump and "crix belli" may be caused by PIs, lipoatrophy by NRTIs. Lipoatrophy may occur shortly after initiation of cART. In a large observational cohort, 62% of the patients who developed lipoatrophy has symptoms within one year. In this cohort a highly significant correlation was found between lipoatrophy and the use of d4T **(40)**. It has been shown in observational cohort studies, clinical trials and in pathologic studies that lipoatrophy is specifically related to the use of NRTI especially d4T and in to a lesser extent to ZVD. Host factors have a modulating effect on the risk and the severity of lipoatrophy **(2).**

The development of lipoatrophy is a serious complication which often leads to a marked decrease of the quality of life. In clinical studies is was shown that lipoatrophy improved by the replacement of ZVD or d4T by ABC **(41)** or TDF **(42).**

Peripheral neuropathy

The occurrence of peripheral neuropathy is a well known complication of HIV-infection itself or due to a toxic effect on mitochondria induced by some NRTIs. Its incidence increases with the extent of immunodeficiency and older age. Patients who develop peripheral neuropathy tend to do so shortly after exposure to antiretroviral therapy and certain subgroup of patients are found to be more susceptible than others **(43).**

With ddI use the incidence of medication related sensoric neuropathy was 6.8 cases per 100 person years. In one study the relatieve risk is 1.4 fold higher in d4T use and 3.5 times higher in the combination of ddI/d4T compared to other NRTIs **(44).** In an other study peripheral neuropathy was reported in 3.0 cases per 100 person-years for ZVD monotherapy and in 2.2 cases per 100 person-years for ZVD/ddl **(43).** Sensoric neuropathy has not been associated with the use of ABC,3TC, FTC and TDF.

Rash (hypersensitivity reaction) and muscle disorders

Drug hypersensitivity reactions are an important cause of morbidity in HIV-infected patients. The hypersensitivity reactions can be caused by each of the antiretroviral drugs in the cART regimen or by other concomitend prescribed drugs.

ABC is known for its hypersensitivity reaction usually appearing in the first six week after starting ABC therapy. Symptoms of this ABC related hypersensitivity reaction are nonspecific and can be difficult to distinguish from reactions to other drugs or conditions and can lead to serious complications and death if not recognized. The presence of HLA-B5701 antigen is highly predictive for the chance of developing this hypersensitivity reaction. ABC hypersensitivity reaction affects 5-8% of patients during the first six weeks of treatment **(18).**

Hypersensitivity reactions to 3TC, FTC, ddI, TDF have been reported but occur very rarely **(45).** Other forms of hypersensitivity reactions and rashes are related to the use of NNRTIs and PIs and are usually mild and self-limiting **(46).**

Other serious adverse events like rhabdomyolysis, myopathy and cardiomyopathy are very rare complications, which are not clearly related to NRTIs. **(46).**

Renal failure

Chronic kidney disease in HIV-positive persons can be caused by both HIV and traditional or non-HIV-related factors and antiretroviral drugs. Tenofovir has been associated with decline in renal funtion **(47,48,49).**

Tenofovir is mainly cleared by glomerular filtration and active tubular secretion through tubular transport proteins. Interactions and competition of different anti-retrovirals with these transport proteins can lead to renal toxicity and increased blood levels. The combination of TDF/ddI leads to ~ 30% increased ddI levels and ddI related toxicity.

Up to February 2006, 27 individual cases of renal failure with or without proteinuria or Fanconi syndrome (renal tubular acidosis) have been described with the use of TDF **(47).**

During a follow-up of 144 weeks of 600 patients in the 903 Study **(17,50)** comparing d4T/3TC/EFV with TDF/3TC/EFV no significant increases in mean creatinine level were seen in the 299 patients treated with tenofovir. In the Heat study **(10)** comparing ABC/3TC and TDF/FTC and in Study 934 **(13)** comparing ZVD/3TC and TDF/FTC during an obserervation period of respectively 96 weeks and 48 weeks no significant difference in renal function could be shown.

In the Swiss HIV Cohort Study **(48)** 363 treatment-naive patients or patients with treatment interruptions of more than 12 months starting either a TDF-based cART and 715 patients on a TDF-sparing regime were compared for the time to reach a 10 ml/min reduction in calculated GFR (cGFR). Apart from diabetes mellitus, higher baseline cGFR (by 10 ml/min), TDF use and boosted PI use were significantly associated with an increased risk for reaching a 10 ml/min reduction in cGFR during an observation time of two years.

During a median follow-up of 3.7 years in the EuroSida Study Group **(49)** 225 (3.3%) persons progressed to chronic kidney disease during 21.482 person-years follow-up, an incidence of 1.05 per 100 person-years follow-up. After adjustment for traditional factors associated with chronic kidney disease, increasing cumulative exposure to TDF and the PIs, indinavir, atazanavir and lopinavir/ritonavir were associated with a significantly increased rate of decline in renal function. No other antiretroviral drugs were associated with increased incidence of chronic kidney disease.

In a prospective observational cohort study at Johns Hopkins **(51)** patients taking both TDF and NRTIs experienced an initial decline in cGFR during the first 180 days of therapy, but cGFR stabilized between 180 and 720 days. In this study there was no difference between TDF and NRTI use in more than 25% or 50% decline in cGFR at 1 or 2 years or in change in cGFR at 6, 12, or 24 months. Those taking TDF and a PI/ritonavir had a greater median decline in cGFR than those taking TDF and a NNRTI at 6 months. There was no difference in median cGFR decline between those on an NRTI/PI/ritonavir versus those on an NRTI/NNRTI regimen.

The reversibility of TDF-related nephrotoxicity in 24 male patients who ceased TDF for renal impairment by retrospective assessment were determined **(52).** Median eGFR pre-TDF was 74 mL/min/1.73 m^2 (using the Modified Diet in Renal Disease equation) and fell to 51 mL/min/1.73 m^2 at TDF cessation and increased to 58 mL/min/1.73 m^2 in a median of 13 months after TDF cessation. This decline in cGFR, most recent versus pre-TDF is significant. Results were similar using the Cockcroft-Gault equation for cGFR. Only 10 patients reached their pre-TDF cGFR.

Many patients on antiretroviral therapy have multiple medical problems and may take other potentially nephrotoxic drugs. It has been clearly shown that taking TDF in combination with PI may increase a decline in renal function.

In a systematic review **(53)** of a total of 17 studies (including 9 randomized, controlled trials) a significantly greater loss of kidney function was seen among patients using TDF, compared with control subjects (mean difference in eGFR was 3.92 mL/min, as well as a greater risk of acute renal failure. There was no evidence that TDF use led to increased risk of severe proteinuria, hypophosphatemia, or fractures.

Thus in some well designed randomized prospective trials **(10,17,50)** no decline in renal function during treatment with TDF has been noted. Some observational stusies have found evidence of mild decrease in kidney function in TDF treated patients and when TDF related renal toxicity was present it was not always fully reversible.

Cardiovascular risk and lipids

The risk of cardio vascular disease (CVD) and other non-AIDS conditions increases with age, but prevalence of these diseases by age is greater in HIV-positive populations. In a case-control study of HIV-infected patients and healthy HIV-negative individuals from an observational database comparing rates of 6 comorbidities,CVD, hypertension, renal failure, osteoporosis, diabetes, and hypothyroidism to be higher in HIV-infected patients **(54).**

Numerous large observational cohort studies in Europe and the USA have found higher rates of acute myocardial infarction (MI) or coronary heart disease (CHD) in patients with HIV. (5-10) In a cross-sectional study of HIV-infected participants and controls without pre-existing CVD preclinical atherosclerosis assessed by carotid intima-medial thickness measurements in the internal/bulb and common carotid regions in HIV-infected participants and controls after adjusting for traditional CVD risk factors showed that HIV infection was accompanied by more extensive atherosclerosis **(61).**

The higher risk among patients with HIV-infected patients held true for every age group analyzed and in multivariate analysis adjusting for demographics and common cardiovascular risk factors confirm that HIV infection is an independent predictor of acute MI, conferring nearly a two-fold risk. The risk of myocardial infarcion is found to be associated with the cumulative use of PIs in these studies **(55,56,59,60).**

In the D.A.D cohort, a lage observational prospective cohort study with more than 30,000 HIV-infected patients in 212 clinics since 1999, it was found that ABC and ddI were associated with a higher risk of acute MI within each CVD risk category defined by the Framingham Risk Score **(62).** Exposure to ABC within the most recent 6 months was associated with a 1.90 relative risk of acute MI. Subsequent analysis suggested cumulative use of ABC may also been associated with increased MI risk, although to a lesser extent than recent use **(63).** Since that first publication, several reports on MI risk associated with ABC have appeared, and some of these analyses have not implicated ABC as an MI risk factor. Several studies have focused on possible mechanisms that may explain the increased risk on MI in patients taking ABC. In the largest analysis, SMART study investigators found higher levels of hsCRP and IL-6 in patients taking ABC than in patients not taking ABC **(64)** However, a study of 13 biomarkers in virologically suppressed patients taking ABC/3TC vs TDF/FTC found no significant change in either group after 48 weeks **(65).** The results of the DAD study **(62)** could have been confounded by te so-called allocation biases such as high cardiovascular risk and renal function. In the Veterans Affairs Study a weak correlation between ABC use and MI was found, disappearing entirely after statistical adjustment for renal disease **(66).**

In November 2008, DHHS guidelines reclassified abacavir from a preferred first-line agent to an alternate agent, partly because of these data on cardiovascular risk.

In the DAD study correcting the increased relative risk for antiretroviral-associated CVD for lipds attenuated this CVD risk by around 10% **(55).** In the ACTG 5202 study **(11,12)** fasting lipids at week 48 had increased more in the ABC/3TC arm than in the TDF/FTC arm (respectively; total cholesterol 0,87 mmol/L versus 0,67 mmol/L and triglycerides 0.28 mmol/L versus 0.03 mmol/L) with no significant difference between groups in the change in the ratio of total cholesterol to HDL cholesterol. In a systemic review of 7 clinical trials with a total of 3,807 paticipants, studying initial treatment in naïve subjects receiving 2NRTIs/efavirenz regimens the mean change in total cholesterol from baseline to 48 weeks was significantly greater in patients taking a non-TDF containing regimen **(67).**

Bone mineral density loss associated with HIV infection and cART

Many studies have documented an increased prevalence of osteopenia in HIV-infected individuals with dual x-ray absorptiometry bone densitometry (DEXA) scans. This finding is important since bone mineral density (BMD) predicts fracture risk **(68).** A higher fracture rate has been demonstrated among HIV-infected subjects compared with controls in a large healthcare system.**(69).** Many factors may play a role in the increased prevalence of osteopenia like vitamine D deficiency, low body mass, aging, corticosteroid use, alcoholism and HIV-infection.

Decreased BMD has been found in both treatment-naive and treated HIV-infected patients. Ongoing BMD loss over time has been observed in some treatment studies, although it is uncertain whether it is due to drug toxicity since it is difficult to differentiate between effects associated with antiretrovirals and other factors. In addition the presence and strength of antiviral-related factors is difficult to ascertain as combinations of classes of antiretroviral drugs are used.

In the GS 903 study comparing d4T/3TC and TDF/3TC, each combined with efavirenz in treatment-naive patients, after an an initial decrease in BMD was found in both study arms but stabilized after 24 weeks. By week 144, the mean decrease in BMD of the spine was significantly different 0.9% in the d4T/3TC arm and 2.2% in the TDF/3TC arm. At baseline there was a relatively high incidence of both osteopenia and osteoporosis in both study arms, but there was no significant difference in rates of new-onset osteopenia or progression to osteoporosis through week 144 **(70).**

In the STEAL study, 360 virologically suppressed patients were randomized to switch their current NRTIs to either ABC/3TC or TDF/FTC. No significant change in spine or hip T scores were observed in the ABC/3TC arm, but BMD at spine and hip decreased in the TDF/FTC arm, and the difference between the regimens was statistically significant at weeks 48 and 96 **(71).**

In a study comparing the effect of TDF versus ABC based regimens on BMD, BMD decreased early during therapy in both arms before stabilizing. The mean loss of BMD was statistically greater with TDF and the loss correlated with biomarkers of bone turnover **(72).** Similar results were obtained in an other study comparing the safety aspects of ABC/3TC and TDF/FTC in 385 treatment-naive patients **(73).**

In the ACTG 5202 metabolic substudy, there was an initial reduction in BMD in all stady arms, which stabilized after 48 weeks. A significantly greater loss of BMD was seen at week 96 with TDF/FTC versus ABC/3TC. This included a significant 2% greater reduction in lumbar spine BMD and a significant 1.5% greater reduction in hip BMD. No difference was found in fracture rates between study arms at week 48 **(74).**

In the bone substudy of this trial, the initiation of antiretroviral therapy was associated with a decrease in bone mass of 2% to 4% that was independent of the regimen selected and stabilized by week 48; this decrease was greatest in patients who started a regimen that contained TDF **(75).**

Thus overall, BMD appears to decline to some degree during the first several months after initiation of cART, regardless of regimen, but the decline may be slightly greater with TDF containing regimens. However, there are no conclusive data showing that therapy-associated reductions in bone mineral density are also associated with an increased rate of fractures.

3.2 Documentation

The clinical documentation of the combinations is summarised in Table 2

	Number of clinical trials*	Years since registration
Zidovudine/Lamivudine or emtricitabine	532/23	>10 Emt: 8
Didanosine/Lamivudine or emtricitabine	165/10	>10 Emt: 8
Abacavir/Lamivudine or emtricitabine	160/15	> 10 Emt: 8
Tenofovir/emtricitabine or Lamivudine	78/115	>10 >10

Table 2. Documentation

* according to the definition of National Institute of Health/PubMed (www.ncbi.nih.gov)

4. Tolerability of anti-retroviral backbones

4.1 Grade 1 and 2, mild to moderate side-effects

The tolerability of a cART regimens is an important predictor of durability and long-term succes. Grade 1(mild adverse event) and grade 2 (moderate adverse event) **(19)** may have a

significant influence on compliance and quality of life **(22,26)** and on the durability of a certain combination. It is not always evident which drug in a cART regimen is responsible for which side-effect. The HIV-infection as such or complications of opportunistic infections may lead to symptoms marked as adverse events of anti-retroviral medication.
General symptoms as fatigue, pain, anorexia, sleep and concentration disturbances occur frequently **(46).**
It is difficult to give a reliable estimation of the relative incidence of different grade of adverse events, based on the EMEA and FDA data **(76)**, because of the relative lack of randomised comparative studies with extended follow-up and asufficient number of participants.
Cohort studies yield better insight as to why patients switch or stop certain antiretroviral drugs and how long they keep using the same regimen, in comparison with randomised studies which usually have a limited follow-up time.
In the older cohort studies high rates of toxicity driven changes in antiretroviral drugs were common. For instance in the Swiss HIV Cohort Study, with 2,674 patients, 35% stopped treatment with at least one drug during the observation period of 3.2 years because of adverse events and/or intolerability and 41% stopped the combination of anti-retroviral drugs at least once or completely changed to another combination **(77).**
In the Italian ICONA-cohort **(78),** 36% of the 862 patients stopped because of side-effects during study period of 45 weeks and only 5% because of virologic failure.
Earlier initiation of cART, lower pill burden and dosing schemes of once or twice daily, together with declining toxicity, have improved tolerability.
In the Athena-cohort the incidence per 100 patient years of toxicity driven changes of cART during the first 3 years after the start of therapy decreased from 29% in 1996 to 15% in 2008. Significant decline in toxicity driven changes of cART started to be apparent after calendar year 2000. The incidence of toxicity driven changes of cART is highest in the first 3 month after initiation.

5. Easy of use

5.1 Ease of use (dosage frequency, number of tablets per day)

The combinations of ABC/3TC, TDF/FTC and ddI/FTC or 3TC can be given once daily. ZVD/3TC (Combivir®)has to be given twice daily. The other combinations are given once or twice daily. The combinations of ABCbacavir/Lamivudine (Kivexa®, Epzicom®) and TDT/FTC (Truvada ®) can be given as one tablet per day. TDT/FTC in combination with efavirenz can be given in one tablet (Atripla ®)
DdI is given 2 hours before or after food. The rest of the drugs can be taken irrespective of food.

6. Applicability

6.1 Availability of different formulations

Liquid or dispersible formulations are available for ddI.

6.2 Drug interactions

Abacavir
Abacavir is not significantly metabolised by CYP450, which makes serious reactions regarding inhibition or induction of CYP450 enzymes unlikely **(80).** No interactions were seen with adefovir, amprenavir, indinavir, ZVD and 3TC **(50).**

Enzymeinducers like rifampicin, phenobarbital and phenytoin may decrease the plasma concentrations of abacavir to a minor extent through an effect on UDP-glucuronyltransferases [72].
Alcohol may decrease the AUC of abacavir by 40% **(81,82).**
Didanosine
The AUC of ddI doubles during simultaneous use of ganciclovir. Didanosine has no significant effect on the pharmacokinetics of zidovudine **(83).**
No clinically relevant interaction occurs between ddI with ritonavir, nevirapine, emtricitabine and nelfinavir **(84).**
Ribavirine may increase intracellular levels of ddI. The relevance of this is unknown.
Didanosine decreases the bioavailability of ciprofloxacin during simultaneous intake. It is recommended to take ciprofloxacin an hour before or at least 4 hours after ddI **(84).** Didanosine showed no interaction with indinavir and fluconazole. Ketoconazole and itraconazole increase the AUC of ddI, maar these interactions do not appear te be very relevant.
The AUC of ddI increases by 50% in combination with tenofovir often leading to ddI toxicity **(3).**
Xanthine oxidase plays a role in the metabolism of didanosine, interactions with inhibitors of xanthine oxidase, like allopurinol, may theoretically decrease the clearance of didanosine.
Emtricitabine
Tenofovir and FTC do not affect each other's pharmacokinetics **(85, 86).** Emtricitabine is metabolised to a limited extent and is excreted unchanged in the urine through glomerular filtration and active tubular secretion**(85).** Interactions regarding to inhibition of active tubular secretion cannot be excluded, maar have not been studied **(85).**
Emcitabrine shows no pharmacokinetic interactions with protease inhibitors or with ddI **(85).**
Lamivudine
Lamivudine shows few metabolic interactions. The drug is excreted in an unchanged form through glomerular filtration and active tubular secretion **(87, 88).**
No interaction is seen with ZVD and ddI **(87, 88).**
Trimethoprim may decrease active tubular secretion, increasing the AUC of lamivudine by 40% **(87, 88).** Applications of high dose co-trimoxazole in pneumocystis carinii infections should not be combined with lamivudine **(87).** There is inadequate documentation on a possible interaction with intravenous ganciclovir or foscarnet. This combination should be avoided.
Tenofovir
Tenofovir is mainly excreted uchanged in the urine through glomerular filtration and active tubular secretion **(90,91).** Interactions regarding to inhibition of active tubular secretion cannot be excluded, but have not been studied **(90).**
Tenofovir and FTC have no effect on each other's pharmacokinetics **(85, 86,91).**
The AUC of TDF increases by 30% in combination with lopinavir and ritonavir or atazanavir **(92,93).** Tenofovir may decrease the AUC of atazanavir by 25%. The AUC of lopinavir increases by 15% by tenofovir. Tenofovir shows no interaction with saquinavir **(91).**
The AUC of ddI increases by 50% in combination with tenofovir **(91).** This may increase the risk of pancreatitis and other ddI related toxicity. The AUC of atazanavir decreases by 25% in combination with TDF **(86).**
Tenofovir showed no interactions with indinavir, methadon, ribavirine or rifampicin **(91,93, 94).**

Zidovudine

Zidovudine is mainly glucuronidated. The drug may theoretically show interactions with a large number of drugs which are also excreted through glucuronidation, like aspirin, NSAIDs, penicillins and oxazepam. Very limited data on the relevance of these possible interactions is available **(95).**

The bioavailability of zidovudine may be decreased to a limited extent (22%) by simultaneouse intake with food **(96).**

The renal clearance of zidovudine decreases by 50% during simultaneous use of co-trimoxazole **(96).** This interaction is only relevant in disturbed glucuronidation of zidovudine.

Rifampicin lowers the AUC of zidovudine by 50%, an interaction with rifabutin is not very relevant, a 14% decrease of the AUC of zidovudine was seen **(96)**.

The AUC of ZVD increases by 75% in combination with fluconazole **(96).**

Zidovudine may cause an unpredictable interaction with phenytoin (increase of decrease of the phenytoin levels). Phenytoin levels have to be checked on a regular basis.

Atovaquone increases the AUC of zidovudine by 35%. Valproic acid and methadone may also lead to an increase in the AUC of zidovudine, but little data are available.

Zidovudine is antagonistic in combination with ribavirine or stavudine.

Nephrotoxic or myelosuppressive drugs may increase potential side-effects of ZVD (SPC on zidovudine).

6.3 Approved indications

There are no major differences in the approved indications. The applicability in children is described in 5.5.

Treatment co-infections

Lamivudine, emtricitabine and tenofovir also have anti hepatitis B virus activity. An advantage of these drugs is that "two in one" treatment is possible It is recommended that lamivudine or emtricitabine should be combined with tenofovir (97) in case of hepatitis B co-infection. Only lamivudine is approved for this indication.

6.4 Contra-indications

All drugs are contra-indicated in case of hypersensitivity.

Hypersensitivity to abacavir may be very serious.

6.5 Use in children and elderly

No dose adjustments are necessary in the elderly.

Zidovudine/lamivudine (Combivir) and abacavir/lamivudine (Kivexa) can be used in children from 12 years. The individual components can be used from 3 months.

Lamivudine can be used from 3 months

Didanosine tablets can be used from 6 years.

Tenofovir and emcitabine are only applicable in adults.

6.6 Use in renal and hepatic disease

A dose reduction is necessary in case of renal function impaiment. Abacavir/Lamivudine should not be used when the creatinine clearance is lower than 50 ml/min. Tenofovir/Emtricitabine should bot be used when the creatinine clearance is lower than 30 ml/min.

No dose adjustments are usually necessary in patients with liver disease.

6.7 Use in pregancy and lactation

A variable extent of mitochondrial damage may occur during in utero exposition to nucleoside-analogues. This may lead to hematologic toxicity or metabolic disturbances.
All drugs should be avoided during lactation. None of the combinations is recommended in case of pregnancy, but they are usually not absolutely contra-indicated.

6.8 Special precautions

Zidovudine/Lamivudine (Combivir)	Monitoring of hematologic parameters (ZVD) Lowering of the dosage of ZVD in abnormal hematologic parameters Therapy cessation during signs of pancreatitis (ZVD and 3TC) Lactic acidosis has been described. Therapy should be stopped in case of hyperlactatemia or metabolic acidosis Use with great caution in case of hepatomegaly, hepatitis or risk factors for liverdiseases (3TC) Cessation of L may lead to increased symptoms in patients who also have hepatitis B.
Didanosine/Lamivudine	Great caution with pancreatitis in the anamnesis (ddI and 3TC) Peripheral neuropathy may occur (ddI) Changes in the retina and N.opticus are to be checked in children (ddI) Use with great caution in case of hepatomegaly, hepatitis or riskfactors for liverdiseases (3TC) Lactic acidosis has been described. Therapy should be stopped in case of hyperlactatemia or metabolic acidosis (ddI and 3TC) Patients with hepatitis B or C have an increased risk on serious hepatic side-effects (ddI) Lipodystrophy may occur (ddI) Cessation of L may lead to increased symptoms in patients who also have hepatitis B.
Abacavir/Lamivudine (Kivexa)	Cessation of therapy during signs of pancreatitis (ABC and 3TC) Lactic acidosis has been described. Therapy should be stopped in case of hyperlactatemia or metabolic acidosis Use with great caution in case of hepatomegaly, hepatitis or risk factors for liverdiseases (3TC) Lipodystrophy may occur (3TC) Patients with hepatitis B or C have an increased risk on serious hepatic side-effects Cessation of 3TC may lead to increased symptoms in patients who also have hepatitis B.
Tenofovir/Lamivudine	Tenofovir may lower the BMD (TDF) No not use in case of the HIV-1 K65R mutation (TDF) Lactic acidosis has been described. Therapy should be stopped in case of hyperlactatemia or metabolic acidosis (TDF) Cessation of L may lead to increased symptoms in patients who

	also have hepatitis B. Use with great caution in case of hepatomegaly, hepatitis or risk factors for liverdiseases (3TC) Renal function should be checked. Combination with nephrotoxic drugs is not recommended (3TC)
Tenofovir/Emtricitabine (Truvada)	Do not combine with lamivudine Combination with a third nucleoside analogue is not recommended beause of possible virologic failure. The tablet contains lactose. Renal function should be checked. Combination with nephrotoxisc drugs is not recommended (TDF) No not use in case of the HIV-1 K65R mutation (TDF) Tenofovir may lower the bone mineral density (TDF) Patients with hepatitis B or C have an increased risk on serious hepatic side-effects (TDF) Cessation of TDF/FTC may lead to increased symptoms in patients who also have hepatitis B.
Didanosine/Emtricitabine	Great caution with pancreatitis in the anamnesis (ddI) Peripheral neuropathy may occur (ddI) Changes in the retina and N.opticus are to be checked in children (ddI) Lactic acidosis has been described. Therapy should be stopped in case of hyperlactatemia or metabolic acidosis (ddI) Lipodystrophy may occur (ddI) Patients with hepatitis B of C have an increased risk on serious hepatic side-effects (ddI) Lipodystrophy may occur (ddI)

7. Acquisition cost

Acquisition cost excluded for VAT in Euro ("vergoedingsprijs", Z-Index July 2011)

		Cost per month in Euro
Zidovudine/Lamivudine (Combivir)	2 dd 300/150 mg	379
Didanosine ER (Videx) Lamivudine (Epivir)	1 dd 400 or 250 mg (weight based) 300 mg in 1-2 doses	306/336
Abacavir/Lamivudine (Kivexa, Epzicom)	1 dd 600/300 mg	422
Tenofovir (Viread) Lamivudine (Epivir)	1 dd 245 mg 300 mg in 1-2 doses	510
Tenofovir/Emtricitabine (Truvada)	1 dd 200/245 mg	510
Didanosine ER (Videx) Emtricitabine (Emtriva)	1 dd 400 or 250 mg (weight based) 200 mg 1 dose	313/343

8. Conclusion

Optimal care requires individualized management and ongoing attention to relevant scientific and clinical information. The availability of new antiretroviral drugs since the introduction of the fist cART has expanded treatment choices. Guidelines are presented as recommendations if the supporting evidence warrants routine use in a particular situation and as considerations if data are preliminary or incomplete but suggestive. But the importance of adherence, emerging long-term complications of therapy, recognition and management of antiretroviral failure is often underestimated and there is but to often little data to guide our choices.

The judgement of the relative efficacy and safety of the various NRTI backbones in the treament of HIV infection is hindered by the fact that there are only few direct comparative studies. This makes it difficult to make firm statements concerning the pros and cons of the individual drugs concerning efficacy and safety.

In this InforMatrix manuscript, no firm conclusions are drawn by the authors. The purpose of this manuscript is to facilitate discussion on the properties of each treatment option for HIV by using only clinically relevant selection criteria by providing an up-to-date overview. The InforMatrix program will be made available in an interactive format on www.informatrix.nl. By means of the program, the user can assign a relative weight to each main selection criterion (with a total of 30 points to be distributed) and can judge the properties of each therapeutic option per criterion on the basis of his own personal expertise and/or the present document. Zero to ten points can be assigned to each treatment option on each criterion. The program is freely accessible.

The present InforMatrix manuscript is specific for the Netherlands, because the Dutch available formulations and Dutch prices were used. The most important part of the paper (efficacy, safety and tolerability) is internationally valid. Local adjustments are necessary for an optimal use of the method in other countries. This could also include price-adjustments for the individual hospitals in other countries.

9. References

[1] Bartlett J FM, DeMasi R, Quinn J, et al. An Updated Meta-analysis of Triple Combination Therapy in Antiretroviral-naive HIV-infected Adults. Abstract 586 12th Conference on Retrovirusses and Oportunistic Infections 2006.

[2] Hammond E, McKinnon E, Nolan D. Human immunodeficiency virus treatment-induced adipose tissue pathology and lipoatrophy: prevalence and metabolic consequences. Clin Infect Dis. 2010;51:591-9.

[3] Torti C, Quiros-Roldan E, Regazzi M, et al. Early virological failure after tenofovir + didanosine + efavirenz combination in HIV-positive patients upon starting antiretroviral therapy. Antivir Ther 2005;10:505-13

[4] Mallewa JE, Wilkins E, Vilar J, et al HIV-associated lipodystrophy: a review of underlying mechanisms and therapeutic options. J Antimicrob Chemother. 2008;62:648-60.

[5] Guidelines for the Use of Antiretroviral agents in HIV-1 infected Adults and Adolescents. DHHS Panel December 1, 2009. wwwaidsinfonihgov.

[6] Guidelines of the European AIDS Clinical Society version 5 November 2009, www.europeanaidsclinicalsociety.org

[7] Thompson MA, Aberg JA, Cahn P, et al. Antiretroviral treatment of adult HIV infection: 2010 recommendations of the International AIDS Society-USA panel. JAMA. 2010;304:321-33.
[8] Gulick RM, Ribaudo HJ, Shikuma CM, et al. Triple-nucleoside regimens versus efavirenz-containing regimens for the initial treatment of HIV-1 infection. N Engl J Med. 2004;350:1850-61.
[9] Gras L, Kesselring AM, Griffin JT, et al. CD4 cell counts of 800 cells/mm3 or greater after 7 years of highly active antiretroviral therapy are feasible in most patients starting with 350 cells/mm3 or greater. J Acquir Immune Defic Syndr. 2007;45:183-92.
[10] Smith K, Patel P, Fine DM, et al Randomized, double-blind, placebo-matched, multicenter trial of abacavir/lamivudine or tenofovir/emtricitabine with lopinavir/ritonavir for initial HIV treatment. AIDS 2009;23:1547-56
[11] Sax P, Tierney C, Collier A, and ACTG A5202 Study Team Abacavir-lamivudine versus tenofovir-emtricitabine for initial HIV-1 therapy New Engl J Med 2009;361:2230-40
[12] Daar E, Tierney C, Fischl M, and ACTG A5202 Study Team, ACTG 5202: Final Results of ABC/3TC or TDF/FTC with either EFV or ATV/r in Treatment-naive HIV-infected Patients, Abstract 59LB 17th Conference on Retroviruses and Opportunistic Infections San Francisco, CA, USA, 2010
[13] Gallant J, DeJesus E, Arribas JR, et al. Tenofovir DF, emtricitabine and efavirenz vs zidovudine, lamivudine and EFV for HIV. N Engl J Med 2006;354:251-60
[14] DeJesus E, Herrera G, Teofilo E, et al Abacavir versus Zidovudine combined with lamivudine and efavirenz, for the treatment of antiretroviral-naive HIV-infected adults Clin Infect Dis 2004;48:1038-46
[15] Berenguer J, Gonzales J, Ribera E, et al. Didanosine, lamivudine, and efavirenz vs zidovudine, lamivudine, and efavirenz, for initial treatment of HIV infection: Final analysis of a prospective randomized noninferiority clinical trial, GESIDA 3903 Clin Infect Dis 2008:47:1083-32
[16] Saag M, Cahn P, Raffi F, et al. Efficacy and safety of emtricitabine vs stavudine in combination therapy in antiretroviral-naive patients: a randomized trial JAMA 2004;292:180-90
[17] Cassetti I, Madruga JV, Suleiman JM, et al The safety and efficacy of tenofovir DF in combination with lamivudine and efavirenz through 6 years in antiretroviral-naïve HIV-1-infected patients. HIV Clin Trials 2007;8:164-72
[18] Mallal S, Phillips E, Caras G, et al HLA-B5701 screening for hypersensitivity to abacavir. New Engl J Med 2008;358:568-79
[19] National Institute of Allrgy and Infectious Diseases, Division of AIDS (DAIDS) table for grading severity of adult adverse experiences http://www.niaid.nih.gov
[20] Pappa K, Hernandez J, Ha1 B, et al Abacavir/lamivudine shows robust virologic responses in ART-naïve patients for baseline viral loads (VL) of >100,000c/mL and <100,000c/mL by endpoint used in ACTG5202, Abstract THABO304, XVII International AIDS Conference 2008
[21] Hill AM, Sawyer WS. Effects of NRTI backbone on efficacy of first-line boosted PI-based HAART--meta-analysis of 12 clinical trials in 4896 patients. Abstract H-1254. 48th Annual International Conference on Antimicrobial Agents and Chemotherapy 2008. Washington DC, USA.

[22] Vervoort SC, Borleffs JC, Hoepelman AI, et al Adherence in antiretroviral therapy: a review of qualitative studies. AIDS 2007;21:271-81
[23] Kantor R, Shafer RW, Follansbee S, et al Evolution of resistance to drugs in HIV-1 infected patients failing antiretroviral therapy. AIDS 2004;18:1503-11
[24] Sethi AK, Cellentano DD, Gange SJ, et al Association between adherence to antiretroviral therapy and human immunodeficiency virus drug resistance. Clin Infect Dis 2003;37:1112-8.
[25] Bartlett JA, DeMasi R, Quinn J,et al. Overview of the effectiveness of triple combination therapy in antiretroviral-naïve HIV-1 infected adults. AIDS (2001) 15: 1369-77.
[26] Ammassari A, Trotta MP, Murri R, et al. Correlates and predictors of adherence to HAART: Overview of published literature. J AIDS (2002) 31:S123-7.
[27] Parienti JJ, Bangsberg DR,Verdon R et al Better adherence with once daily antiretroviral therapy Clin Infect Dis 2009;48: 484-8
[28] Spaulding A, Rutherford GW, Siegfried N. Tenofovir or zidovudine in three-drug combination therapy with one nucleoside reverse transcriptase inhibitor and one non-nucleoside reverse transcriptase inhibitor for initial treatment of HIV infection in antiretroviral-naïve individuals. Cochrane Database Syst Rev. 2010:CD008740. Review.
[29] Gottesman BS, Leibovici L, Schapiro JM,et al. Nucleoside reverse transcriptase inhibitors in combination therapy for HIV patients: systematic review and meta-analysis. Eur J Clin Microbiol Infect Dis. 2010;29:779-86.
[30] Elzi L, Marzolini C, Furrer H, et al Swiss HIV Cohort Study.Treatment modification in human immunodeficiency virus-infected individuals starting combination antiretroviral therapy between 2005 and 2008. Arch Intern Med. 2010;170:57-65.
[31] Gill CJ, Griffith JL, Jacobson D, et alRelationship of HIV viral loads, CD4 counts, and HAART use to health-related quality of life. J Acquir Immune Defic Syndr. 2002;30:485-92.
[32] Harrigan PR, Hogg RS, Dong WW, et al Predictors of HIV drug-resistance mutations in a large antiretroviral-naive cohort initiating triple antiretroviral therapy. J Infect Dis 2005;191:339-47.
[33] Van Sighum Virologic failure and drug resistance. Chapter 5 Annual Report 2010 Monitoring of HIV infection in the Netherlands. Stichting HIV Monitoring (Athena cohort) www.hiv-monitoring.nl
[34] Nolan D, Mallal S. Complications associated with NRTI therapy: update on clinical features and possible pathogenic mechanisms. Antivir Ther 2004;9:849-63.
[35] White AJ. Mitochondrial toxicity and HIV therapy. Sex Transm Infect 2001;77:158-73.
[36] Kirian MA, Higginson RT, Fulco PP. Acute onset of pancreatitis with concomitant use of tenofovir and didanosine. Ann Pharmacother 2004;38:1660-63.
[37] Reisler RB, Murphy RL, Redfield RR, Parker RA Incidence of pancreatitis in HIV-1-infected individuals enrolled in 20 adult AIDS clinical trials group studies: lessons learned.J. Acquir Immune Defic Syndr 2005 ;39:159-66.
[38] Smith CJ, Olsen CH, Mocroft A, et al The role of antiretroviral therapy in the incidence of pancreatitis in HIV-positive individuals in the EuroSIDA study. AIDS. 2008 Jan 2;22:47-56.
[39] Kakuda TN. Pharmacology of nucleoside and nucleotide reverse transcriptase inhibitor-induced mitochondrial toxicity. Clin Ther 2000;22:685-708.

[40] Saves M, Raffi F, Capeau J, et al Factors related to lipodystrophy and metabolic alterations in patients with human immunodeficiency virus infection receiving highly active antiretroviral therapy. Clin Infect Dis 2002 34:1396-1405.

[41] Martin A, Smith DE, Carr A, et al Reversibility of lipoatrophy in HIV-infected patients 2 years after switching from a thymidine analogue to abacavir: the MITOX Extension Study. AIDS 2004;18:1029-36.

[42] Moyle G, Sabin C, Cartledge J, et al. A randomized trial of tenofovir DF abacavir as replacement for thymidine analog in persons with lipoatrophy. AIDS 2006;20:2043-50

[43] Arenas-Pinto A, Bhaskaran K, Dunn D, et al. The risk of developing peripheral neuropathy induced by nucleoside reverse transcriptase inhibitors decreases over time: evidence from the Delta trial. Antivir Ther. 2008;13:289-95.

[44] Moore RD, Wong WM, Keruly JC, et al Incidence of neuropathy in HIV-infected patients on monotherapy versus those on combination therapy with didanosine, stavudine and hydroxyurea. AIDS 2000;14:273-78.

[45] Davis CM, Shearer WT. Diagnosis and management of HIV drug hypersensitivity. J. Allergy Clin Immunol 2008;121:826-32

[46] Schiller DS. Identification, management, and prevention of adverse effects associated with highly active antiretroviral therapy. Am J Health Syst Pharm. 2004;61:2507-22.

[47] Zimmermann, A.E, Pizzoferrato T, Bedford J et al., Tenofovir-associated acute and chronic kidney disease: a case of multiple drug interactions. Clin Infect Dis. 2006;42:283-90.

[48] Fux CA, Simcock M, Wolbers M, et al Swiss HIV Cohort Study. Tenofovir use is associated with a reduction in calculated glomerular filtration rates in the Swiss HIV Cohort Study.Antivir Ther. 2007;12:1165-73.

[49] Mocroft A, Kirk O, Reiss P, De Wit S, Sedlacek D, Beniowski M, Gatell J, Phillips AN, Ledergerber B, Lundgren JD; EuroSIDA Study Group. Estimated glomerular filtration rate, chronic kidney disease and antiretroviral drug use in HIV-positive patients. AIDS 2010;24:1667-78.

[50] Izzedine, H.Hulot JS, Vittecoq D, et al. Long-term renal safety of tenofovir disoproxil fumarate in antiretroviral-naive HIV-1-infected patients. Data from a double-blind randomized active-controlled multicentre study. Nephrol Dial Transplant 2005;20:743-6.

[51] Gallant JE, Moore RD. Renal function with use of tenofovir-containing initial antiretroviral regimen. AIDS 2009;23:1971-75

[52] Wever K, van Agtmael MA, Carr A. Incomplete reversibility of tenofovir-related renal toxicity in HIV-infected men. J Acquir Immune Defic Syndr. 2010;55:78-81

[53] Cooper RD, Wiebe N, Smith N, et al Systematic review and meta-analysis: renal safety of tenofovir disoproxil fumarate in HIV-infected patients.Clinical Infect Dis 2010;51:496-505

[54] Guaraldi G, Zona S, Roverato A, et al. Prevalence of poly-pathology is more common in HIV-infected patients than in HIV-negative controls in any age strata. Program and abstracts of the 17th Conference on Retroviruses and Opportunistic Infections; February 16-19, 2010; San Francisco, California. Abstract 727.

[55] DAD Study Group, Friis-Møller N, Reiss P, et al. Class of antiretroviral drugs and the risk of myocardial infarction. N Engl J Med. 2007;356:1723-1735.

[56] Currier JS, Taylor A, Boyd F, et al. Coronary heart disease in HIV-infected individuals. J Acquir Immune Defic Syndr. 2003;33:506-512.
[57] Klein D, Hurley LB, Quesenberry CP Jr, Sidney S. Do protease inhibitors increase the risk for coronary heart disease in patients with HIV-1 infection? J Acquir Immune Defic Syndr. 2002;30:471-7.
[58] Triant VA, Lee H, Hadigan C, et al Increased acute myocardial infarction rates and cardiovascular risk factors among patients with human immunodeficiency virus disease. J Clin Endocrinol Metab. 2007;92:2506-12.
[59] Mary-Krause M, Cotte L, Simon A, et al. Increased risk of myocardial infarction with duration of protease inhibitor therapy in HIV-infected men. AIDS. 2003;17:2479-86.
[60] Bozzette SA, Ake CF, Tam HK, et al Cardiovascular and cerebrovascular events in patients treated for human immunodeficiency virus infection. N Engl J Med. 2003;348:702-10.
[61] Grunfeld C, Delaney JA, Wanke C, et al Preclinical atherosclerosis due to HIV infection: carotid intima-medial thickness measurements from the FRAM study. AIDS. 2009;23:1841-9.
[62] D:A:D Study Group, Sabin CA, Worm SW, et al. Use of nucleoside reverse transcriptase inhibitors and risk of myocardial infarction in HIV-infected patients enrolled in the D:A:D study: a multi-cohort collaboration. Lancet. 2008;371:1417-26.
[63] Worm SW, Sabin C, Weber R, et al. Risk of myocardial infarction in patients with HIV infection exposed to specific individual antiretroviral drugs from the 3 major drug classes: the Data Collection on Adverse Events of Anti-HIV Drugs (D:A:D) study. J Infect Dis. 2010;201:318-30.
[64] Strategies for Management of Anti-Retroviral Therapy/INSIGHT; DAD Study Groups. Use of nucleoside reverse transcriptase inhibitors and risk of myocardial infarction in HIV-infected patients. AIDS. 2008;22:F17-F24.
[65] Martínez E, Larrousse M, Podzamczer D, et al. Abacavir-based therapy does not affect biological mechanisms associated with cardiovascular dysfunction. AIDS. 2010;24:F1-F9.
[66] Bedimo R, Westfall A, Drechsler H, et al Abacavir use and risk of acute myocardial infarction and cerebrovascular disease in the HAART era. Program and abstracts of the 5th International AIDS Society Conference on HIV Pathogenesis, Treatment and Prevention; July 19-22, 2009; Cape Town, South Africa. Abstract MOAB202.
[67] Bartlett JA, Chen SS, Quinn JB. Comparative efficacy of nucleoside/nucleotide reverse transcriptase inhibitors in combination with efavirenz: results of a systematic overview. HIV Clin Trials. 2007;84:221-6. Review.
[68] Brown TT, Qaqish RB. Antiretroviral therapy and the prevalence of osteopenia and osteoporosis: a meta-analytic review. AIDS 2006;20:2165-74
[69] Womack J, Goulet J, Gibert C, and Veterans Aging Cohort Project Team. HIV infection and fragility fracture risk among male veterans. Program and abstracts of the 17th Conference on Retroviruses and Opportunistic Infections; February 16-19, 2010; San Francisco, California. Abstract 129.
[70] Gallant JE, Staszewski S, Pozniak AL, et al. Efficacy and safety of tenofovir DF vs stavudine in combination therapy in antiretroviral-naive patients: a 3-year randomized trial. JAMA. 2004;292:191-201.

[71] Martin A, Bloch M, Amin J, et al. Simplification of antiretroviral therapy with tenofovir-emtricitabine or abacavir-lamivudine: a randomized, 96-week trial. Clin Infect Dis. 2009;49:1591-1601.

[72] Moyle G, Givens N, Pearce H, Compston J. Effects of ART on bone turnover markers and bone density in HIV-infected patients. Antivir Ther. 2009;14(suppl 2):A14.

[73] Stellbrink HJ, Orkin C, Arribas JR, et al. Comparison of changes in bone density and turnover with abacavir-lamivudine versus tenofovir-emtricitabine in HIV-infected adults: 48-week results from the ASSERT study. Clin Infect Dis. 2010;51:963-972.

[74] McComsey G, Kitch D, Daar E, et al. Bone and limb fat outcomes of ACTG A5224s, a substudy of ACTG A5202: a prospective, randomized, partially blinded phase III trial of ABC/3TC or TDF/FTC with EFV or ATV/r for initial treatment of HIV-1 infection. Program and abstracts of the 17th Conference on Retroviruses and Opportunistic Infections; February 16-19, 2010a; San Francisco, California. Abstract 106LB.

[75] Huang J, Hughes M, Riddler S, et al. Effects of randomized regimen and nucleoside reverse transcriptase inhibitor (NRTI) selection on 96 week bone mineral density (BMD): results from ACTG 5142. Program and abstracts of the 18th International AIDS Conference; Vienna, Austria; July 18-23, 2010. Abstract WEAB0304.
www.emea.eu and www.fda.gov (latest assessed December 2010)

[76] Opravil M, Ledergerber B, Furrer H, et al Clinical efficacy of early initiation of HAART in patients with asymptomatic HIV infection and CD4 cell l count > 350 x 106/L. AIDS 2002:16:1371-81

[77] d'Arminio Monforte A, Lepri AC, Rezza G, et al Insight into reasons for discontinuation of the first highly active antiretroviral therapy regimen in a cohort of antiretroviral naïve patients. AIDS 2000;14:499-507

[78] Gras L, Smit C. Effects of cART on HIV RNA concentration in plasma, CD4 cell count and toxicity driven therapy changes. Chapter 4 Annual Report 2010 Monitoring of HIV infection in the Netherlands. Stichting HIV Monitoring (Athena cohort) www.hiv-monitoring.nl

[79] Dando TM, Scott LJ. Abacavir plus lamivudine: a review of their combined use in the management of HIV infection. Drugs 2005;65:285-302.

[80] Hervey PS, Perry CM. Abacavir: a review of its clinical potential in patients with HIV infection.Drugs 2000;60:447-79.

[81] Foster RH, Faulds D. Abacavir. Drugs 1998;55:729-736.

[82] Perry CM, Balfour JA. Didanosine. An update on its antiviral activity, pharmacokinetic properties and therapeutic efficacy in the management of HIV disease. Drugs 1996;52:928-62.

[83] Perry CM, Noble S. Didanosine: an updated review of its use in HIV infection. Drugs 1999;58:1099-1135.

[84] Bang LM, Scott LJ. Emtricitabine: an antiretroviral agent for HIV infection. Drugs 2003;63:2413-24.

[85] Dando TM, Wagstaff AJ. Emtricitabine/tenofovir disoproxil fumarate. Drugs 2004;64:2075-82.

[86] Johnson MA, Moore KH, Yuen GJ et al. Clinical pharmacokinetics of lamivudine. Clin Pharmacokinet 1999;36:41-66.

[87] Perry CM, Faulds D. Lamivudine. A review of its antiviral activity, pharmacokinetic properties and therapeutic efficacy in the management of HIV infection. Drugs 1997;53:657-80.
[88] Lea AP, Faulds D. Stavudine: a review of its pharmacodynamic and pharmacokinetic properties and clinical potential in HIV infection. Drugs 1996;51:846-64.
[89] Rana KZ, Dudley MN. Clinical pharmacokinetics of stavudine. Clin Pharmacokinet 1997;33:276-284.
[90] Kearney BP, Flaherty JF, Shah J. Tenofovir disoproxil fumarate: clinical pharmacology and pharmacokinetics. Clin Pharmacokinet 2004;43:595-612.
[91] Chapman T, McGavin J, Noble S. Tenofovir disoproxil fumarate. Drugs 2003;63:1597-1608.
[92] Lyseng-Williamson KA, Reynolds after et al. Tenofovir disoproxil fumarate: a review of its use in the management of HIV infection. Drugs 2005;65:413-32.
[93] Fung HB, Stone EA, Piacenti FJ. Tenofovir disoproxil fumarate: a nucleotide reverse transcriptase inhibitor for the treatment of HIV infection. Clin Ther 2002;24:1515-48.
[94] Wilde MI, Langtry HD. Zidovudine. An update of its pharmacodynamic and pharmacokinetic properties, and therapeutic efficacy. Drugs 1993;46:515-78.
[95] Acosta EP, Page LM, Fletcher CV. Clinical pharmacokinetics of zidovudine. An update. Clin Pharmacokinet 1996;30:251-62.
[96] EASL Clinical Practice Guidelines : Management of chronic hepatitis B. J of Hepatology 2009;50:227-42

Part 7

New Therapy Strategies

19

Crippling of HIV at Multiple Stages with Recombinant Adeno-Associated Viral Mediated RNA Interference

Ramesh B. Batchu[1,2] et al.*
[1]*Laboratory of Surgical Oncology & Developmental Therapeutics, Department of Surgery, Wayne State University, Detroit, MI*
[2]*John D. Dingell VA Medical Center, Detroit, MI*
USA

1. Introduction

Acquired immunodeficiency syndrome (AIDS) is a disease caused by the infection of human immunodeficiency virus-1 (HIV-1) that primarily impairs immune function by reducing the CD4 T-lymphocyte count. More than two decades after the first clinical evidence of AIDS was reported, AIDS continues to be a major public health problem worldwide with millions of people infected and new infections rising in an alarming rate in third world countries especially in Asia and sub-Saharan Africa.(1, 2) AIDS has become one of the most devastating diseases that the scientific community has ever faced, struggling till today to come up with a therapeutic strategy that successfully controls the disease. AIDS is now the leading cause of death in sub-Saharan Africa, and is presently the fourth biggest killer worldwide. AIDS-related deaths totaled over 5 million by 2009 reaching a cumulative death toll of over 30 million since the beginning of the epidemic. More than 75 million people have been infected with HIV-1, and roughly 2.7 million new HIV-1 infections were diagnosed in 2009(3) even though this rate has decreased from one decade ago.

To date, there is no effective treatment and the number of individuals infected with HIV-1 is growing dramatically in the eastern part of the world. Considering its infection rate, it is imperative to devise newer strategies to control progression of the disease. Although newer approaches such as highly active antiretroviral therapy (HAART) have proven to be effective in prolonging life, other constraints associated with their use underscores the need for development of other effective therapies. Protease inhibitors appear to be successful at controlling the viral replication immediately following budding of immature virus particle, but the development of drug resistant viral mutants and toxicity after prolonged therapy contributes to their failure.(4) HAART has considerable toxicity and its inability to

---

*Oksana V. Gruzdyn[1], Aamer M. Qazi[1,2], Assaad Y. Semaan[1], Shelly M. Seward[1], Christopher P. Steffes[1], David L. Bouwman[1], Donald W. Weaver[1] and Scott A. Gruber[2]
[1]*Laboratory of Surgical Oncology & Developmental Therapeutics, Department of Surgery, Wayne State University, Detroit, MI, USA*
[2]*John D. Dingell VA Medical Center, Detroit, MI, USA*

effectively act on virus in secondary lymphoid tissue is a significant drawback. Vast majority of people with AIDS live in poorer countries. HAART is expensive and unreachable to low and middle-income countries.(5) Many of these places do not have access to HAART, or if they do, supply can be intermittent. The finding that infections with drug-resistant HIV-1 are increasing further underscores the need to develop inhibitors of HIV-1 that are effective, affordable and universally accessible.

With the discovery of RNA interference (RNA*i*) phenomenon, that operates in mammalian cells and is highly effective in selective gene silencing, new, potent, small interfering RNA (siRNA) molecules have become available to add to control HIV-1. By analyzing the challenges of HIV-1 drug development, we review novel and multi-faceted therapies by simultaneously targeting multiple regions of HIV-1 so as to effectively cripple of the virus. The targets include essential cellular genes to avoid viral escape through mutations; multiple regions at various phases of the viral life cycle for a synergistic effect; and anti-sense approach as well to avoid viral escape strategies of HIV-1 against RNA*i*. Current challenges facing the advancement of RNA*i* therapy are its safety and inefficient delivery *in vivo*. Self-complimentary recombinant adeno-associated viral (rAAV-sc) vectors can overcome shortcomings associated with RNA*i*-mediated gene silence therapy.(6) AAV vectors are safe and clinically proven. New generation vectors with mutant capsids circumvent pitfalls of ubiquitin-proteasome mediated degradation leading to high-efficiency transduction at low doses ideally suited to be part of a new arsenal for in vivo RNA*i* delivery to fight HIV-1.(7) Unlike present drugs in the clinical trial or R&D stage, the multi-targeted AAV mediated RNA*i* approach not only kills the virus but also prevents the development of escape strategies and emergence of resistant viruses by simultaneous attack at multiple targets employing multiple technologies.

2. Traditional AIDS therapies

Anti-retroviral drugs such as nucleoside reverse transcriptase inhibitors and non-nucleoside inhibitors are first generation drugs successful in reducing the viral burden.(8-13) Although they prolong life in selected patients, these agents have significant side effects and generate drug resistant viral mutants. Protease inhibitors appear to be most effective at blocking HIV-1 replication, substantially reducing AIDS-related hospital admissions and death rates.(14)

Present-day therapy uses a combination of nucleoside analogues and protease inhibitors known as HAART.(15) HAART has been shown to be effective in controlling the spread of the virus by reducing the plasma viral load to undetectable levels and to some extent depleting the pool of virus in lymphoid tissues. In the past decade, HAART has become more effective with the introduction of several protease inhibitors, but the treatment is expensive and unavailable in poor countries.(5, 15) Approximately 30 million HIV-1 positive people of whom the vast majority live in low- and middle-income countries do not have access to proper treatment. This underscores the need for the development of inexpensive, yet effective drugs that can reach the majority of patients. Despite the apparent success of HAART therapy, the capacity of HIV-1 to establish latent infection of $CD4^+$ T cells allows viral particles to persist in tissues. Some studies indicated that the therapy does not completely eliminate viral replication in secondary lymphoid tissues. HIV-1 was routinely isolated from lymphoid organs of patients even after years of therapy due to continued replication.(16) Moreover, the initiation of HAART even as early as days after the onset of AIDS symptoms, could not prevent the establishment of a pool of latently-infected T lymphocytes.(17)These observations clearly indicate that traditional combinatorial therapies with protease inhibitors and nucleoside analogs for HIV-1, though effective in selected patients in prolonging life, unfortunately generate drug resistant viral mutants, unacceptable levels of drug toxicity, and are ineffective against virus in secondary lymphoid tissue.

3. Newer approaches to therapy

Introduction of molecules that are able to dominantly interfere with intracellular replication of HIV-1 is known as "intracellular immunization". Intracellular immunization by gene therapy strategies offers a promising alternative approach for controlling and managing HIV-1 disease. These include protein-based approaches such as trans-dominant strategies to inhibit HIV-1: toxins, zinc finger nucleases and single-chain antibodies.(18) Protein-based strategies have been the single largest area of anti-HIV-1 gene transfer trials in humans in the recent past.(19) Other RNA-based intracellular immunization approaches include the use of ribozymes and decoys. These second generation ribozymes are RNA molecules that cleave viral transcripts such as *tat, rev,* and *gag* at specific sequences targeting HIV-1 at critical stages, and have been shown to reduce HIV-1 levels *in vitro*.(20-22) RNA decoys are RNA homologues, such as TAR and RRE that bind viral proteins and compete with native ligands necessary for replication. They were also shown to inhibit HIV-1 *in vitro*.(20, 23, 24) In comparison with protein-based strategies, RNA-based approaches may have the advantage of not being immunogenic. Both viral or host cellular factors can be targeted, the latter potentially mitigating the possibility of escape mutants, but nevertheless, these trans-dominant approaches had shown initial promise but fell short of practical utility in providing adequate protection. DNA-based vaccines have shown partial success.(23, 25, 26) Anti-sense molecules were shown by several groups to inhibit HIV-1 *in vitro* when targeted towards critical HIV-1 genes such as *tat, rev,* and integrase, but the need for large amounts for *in vivo* studies apart from the problems associated with stability contributed to their failure to enter the clinic.(27)

4. RNA interference (RNA*i*): A natural way of gene silencing

Diseases, for which a foreign gene can be identified as the cause, such as in the case of viral infections, are potentially treatable by blocking its expression that will cripple the causative agent. Over the last decade, small non-coding RNA molecules such as short interfering RNA (siRNA), micro RNA (miRNA) and piwi RNA (*pi*RNA), collectively known as RNA interference (RNA*i*), emerged as critical regulators in mammalian gene expression and hold the promise of selectively inhibiting expression of disease-causing genes.(28, 29) RNA*i* is an evolutionarily conserved mechanism of gene inhibition or silencing first described in Caenorhabditis elegans and was shown to produce sequence-specific gene silencing.(30) In 1999, it was recognized as the natural cellular process to destroy unwanted foreign genes such as those causing viral infections(31). In 2001, for the first time, *the use of synthetic siRNA to silence genes in mammalian cells was demonstrated, and was referred to* as 'Biotech's billion dollar break through.(32) In short, RNA*i* has the potential to revolutionize the treatment approach to various diseases. Over the years, it has become clear that RNA*i* is a highly conserved molecular mechanism used by eukaryotic organisms to control gene expression during development and to defend their genomes against invaders, such as transposons and RNA viruses. siRNAs are primarily exogenous in origin, derived directly from the virus or transposon. siRNAs are 21 to 23 double-stranded RNA molecules that recognize the cognate mRNA with complementary sequence and cleave by naturally occurring cellular mechanisms.(31) *In vivo* silencing occurs after the formation of long double-stranded RNAs that are processed into short interfering RNAs (siRNAs) by an enzyme called Dicer, forming a ribonucleo-protein complex called RNA induced silencing complex (RISC). In the RISC, the anti-sense strand of the siRNA serves as a guide for the degradation of the homologous RNA target. In recent years, siRNA has emerged as a method of choice for specific and efficient gene silencing.

Since discovery of their mechanism, chemically synthesized siRNA molecules are being used to target abnormally elevated genes in many diseases. Since siRNA is a natural biological mechanism against viruses, it can elicit specific intracellular antiviral resistance that may provide a therapeutic strategy against human viruses. siRNAs have been shown to inhibit viral replication or block gene expression in cell culture systems for several viruses. In one study, pre-treatment of cells siRNAs specific to the poliovirus genome promoted the clearance of the virus from most of the infected cells.(33) Shlomai et al observed significant reduction in hepatitis B virus (HBV) by siRNA-producing vectors.(34) A number of groups have demonstrated that siRNAs interfere with hepatitis C virus (HCV) gene expression and replication.(35-39) Over 90% of human cervical cancers are positive for human papilloma virus (HPV) and siRNA-mediated silencing of E6 and E7, the viral genes necessary for the HPV life cycle, completely inhibited them in mammalian cells.(40)

5. Targeting HIV-1 with RNA*i*

Since siRNA can elicit specific knockdown of transcripts and they have been successfully used against human viruses, this ancient defense mechanism can be recruited as a weapon in the fight against HIV-1. Several laboratories have shown that the introduction of siRNAs specific for HIV-1 transcripts has shown viral RNA degradation and inhibition of replication. (41-43) Stable and modified promoters for the expression of siRNA molecules have further shown to increase the potency of HIV *in vitro*.(44) The successful silencing of HIV-1 replication by several investigators through siRNA-mediated targeted knockdown of viral proteins made RNA interference a weapon of choice against HIV-1. (41, 45, 46)

HIV-1 has a total of 15 proteins encoded by 9 genes.(47) Essentially, these can be grouped into four potential target sets for siRNA knockdown. The first potential target for gene silencing is the viral genomic RNA upon viral entry. Jacque et al demonstrated siRNA-mediated destruction of incoming HIV-1(48), although other studies of RNA*i* inhibition of retroviral infection suggested that incoming genomic RNA may not be the best target for siRNAs.(49) Once viral DNA is integrated, the viral mRNA transcripts as well as the un-spliced genomic RNA can be potential target. Early transcripts of HIV-1 such as *rev*, *nef* and *tat* are an important second group of targets for gene silencing with RNA*i* because they not only regulate the subsequent expression of the structural genes, *gag*, *pol*, and *env* but also the synthesis of full length viral genomic RNA. siRNA targeting the *nef* gene has been demonstrated to provide efficient silencing in a transient-transfection system.(50) There have been efficient demonstrations of silencing of the expression of various regulatory genes in a transient-transfection system.(44, 51, 52) siRNAs targeted to the TAR regulatory region and nef of the HIV-1 genome have also been shown to be effective at silencing the level of virus replication and inhibiting reverse transcription intermediates.(53, 54) After regulatory genes, structural genes also represent a potential target group.(55-57) It was found that inhibition was more significant when the siRNA

were present before the viral infection. This is because the vulnerability of genomic HIV RNA for RNA*i*-mediated knockdown is much greater immediately after viral entry into the cytoplasm due to the availability of target transcripts.
A crucial finding was that a high degree of specificity of the RNA*i* for the sequence of its target was required. Even one base pair change dramatically lowers the potency of RNA*i*-mediated inhibition.(58)This becomes important, given the high error rate of HIV-1 reverse transcriptase that leads to the emergence of RNA*i* escape mutants. The HIV-1 virus often becomes resistant to RNAi therapy as a result of the appearance of mutant variants. Because of these mutations, although siRNA directed against various HIV-1 genes shows initial success, the virus may soon escape inhibition within weeks. (44) Silencing evasion can also result from loss of target sequences within viral genomes, owing to the high viral mutation rates. In lymphocytes, for example, the effects of anti-HIV-1 siRNAs were progressively dampened by the emergence of viral quasi species that harbor mutations within the siRNA target sequence.(59) RNA*i*-mediated inhibition with single target has not yet been shown to protect cells against HIV-1 in long-term. RNA*i* could become a realistic therapeutic option, however, if used in a combined fashion while targeting multiple genes to prevent the emergence of mutant viruses. Simultaneous attacks by siRNA on various targets will minimize the escape of the resistant virus.

6. Cellular targets of HIV for RNA*i*

An essential cellular HIV receptor or co-receptor target may have more appeal than viral targets, which are prone to mutations. Cellular mRNAs that encode critical proteins involved in HIV-1 replication may circumvent pitfalls associated with viral escape mechanisms. Targeting cellular genes that are an essential part of the HIV-1 life cycle could therefore be advantageous. CD4 is the primary cellular receptor for HIV-1 entry on T lymphocytes. In addition to the CD4 primary receptor, the cellular chemokine receptors CCR5 and CXCR4, which function as co-receptors for HIV-1, have provided new therapeutic targets and a better understanding of the progression of viral infection. Several investigators targeted cellular proteins necessary for the HIV-1 life cycle by siRNAs and produced decreased levels of virus production.(60, 61) Preliminary observations from various laboratories have demonstrated that siRNAs specific for CD4 receptor do indeed inhibit HIV-1 replication.(62, 63) After transfection of cultured T cells with siRNA against the mRNA for CD4, HIV production, after exposure of the cells to the virus, decreased substantially. (64) CCR5, an HIV-1 co-receptor for the M-tropic HIV-1 variant, providing an attractive cellular target for siRNAs since homozygous deletions of CCR5 effectively confer protection from HIV-1 without any serious deleterious effects in immune function.(65) At least one group has taken advantage of this target for RNA*i*-mediated gene silencing, demonstrating that in vitro knockdown of CCR5 by siRNAs provided marked protection from HIV-1 infection.(63)
Although suppression of the primary receptor CD4 may be restricted by its normal role in the immune system, CCR5 seems dispensable for normal life.(66) Unfortunately, not all HIV-1 strains require CCR5, and the inhibition of CCR5 may result in the selection of HIV-1 variants that use CXCR4 as a co-receptor. It is critical to identify this particular aspect by studying strain variants.

7. Escape strategies of HIV-1 from siRNA

One of the hallmarks of RNA*i* is its sequence-specific knockdown of the target transcript, but unfortunately, it also presents a way out for HIV-1, since single nucleotide substitutions in the target region can drastically decrease the efficiency of the knockdown. HIV-1 has a high mutation rate, and this is one of the reasons why RNA*i* gene silencing has not yet been shown to protect cells against HIV-1 in long-term virus replication assays although they were successful in the short term. For example, the effects of anti-HIV-1 siRNAs in lymphocytes were progressively dampened by the emergence of viral mutant genes *tat* and *nef* through nucleotide substitution or deletions within the siRNA target sequences.(44, 59) HIV-1 can also escape from RNA*i*-mediated inhibition through mutations that alter the local RNA secondary structure.(67) This emergence of escape mutants occurs even without necessarily changing the encoded protein after prolonged culturing. In order to circumvent the emergence of resistant viruses, targeting of conserved sequences and the simultaneous use of multiple siRNAs have been suggested. Further strategies to prevent this siRNA escape strategy by HIV-1 suggested the use of anti-sense for *tat* and *nef* genes. Unlike siRNA, the anti-sense approach is not a natural phenomenon occurring in the cells and no escape strategies have been developed by HIV-1. By the combination of gene knockout by two approaches, an effective and complete suppression of HIV-1 can be achieved.

8. Multi-targeted knockdown of HIV-1 genes

Although targeting a single HIV-1 sequence can result in strong inhibition of viral replication, it is likely followed by viral escape. Thus far, studies establishing the utility of siRNAs in suppressing HIV-1 infection failed in the long run because of the high mutation rate of HIV-1 replication. There are considerable challenges in achieving this long-term inhibition, preventing the transient success achieved from translating into clinical advantage. Therefore, approaches that not only target different stages of the viral life cycle but also simultaneously target specific sets of cellular genes that are needed for viral entry should be explored. In fact, it has been clearly demonstrated that the introduction of multiple siRNAs specific for HIV-1 could lead to viral RNA degradation and replication during different stages of the viral life cycle.(59) This multi-frontal RNA*i*-mediated attack on HIV-1 potentially inhibits the mutation escape mechanism. There have been several successful demonstrations of inhibition of HIV-1 replication using siRNA targeting distinct steps of the viral life cycle. HIV RNA in the post entry complex was successfully degraded abolishing the integration of proviral DNA when siRNAs targeted more than one region.(43) Dual-specific short hairpin siRNA constructs containing an intervening bridge, targeted against both receptors were demonstrated to successfully inhibit HIV-1 replication, thus demonstrating the practical utility of an siRNA multi-frontal attack on HIV-1.(60)

It has been previously established that if the length of siRNA exceeds 30 bp, there is an induction of nonspecific antiviral interferon responses.(33) Contrary to this belief, it was shown recently that this phenomenon might not be applicable to all sequences. Chang et al. generated 38 bp siRNAs that can induce targeted gene silencing of more than one gene without nonspecific antiviral responses. This structural flexibility of gene silencing with siRNAs needs to be further explored in order to achieve complete inhibition of HIV-1 by targeting simultaneously several regions.(68) By targeting two separate regions to knockout transcription of the gene *rev*, the highest degree of inhibition of viral replication was achieved.(69)

These newer drug designs had shown initial promise, but fell short of practical utility in providing adequate protection in every case. Since no effective therapy is currently available for prevention, new and innovative therapies are urgently needed to control, prevent and

eradicate HIV-1 disease. With this backdrop of HIV-1 drug development research, we propose to develop a cocktail of HIV-1 drug analogous to the current clinical use of combinations of antiviral drugs that target the reverse transcriptase and protease enzymes. These combinatorial approaches attacking multiple targets were designed essentially to prevent escape strategies observed by HIV-1 by various labs.
Analogous to the current clinical practice of HAART therapy, RNA*i* approaches should also be administered in a combined fashion to prevent HIV-1 escape strategies.

9. Limitations and hurdles of *in vivo* delivery of RNA*i*

Although RNA*i* mediated inhibition through siRNAs to knockdown HIV-1 genes in the laboratory has been successful, transfection of these purchased siRNA from commercial sources is impractical and has little value for translational work. siRNA is highly labile and often requires exceptionally high levels to achieve gene silencing *in vivo*. Further, the gene-silencing effect of siRNA is directly dependent on the number of molecules available in the cells, underscoring the need for development of plasmid vectors for the continuous synthesis of siRNA inside the cell. Current challenges facing the *in vivo* application of siRNA are the maintenance of duplex stability to avoid endonuclease degradation, need for improved delivery and the need to minimize immunological responses.(70) Though successful *in vivo* application of siRNA was demonstrated in liver through high-pressure tail vein injection in a murine model, its applicability to humans is limited.(71, 72) The quantity of siRNA necessary for efficient silencing is incompatible with scale-up to larger preclinical models.(73) Liposomal packaging(74) and chemical modification of the RNA and polyethylene glycol (PEG)(75) conjugated methods give stability to siRNA molecules, but still require large amounts of RNA*i* and are financially non-viable techniques. Hydrodynamic transfection of siRNA has been successful in targeting organs in mice, but this approach is not practical for clinical use. (76, 77)
One way to address this problem is to construct a siRNA sequence for insertion in a vector for intracellular expression of siRNA. Here the siRNA cassette is driven by RNA polymerase III promoter such as U6 that express sense and antisense strands separated by short "hairpin" RNAs (shRNAs) that are cleaved by the dicer to produce siRNA. In some cases both the sense and anti-sense siRNA strands are transcribed separately, which then hybridize *in vivo* to make the siRNA. Expression from a DNA plasmid or a viral vector such as shRNA enhances stability and safe delivery of siRNA apart from providing continuous production *in vivo*. It has been demonstrated that the transfection of human cells with plasmid encoding shRNA against HIV-1 *rev* drastically inhibited viral replication over a period of several days. Further, the highest degree of inhibition of viral replication was achieved by simultaneously targeting two distinct sites within *rev*.(51, 69)
Selection of highly accessible targets within the HIV-1 RNA genome should be determined first with antisense DNA oligonucleotide arrays before designing shRNA.(78, 79) There is recent evidence that the efficacy of siRNAs is similarly influenced by secondary structure in the target transcript.(80). These selection criteria should be used in the design of the siRNA molecule in order to get optimal inhibition.

10. Efficient delivery and expression of shRNA by viral vectors

One of the important limitations of siRNA-mediated drug delivery is the vehicle to carry the inhibitory molecules to the target cells. Viral vectors are generally more efficient vehicles for shRNA *in vivo* than nonviral vectors.(81) Adenovirus, retro- or lentivirus, and AAV have been successfully used for this purpose. Retroviral/lentiviral vectors can potentially generate insertional mutagenesis, while adenoviral vectors trigger unacceptable levels of immune responses with concerns of safety.(82) shRNA can be packaged as recombinant viral vectors for better delivery in the whole organism. Retroviral vectors are successfully used for shRNA delivery, derived from moloney murine leukemia virus (MMLV). Lentiviral vectors are derived from HIV itself and can infect all the cells without the need for receptor interaction. Studies with lentiviral vectors silencing CCR5 have been performed but showed that the down regulating effect of CCR5 alone was insufficient. However, combinatorial constructs targeted to both CXCR4 and CCR5 and have shown better efficacy.(61) Retroviral/lentiviral vectors randomly integrate into the genome, generate insertional mutagenesis, and are derived from pathogenic viruses.

Dual-specific short hairpin siRNA constructs containing an intervening spacer, targeting receptor and co-receptor, demonstrated the practical utility of shRNA constructs synthesized as a single transcript. Since the shRNA design will permit tandem assembly of multiple motifs, it is now possible to introduce promising multivalent siRNA constructs into viral vectors for *in vivo* gene therapeutic applications. Based on this rationale, recent work with synthetic siRNAs demonstrated that down regulating either CXCR4 or CCR5 will protect cells from X4 or R5 HIV-1 strains, respectively, at the level of viral entry.(83) As mentioned earlier, CCR5 is a co-receptor, necessary for cellular entry by HIV-1 (R5 tropic viral strain), but is dispensable for normal human physiology. Owing to its crucial role in HIV-1 infection, the CCR5 co-receptor has been the subject of many therapeutic approaches, including RNA*i*-mediated gene silence therapy. siRNA targeting was shown to be effective; however, complete knockdown remained an elusive goal. In one study, transgenic macrophages expressing high levels of CCR5 were used for testing the efficacy of lentiviral vectors carrying CCR5 shRNA. Lentiviral delivery of longer (28-mer) shRNA were shown to be very effective in gene knockdown.(84) Thus, anti-CCR5 shRNA viral delivery is a promising candidate for clinical application.

We have tested retroviral vectors for gene therapy(85, 86); however, retroviral-mediated gene therapy is limited by a variety of practical and theoretical concerns, such as the immunogenicity of viral capsid proteins and insertional mutagenesis, which limit their utility for clinical purposes.(87)

Adenoviral vectors have also been successfully used for the delivery of shRNA(88) but they are well known to trigger unacceptable levels of immune responsiveness due to their large size and thereby limit repeat administration. Stability and efficiency is not the concern with viral vectors, but safety is a primary concern.

11. Recombinant Adeno-Associated Virus (rAAV) – Ideal RNA*i* gene silence therapy vectors

AAV belongs to the parvovirus family and is the only viral vector not known to be associated with any human disease(89) and the smallest vector suitable for RNA*i*-mediated gene silencing. Due to the safety(90), efficacy and potency provided by rAAV vectors, they make better alternative to the more commonly-used retroviral, lentiviral and adenovirus based vectors for gene therapy. rAAV vectors are easy to propagate and have many characteristics that make them a better choice for somatic gene therapy with RNA*i*-mediated gene silencing.(91, 92) rAAV vectors have long been established to transduce a wide variety of tissues.(93-95) First generation rAAV vectors were single stranded, but the development of self-complimentary (double stranded) rAAV vectors helped to avoid delay in trans-gene expression.(96) Multiple administration of the rAAV vectors is possible to overcome neutralization by the antibody produced following the initial administration due to the availability of multiple serotypes with significantly higher trans-gene expression levels than that of prototype single stranded-vectors.(97) rAAV-based vectors have the potential for stable long-term trans-gene expression. rAAV is naturally gutless vector, which do not express any viral genes or cause a cytotoxic cellular immune response in the host. Furthermore, rAAV vectors show only a modest frequency of integration into host genome, thus avoiding insertional mutagenesis.(89) Overall, rAAV vectors fulfill the requirements for an ideal *in vivo* RNA*i* delivery vehicle.

12. Capsid mutant rAAV for enhanced transduction

One of the shortcomings of the traditional rAAV vectorology is low transduction efficiency, which requires large doses of vectors to achieve the desired effect. This is due to the phosphorylation of AAV capsids at tyrosine residues in the cell, which leads to a ubiquitin-proteasome-mediated destruction of the majority of rAAV particles and a decrease in transduction efficiency.(98) Gene therapy with these traditional rAAV vectors necessitates the delivery of undesirably high doses of the virus in order to achieve therapeutic benefit.(99) Recent advances have lead to the generation of rAAV vectors with mutant capsids protecting them from ubiquitin-proteasome-mediated degradation in the cytosol, eventually leading to an increase in DNA transduction efficiency.(7) We acquired these next generation rAAV vectors from Dr. Srivastava's laboratory consisting of a variant of rAAV-2/8 with a mutated capsid making the vector resistant to degradation in the cytosol.(7) By using triple-capsid mutant, pACG2-3M (Y444F, Y500F & Y730F)(7), along with the self-complimentary rAAV vector, we achieved a significant enhancement in rAAV2-sc green fluorescent protein (GFP) mediated transduction (Fig-1). With pseudo-typed rAAV vectors and capsid mutations, even greater *in vivo* transduction efficiency has been demonstrated.(7)

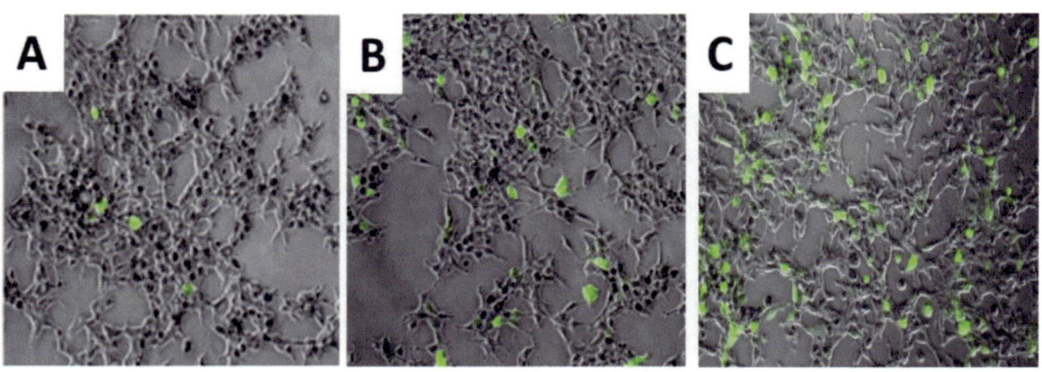

Fig. 1. HEK-293 cells transduced with various preparations of rAAV-GFP showing transduction efficiency based on green fluorescence intensity. A. Wild type rAAV-GFP; B. rAAV double stranded-GFP; C. rAAV-Capsid mutant.

13. rAAV vectors for siRNA delivery *in vivo* as short hairpin RNA (shRNA)

An ideal vector system for RNA*i* expression should be efficient and allow stable expression of the shRNA cassette without causing insertional mutagenesis or undesired immune responses. AAV is a small virus of 4.7 kb and relatively simple in its organization, comprising only two genes *Rep* and *Cap*. AAV vectors are extremely efficient tools for gene delivery *in vitro* and *in vivo*, as demonstrated by a number of laboratories. rAAV vectors have been shown to efficiently transduce hematopoietic cells.(100-102) Moreover, rAAV only retain inverted terminal repeats but do not express any viral genes and thus are gutless by design and definition more over it has not been associated with any human pathogenic, making it the vector of choice for human gene therapy. Because of their efficient transcription and inability to recombine with HIV-1, rAAV vectors represent a promising form of anti-retroviral gene therapy.(100)

One of the first studies using rAAV vector to deliver shRNA by Tomar et al. provided initial proof of principle that rAAV vector particles can be engineered to express shRNA.(88) They showed efficient knockdown of p53 and caspase 8 proteins. Subsequent studies by several investigators further demonstrated the usefulness of the rAAV vectors to express the shRNA cassette.(103-106) rAAV vectors have also been successfully used for a variety of gene silence experiments.(103-105) Use of rAAV vector encoding an anti-sense RNA against HIV-1 has been well documented by various labs.(23, 27, 100, 107) We studied the effect of anti-sense p53 gene transduction in a multiple myeloma cell line, ARH77, using AAV vector, where we delivered p53 cDNA in an anti-sense orientation.(108) *In vivo* studies in mice showed persistent knockdown of the target tyrosine hydroxylase in a Parkinson's disease model. They further demonstrated that reduction in the target elicited behavioral defects in the treated mice and created a phenotype reminiscent of rodent models of Parkinson's disease.

rAAV-mediated transduction is very efficient, particularly when compared with passive entry of simple siRNA or plasmid DNA.(109-111) rAAV siRNA delivery has been recently tested by several groups and shown to be highly efficient. Specific and efficient inhibition of HIV-1 replication was demonstrated in cultures.(91, 112) Together, this underscores the great promise of pseudo-typing shRNA-expressing AAV vectors to achieve targeted and controlled siRNA induction *in vivo*. Although the targeting of a single HIV-1 sequence can result in strong inhibition of viral replication, it is likely to be followed by viral escape. In fact, in most *in vitro* tests, siRNA did not stand the test of long-term protection against HIV-1. To overcome this escape strategy by HIV-1, we have a multi-pronged attack on HIV-1. First, HIV-1 is targeted at multiple genes for inhibition. Second, HIV-1 entry is inhibited by targeting siRNA to its cellular receptor CCR5 that is resistant to mutation. Third, we are introducing an anti-sense approach to knockdown HIV-1 *tat*, shown to be responsible for siRNA escape. Synthetic bi-specific or combinatorial constructs targeting both CXCR4 and CCR5 receptors have shown to confer resistance to HIV-1 infection much stronger than that conferred by targeting each one alone, giving a clear indication that multiple targeting is better than a single target.(22, 43, 61, 113)

14. Conclusion

Gene silencing therapy has the potential to inhibit HIV-1 replication and increase patient quality of life as an additional therapeutic class, and may serve as an adjuvant to current HAART treatment. This review gives a brief introduction regarding the emergence of RNAi, the hurdles to overcome to proceed to the next stage, and possible solutions. Although RNA*i* molecules can be introduced into cells as double stranded or expressed from a plasmid to inhibit abnormally elevated genes, transfection of these purchased molecules from commercial sources is impractical and has little value for translational work. The main difficulty thus far in extending the power of RNA interference (RNA*i*) to clinical practice has been the development of safe vectors coding for shRNAs to achieve persistent knockdown *in vivo*. rAAV vectors are different from other vectors, since the only gene expressed from recombinant vector is the trans-gene itself, naturally gutless by design and thus avoiding any cytotoxic cellular immune responses in the host. Furthermore, rAAV vectors show only a modest frequency of integration into the host genome, thus avoiding insertional mutagenesis, which has been a stumbling block for the clinical use of retroviral or lentiviral vectors. Development of self-complimentary (also known as double stranded) vectors to avoid delay in trans-gene expression(96, 114) and packaging with capsid mutants(115) to increase transduction efficiency has further contributed to rAAV vectorology. Recent advances in our understanding of RNA*i* make rAAV an especially attractive candidate for anti-HIV-1 gene therapy, and rAAV-based RNA*i* approaches can be combined with other therapeutic modalities to make a combinatorial therapy akin to HAART.

15. Acknowledgments

This work has been conducted at the John D Dingell VA Medical Center, Detroit, MI 48201 and Karmanos Cancer Institute, Detroit, MI 48201. Ariel J. Harden helped with manuscript corrections.

16. References

[1] C.J. Liand C.J. Li. Therapeutic biology: checkpoint pathway activation therapy, HIV Tat, and transkingdom RNA interference. Journal of Cellular Physiology. 209:695-700 (2006).
[2] Q.E. Yang. Eradication of HIV in infected patients: some potential approaches. Medical Science Monitor. 10:RA155-165 (2004).
[3] J. Ambrosioni, A. Calmy, and B. Hirschel. HIV treatment for prevention. Journal of the International AIDS Society. 14:28 (2011).
[4] M. Harringtonand J. Hidalgo. HIV TREATMENT FAILURE: A REVIEW OF CURRENT CLINICAL RESEARCH, Vol. 1, 2010.
[5] T. Gonzalo, M.G. Goñi, and M.Á. Muñoz-Fernández. Socio-economic impact of antiretroviral treatment in HIV patients. An economic review of cost savings after introduction of HAART. AIDS Reviews. 11:79-90 (2009).
[6] C. Muellerand T. Flotte. Clinical gene therapy using recombinant adeno-associated virus vectors. Gene Therapy. 15:858-863 (2008).
[7] L. Zhong, B. Li, C.S. Mah, L. Govindasamy, M. Agbandje-McKenna, M. Cooper, R.W. Herzog, I. Zolotukhin, K.H. Warrington, and K.A. Weigel-Van Aken. Next generation of adeno-associated virus 2 vectors: point mutations in tyrosines lead to high-efficiency transduction at lower doses. Proceedings of the National Academy of Sciences. 105:7827 (2008).
[8] S. Beckerand L. Thornton. Fosamprenavir: advancing HIV protease inhibitor treatment options. Expert Opinion on Pharmacotherapy. 5:1995-2005 (2004).

[9] M. Boffito, D. Maitland, Y. Samarasinghe, and A. Pozniak. The pharmacokinetics of HIV protease inhibitor combinations. Current Opinion in Infectious Diseases. 18:1-7 (2005).

[10] B.A. Boyle, R.A. Elion, G.J. Moyle, and C.J. Cohen. Considerations in selecting protease inhibitor therapy. AIDS Reviews. 6:218-225 (2004).

[11] R. Hazra, F.M. Balis, A.N. Tullio, E. DeCarlo, C.J. Worrell, S.M. Steinberg, J.F. Flaherty, K. Yale, M. Poblenz, B.P. Kearney, L. Zhong, D.F. Coakley, S. Blanche, J.L. Bresson, J.A. Zuckerman, and S.L. Zeichner. Single-dose and steady-state pharmacokinetics of tenofovir disoproxil fumarate in human immunodeficiency virus-infected children. Antimicrobial Agents & Chemotherapy. 48:124-129 (2004).

[12] B.L. Musial, J.K. Chojnacki, and C.I. Coleman. Atazanavir: a new protease inhibitor to treat HIV infection.[erratum appears in Am J Health Syst Pharm. 2004 Nov 1;61(21):2243]. American Journal of Health-System Pharmacy. 61:1365-1374 (2004).

[13] A. Winstonand M. Boffito. The management of HIV-1 protease inhibitor pharmacokinetic interactions. Journal of Antimicrobial Chemotherapy. 56:1-5 (2005).

[14] P. Braitstein, M. Brinkhof, F. Dabis, M. Schechter, A. Boulle, P. Miotti, R. Wood, C. Laurent, E. Sprinz, and C. Seyler. Mortality of HIV-1-infected patients in the first year of antiretroviral therapy: comparison between low-income and high-income countries. Lancet. 367:817 (2006).

[15] K.M. Johnston, A.R. Levy, V.D. Lima, R.S. Hogg, M.W. Tyndall, P. Gustafson, A. Briggs, and J.S. Montaner. Expanding access to HAART: a cost-effective approach for treating and preventing HIV. AIDS. 24:1929 (2010).

[16] D. Finzi, M. Hermankova, T. Pierson, L.M. Carruth, C. Buck, R.E. Chaisson, T.C. Quinn, K. Chadwick, J. Margolick, R. Brookmeyer, J. Gallant, M. Markowitz, D.D. Ho, D.D. Richman, and R.F. Siliciano. Identification of a reservoir for HIV-1 in patients on highly active antiretroviral therapy.[see comment]. Science. 278:1295-1300 (1997).

[17] J. Uy, C. Armon, K. Buchacz, K. Wood, and J.T. Brooks. Initiation of HAART at higher CD4 cell counts is associated with a lower frequency of antiretroviral drug resistance mutations at virologic failure. JAIDS Journal of Acquired Immune Deficiency Syndromes. 51:450 (2009).

[18] G.P. Symonds, H.A. Johnstone, M.L. Millington, M.P. Boyd, B.P. Burke, and L.R. Breton. The use of cell-delivered gene therapy for the treatment of HIV/AIDS. Immunologic Research:1-15 (2010).

[19] M. Giacca. Gene therapy to induce cellular resistance to HIV-1 infection: lessons from clinical trials. Advances in Pharmacology. 56:297-325 (2008).

[20] R. Akkina, A. Banerjea, J. Bai, J. Anderson, M.J. Li, and J. Rossi. siRNAs, ribozymes and RNA decoys in modeling stem cell-based gene therapy for HIV/AIDS. Anticancer Research. 23:1997-2005 (2003).

[21] J. Bai, S. Gorantla, N. Banda, L. Cagnon, J. Rossi, and R. Akkina. Characterization of anti-CCR5 ribozyme-transduced CD34+ hematopoietic progenitor cells in vitro and in a SCID-hu mouse model in vivo. Molecular Therapy: the Journal of the American Society of Gene Therapy. 1:244-254 (2000).

[22] Y. Feng, M. Leavitt, R. Tritz, E. Duarte, D. Kang, M. Mamounas, P. Gilles, F. Wong-Staal, S. Kennedy, J. Merson, M. Yu, and J.R. Barber. Inhibition of CCR5-dependent HIV-1 infection by hairpin ribozyme gene therapy against CC-chemokine receptor 5. Virology. 276:271-278 (2000).

[23] S.F. Ding, R. Lombardi, R. Nazari, and S. Joshi. A combination anti-HIV-1 gene therapy approach using a single transcription unit that expresses antisense, decoy, and sense RNAs, and trans-dominant negative mutant Gag and Env proteins. Frontiers in Bioscience. 7:a15-28 (2002).
[24] A. Michienzi, S. Li, J.A. Zaia, and J.J. Rossi. A nucleolar TAR decoy inhibitor of HIV-1 replication. Proceedings of the National Academy of Sciences of the United States of America. 99:14047-14052 (2002).
[25] M.L. Bonyhadi, K. Moss, A. Voytovich, J. Auten, C. Kalfoglou, I. Plavec, S. Forestell, L. Su, E. Bohnlein, and H. Kaneshima. RevM10-expressing T cells derived in vivo from transduced human hematopoietic stem-progenitor cells inhibit human immunodeficiency virus replication. Journal of Virology. 71:4707-4716 (1997).
[26] M.H. Malim, W.W. Freimuth, J. Liu, T.J. Boyle, H.K. Lyerly, B.R. Cullen, and G.J. Nabel. Stable expression of transdominant Rev protein in human T cells inhibits human immunodeficiency virus replication. Journal of Experimental Medicine. 176:1197-1201 (1992).
[27] J. Goodchild, S. Agrawal, M.P. Civeira, P.S. Sarin, D. Sun, and P.C. Zamecnik. Inhibition of human immunodeficiency virus replication by antisense oligodeoxynucleotides.[erratum appears in Proc Natl Acad Sci U S A 1989 Mar;86(5):1504]. Proceedings of the National Academy of Sciences of the United States of America. 85:5507-5511 (1988).
[28] M.T. McManusand P.A. Sharp. Gene silencing in mammals by small interfering RNAs. Nature Reviews Genetics. 3:737-747 (2002).
[29] N.J. Caplen, S. Parrish, F. Imani, A. Fire, and R.A. Morgan. Specific inhibition of gene expression by small double-stranded RNAs in invertebrate and vertebrate systems. Proceedings of the National Academy of Sciences of the United States of America. 98:9742-9747 (2001).
[30] A. Fire, S. Xu, M.K. Montgomery, S.A. Kostas, S.E. Driver, and C.C. Mello. Potent and specific genetic interference by double-stranded RNA in Caenorhabditis elegans.[see comment]. Nature. 391:806-811 (1998).
[31] A.J. Hamiltonand D.C. Baulcombe. A species of small antisense RNA in posttranscriptional gene silencing in plants.[comment]. Science. 286:950-952 (1999).
[32] D. Stipp. Biotech's Billion Dollar Breakthrough. Fortune (2003).
[33] L. Gitlin, S. Karelsky, and R. Andino. Short interfering RNA confers intracellular antiviral immunity in human cells.[see comment]. Nature. 418:430-434 (2002).
[34] A. Shlomaiand Y. Shaul. Inhibition of hepatitis B virus expression and replication by RNA interference. Hepatology. 37:764-770 (2003).
[35] T. Hugleand A. Cerny. Current therapy and new molecular approaches to antiviral treatment and prevention of hepatitis C. Reviews in Medical Virology. 13:361-371 (2003).
[36] C. Martinand-Mari, B. Lebleu, and I. Robbins. Oligonucleotide-based strategies to inhibit human hepatitis C virus. Oligonucleotides. 13:539-548 (2003).
[37] G. Randalland C.M. Rice. Interfering with hepatitis C virus RNA replication. Virus Research. 102:19-25 (2004).
[38] P.D. Zamoreand N. Aronin. siRNAs knock down hepatitis.[comment]. Nature Medicine. 9:266-267 (2003).
[39] J.A. Wilson, S. Jayasena, A. Khvorova, S. Sabatinos, I.G. Rodrigue-Gervais, S. Arya, F. Sarangi, M. Harris-Brandts, S. Beaulieu, and C.D. Richardson. RNA interference blocks gene expression and RNA synthesis from hepatitis C replicons propagated

in human liver cells. Proceedings of the National Academy of Sciences of the United States of America. 100:2783-2788 (2003).
[40] M. Jiangand J. Milner. Selective silencing of viral gene expression in HPV-positive human cervical carcinoma cells treated with siRNA, a primer of RNA interference. Oncogene. 21:6041-6048 (2002).
[41] B. Berkhout. RNA interference as an antiviral approach: targeting HIV-1. Current Opinion in Molecular Therapeutics. 6:141-145 (2004).
[42] C. Chakrabortyand C. Chakraborty. Potentiality of small interfering RNAs (siRNA) as recent therapeutic targets for gene-silencing. Current Drug Targets. 8:469-482 (2007).
[43] M.A. Martinez, B. Clotet, and J.A. Este. RNA interference of HIV replication. Trends in Immunology. 23:559-561 (2002).
[44] A.T. Das, T.R. Brummelkamp, E.M. Westerhout, M. Vink, M. Madiredjo, R. Bernards, and B. Berkhout. Human immunodeficiency virus type 1 escapes from RNA interference-mediated inhibition. Journal of Virology. 78:2601-2605 (2004).
[45] J. Capodici, K. Kariko, and D. Weissman. Inhibition of HIV-1 infection by small interfering RNA-mediated RNA interference. Journal of Immunology. 169:5196-5201 (2002).
[46] J.M. Jacque, K. Triques, and M. Stevenson. Modulation of HIV-1 replication by RNA interference. Cell. 15:20.
[47] B.M. Peterlinand D. Trono. Hide, shield and strike back: how HIV-infected cells avoid immune eradication. Nature Reviews Immunology. 3:97-107 (2003).
[48] J.M. Jacque, K. Triques, and M. Stevenson. Modulation of HIV-1 replication by RNA interference.[see comment]. Nature. 418:435-438 (2002).
[49] W.Y. Hu, F.D. Bushman, and A.C. Siva. RNA interference against retroviruses. Virus Research. 102:59-64 (2004).
[50] R. Kretschmer-Kazemi Farand G. Sczakiel. The activity of siRNA in mammalian cells is related to structural target accessibility: a comparison with antisense oligonucleotides. Nucleic Acids Research. 31:4417-4424 (2003).
[51] N.S. Lee, T. Dohjima, G. Bauer, H. Li, M.J. Li, A. Ehsani, P. Salvaterra, and J. Rossi. Expression of small interfering RNAs targeted against HIV-1 rev transcripts in human cells.[see comment]. Nature Biotechnology. 20:500-505 (2002).
[52] R.M. Surabhiand R.B. Gaynor. RNA interference directed against viral and cellular targets inhibits human immunodeficiency Virus Type 1 replication. Journal of Virology. 76:12963-12973 (2002).
[53] C.D. Novina, M.F. Murray, D.M. Dykxhoorn, P.J. Beresford, J. Riess, S.K. Lee, R.G. Collman, J. Lieberman, P. Shankar, and P.A. Sharp. siRNA-directed inhibition of HIV-1 infection.[see comment]. Nature Medicine. 8:681-686 (2002).
[54] H. Takaku. Gene silencing of HIV-1 by RNA interference. Antiviral Chemistry & Chemotherapy. 15:57-65 (2004).
[55] E. Song, P. Zhu, S.K. Lee, D. Chowdhury, S. Kussman, D.M. Dykxhoorn, Y. Feng, D. Palliser, D.B. Weiner, P. Shankar, W.A. Marasco, and J. Lieberman. Antibody mediated in vivo delivery of small interfering RNAs via cell-surface receptors.[see comment]. Nature Biotechnology. 23:709-717 (2005).
[56] W. Han, M. Wind-Rotolo, R.L. Kirkman, and C.D. Morrow. Inhibition of human immunodeficiency virus type 1 replication by siRNA targeted to the highly conserved primer binding site. Virology. 330:221-232 (2004).

[57] W.S. Park, M. Hayafune, N. Miyano-Kurosaki, and H. Takaku. Specific HIV-1 env gene silencing by small interfering RNAs in human peripheral blood mononuclear cells. Gene Therapy. 10:2046-2050 (2003).
[58] L. Scherer, J. Rossi, and M. Weinberg. Progress and prospects: RNA-based therapies for treatment of HIV infection. Gene Therapy. 14:1057-1064 (2007).
[59] D. Boden, O. Pusch, F. Lee, L. Tucker, and B. Ramratnam. Human immunodeficiency virus type 1 escape from RNA interference. Journal of Virology. 77:11531-11535 (2003).
[60] J. Anderson, A. Banerjea, and R. Akkina. Bispecific short hairpin siRNA constructs targeted to CD4, CXCR4, and CCR5 confer HIV-1 resistance. Oligonucleotides. 13:303-312 (2003).
[61] X.F. Qin, D.S. An, I.S. Chen, and D. Baltimore. Inhibiting HIV-1 infection in human T cells by lentiviral-mediated delivery of small interfering RNA against CCR5. Proceedings of the National Academy of Sciences of the United States of America. 100:183-188 (2003).
[62] C.D. Novina, M.F. Murray, D.M. Dykxhoorn, P.J. Beresford, J. Riess, S.K. Lee, R.G. Collman, J. Lieberman, P. Shankar, and P.A. Sharp. siRNA-directed inhibition of HIV-1 infection. Nature Medicine. 8:681-686 (2002).
[63] M.A. MartÌnez, A. GutiÈrrez, M. Armand-UgÛn, J. Blanco, M. Parera, J. GÛmez, B. Clotet, and J.A. EstÈ. Suppression of chemokine receptor expression by RNA interference allows for inhibition of HIV-1 replication. AIDS. 16:2385 (2002).
[64] M.A. Martinez, B. Clotet, and J.A. Este. RNA interference of HIV replication. Trends in Immunology. 23:559-561 (2002).
[65] J. Rucker, M. Samson, B.J. Doranz, F. Libert, J.F. Berson, Y. Yi, R.J. Smyth, R.G. Collman, C.C. Broder, and G. Vassart. Regions in [beta]-chemokine receptors CCR5 and CCR2b that determine HIV-1 cofactor specificity. Cell. 87:437-446 (1996).
[66] Q.H. Liu, D.A. Williams, C. McManus, F. Baribaud, R.W. Doms, D. Schols, E. De Clercq, M.I. Kotlikoff, R.G. Collman, and B.D. Freedman. HIV-1 gp120 and chemokines activate ion channels in primary macrophages through CCR5 and CXCR4 stimulation. Proceedings of the National Academy of Sciences of the United States of America. 97:4832 (2000).
[67] E.M. Westerhout, M. Ooms, M. Vink, A.T. Das, and B. Berkhout. HIV-1 can escape from RNA interference by evolving an alternative structure in its RNA genome. Nucleic Acids Research. 33:796 (2005).
[68] C.I. Chang, H.S. Kang, C. Ban, S. Kim, and D. Lee. Dual-target gene silencing by using long, synthetic siRNA duplexes without triggering antiviral responses. Molecules and cells. 27:689-695 (2009).
[69] K.V. Morrisand J.J. Rossi. Anti-HIV-1 gene expressing lentiviral vectors as an adjunctive therapy for HIV-1 infection. Current HIV Research. 2:185-191 (2004).
[70] Y. Higuchi, S. Kawakami, and M. Hashida. Strategies for in vivo delivery of siRNAs: recent progress. Biodrugs. 24:195-205 (2010).
[71] D.L. Lewis, J.E. Hagstrom, A.G. Loomis, J.A. Wolff, and H. Herweijer. Efficient delivery of siRNA for inhibition of gene expression in postnatal mice. Nature Genetics. 32:107-108 (2002).
[72] A. McCaffrey, L. Meuse, T. Pham, D. Conklin, G. Hannon, and M. Kay. Gene expression: RNA interference in adult mice. Nature. 418:38-39 (2002).

[73] T. Zimmermann, A. Lee, A. Akinc, B. Bramlage, D. Bumcrot, M. Fedoruk, J. Harborth, J. Heyes, L. Jeffs, and M. John. RNAi-mediated gene silencing in non-human primates. Nature. 441:111-114 (2006).

[74] J. Yano, K. Hirabayashi, S.-I. Nakagawa, T. Yamaguchi, M. Nogawa, I. Kashimori, H. Naito, H. Kitagawa, K. Ishiyama, T. Ohgi, and T. Irimura. Antitumor activity of small interfering RNA/cationic liposome complex in mouse models of cancer. Clinical Cancer Research. 10:7721-7726 (2004).

[75] S.H. Kim, J.H. Jeong, S.H. Lee, S.W. Kim, and T.G. Park. PEG conjugated VEGF siRNA for anti-angiogenic gene therapy. Journal of Controlled Release. 116:123-129 (2006).

[76] A. Inoue, S.Y. Sawata, and K. Taira. Molecular design and delivery of siRNA. Journal of Drug Targeting. 14:448-455 (2006).

[77] Z. Parooand D.R. Corey. Challenges for RNAi in vivo. Trends in Biotechnology. 22:390-394 (2004).

[78] B. Berkhout, M. Ooms, N. Beerens, H. Huthoff, E. Southern, and K. Verhoef. In vitro evidence that the untranslated leader of the HIV-1 genome is an RNA checkpoint that regulates multiple functions through conformational changes. Journal of Biological Chemistry. 277:19967-19975 (2002).

[79] M. Ooms, K. Verhoef, E. Southern, H. Huthoff, and B. Berkhout. Probing alternative foldings of the HIV-1 leader RNA by antisense oligonucleotide scanning arrays. Nucleic Acids Research. 32:819-827 (2004).

[80] E.A. Bohula, A.J. Salisbury, M. Sohail, M.P. Playford, J. Riedemann, E.M. Southern, and V.M. Macaulay. The efficacy of small interfering RNAs targeted to the type 1 insulin-like growth factor receptor (IGF1R) is influenced by secondary structure in the IGF1R transcript. Journal of Biological Chemistry. 278:15991-15997 (2003).

[81] D. Bouard, N. Alazard-Dany, and F. Cosset. Viral vectors: from virology to transgene expression. British Journal of Pharmacology. 157:153-165 (2009).

[82] K. Park, W.J. Kim, Y.H. Cho, Y.I. Lee, H. Lee, S. Jeong, E.S. Cho, S.I. Chang, S.K. Moon, B.S. Kang, Y.J. Kim, S.H. Cho, K. Park, W.-J. Kim, Y.-H. Cho, Y.-I. Lee, H. Lee, S. Jeong, E.-S. Cho, S.-I. Chang, S.-K. Moon, B.-S. Kang, Y.-J. Kim, and S.-H. Cho. Cancer gene therapy using adeno-associated virus vectors. Frontiers in Bioscience. 13:2653-2659 (2008).

[83] J. Andersonand R. Akkina. HIV-1 resistance conferred by siRNA cosuppression of CXCR 4 and CCR 5 coreceptors by a bispecific lentiviral vector. AIDS Research and Therapy. 2:1 (2005).

[84] J. Andersonand R. Akkina. Complete knockdown of CCR5 by lentiviral vector-expressed siRNAs and protection of transgenic macrophages against HIV-1 infection. Gene Therapy. 14:1287-1297 (2007).

[85] Batchu RB, Moreno AM, Szmania S, Gupta SK, Zhan F, Rosen N, Kozlowski M, Spencer T, Spagnoli GC, Shaughnessy J, Barlogie B, Tricot G, and V.R. F. High-Level Expression of Cancer/Testis Antigen NY-ESO-1 and Human Granulocyte-Macrophage Colony-Stimulating Factor in Dendritic Cells with a Bicistronic Retroviral Vector. Human Gene Therapy. 14:1333-1345 (2003).

[86] L. Ding, S. Lu, R. Batchu, R.S. Iii, and N. Munshi. Bone marrow stromal cells as a vehicle for gene transfer. Gene Ther. 6:1611-1616. (1999).

[87] I.M. Vermaand N. Somia. Gene therapy -- promises, problems and prospects. Nature. 389:239-242 (1997).

[88] R.S. Tomar, H. Matta, and P.M. Chaudhary. Use of adeno-associated viral vector for delivery of small interfering RNA. Oncogene. 22:5712-5715 (2003).

[89] K.I. Bernsand C. Giraud. Biology of adeno-associated virus. Current Topics in Microbiology & Immunology. 218:1-23 (1996).
[90] L. Tenenbaum, E. Lehtonen, and P.E. Monahan. Evaluation of risks related to the use of adeno-associated virus-based vectors. Current Gene Therapy. 3:545-565 (2003).
[91] M. Hallekand C.M. Wendtner. Recombinant adeno-associated virus (rAAV) vectors for somatic gene therapy: recent advances and potential clinical applications. Cytokines & Molecular Therapy. 2:69-79 (1996).
[92] A. Handa, S. Muramatsu, J. Qiu, H. Mizukami, and K.E. Brown. Adeno-associated virus (AAV)-3-based vectors transduce haematopoietic cells not susceptible to transduction with AAV-2-based vectors.[see comment]. Journal of General Virology. 81:2077-2084 (2000).
[93] T.R. Flotte, S.A. Afione, C. Conrad, S.A. McGrath, R. Solow, H. Oka, P.L. Zeitlin, W.B. Guggino, and B.J. Carter. Stable in vivo expression of the cystic fibrosis transmembrane conductance regulator with an adeno-associated virus vector. Proceedings of the National Academy of Sciences of the United States of America. 90:10613-10617 (1993).
[94] R.O. Snyder, C.H. Miao, G.A. Patijn, S.K. Spratt, O. Danos, D. Nagy, A.M. Gown, B. Winther, L. Meuse, L.K. Cohen, A.R. Thompson, and M.A. Kay. Persistent and therapeutic concentrations of human factor IX in mice after hepatic gene transfer of recombinant AAV vectors. Nat Genet. 16:270-276. (1997).
[95] X. Xiao, J. Li, and R.J. Samulski. Efficient long-term gene transfer into muscle tissue of immunocompetent mice by adeno-associated virus vector. Journal of Virology. 70:8098-8108 (1996).
[96] D. McCarty, P. Monahan, and R. Samulski. Self-complementary recombinant adeno-associated virus(scAAV) vectors promote efficient transduction independently of DNA synthesis. Gene therapy(Basingstoke). 8:1248-1254 (2001).
[97] H. Nakai, S. Yant, T. Storm, S. Fuess, L. Meuse, and M. Kay. Extrachromosomal recombinant adeno-associated virus vector genomes are primarily responsible for stable liver transduction in vivo. Journal of Virology. 75:6969-6976 (2001).
[98] W. Ding, L. Zhang, Z. Yan, and J. Engelhardt. Intracellular trafficking of adeno-associated viral vectors. Gene Therapy. 12:873-880 (2005).
[99] J. Hansen, K. Qing, and A. Srivastava. Adeno-associated virus type 2-mediated gene transfer: altered endocytic processing enhances transduction efficiency in murine fibroblasts. Journal of Virology. 75:4080-4090 (2001).
[100] S. Chatterjee, P.R. Johnson, and K.K. Wong, Jr. Dual-target inhibition of HIV-1 in vitro by means of an adeno-associated virus antisense vector. Science. 258:1485-1488 (1992).
[101] A. Srivastava. Obstacles to human hematopoietic stem cell transduction by recombinant adeno-associated virus 2 vectors. Journal of Cellular Biochemistry - Supplement. 38:39-45 (2002).
[102] V.F. Van Tendeloo, P. Ponsaerts, F. Lardon, G. Nijs, M. Lenjou, C. Van Broeckhoven, D.R. Van Bockstaele, and Z.N. Berneman. Highly efficient gene delivery by mRNA electroporation in human hematopoietic cells: superiority to lipofection and passive pulsing of mRNA and to electroporation of plasmid cDNA for tumor antigen loading of dendritic cells. Blood. 98:49-56 (2001).
[103] M.D. Moore, M.J. McGarvey, R.A. Russell, B.R. Cullen, and M.O. McClure. Stable inhibition of hepatitis B virus proteins by small interfering RNA expressed from viral vectors. Journal of Gene Medicine. 7:918-925 (2005).

[104] O. Pinkenburg, J. Platz, C. Beisswenger, C. Vogelmeier, and R. Bals. Inhibition of NF-kappaB mediated inflammation by siRNA expressed by recombinant adeno-associated virus. Journal of Virological Methods. 120:119-122 (2004).

[105. H. Xia, Q. Mao, S.L. Eliason, S.Q. Harper, I.H. Martins, H.T. Orr, H.L. Paulson, L. Yang, R.M. Kotin, and B.L. Davidson. RNAi suppresses polyglutamine-induced neurodegeneration in a model of spinocerebellar ataxia.[see comment]. Nature Medicine. 10:816-820 (2004).

[106] D. Boden, O. Pusch, F. Lee, L. Tucker, P.R. Shank, and B. Ramratnam. Promoter choice affects the potency of HIV-1 specific RNA interference. Nucleic Acids Research. 31:5033-5038 (2003).

[107] A. Horster, B. Teichmann, R. Hormes, D. Grimm, J. Kleinschmidt, and G. Sczakiel. Recombinant AAV-2 harboring gfp-antisense/ribozyme fusion sequences monitor transduction, gene expression, and show anti-HIV-1 efficacy. Gene Ther. 6:1231-1238. (1999).

[108] R. Iyer, L. Ding, R.B. Batchu, S. Naugler, M.A. Shammas, and N.C. Munshi. Antisense p53 transduction leads to overexpression of bcl-2 and dexamethasone resistance in multiple myeloma. Leukemia Research. 27:73-78 (2003).

[109] M.L. Aitken, R.B. Moss, D.A. Waltz, M.E. Dovey, M.R. Tonelli, S.C. McNamara, R.L. Gibson, B.W. Ramsey, B.J. Carter, and T.C. Reynolds. A phase I study of aerosolized administration of tgAAVCF to cystic fibrosis subjects with mild lung disease. Human Gene Therapy. 12:1907-1916 (2001).

[110] S.C. Jung, I.P. Han, A. Limaye, R. Xu, M.P. Gelderman, P. Zerfas, K. Tirumalai, G.J. Murray, M.J. During, R.O. Brady, and P. Qasba. Adeno-associated viral vector-mediated gene transfer results in long-term enzymatic and functional correction in multiple organs of Fabry mice. Proceedings of the National Academy of Sciences of the United States of America. 98:2676-2681 (2001).

[111] M.Y. Mastakov, K. Baer, R. Xu, H. Fitzsimons, and M.J. During. Combined injection of rAAV with mannitol enhances gene expression in the rat brain. Molecular Therapy: the Journal of the American Society of Gene Therapy. 3:225-232 (2001).

[112] D. Boden, O. Pusch, F. Lee, L. Tucker, B. Ramratnam, D. Boden, O. Pusch, F. Lee, L. Tucker, and B. Ramratnam. Efficient gene transfer of HIV-1-specific short hairpin RNA into human lymphocytic cells using recombinant adeno-associated virus vectors. Molecular Therapy: the Journal of the American Society of Gene Therapy. 9:396-402 (2004).

[113] E. Song, S.K. Lee, D.M. Dykxhoorn, C. Novina, D. Zhang, K. Crawford, J. Cerny, P.A. Sharp, J. Lieberman, N. Manjunath, and P. Shankar. Sustained small interfering RNA-mediated human immunodeficiency virus type 1 inhibition in primary macrophages. Journal of Virology. 77:7174-7181 (2003).

[114] D. Xu, D. McCarty, A. Fernandes, M. Fisher, R.J. Samulski, and R.L. Juliano. Delivery of MDR1 small interfering RNA by self-complementary recombinant adeno-associated virus vector. Molecular Therapy: the Journal of the American Society of Gene Therapy. 11:523-530 (2005).

[115] L. Zhong, B. Li, G. Jayandharan, C.S. Mah, L. Govindasamy, M. Agbandje-McKenna, R.W. Herzog, K.A. Weigel-Van Aken, J.A. Hobbs, S. Zolotukhin, N. Muzyczka, A. Srivastava, L. Zhong, B. Li, G. Jayandharan, C.S. Mah, L. Govindasamy, M. Agbandje-McKenna, R.W. Herzog, K.A. Weigel-Van Aken, J.A. Hobbs, S. Zolotukhin, N. Muzyczka, and A. Srivastava. Tyrosine-phosphorylation of AAV2 vectors and its consequences on viral intracellular trafficking and transgene expression. Virology. 381:194-202 (2008).

20

Cell-Delivered Gene Therapy for HIV

Scott Ledger[1], Borislav Savkovic[2], Michelle Millington[3], Helen Impey[3], Maureen Boyd[3], John M. Murray[2,4,5] and Geoff Symonds[3,5]
[1]*The Faculty of Medicine, The University of New South Wales, Sydney*
[2]*The School of Mathematics and Statistics, The University of New South Wales, Sydney*
[3]*Calimmune Australia, 405 Liverpool St Darlinghurst, NSW*
[4]*The Kirby Institute, The University of New South Wales, Sydney NSW*
[5]*St Vincent's Institute for Applied Medical Research*
405 Liverpool St Darlinghurst, NSW
Australia

1. Introduction

Gene therapy involves the transfer of genetic material into cells of an individual to treat an underlying illness either through the expression of advantageous genes or the silencing of disadvantageous ones (Flotte 2007; Kohn and Candotti 2009). Gene therapy has been used successfully to treat several diseases, for example SCID-X1 (Cavazzana-Calvo, Hacein-Bey et al. 2000) and SCID-ADA (Aiuti 2004) and holds out promise as a more general treatment regimen (Flotte 2007). One of the driving forces behind the area of research into the treatment of HIV is the resistance to, and side effects of, the current drugs being used. This development of resistance and the need for continuous and ongoing daily medication have been major shortcomings of conventional highly active antiretroviral therapy (HAART) when employed as a treatment against HIV (Perno, Moyle et al. 2008). An additional driving force behind interest in gene therapy is the potential for a one-off treatment that would continue to work for the life of the individual (Symonds, Johnstone et al. 2010). One can envisage gene therapy as a full or partial replacement for HAART, that may help to overcome issues of viral resistance, co-morbidity and attendant compliance (i.e. daily administration of HAART for life).

While HAART is a systemic form of treatment which provides a substantial level of protection to HIV susceptible cells in the body for many years, it is highly susceptible to the development of a resistant HIV quasispecies, that may selectively expand due to the strong evolutionary pressure exerted by HAART (Perno, Moyle et al. 2008). Whereas HAART-based treatments bathe each cell in some level of drug, gene-therapy results in a polar population dynamic consisting of gene protected and unprotected cells. This is due to the fact that it is neither practical nor possible to have a protective gene against HIV introduced into all cells of the body, but rather only a subset of the total cell population is afforded protection (Symonds, Johnstone et al. 2010). This polar dynamic is predicted to provide additional pressures to the suriviving HIV population (Applegate, Birkett et al. 2010). Cells that might be afforded protection include CD4+ T cells and macrophages, which are known to be targets of HIV infection, as well as other cell populations susceptible to HIV infection.

In this chapter we describe the biological and clinical underpinnings of gene-therapy including the therapeutic genes employed for protection against HIV, delivery methods of the vectors carrying these protective genes into the cells, expression cassettes and finally the target cells into which the protective genes are introduced. We then estimate the potential in-vivo protective effects of gene-therapy against HIV.

2. Biological and clinical aspects of gene-therapy

In this section we look at the biological and clinical aspects of gene-therapy. Observations associated with natural immunity that may be utilized in gene-therapy against HIV are discussed in section 2.1. Stages of the HIV infection cycle that may be inhibited by gene-therapy, and the various gene therapeutic that may be employed to this aim, are the subject of section 2.2. Various delivery vectors and promoters that can achieve effective delivery and transcription of the protective gene into the cell to be transduced are the subject of section 2.3. The biological underpinnings of the target cell to be transduced with a protective gene, either CD4+ T cells or Hematopoietic Stem Cells (HSC) are discussed in section 2.4. The clinical aspects of collection of cells for transduction via apheresis and associated preparation regimens are discussed in section 2.5. Finally, Section 2.6 is concerned with clinical trials to-date of anti-HIV gene-therapy and results reported therein.

2.1 CCR5 and the 32-nucleotide deletion mutation: A strong case for gene therapy

Recent additional impetus for gene-therapy for HIV is based upon the earlier observation that some individuals do not become infected upon repeated exposure to HIV (Zimmerman, Buckler-White et al. 1997). Studies of these individuals led to the discovery of a mutation in CCR5, an important co-receptor for HIV attachment to target cells prior to infection. Such a mutation was found to confer natural immunity against HIV (Zimmerman, Buckler-White et al. 1997).

The mutation discovered was found to be a 32 nucleotide deletion (CCR5d32) within the CCR5 gene (Zimmerman, Buckler-White et al. 1997). This mutation was observed to be very common among individuals of European background and it has subsequently been determined that of Caucasian individuals, approximately 10% are heterozygous and 1-3% homozygous for this mutation (Dean, Carrington et al. 1996; Liu, Paxton et al. 1996; Samson, Libert et al. 1996; Agrawal, Lu et al. 2004), with the mutation being almost non-existent in all other populations. There has been considerable speculation regarding the origin and purpose of the mutation. It has been shown that the percentage of CCR5d32 mutation occurring in today's population is roughly comparable to that found in samples from individuals of the Bronze Age (approximately 3000 years ago) (Hummel, Schmidt et al. 2005; Hedrick and Verrelli 2006). There is evidence suggesting that smallpox provided a selective advantage for CCR5d32 (Galvani and Slatkin 2003), indicating that there may be other selective advantages associated with the mutation. The mutation does not seem to present any significant disadvantages to the individuals other than an increased risk of West-Nile disease (Glass, McDermott et al. 2006). Such observations led to an interest in mimicking this natural mutation for HIV-infected individuals via genetic manipulation (i.e. transduction) of cells vulnerable to HIV infection. (see below)

It has been noted that the 32 nucleotide deletion results in 31 new amino acids being coded for, resulting in an active CCR5d32 protein. This protein instead of presenting as CCR5 receptors on the cell surface like the wild-type counterpart, CCR5d32 actually binds to and interacts with CXCR4 receptors (Agrawal, Lu et al. 2004), the other major coreceptor for HIV attachment. This provides an additional protection against HIV infection beyond the mere absence of a functional CCR5 co-receptor, especially when concerning strains capable of utilizing the CXCR4 coreceptor (Agrawal, Lu et al. 2004; Jin, Agrawal et al. 2008). Further evidence towards the beneficial effect of the CCR5d32 protein comes from evidence that a polymorphism in the promoter region in CCR5-/- individuals can affect the protective capabilities of the d32 mutation. It has been demonstrated that an increase in CCR5d32 protein expression will improve resistance to HIV, while decreased CCR5d32 expression reduces the protective effect (Jin, Agrawal et al. 2008).

This CCR5d32 mutation has been successfully utilized in a patient, who suffered from both HIV/AIDS and leukaemia (Hutter, Nowak et al. 2009; Allers, Hutter et al. 2010). This individual, termed the "Berlin patient", had complete ablation of their immune system (to treat the leukemia) before matched allogeneic donor hematopoietic stem cells (HSC) homozygous for the CCR5d32 mutation were transfused into the patient. After one recurrence of leukaemia and a repeat of the treatment (ablation and reconstitution), the patient has had undetectable levels of HIV (and no recurring leukaemia) for more than 3 years without the use of any antiretroviral drugs (Hutter, Nowak et al. 2009; Allers, Hutter et al. 2010). This unique result of "functional" cure of HIV indicates significant potential for the use of gene-therapy to mimic this result by down-regulation of CCR5.

2.2 Choosing a stage of HIV infection cycle to inhibit: Which therapeutic genes hold out promise?

2.2.1 Classes and methods of HIV inhibition

Gene-therapy may be aimed to target various stages of the HIV infection cycle as shown in Figure 1. Class 1 therapy inhibits all steps prior to viral integration into the cellular genome, Class 2 inhibits expression of viral genes and Class 3 inhibits production of new virions once integration and expression has taken place (von Laer, Hasselmann et al. 2006). According to predictions from mathematical modelling, as discussed in section 3.1, Class 1 gene therapies are likely to be the most effective as they inhibit HIV at the first steps, and provide a selective advantage to these cells by avoiding any viral or immunological induced death from infection. Hence many gene therapeutics currently under investigation include components that impair attachment or fusion stages of the viral life-cycle (Symonds, Johnstone et al. 2010).

While all these classes are potential HIV gene therapeutics, practically, the use of multiple therapeutics in combination is likely to be the most effective method. This is analogous to the antiretroviral situation where it does not take long for HIV resistance to emerge against single antiretroviral drugs. These antiretroviral drugs have been shown to be far more effective when used in combination. It is for this reason that gene therapy research has often been focused on the use of multiple gene therapuetics used in conjunction with one-another.

As well as the variety of targets being investigated, there is additionally a wide range of methods to achieve inhibition of these targets. The most commonly employed methods to-date include the following:

Antisense (Class 2): Antisense RNA is a synthetic nucleotide sequence that binds to mRNA in order to inhibit its function. This method can be used against a wide range of targets, including the HIV envelope (Levine, Humeau et al. 2006).

Aptamers (Class 2 or 3): Aptamers are single-stranded RNAs or DNAs. They disrupt at the protein level by tightly binding to their target ligand (Que-Gewirth and Sullenger 2007). Aptamers can be used to target a wide array of proteins and as such have potential to be used in multiple settings.

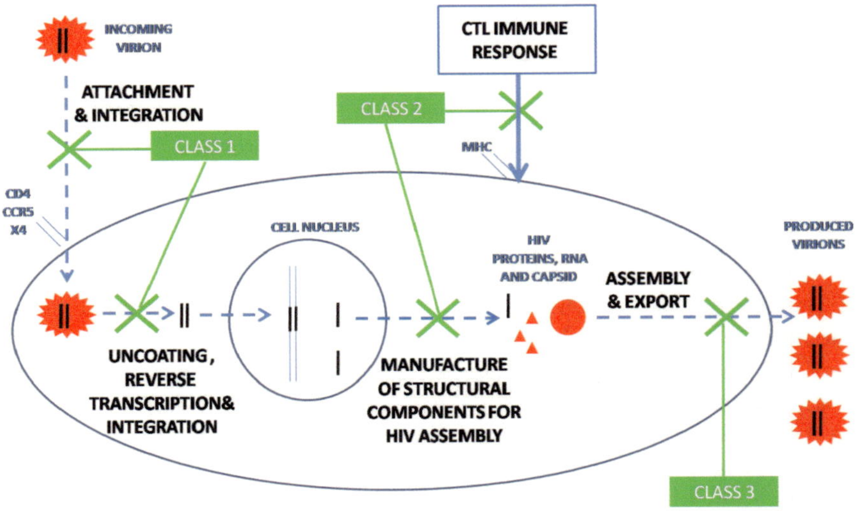

Fig. 1. The three Classes of gene-therapy according to cycle of HIV infection inhibited as defined by von Laer et al(von Laer, Hasselmann et al. 2006; von Laer, Hasselmann et al. 2006). Class 1 inhibits all steps in the infection cycle prior to integration of the HIV RNA into the cellular genome. In particular, Class 1 inhibits either the entry of the HIV virion into the cell (i.e. inhibition of attachment/integration of the HIV virion through the CD4, CCR5 and X4 receptors/coreceptors) or inhibits integration into the cellular genome once a virion has entered the cell (i.e. blocks uncoating, reverse transcription or integration). Class 2 inhibits gene expression and the production of structural components required for the assembly of new HIV virions. Class 2 also results in lower susceptitibliy to cell death through the cytotoxic T lymphocyte (CTL) immune response, as a result of reduced recongnition via the Major Histocompatiblity Complex (MHC). Finally, Class 3 inhibits the assembly and export of virions from the infected cell.

Intracellular Antibodies (Class 1 or 3): Intracellular antibodies, or "intrabodies", are designed to bind to and inactivate target molecules inside host cells (Chen, Bagley et al. 1994). One target which has been used by intrabodies is CCR5, whereby the intrabodies bind to CCR5 and block surface expression (Rossi, June et al. 2007).

Ribozymes (Class 2): Ribozymes are catalytic RNA molecules that have the ability to degrade RNA in a sequence-specific manner (Sun, Wang et al. 1995). When used as anti-HIV agents, they have the potential to target multiple steps, affecting incoming RNA (during infection, in this sense they can act in part as Class1), primary RNA transcripts (from integrated provirus), spliced mRNAs and mature RNA being packaged into virions. These are primarily Class 2 inhibitors and examples are those designed to target the conserved regions of HIV such as the overlapping regions of *vpr* and *tat* reading frames (Mitsuyasu, Merigan et al. 2009). Highly conserved regions are desirable as targets so that sequence specificity is more likely to be maintained.

Short hairpin RNA (Class 1 or 2): Short hairpin RNA is a sequence of RNA that folds back upon itself in a hairpin turn; it can be used to initiate RNA interference and consequently silence gene expression (McIntyre and Fanning 2006). shRNA expression vectors utilise a promoter to drive expression of the shRNA. As an integrated vector, this expression cassette will be passed on to daughter cells, allowing the gene silencing to be maintained *in vivo*. The shRNA hairpin structure is cleaved by the cellular machinery into siRNA which is then bound to the RNA-induced silencing complex. This complex binds to and cleaves mRNAs which match the siRNA that is bound to it (Hannon and Rossi 2004). The use of siRNA for gene silencing has become a method of choice and can be potentially applied to many targets, including down-regulation of CCR5 that will decrease target cell infectivity by HIV and other host receptors as the removal or impairment of these receptors will render HIV non-infectious (Class 1).

Class	Target Site	Why	Goal	How
1	CCR5	Important co-receptor	Remove/prevent expression of CCR5	Zinc-finger, siRNA
1	CD4	Essential receptor for HIV attachment	Remove/prevent expression of CD4	Zinc-finger, siRNA
1	CXCR4	Important co-receptor	Remove/prevent expression of CXCR4	Zinc-finger, siRNA, ribozyme
1	Membrane Fusion (HIV heptad repeat)	Essential for viral entry	Prevent entry of HIV through host-cell membrane	siRNA
2	Tat	Important for Transcription	Disrupt *tat* gene	Tar decoy, siRNA, ribozyme
2	Rev	Important for virion Translation	Disrupt *rev* gene	siRNA, REV mutants
3	Env, Protease, Helicase	Important for virion maturation	Prevent virion maturation	siRNA, Antisense RNA,
3	Gag	Important for virion assembly	Disrupt gag gene	Ribozyme, siRNA

Table 1. A list of some HIV gene therapy targets, the goals and the mechanics of how they are being explored. This table shows a variety of Class 1, 2 and 3 therapies and the range of approaches against targets.

Fusion Inhibitors (Class 1): One fusion inhibitor which has been researched in detail is the maC46 peptide (C46) (Zahn, Hermann et al. 2008). It inhibits viral fusion by interacting with the N-terminal hydrophobic alpha-helix. This prevents changes essential for membrane fusion of the virus and host cell. This fusion inhibitor has been found to be highly effective at blocking HIV replication (Zahn, Hermann et al. 2008).

Zinc Finger Nucleases (ZFNs) (Class 1 or 2): ZFNs bind to targeted open reading frames. Two juxtaposed ZFN's on DNA results in dimerisation of the endonuclease domains, generating a double-stranded break at the targeted DNA (Porteus and Carroll 2005). The mutagenic pathways relied on to repair the DNA breaks result in nucleotide mutations at the break-sites, thus permanently disrupting the gene (Porteus and Carroll 2005). While experiments in mice have shown this method to be effective, there is still a risk of non-target directed mutagenesis. Another limitation of this technique is the inability to add protective genes, as only the effective deletion/inactivation of genes can be performed, thus limiting the applications for the use of ZFNs to applications such as inactivation of CCR5 (Class 1).

2.2.2 Strong arguments for gene-therapy based entry inhibition

Class 1 inhibitors generally act at the level of HIV binding to the target cell (von Laer, Hasselmann et al. 2006). It is expected that this would be the most effective as HIV is blocked from entry to the target cell and any subsequent replication steps cannot take place. An important recent contribution to the argument for Class 1 inhibitors is the discovery of the cause of the so-called 'bystander effect' where apparently non HIV infected cells also succumb to HIV pathogenesis (Doitsh, Cavrois et al. 2010). The observation that productively infected cells are not the only contributors to host-cell death has been noted previously, however the cause of this cell death had remained unknown until Doitsh et al discovered abortive/nonproductive HIV infection in host-cells (approximately 95% of infected cells) and the induction of apoptosis in these cells (Doitsh, Cavrois et al. 2010). This "bystander effect" is likely to have contributed to the lack of success of some antiretroviral therapy methods, including a variety of clinical trials whereby HIV infection was only inhibited after HIV entry, as host-induced apoptosis would greatly reduce the effectiveness of treatment. This effect indicates a crucial additional benefit of entry-inhibitors over other classes of antiviral treatment.

One of the resistance mechanisms developed by HIV against the antiretroviral CCR5 antagonists, such as maraviroc, is not just the use of other co-receptors such as CXCR4, it is the use of maraviroc-bound CCR5 receptors (Westby, Smith-Burchnell et al. 2007). This mechanism of resistance would not be available against cells containing a down-regulation, or mutation-mediated deletion of the CCR5 receptor produced by gene therapy. An added bonus of the use of attachment and/or fusion inhibitors is that they do not provide cross-resistance with other treatment methods such as protease and integration inhibitors.

2.3 Vectors, delivery methods and promoters: Delivering the protective gene into the cell

The therapeutic used in gene therapy must be carried within a suitable vector or delivery system; for HIV gene therapy these vectors should generally be capable of integrating into the host cells with minimal risk of generation of replication competent lentivirus or insertional mutagenesis (Wu, Wakefield et al. 2000; Symonds, Johnstone et al. 2010). The vector must also be non-toxic to the host while allowing the expression of the relevant gene(s). There are many techniques and delivery vectors which can be utilized for this purpose. Examples of the most commonly used delivery vectors are shown in Table 2.

Transposon-based delivery systems consist of a synthetic transposon and an associated transposase and work via a cut-and-paste mechanism whereby the transposase recognises the inverted direct sequences in the transposon, and then the transposon is excised and later integrated into a target DNA region (Tamhane and Akkina 2008). They can, for example, be used to carry shRNAs.

Delivery Vector	Advantage	Disadvantage
Transposons	Can provide permanent expression of multiple genes	Potential for insertional mutagenesis
Plasmid DNA Nucleofection	Treatment has been highly effective (Holt, Wang et al. 2010)	Slight increase in apoptosis of HSCs (Holt, Wang et al. 2010)
Murine Leukaemia Virus	Little/no adverse effects (Amado, Mitsuyasu et al. 2004; Macpherson, Boyd et al. 2005)	Can only infect actively replicating cells (Roe, Reynolds et al. 1993) May induce insertional mutagenesis (Symonds, Johnstone et al. 2010)
Adenovirus	Can infect non-replicating cells (Zhang, Sankar et al. 1998)	Innate immune response (Liu and Muruve 2003)
Lentivirus	Can infect non-replicating cells (Zufferey, Dull et al. 1998), Does not effect proliferation or differentiation of HSCs (Gervaix, Schwarz et al. 1997)	Slight risk of insertional mutagenesis (Philippe, Sarkis et al. 2006)
Conditionally replicating virus	Higher transduction efficiency	Risk of mutation/recombination

Table 2. A variety of commonly used delivery vectors and their associated advantages and disadvantages.

Nucleofection of DNA involves directly adding the DNA into the targeted cells by disrupting the cell membrane through electroporation. While this is not an ever-present biological vector as those mentioned above, it is more of an event-based vector which can provide a method of entry either for less entry-capable vectors, or plasmid DNA (Aluigi, Fogli et al. 2006).

Viral delivery vectors are typically made from the backbone of suitable viruses, whereby pathogenic, and (often) replication-mediating genes are removed, and only the essential genes remain (Kootstra and Verma 2003). The therapeutic gene(s) being used is/are then added to the viral backbone. The virus is then able to infect host cells as would its natural counterpart. However without the ability to replicate or express harmful genes. It is used only to integrate into the host genome and allow the therapeutic gene to be active.

One of the main concerns regarding gene therapies is the potential for insertional mutagenesis. This has been shown to occur in SCID-X1 trials (Howe, Mansour et al. 2008) where the insertional mutagenesis led to myeloproliferation/leukemia (Howe, Mansour et al. 2008). While insertional mutagenesis events have occurred in this and a few other gene therapy trials eg CGD (Stein, Ott et al. 2010), they have not occurred in HIV gene therapy trials, and a great deal of effort is undertaken to ensure that this event does not occur.

To ensure efficient transcription of the therapeutic gene, a suitable promoter is required. A promoter is a region of DNA that facilitates the transcription of nearby downstream gene(s), and is essential for the efficient expression of the desired gene(s). The choice of the promoter to be used in gene therapies is highly important, and various promoters have been tested in laboratory studies and clinical trials. Promoters currently in use in HIV gene therapy studies are quite diverse and include U6 (human derived), T7 (bacteriophage derived), and Ubc (Human ubiquitin c) (Anderson, Banerjea et al. 2003; Boden, Pusch et al. 2003; Weber and Cannon 2007):

There have been studies using different promoters in HIV gene therapy work-up and many have been shown to be effective. However, due to the many different therapeutic genes, their delivery vectors, and the cells targeted for transduction, it is difficult to determine which promoters are the most effective and as such, each needs to be tested.

It has been noted that a highly expressive promoter may not be the ideal candidate, as many highly efficient promoters can have other side-effects. As noted above, of key concern is the trans-activation (insertional mutagenesis) of nearby cellular genes (Weber and Cannon 2007), potentially leading to oncogenic effects by over-expression of important proteins.

2.4 Transduction targets: Which cells should be protected against HIV?

HIV infection is typically characterized by CD4+ T cell infection and depletion. In addition, other cells are also infected by HIV, including macrophages and monocytes and most recently there have been reports of hematopoietic stem cell (HSC) infection (Stanley, Kessler et al. 1992; Carter, Onafuwa-Nuga et al. 2010; Carter, McNamara et al. 2011). In the case of gene therapy for HIV the two most common cell types that have been transduced to date with the therapeutic relevant gene are CD4+ T lymphocytes and HSC. Transduction of these cells is expected to provide the best outcome due to CD4+ T cells being the main targets of HIV infection and the ability of HSC to differentiate into all susceptible cells. In this subsection we discuss the biological aspects of transducing either CD4+ T cells or HSC with a protective gene.

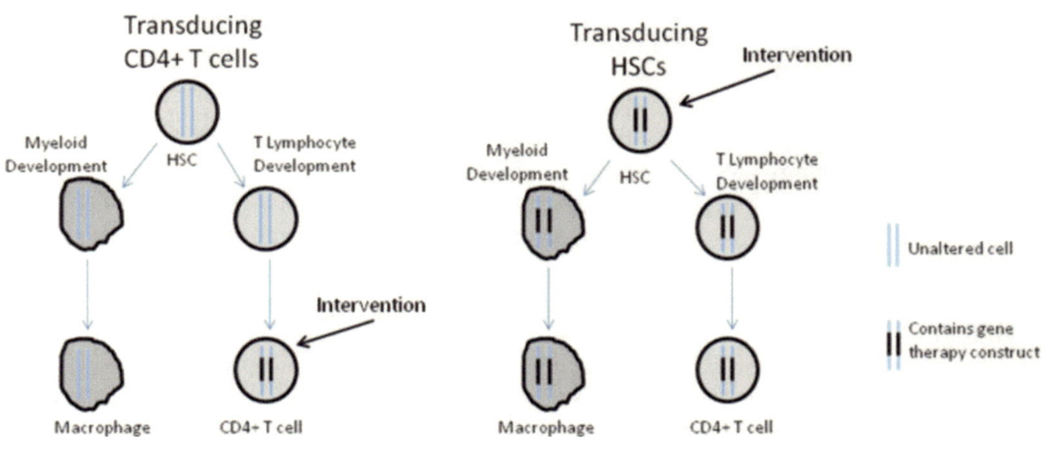

Fig. 2. Two ways of achieving cell populations protected against HIV as a result of either transducing CD4+ T cells or HSC. If the CD4+ T cell population is transduced with a protective gene (left), then protection against HIV is only afforded to CD4+ T cells. If on the other hand HSC are transduced with a protective gene (right), then the protected gene is retained by all cells derived from the HSC via differentiation through the myeloid (e.g macrophage) and lymphoid lineages (e.g CD4+ T cell). The approach of transducing HSC thus provides protection against HIV to a broader class of cells.

2.4.1 Transduction of CD4+ T cells

The use of CD4+ T cells as target cells for HIV gene therapy has been explored in several studies (see section relating to clinical trials). Isolation and transduction of CD4+ T cells is relatively simple. The key advantage of targeting CD4+ T cells is the ease with which they may be accessed. As they largely populate and regularly traffic through peripheral blood, no stimulatory factors are required to mobilize them prior to collection. Conceptually it can be envisaged that the introduction of a protected population of CD4+ T lymphocytes should have impact as these are the cells specifically depleted by HIV infection; the greater the severity of HIV infection the greater the CD4+ T lymphocyte decline.

One such study involving the therapy of CD4+ T cells was performed by Levine in 2006 (Levine, Humeau et al. 2006) whereby peripheral blood CD4+ T cells were harvested from each subject by apheresis. The collected samples were then depleted of CD8+ cells and monocytes, transduced with the gene construct *ex vivo*, activated via CD3 and CD28 costimulation and expanded before being re-infused into the patients. This method of therapy was shown to be both safe in treatment, and effective in delivery of the therapeutic gene (Levine, Humeau et al. 2006; Brunstein, Miller et al. 2011).

Predicted in-vivo dynamics of CD4+ T cell transduction, based on mathematical modelling, are discussed in section 3.2.1.

2.4.2 Transduction of hematopoietic stem cells (HSC)

Due to the range of cells which HIV infects, it is thought to be a significant advantage to transduce HSC, as these cells provide a continuous supply (following differentiation) into a range of immunological cells (monocytes, macrophages, CD4+ T cells, CD8+ cells, dendritic cells, microglial cells) which may thus be protected against HIV infection (Carter and Ehrlich 2008). A delay in the newly 'protected cell' production would be expected, thus delaying the effect of the therapeutic gene(s). However, there can still be a significant production of CD4+ T lymphocytes, the supply of which has been predicted to be a rate of approximately 1.65 cells/μL of blood/day (due to thymic reconstitution) (Murray, Kaufmann et al. 2003). This results in the production of a stable population of protected cells which could impact on CD4+ T cell number and viral load.

While CD4+ T cells (and other cell types common in peripheral blood) can be obtained relatively simply prior to transduction by apheresis from peripheral blood, HSC must first be mobilised from the bone marrow (discussed in detail below). This creates an additional component to the treatment process. Currently the most common method for the mobilisation of HSC is the use of granulocyte colony stimulating factor (G-CSF), a treatment that usually spans 4-5 days before the apheresis of peripheral blood can begin. Predicted in-vivo dynamics of HSC transduced with a protective gene are discussed in section 3.2.2.

2.5 Collection of cells for transduction: Apheresis and treatment methods for optimized and high-volume cell collection

Current gene therapy protocols for HIV require the isolation of the relevant cells to be transduced, generally following apheresis (Symonds, Johnstone et al. 2010). Apheresis is the process of removing mononuclear cells from blood and returning neutrophils, platelets, plasma and red blood cells to the donor, in order to collect more of one particular part of the blood than could be separated from a unit of whole blood. Apheresis allows for the collection of large quantities of cells, and in the case of gene therapies for HIV, total lymphocytes, CD4+ cells, or HSC are the cell types collected.

It is common practice to use a stimulating agent such as G-CSF in order to increase the quantity of HSC in the peripheral blood. The resulting increase in cell numbers in peripheral blood is due to redistribution of cells from other compartments of the body (i.e bone marrow and lymph tissue). The use of G-CSF and other stimulating factors is essential when HSC (largely inhabiting the bone marrow) are to be transduced with the therapeutic gene. Various trials have shown HSC cell counts in peripheral blood increase 20-50-fold over the course of GCSF administration (Lane, Law et al. 1995; Law, Lane et al. 1999; Valgimigli, Rigolin et al. 2005).

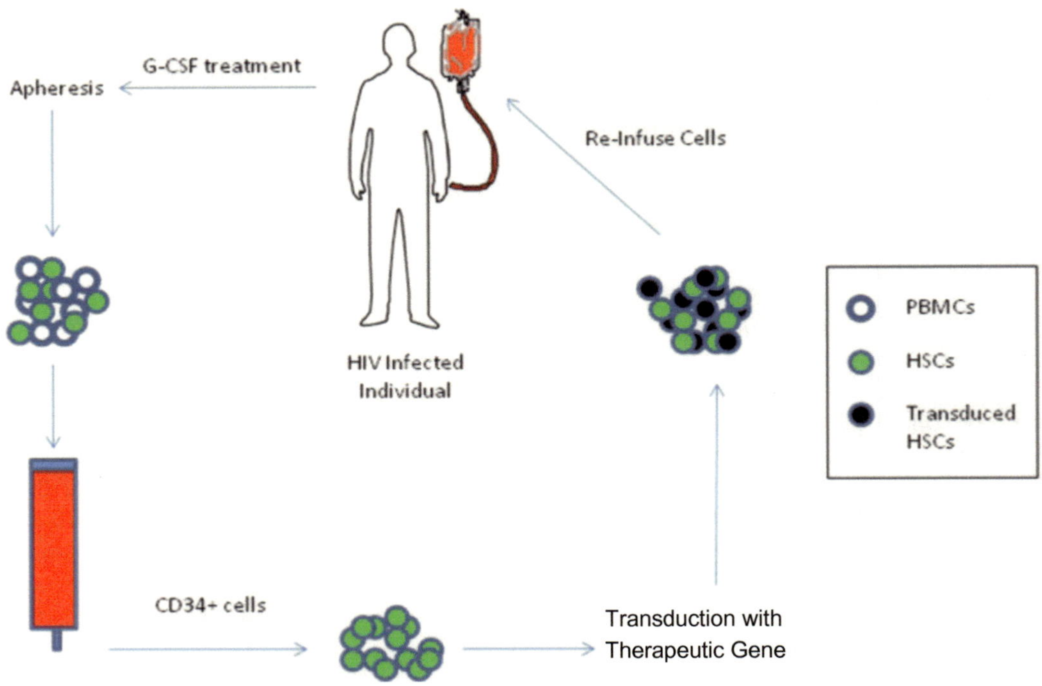

Fig. 3. Illustration of the clinical aspects of therapeutic apheresis (for HSC harvesting), and the subsequent processes of transduction and reinfusion. The HIV infected individual is first administered G-CSF in order to effect mobilization of HSC from bone marrow into peripiheral blood. The mobilized HSC are then collected from peripheral blood and subsequently transduced with a protective gene. The transduced HSC are then reinfused into the patient.

A technique known as myeloablation has been utilized in some clinical trials (before the transduced cell infusion) in order to improve engraftment of the gene-containing cells (Strayer, Akkina et al. 2005). This procedure involves the killing of HSC, thereby reducing the endogenous non-transduced cells, thereby creating more space for the transduced cell population.

2.6 Important studies involving gene-therapy: Promising results and insights

Several mouse studies and clinical trials have been conducted in the area of HIV gene therapy, with several different therapuetic targets.

Target/Mechanism of Action	Construct	Results	Reference
Rev	Inhibitory Rev protein, Rev M10, delivered to CD4+ cells by gold particles	Preferential survival of cells with construct. Limited duration of engraftment.	(Woffendin, Ranga et al. 1996)
Rev	Inhibitory Rev protein, Rev M10, delivered to CD4+ cells by retroviral vector	More persistent engraftment compared with gold particle delivery. No change	(Ranga, Woffendin et al. 1998)
Rev	"Humanized" dominant-negative REV protein (huM10) and nontranslated marker gene (FX) as an internal control in retroviral vector	Gene marking in first months, then low or undetectable except in one patient when viral load increased. No serious adverse events.	(Podsakoff, Engel et al. 2005)
rev/TAR	Trans-dominant rev with or without antisense TAR and control (neo) gene in CD4+ T lymphocytes	Long term survival of cells at low level. Preferential survival of gene-containing cells in a patient with high viral load.	(Morgan, Walker et al. 2005)
RRE decoy	Retroviral-mediated transfer of an RRE decoy gene into bone marrow CD34+ cells	No adverse effects. 2 subjects' cells detected containing both the RRE and LN vectors on the day after cell infusion. All subsequent samples negative for the L-RRE-neo vector. Cells containing the control LN vector detected up to 330 days.	(Kohn, Bauer et al. 1999; Bauer, Selander et al. 2000)
Env antisense	Single infusion of VRX496™, a lentiviral construct encoding an antisense targeting HIV env, in CD4+ T cells	CD4+ counts increased in 4/5 patients, viral loads stable, prolonged engraftment. Well tolerated. Transient vector mobilization. Safe to date.	(Levine, Humeau et al. 2006)
rev/tat ribozyme	tat and tat/rev ribozyme in CD34+cells in autologous CD34+ cells and empty vector backbone in two patient groups with and without ablation	Trial 1 - 3/5 patients showed low-frequency marking of PBMC with ribozyme and vector backbone. Trial 2 – gene marked cells detected after infusion and to one year, and RNA expression detected.	(Michienzi, Castanotto et al. 2003)

Target/Mechanism of Action	Construct	Results	Reference
tat/vpr ribozyme	Phase I study: Moloney murine leukaemia retroviral vector encoding a ribozyme vs control LNL6 vector in CD34+ HPSC	de novo production of myeloid and lymphoid cells. Degree of persistence of gene-containing cells dependent on transduced cell dose	(Amado, Mitsuyasu et al. 1999; Amado, Mitsuyasu et al. 2004)
tat/vpr ribozyme	Retroviral vector encoding a ribozyme vs control LNL6 vector to transduce T lymphocytes, predominantly CD4+ T lymphocytes	Safe and feasible procedure. Long-term survival of genetically modified T-lymphocytes.	(Macpherson, Boyd et al. 2005)
tat/vpr ribozyme	Phase II study: Moloney murine leukaemia virus-based, replication-incompetent gamma retroviral vector with gene encoding a ribozyme vs placebo in CD34+ cells	No significant difference mean plasma viral load at primary end-point but lower TWAUC. No safety concerns.	(Mitsuyasu, Merigan et al. 2009)
Fusion inhibitor	Gene encoding membrane anchored peptide C46 fusion inhibitor delivered by retroviral vector in T cells.	Increased CD4. No significant change in viral load (except after treatment change). Modified cells detected at one year. Low level marking. No major toxicity	(van Lunzen, Glaunsinger et al. 2007)
CCR5	CCR5-specific zinc finger nuclease based product, SB-728-T, in autologous CD4+ T cells. Two phase 1 trials with various dosing regimens in different patient groups.	Preliminary data on 1 patient only ZFN-modified cells persisted in circulation and observed in GALT. Suggested delay in return of viral load after structured treatment interruption.	(2009)
Tat/rev, CCR5, TAR decoy	Tat/rev short hairpin RNA, TAR decoy and CCR5 ribozyme expressed from a self-inactivating lentiviral vector transduced in CD34+ cells, along with standard unmanipulated HPCs in 4 patients with HIV and non-Hodgkin's lymphoma	Engraftment by 11 days. Low levels of gene marking observed up to 24 months as was expression of siRNA and CCR	(DiGiusto, Krishnan et al. 2010)

Target/Mechanism of Action	Construct	Results	Reference
Modified T-cell receptor	Autologous infusion of CD4+ and CD8+ T cells modified by CD4ζ in a murine moloney leukaemia virus backbone given +/- IL-2.	Gene-modified cells followed and detected to 12 months with no difference due to IL-2. No significant change in plasma viral load. CD4ζ signal detected in rectal biopsy.	(Mitsuyasu, Anton et al. 2000)

Table 3. (Apapted from Symonds et al (Symonds, Johnstone et al. 2010)): A list of HIV gene therapy clinical trials and their outcomes. Each of these studies vary in their gene therapy target, and method of targeting the specific region.

To date, as shown in Table 3, several different gene therapies have entered Phase 1 clinical trials, (and some into Phase 2) indicating the safety of a range of HIV gene therapeutics including antisense, ribozymes, decoys, intracellular antibodies and zinc fingers targeting CCR5.

3. Protective effects of anti-HIV gene-therapy: Predictions from mathematical modeling

In gene-therapy research, mathematical modelling has been employed to predict the protective effects of anti-HIV gene-therapy (von Laer, Hasselmann et al. 2006; von Laer, Hasselmann et al. 2006). In this section we review current results on mathematical modelling, with respect to predictions of the *in-vivo* anti-HIV protective effects. Mathematical models deal with the complex interactions between gene-therapy, the immune system and HIV infection (Perelson, Essunger et al. 1997). Given the relative sparsity of current clinical trial data of gene-therapy for HIV, and the long time-spans over which predictions are to be made (i.e. over many years) mathematical modelling can provide predictions on the likely *in-vivo* effectiveness of current and future gene-therapies. Modelling work to-date has led to important insights regarding key design factors as well as parameters that should be optimized in order to maximize the effectiveness of therapy (von Laer, Hasselmann et al. 2006; von Laer, Hasselmann et al. 2006). In this section we review current results and key insights.

3.1 Why is Class 1 gene-therapy the most promising approach?

As discussed previously, three different broad stages of the HIV infection cycle may be targeted for inhibition of HIV infection (Figure 1) with the inhibitors referred to as Class 1, 2, and 3 (von Laer, Hasselmann et al. 2006; von Laer, Hasselmann et al. 2006). It is of interest whether inhibiting earlier stages (via Class 1), intermediate stages (via Class 2) or later stages (via Class 3) of the infection cycle might provide maximum effectiveness of the therapy. Is it more desirable to prevent HIV entry and integration into the cellular genome via Class 1, to inhibit the production of structural components for HIV assembly via Class 2, or to inhibit the assembly/export of new HIV virions via Class 3? This question has been addressed by a number of investigators (von Laer, Hasselmann et al. 2006; von Laer, Hasselmann et al. 2006; Applegate, Birkett et al. 2010), subject to a variety of modelling assumptions reflecting differing levels of complexity of the interaction between HIV, gene-therapy and the immune system.

Investigations to-date have demonstrated that Class 1 protection appears to be highly desirable in terms of reducing viral loads and increasing CD4+ T cell counts (von Laer, Hasselmann et al. 2006; Applegate, Birkett et al. 2010; Aviran, Shah et al. 2010). The underlying reason for the superiority of Class 1 therapy (over Class 2 and Class 3) has been attributed to the high selective advantage of the protected cell population conferred by Class 1 inhibition (von Laer, Hasselmann et al. 2006; von Laer, Hasselmann et al. 2006; Applegate, Birkett et al. 2010). Since Class 1 inhibits all steps prior to viral integration into the cellular genome (Figure 1), any cell containing the protective gene is less likely to be infected than a non-protected cell. Consequently, Class 1 promotes the survival and expansion of the protected non-infected cells, whereas the non-protected cells are more prone to infection and selective killing through cytopathic effects associated either with the virus or the CTL immune response (von Laer, Hasselmann et al. 2006; von Laer, Hasselmann et al. 2006).

In contrast to Class 1 agents, Class 2 and Class 3 therapies have been shown to require much higher degrees of inhibition in order to achieve clinically significant effects (von Laer, Hasselmann et al. 2006; von Laer, Hasselmann et al. 2006; Applegate, Birkett et al. 2010). Class 2 inhibits cytopathic effects associated with the viral infection and the CTL immune response (Figure 1). Any infected cell with Class 2 protection is therefore longer-lived and also has a reduced viral production rate compared to an unprotected and infected cell (von Laer, Hasselmann et al. 2006; von Laer, Hasselmann et al. 2006; Applegate, Birkett et al. 2010). Class 2 consequently confers a selective survival advantage to the infected cells containing the protective gene relative to other infected cells, but not to non-infected cells containing the protective gene (as is the case with Class 1). In contrast, Class 3 only inhibits the export of new HIV virions from an infected cell and thus provides minimal selective advantage (von Laer, Hasselmann et al. 2006; von Laer, Hasselmann et al. 2006). Hence Class 1 is the only class that confers a selective survival advantage to non-infected cells containing the protective gene (von Laer, Hasselmann et al. 2006; von Laer, Hasselmann et al. 2006; Applegate, Birkett et al. 2010).

Collectively therefore, modelling work to-date implies that Class 1 is essential due to the selective survival advantage conferred to the protected and non-infected cells. Still, it is important to note that augmenting Class 1 with Class 2 and/or Class 3 protection might further increase the effectiveness of therapy (von Laer, Hasselmann et al. 2006; von Laer, Hasselmann et al. 2006; Applegate, Birkett et al. 2010). Recent findings relating to the "Bystander Effect", as discussed previously in section 2.2.2, have lent further support to arguments relating to Class 1 inhibition (Doitsh, Cavrois et al. 2010), as abortive infections (HIV virion enters the cell, but does not integrate into cellular genome) comprise 95% of all cell death resulting from HIV infection.

3.2 Two different transduction approaches: To transduce CD4+ T cells or HSC with a protective gene?

As discussed previously in section 2.4, it is possible to either transduce CD4+ T cells with a protective gene (for an immediately protected population of CD4+ T cells) or to transduce HSC, that provide protection to CD4+ T cells following differentiation through the lymphoid line and to monocyte/macrophages following differentiation throught the myeloid line. While the relative merits of each approach have attracted substantial interest, the long-term quantitative advantages and disadvantages of each approach in the clinical setting remain to be elucidated. Consequently, investigators have turned to predictions from mathematical modelling in order to shed light on the in-vivo dynamics of the two approaches. In this section, we review the predictions from such modelling work to-date.

3.2.1 Transducing CD4+ T cells with a protective gene: Can we achieve establishment of a sufficiently large and sufficiently "receptor-diverse" CD4+ T cell population that is protected against HIV?

Expansion of numbers of CD4+ T cells containing a protective gene is subject to the rate-limiting step of homeostatic cell division and proliferation (von Laer, Hasselmann et al. 2006). Thus it is important to determine how quickly a substantial CD4+ T cell population could expand from a small initial fraction of protected cells. Such considerations are motivated by the fact that it is currently feasible and practical to transduce only a portion of the total CD4+ T cell population (Dropulic and June 2006; von Laer, Baum et al. 2009), so that expansion of the protected CD4+ T cell population will have to rely on in vivo mechanisms.

While modelling has shown that a small fraction of initially transduced cells could potentially result in significant expansion of the protected CD4+ T cell population, reductions of viral load, and also a delay in the onset of AIDS (Lund, Lund et al. 1997; Leonard and Schaffer 2006; von Laer, Hasselmann et al. 2006; Aviran, Shah et al. 2010), most of these models have assumed a strong feedback mechanism upregulating cellular proliferation when numbers fall below a normal level. Whereas such homeostatic mechanisms are believed to contribute to the maintenance of T cell numbers in healthy individuals (Khaled and Durum 2002), the speed with which they occur is likely to be significantly slower in practice. Current clinical trials have not produced CD4+ T cell expansions at rates as fast as predicted by mathematical modelling (Dropulic and June 2006; von Laer, Baum et al. 2009).

Current estimates of T lymphocyte division put the normal rate at approximately 1 division every 3.5 years for naive T cells and 1 division every 22 weeks for memory T cells (McLean and Michie 1995). If the transduced CD4+ T cells are to expand in vivo, then such time-scales should provide an indication of the slow nature of any in vivo expansion of the transduced CD4+ T cell population unless driven by strong selective pressure by HIV.

More realistic upper bounds on rates of CD4+ T cell expansion in-vivo under gene-therapy may be obtained by consideration of CD4+ T cell reconstitution on HAART (Byakwaga, Murray et al. 2009). Reconstitution of the CD4+ T cell population under HAART appears relatively slow with average increases of approximately 300 cells/μL observed after about 6 years (Byakwaga, Murray et al. 2009). Given that reconstitution on HAART usually only takes place under complete viral suppression (as opposed to gene-therapy where a measurable viral population may be present), it appears likely that the expansion rates of the protected CD4+ T cell population under gene-therapy may be substantially slower. Unlike the situation with HAART high viral levels may be preferable in early stages of gene therapy to act as a driving force for the expansion of a protected CD4+ T cell population via a selective mechanism.

Several additional factors might further inhibit the expansion of the protected CD4+ T cell population in-vivo. First, unless sufficient selective survival advantage is conferred to the protected CD4+ T cell population, the protected cell population might not expand substantially in-vivo. Second, the transduced CD4+ T-cells might have increased death rates or decreased proliferative ability due to interference of the protective gene with normal cell functionality (Dropulic and June 2006; von Laer, Baum et al. 2009; Tayi, Bowen et al. 2010). Third, the unprotected de-novo CD4+ T-cells exported from the thymus might effectively dilute the transduced CD4+ T-cells in the periphery (Aviran, Shah et al. 2010). This latter problem may potentially be addressed by subsequent "booster" treatments involving repeated infusions of transduced CD4+ T cells or by also using HSC.

An additional disadvantage associated with the direct transduction of CD4+ T cells is that peripheral expansion of their number does not necessarily correspond to an equivalent expansion in the T cell repertoire (Nikolich-Zugich, Slifka et al. 2004; Allen, Turner et al. 2011; Wiegers, Kaufmann et al. 2011). This is important as any resulting "gaps" in the T cell repertoire may result in increased probability of immune system evasion by pathogens and consequently in increased risk of infection or morbidity (Nikolich-Zugich, Slifka et al. 2004; Allen, Turner et al. 2011; Wiegers, Kaufmann et al. 2011).

Hence although direct transduction of CD4+ T cells results in a faster appearance in peripheral blood of a protected component of this susceptible population, there may be disadvantages in that these may not provide a diverse immune response and other cell populations will not protected.

3.2.2 Transducing HSC with a protective gene: Increasing T cell receptor repertoire and broadening class of protected cells

An alternative to transducing CD4+ T cells directly is to instead transduce HSC. In this case, the production of de-novo CD4+ T cells containing the protective gene occurs as a result of HSC differentiation through the lymphoid line and subsequent export from the thymus (Symonds, Johnstone et al. 2010).

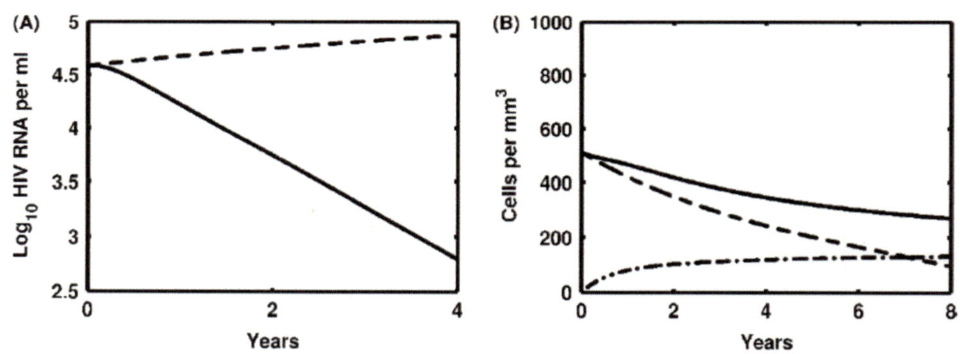

Fig. 4. Modelling predictions by Murray et al.(Murray, Fanning et al. 2009) regarding comparison of the scenario that 20% of all HSC in the bone marrow are transduced with a tat-vpr specific anti-HIV ribozyme (OZ1) versus the scenario that no gene-therapy treatment is received. Reproduced with permission from Murray et al.(Murray, Fanning et al. 2009). The patient was assumed HAART-naive. The time-scale on the horizontal ordinate denotes the time since receiving gene-therapy at year 0. (A) Treatment with OZ1, $\log_{10}$ HIV RNA copies/ml (solid line); No treatment, $\log_{10}$ HIV RNA copies/ml (dashed line). (B) Treatment with OZ1, total CD4+ T lymphocytes/mm^3 (solid line), OZ1+CD4+ T lymphocytes/mm^3 (dash-dot line); No treatment , total CD4+ T lymphocytes/mm^3 (dashed line).

Transducing HSC with a protective gene has two distinct advantages. First, the export of protected de-novo CD4+ T cells from the thymus results in a diversification of the T cell receptor repertoire (Allen, Turner et al. 2011; Wiegers, Kaufmann et al. 2011). Consequently the expanded CD4+ T cell population containing the protective gene exhibits more "extensive" TCR coverage over time, reducing the risk that pathogens might evade the immune response (Nikolich-Zugich, Slifka et al. 2004; Allen, Turner et al. 2011; Wiegers, Kaufmann et al. 2011). Secondly, HSC differentiate into a broad range of cells (besides CD4+ T cells), including macrophages that are susceptible to HIV infection and that may represent important latent HIV reservoirs (Chun, Carruth et al. 1997; Chun, Stuyver et al. 1997; Crowe and Sonza 2000). Consequently, HSC transduction provides protection against HIV to a broader class of cells than just CD4+ T cells.

The transduction of HSC does not immediately provide a protected population of CD4+ T cells in the periphery, but rather the protected CD4+ T cell population is established relatively slowly as HSC differentiate and are exported from the thymus (Symonds, Johnstone et al. 2010). Thymic production of CD4+ T cells has been estimated at approximately 1.65 cells/μL/day (Murray, Kaufmann et al. 2003) in peripheral blood. Assuming that a percentage P of total HSC in the bone marrow is transduced, then one would correspondingly expect that CD4+ T cells containing the protective gene would be exported at a rate of 1.65 x P cells/μL/day from the thymus (Murray, Fanning et al. 2009). Such numbers provide estimates of rates at which the establishment of a protected CD4+ T cell population might take place in-vivo in peripheral blood.

Achieving high engraftment efficiencies of HSC in the bone marrow is important. While a number of clinical trials in which HSC were transduced reported indications of clinical effect against HIV (Symonds, Johnstone et al. 2010), engraftment percentages in the bone marrow have been relatively low (Dropulic and June 2006; Mitsuyasu, Merigan et al. 2009; von Laer, Baum et al. 2009; Symonds, Johnstone et al. 2010). Such results underscore the need for more effective methods of cell harvesting, transduction and homing, that achieve higher engraftment efficiencies. Increased engraftment percentages should lead to more substantial clinical effects in terms of protection against HIV (Mitsuyasu, Merigan et al. 2009; Murray, Fanning et al. 2009).

Despite relatively low engraftment efficiencies to-date, it is of practical interest for future research directions to determine what engraftment percentages might suffice for clinically meaningful effects of the therapy. This question was addressed in recent modelling work (Murray, Fanning et al. 2009), that considered HSC transduction with a *tat-vpr* specific anti-HIV ribozyme (OZ1) employed in a recent phase 2 clinical trial (Mitsuyasu, Merigan et al. 2009). Under the assumption that 20% of all HSC in the bone marrow are transduced (i.e. engraftment percentage P = 20%), and that correspondingly 20% of CD4+ T cells exported from the thymus contain the protective gene, the modelling predicted reductions of 0.5 log_{10} in viral load for a HAART-naive individual after 1 year (Figure 4 A). Benefits in terms of forestalment of onset of AIDS at 8 years post-infection were also estimated (Figure 4 B). Slighly less prononunced effects were observed for patients that were concurrently enrolled on HAART (Murray, Fanning et al. 2009). Such results are encouraging and indicate that relatively modest engraftment percentages could achieve a clinically relevant effect. Consequently full bone marrow ablation may be unnecessary.

3.3 Resistance development under gene-therapy: How does it differ from HAART?

Systemic antiretroviral therapy bathes each cell in some level of the drugs being used depending on the penetration of the individual drugs to that region of the body, their concentration, pharmacokinetics and timing between dosages (Abdel-Rahman and Kauffman 2004). The clinical management of the combinations of drugs used in a regimen is an important part of successful treatment through suppressing the development of drug resistance. Early in the development of antiretroviral drugs there were few agents available and by necessity these were applied as monotherapy leading to the failure of these and subsequent drugs from the same class. Current HAART regimens involve three drugs from at least 2 drug classes to limit the likelihood that mutations in the HIV quasispecies will be present prior to the commencement of therapy or will develop subsequently.

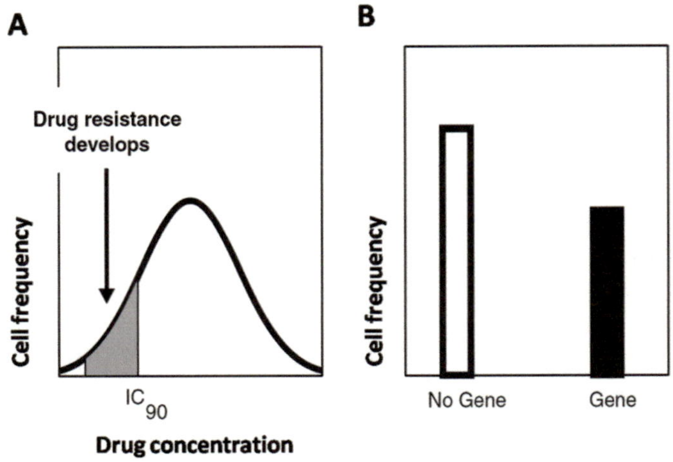

Fig. 5. Illustration of principles behind selection pressures driving the development of resistance with antiretroviral therapy and with gene-therapy. Adapted with permission from Applegate et al.(Applegate, Birkett et al. 2010). (A) The horizontal ordinate denotes the concentration of antiretroviral drug received, and the vertical ordinate denotes the frequency of cells receiving the antiretroviral drug concentration. The selection pressure driving resistance in systemic antiretroviral therapy results from bathing each cell in some drug concentration. This provides a "continuous spectrum" for selection of HIV escape mutants, since many cells will receive suboptimal drug concentrations allowing viral replication and the preferential development of drug-resistant strains (as shown by shaded region indicated by the arrow). (B) The horizontal ordinate splits the cell population into two parts of either having a protective gene or not. The vertical ordinate denotes the frequency of cells containing the gene and not containing the gene. The bipartite distribution of protected and unprotected results provides a different selection environment whereby sufficient wild-type replication takes place in the non-protected population (i.e. no gene), thus mitigating the escape of viral mutants.

Similar concerns exist for the development of resistance to HIV gene therapy (Leonard and Schaffer 2006; Applegate, Birkett et al. 2010). The quasispecies nature of HIV and its high mutation rate imply the existence of every single mutation to any agent prior to the start of therapy. If there is sufficient viral replication under therapy, even for a reasonably short period, there is the chance that these singly resistant clones will evolve into variants with additional mutations and that are highly resistant to therapy. HIV gene therapy seems to fall into the classification of approaches that lend themselves to the development of resistance: not all cells will contain the therapy and so there will be considerable viral replication, and this will be even more evident for gene therapy delivered to HSC since it will take some time for the protected CD4+ T cells to mature from the HSC and appear in the periphery (Applegate, Birkett et al. 2010). However there is a considerable difference between gene therapy and a systemic treatment that is not suitably suppressive.

Unless myeloablation is conducted to eliminate endogenous non-gene containing HSC and T cells, it is expected that there will always be a sizeable proportion of HSC and CD4+ T cells that do not contain the therapy. Achieving 20% gene transduced HSC without ablation may be an upper bound (this remains to be tested). Similar limitations exist for those trials that instead transduce peripheral CD4+ T cells. At any time there is an estimated 2% of total T cells in peripheral blood and not all T cells are likely to traffic to this compartment. So large-scale apheresis of CD4+ T cells from peripheral blood will remove, and be able to infuse, only a fraction of their total.

Hence gene therapy will partition HIV-susceptible cells into a bipartite population: those containing the therapy and those that do not. This 0-1 distribution is very different from the continuous distribution of drug concentration within cells for an individual receiving antiretroviral therapy (Figure 5). In this situation gene therapy is less likely to lead to the development of resistance (Applegate, Birkett et al. 2010). However there is a trade-off in that it is also less suppressive for the same reason. As cells containing gene therapy become more widespread in the body of an infected individual they will exert more pressure on the virus and select for resistance (Leonard and Schaffer 2006). For this reason the same general principles that apply to antiretroviral therapy are also valid in this context. Gene therapy should target multiple viral and cellular mechanisms.

Mathematical modelling of gene therapy delivered to HSC that targets multiple mechanisms with reasonable efficacy and where the resistant virus is also less fit than wild-type determined that this therapy will reduce virus and maintain a viable T cell population for extended periods without the expansion of resistant virus (Applegate, Birkett et al. 2010). However there were important qualifications to the extent of this success. Primarily the gene therapy needs to be Class 1 and inhibit infection of cells. Additionally the likelihood of resistance to a particular component of the therapy and the fitness cost that incurs will also contribute to the speed at which virus overcomes the therapy.

3.4 Future perspectives: What can we expect from gene-therapy against HIV?

Gene therapy holds out high promise as an effective therapy against HIV. The definition of success of gene-therapy treatment may vary, depending on a variety of circumstances. As discussed in Section 2.1, an obvious success would be one similar to that of the Berlin Patient whereby an individual would be completely and sustainably cured of HIV and have their immune system restored to "normal" levels. It is however important to provide more practical goals, as it is not likely that a "cure" will be achieved with all patients, and as such, more "modest" goals might be more practical and more realistic. Removing the need for an individual to be on HAART would be defined as success, as this can save the individual from life-long drug regimens often with considerable side-effects (Yeni 2006). Another "successful" outcome might consists in preservation of immune system functionality depite the presence of measurable viral loads, as observed during SIV infection in its natural hosts (Liovat, Jacquelin et al. 2009; Pandrea, Silvestri et al. 2009).

As discussed in section 3.2.2 above, predictions from mathematical modelling indicate that full ablation of the immune system need not be necessary in order for clinically significant effects to be observed (Murray, Fanning et al. 2009). Assuming HSC engraftment percentages of about 20%, it has been predicted that substantial viral control may be achieved and CD4+ T cell counts maintained above the critical limit of 200 cells/μL (Murray, Fanning et al. 2009). The major challenge to achieving substantial clinical effect thus relates to achieving sufficient engraftment percentages.

Gene therapy will have varying degrees of effectiveness depending on the circumstances of the individual. The length of time for which an individual has been infected with HIV is an important factor to consider when providing gene therapy treatment. Due to the tropism of HIV in an infected individual changing over the duration of infection from CCR5-tropic to CXCR4-tropic, any treatment targeting CCR5 would be best used on patients in fairly early-phase infection (Mosier 2009). For gene-therapy aiming to transduce HSC, it also appears reasonable to expect that the therapeutic effects in younger patients will be more pronounced due to their greater rates of thymic activity (Pido-Lopez, Imami et al. 2001). Futhermore, patients on HAART, patients for whom available antiretroviral therapies have been exhausted and patients suffering severe HAART-associated side-effects should also benefit, given that gene-therapy provides an alternative layer of protection via cell-mediated immunity in addition to antiretroviral therapies (Symonds, Johnstone et al. 2010).

Finally, as discussed in section 3.2, both HSC and CD4+ T cells represent feasible targets for transduction. While CD4+ T cell transduction may suffer from limitations due to a restricted T cell receptor repertoire and not protecting other susceptible cell population, it will however provide an immediate protected population. Conversely HSC are limited by the degree of thymic production and bone marrow engraftment, yet have the potential to generate a long-lasting array of HIV protected immune cells. Thus it appears that most effective therapies might employ a combination of these two approaches in order to provide optimum protection, possibly employing infusions of transduced cells.

4. Conclusion

In this chapter we discussed the current biological underpinnings of gene-therapy against HIV, as well as predictions from mathematical modelling of the clinical effects achievable through gene-therapy.

We discussed the various biological and clinical aspects relating to HIV gene therapy. An indication of the possible effectiveness of gene therapy was provided in terms of the naturally occurring mutation, CCR5d32, which provides extremely high levels of resistance against HIV infection. Most importantly however, the utilisation of this mutation in a bone marrow transplant, ridding an individual of any measurable HIV levels, indicates the capability of using gene therapy to functionally "cure" people of HIV. An assessment of the target areas of HIV gene therapy was conducted, indicating not only the possibility, but also a clear need to target multiple aspects of HIV infection (favourably entry stage), in order to prevent the emergence of resistance. The various options for delivery methods were discussed, indicating a range of techniques by which to introduce the therapeutic gene. Each of these methods exhibit their own advantages and disadvantages, however all are valid options in a variety of situations, with lentiviral vectors showing some of the most promise. The options for the ideal cell-type to target were discussed, indicating validity of using either CD4+ T cells for their immediate effect or HSC for the more sustained and broad spectrum protection. However it is also critical to consider the combination of these as an option in gene therapy. The aspects and priniciples of apheresis, ablation, and G-CSF-induced mobilisation were discussed, indicating their role in treatments. With mobilisation being crucial for the efficient transduction of HSC, and ablation of non-tranduced cells having the potential to provide a significant proportional increase in the amount of protected cells, both are critical when designing treatment regimens. Finally, clinical trials whereby HIV gene therapy has been conducted, and the outcomes of these trials were summarised, highlighting the high safety levels associated with gene therapuetics. Due to the observed high safety in these studies, with the promise of reasonable levels of efficacy and a proof of concept (in the Berlin Patient), HIV gene therapies are a very promising area of HIV research.

In the final sections we discussed predictions obtained from mathematical modelling regarding the in-vivo effectiveness of gene-therapy. We outlined why HIV virion entry inhibition via Class 1 gene-therapy has been shown to be essential in terms of achieving clinically meaningful effects. We explained how the selective survival advantage conferred to non-infected cells containing the Class 1 protective gene is the key factor contributing to the success of Class 1 therapy. We saw that transduction of CD4+ T cells provides an immediately protected CD4+ T cell population, but that in-vivo expansion of the protected cells may be a slow process and does not result in increased T cell receptor diversity in the expanded population. In contrast, transduction of HSC results in higher T cell receptor diversity, and in protection of a broader range of cells than solely CD4+ T cells. We also discussed the differences in viral resistance development under HAART and under gene-therapy. While HAART bathes each cell in some drug concentration, resulting in suboptimal dosages for many cells and consequent promotion in escape of viral mutants, gene-therapy partitions the cell population into protected (contains gene) and unprotected (does not contain gene) cell populations. We outlined how this bi-partite distribution promotes the expansion of a cell population protected against HIV, while at the same time mitigating risks of viral mutation escape as a result of sufficient wild-type viral replication in the non-protected cell population. Finally, we discussed future perspectives outlining how gene-therapy promises to achieve sufficient preservation of immune system functionality (without HAART-associated toxicity and non-adherence issues) resulting in forestallement of AIDS and thereby achieving similar effects as observed during SIV infection in its natural hosts. We also outlined how gene-based therapies may be employed in conjunction or disjunction with HAART depending on individual patient circumstances and viral tropism in the infected individual.

In conclusion, based on the clinical results and mathematical modeling work to-date, further clinical investigation of gene-therapy is more than justified, as gene-therapy holds high promise in terms of controlling HIV infection, preserving immune system functionality, and prevention of the onset of AIDS.

5. References

(2009). "Trial watch: novel HIV gene therapy enters Phase I trial." Nat Rev Drug Discov 8(4): 267.

Abdel-Rahman, S. M. and R. E. Kauffman (2004). "The integration of pharmacokinetics and pharmacodynamics: understanding dose-response." Annu Rev Pharmacol Toxicol 44: 111-136.

Agrawal, L., X. Lu, et al. (2004). "Role for CCR5Delta32 protein in resistance to R5, R5X4, and X4 human immunodeficiency virus type 1 in primary CD4+ cells." J Virol 78(5): 2277-2287.

Aiuti, A. (2004). "Gene therapy for adenosine-deaminase-deficient severe combined immunodeficiency." Best Pract Res Clin Haematol 17(3): 505-516.

Allen, S., S. J. Turner, et al. (2011). "Shaping the T-cell repertoire in the periphery." Immunol Cell Biol 89(1): 60-69.

Allers, K., G. Hutter, et al. (2010). "Evidence for the cure of HIV infection by CCR5{Delta}32/{Delta}32 stem cell transplantation." Blood.

Aluigi, M., M. Fogli, et al. (2006). "Nucleofection is an efficient nonviral transfection technique for human bone marrow-derived mesenchymal stem cells." Stem Cells 24(2): 454-461.

Amado, R. G., R. T. Mitsuyasu, et al. (2004). "Anti-human immunodeficiency virus hematopoietic progenitor cell-delivered ribozyme in a phase I study: myeloid and lymphoid reconstitution in human immunodeficiency virus type-1-infected patients." Hum Gene Ther 15(3): 251-262.

Amado, R. G., R. T. Mitsuyasu, et al. (1999). "A phase I trial of autologous CD34+ hematopoietic progenitor cells transduced with an anti-HIV ribozyme." Hum Gene Ther 10(13): 2255-2270.

Anderson, J., A. Banerjea, et al. (2003). "Potent suppression of HIV type 1 infection by a short hairpin anti-CXCR4 siRNA." AIDS Res Hum Retroviruses 19(8): 699-706.

Applegate, T. L., D. J. Birkett, et al. (2010). "In silico modeling indicates the development of HIV-1 resistance to multiple shRNA gene therapy differs to standard antiretroviral therapy." Retrovirology 7: 83.

Aviran, S., P. S. Shah, et al. (2010). "Computational models of HIV-1 resistance to gene therapy elucidate therapy design principles." PLoS Comput Biol 6(8).

Bauer, G., D. Selander, et al. (2000). "Gene therapy for pediatric AIDS." Ann N Y Acad Sci 918: 318-329.

Boden, D., O. Pusch, et al. (2003). "Promoter choice affects the potency of HIV-1 specific RNA interference." Nucleic Acids Res 31(17): 5033-5038.

Brunstein, C. G., J. S. Miller, et al. (2011). "Infusion of ex vivo expanded T regulatory cells in adults transplanted with umbilical cord blood: safety profile and detection kinetics." Blood 117(3): 1061-1070.

Byakwaga, H., J. M. Murray, et al. (2009). "Evolution of CD4+ T cell count in HIV-1-infected adults receiving antiretroviral therapy with sustained long-term virological suppression." AIDS Res Hum Retroviruses 25(6): 756-776.

Carter, C. A. and L. S. Ehrlich (2008). "Cell biology of HIV-1 infection of macrophages." Annu Rev Microbiol 62: 425-443.

Carter, C. C., L. A. McNamara, et al. (2011). "HIV-1 utilizes the CXCR4 chemokine receptor to infect multipotent hematopoietic stem and progenitor cells." Cell Host Microbe 9(3): 223-234.

Carter, C. C., A. Onafuwa-Nuga, et al. (2010). "HIV-1 infects multipotent progenitor cells causing cell death and establishing latent cellular reservoirs." Nat Med 16(4): 446-451.

Cavazzana-Calvo, M., S. Hacein-Bey, et al. (2000). "Gene therapy of human severe combined immunodeficiency (SCID)-X1 disease." Science 288(5466): 669-672.

Chen, S. Y., J. Bagley, et al. (1994). "Intracellular antibodies as a new class of therapeutic molecules for gene therapy." Hum Gene Ther 5(5): 595-601.

Chun, T. W., L. Carruth, et al. (1997). "Quantification of latent tissue reservoirs and total body viral load in HIV-1 infection." Nature 387(6629): 183-188.

Chun, T. W., L. Stuyver, et al. (1997). "Presence of an inducible HIV-1 latent reservoir during highly active antiretroviral therapy." Proc Natl Acad Sci U S A 94(24): 13193-13197.

Crowe, S. M. and S. Sonza (2000). "HIV-1 can be recovered from a variety of cells including peripheral blood monocytes of patients receiving highly active antiretroviral therapy: a further obstacle to eradication." J Leukoc Biol 68(3): 345-350.

Dean, M., M. Carrington, et al. (1996). "Genetic restriction of HIV-1 infection and progression to AIDS by a deletion allele of the CKR5 structural gene. Hemophilia Growth and Development Study, Multicenter AIDS Cohort Study, Multicenter Hemophilia Cohort Study, San Francisco City Cohort, ALIVE Study." Science 273(5283): 1856-1862.

DiGiusto, D. L., A. Krishnan, et al. (2010). "RNA-based gene therapy for HIV with lentiviral vector-modified CD34(+) cells in patients undergoing transplantation for AIDS-related lymphoma." Sci Transl Med 2(36): 36ra43.

Doitsh, G., M. Cavrois, et al. (2010). "Abortive HIV infection mediates CD4 T cell depletion and inflammation in human lymphoid tissue." Cell 143(5): 789-801.

Dropulic, B. and C. H. June (2006). "Gene-based immunotherapy for human immunodeficiency virus infection and acquired immunodeficiency syndrome." Hum Gene Ther 17(6): 577-588.

Flotte, T. R. (2007). "Gene therapy: the first two decades and the current state-of-the-art." J Cell Physiol 213(2): 301-305.

Galvani, A. P. and M. Slatkin (2003). "Evaluating plague and smallpox as historical selective pressures for the CCR5-Delta 32 HIV-resistance allele." Proc Natl Acad Sci U S A 100(25): 15276-15279.

Gervaix, A., L. Schwarz, et al. (1997). "Gene therapy targeting peripheral blood CD34+ hematopoietic stem cells of HIV-infected individuals." Hum Gene Ther 8(18): 2229-2238.

Glass, W. G., D. H. McDermott, et al. (2006). "CCR5 deficiency increases risk of symptomatic West Nile virus infection." J Exp Med 203(1): 35-40.

Hannon, G. J. and J. J. Rossi (2004). "Unlocking the potential of the human genome with RNA interference." Nature 431(7006): 371-378.

Hedrick, P. W. and B. C. Verrelli (2006). ""Ground truth" for selection on CCR5-Delta32." Trends Genet 22(6): 293-296.

Holt, N., J. Wang, et al. (2010). "Human hematopoietic stem/progenitor cells modified by zinc-finger nucleases targeted to CCR5 control HIV-1 in vivo." Nat Biotechnol.

Howe, S. J., M. R. Mansour, et al. (2008). "Insertional mutagenesis combined with acquired somatic mutations causes leukemogenesis following gene therapy of SCID-X1 patients." J Clin Invest 118(9): 3143-3150.

Hummel, S., D. Schmidt, et al. (2005). "Detection of the CCR5-Delta32 HIV resistance gene in Bronze Age skeletons." Genes Immun 6(4): 371-374.

Hutter, G., D. Nowak, et al. (2009). "Long-term control of HIV by CCR5 Delta32/Delta32 stem-cell transplantation." N Engl J Med 360(7): 692-698.

Jin, Q., L. Agrawal, et al. (2008). "CCR5Delta32 59537-G/A promoter polymorphism is associated with low translational efficiency and the loss of CCR5Delta32 protective effects." J Virol 82(5): 2418-2426.

Khaled, A. R. and S. K. Durum (2002). "Lymphocide: cytokines and the control of lymphoid homeostasis." Nat Rev Immunol 2(11): 817-830.

Kohn, D. B., G. Bauer, et al. (1999). "A clinical trial of retroviral-mediated transfer of a rev-responsive element decoy gene into CD34(+) cells from the bone marrow of human immunodeficiency virus-1-infected children." Blood 94(1): 368-371.

Kohn, D. B. and F. Candotti (2009). "Gene therapy fulfilling its promise." N Engl J Med 360(5): 518-521.

Kootstra, N. A. and I. M. Verma (2003). "Gene therapy with viral vectors." Annu Rev Pharmacol Toxicol 43: 413-439.

Lane, T. A., P. Law, et al. (1995). "Harvesting and enrichment of hematopoietic progenitor cells mobilized into the peripheral blood of normal donors by granulocyte-macrophage colony-stimulating factor (GM-CSF) or G-CSF: potential role in allogeneic marrow transplantation." Blood 85(1): 275-282.

Law, P., T. A. Lane, et al. (1999). "Mobilization of peripheral blood progenitor cells for human immunodeficiency virus-infected individuals." Exp Hematol 27(1): 147-154.

Leonard, J. N. and D. V. Schaffer (2006). "Antiviral RNAi therapy: emerging approaches for hitting a moving target." Gene Ther 13(6): 532-540.

Levine, B. L., L. M. Humeau, et al. (2006). "Gene transfer in humans using a conditionally replicating lentiviral vector." Proc Natl Acad Sci U S A 103(46): 17372-17377.

Liovat, A. S., B. Jacquelin, et al. (2009). "African non human primates infected by SIV - why don't they get sick? Lessons from studies on the early phase of non-pathogenic SIV infection." Curr HIV Res 7(1): 39-50.

Liu, Q. and D. A. Muruve (2003). "Molecular basis of the inflammatory response to adenovirus vectors." Gene Ther 10(11): 935-940.

Liu, R., W. A. Paxton, et al. (1996). "Homozygous defect in HIV-1 coreceptor accounts for resistance of some multiply-exposed individuals to HIV-1 infection." Cell 86(3): 367-377.

Lund, O., O. S. Lund, et al. (1997). "Gene therapy of T helper cells in HIV infection: mathematical model of the criteria for clinical effect." Bull Math Biol 59(4): 725-745.

Macpherson, J. L., M. P. Boyd, et al. (2005). "Long-term survival and concomitant gene expression of ribozyme-transduced CD4+ T-lymphocytes in HIV-infected patients." J Gene Med 7(5): 552-564.

McIntyre, G. J. and G. C. Fanning (2006). "Design and cloning strategies for constructing shRNA expression vectors." BMC Biotechnol 6: 1.

McLean, A. R. and C. A. Michie (1995). "In vivo estimates of division and death rates of human T lymphocytes." Proc Natl Acad Sci U S A 92(9): 3707-3711.

Michienzi, A., D. Castanotto, et al. (2003). "RNA-mediated inhibition of HIV in a gene therapy setting." Ann N Y Acad Sci 1002: 63-71.

Mitsuyasu, R. T., P. A. Anton, et al. (2000). "Prolonged survival and tissue trafficking following adoptive transfer of CD4zeta gene-modified autologous CD4(+) and CD8(+) T cells in human immunodeficiency virus-infected subjects." Blood 96(3): 785-793.

Mitsuyasu, R. T., T. C. Merigan, et al. (2009). "Phase 2 gene therapy trial of an anti-HIV ribozyme in autologous CD34+ cells." Nat Med 15(3): 285-292.

Morgan, R. A., R. Walker, et al. (2005). "Preferential survival of CD4+ T lymphocytes engineered with anti-human immunodeficiency virus (HIV) genes in HIV-infected individuals." Hum Gene Ther 16(9): 1065-1074.

Mosier, D. E. (2009). "How HIV changes its tropism: evolution and adaptation?" Curr Opin HIV AIDS 4(2): 125-130.

Murray, J. M., G. C. Fanning, et al. (2009). "Mathematical modelling of the impact of haematopoietic stem cell-delivered gene therapy for HIV." J Gene Med 11(12): 1077-1086.

Murray, J. M., G. R. Kaufmann, et al. (2003). "Naive T cells are maintained by thymic output in early ages but by proliferation without phenotypic change after age twenty." Immunol Cell Biol 81(6): 487-495.

Nikolich-Zugich, J., M. K. Slifka, et al. (2004). "The many important facets of T-cell repertoire diversity." Nat Rev Immunol 4(2): 123-132.

Pandrea, I., G. Silvestri, et al. (2009). "AIDS in african nonhuman primate hosts of SIVs: a new paradigm of SIV infection." Curr HIV Res 7(1): 57-72.

Perelson, A. S., P. Essunger, et al. (1997). "Dynamics of HIV-1 and CD4+ lymphocytes in vivo." AIDS 11 Suppl A: S17-24.

Perno, C. F., G. Moyle, et al. (2008). "Overcoming resistance to existing therapies in HIV-infected patients: the role of new antiretroviral drugs." J Med Virol 80(4): 565-576.

Philippe, S., C. Sarkis, et al. (2006). "Lentiviral vectors with a defective integrase allow efficient and sustained transgene expression in vitro and in vivo." Proc Natl Acad Sci U S A 103(47): 17684-17689.

Pido-Lopez, J., N. Imami, et al. (2001). "Both age and gender affect thymic output: more recent thymic migrants in females than males as they age." Clin Exp Immunol 125(3): 409-413.

Podsakoff, G. M., B. C. Engel, et al. (2005). "Selective survival of peripheral blood lymphocytes in children with HIV-1 following delivery of an anti-HIV gene to bone marrow CD34(+) cells." Mol Ther 12(1): 77-86.

Porteus, M. H. and D. Carroll (2005). "Gene targeting using zinc finger nucleases." Nat Biotechnol 23(8): 967-973.

Que-Gewirth, N. S. and B. A. Sullenger (2007). "Gene therapy progress and prospects: RNA aptamers." Gene Ther 14(4): 283-291.

Ranga, U., C. Woffendin, et al. (1998). "Enhanced T cell engraftment after retroviral delivery of an antiviral gene in HIV-infected individuals." Proc Natl Acad Sci U S A 95(3): 1201-1206.

Roe, T., T. C. Reynolds, et al. (1993). "Integration of murine leukemia virus DNA depends on mitosis." EMBO J 12(5): 2099-2108.

Rossi, J. J., C. H. June, et al. (2007). "Genetic therapies against HIV." Nat Biotechnol 25(12): 1444-1454.

Samson, M., F. Libert, et al. (1996). "Resistance to HIV-1 infection in caucasian individuals bearing mutant alleles of the CCR-5 chemokine receptor gene." Nature 382(6593): 722-725.

Stanley, S. K., S. W. Kessler, et al. (1992). "CD34+ bone marrow cells are infected with HIV in a subset of seropositive individuals." J Immunol 149(2): 689-697.

Stein, S., M. G. Ott, et al. (2010). "Genomic instability and myelodysplasia with monosomy 7 consequent to EVI1 activation after gene therapy for chronic granulomatous disease." Nat Med 16(2): 198-204.

Strayer, D. S., R. Akkina, et al. (2005). "Current status of gene therapy strategies to treat HIV/AIDS." Mol Ther 11(6): 823-842.

Sun, L. Q., L. Wang, et al. (1995). "Target sequence-specific inhibition of HIV-1 replication by ribozymes directed to tat RNA." Nucleic Acids Res 23(15): 2909-2913.

Symonds, G. P., H. A. Johnstone, et al. (2010). "The use of cell-delivered gene therapy for the treatment of HIV/AIDS." Immunol Res 48(1-3): 84-98.

Tamhane, M. and R. Akkina (2008). "Stable gene transfer of CCR5 and CXCR4 siRNAs by sleeping beauty transposon system to confer HIV-1 resistance." AIDS Res Ther 5: 16.

Tayi, V. S., B. D. Bowen, et al. (2010). "Mathematical model of the rate-limiting steps for retrovirus-mediated gene transfer into mammalian cells." Biotechnology and Bioengineering 105(1): 195-209.

Valgimigli, M., G. M. Rigolin, et al. (2005). "Use of granulocyte-colony stimulating factor during acute myocardial infarction to enhance bone marrow stem cell mobilization in humans: clinical and angiographic safety profile." Eur Heart J 26(18): 1838-1845.

van Lunzen, J., T. Glaunsinger, et al. (2007). "Transfer of autologous gene-modified T cells in HIV-infected patients with advanced immunodeficiency and drug-resistant virus." Mol Ther 15(5): 1024-1033.

von Laer, D., C. Baum, et al. (2009). "Antiviral gene therapy." Handb Exp Pharmacol(189): 265-297.

von Laer, D., S. Hasselmann, et al. (2006). "Gene therapy for HIV infection: what does it need to make it work?" The Journal of Gene Medicine 8(6): 658-667.

von Laer, D., S. Hasselmann, et al. (2006). "Impact of gene-modified T cells on HIV infection dynamics." J Theor Biol 238(1): 60-77.

Weber, E. L. and P. M. Cannon (2007). "Promoter choice for retroviral vectors: transcriptional strength versus trans-activation potential." Hum Gene Ther 18(9): 849-860.

Westby, M., C. Smith-Burchnell, et al. (2007). "Reduced maximal inhibition in phenotypic susceptibility assays indicates that viral strains resistant to the CCR5 antagonist maraviroc utilize inhibitor-bound receptor for entry." J Virol 81(5): 2359-2371.

Wiegers, G. J., M. Kaufmann, et al. (2011). "Shaping the T-cell repertoire: a matter of life and death." Immunol Cell Biol 89(1): 33-39.

Woffendin, C., U. Ranga, et al. (1996). "Expression of a protective gene-prolongs survival of T cells in human immunodeficiency virus-infected patients." Proc Natl Acad Sci U S A 93(7): 2889-2894.

Wu, X., J. K. Wakefield, et al. (2000). "Development of a novel trans-lentiviral vector that affords predictable safety." Mol Ther 2(1): 47-55.

Yeni, P. (2006). "Update on HAART in HIV." J Hepatol 44(1 Suppl): S100-103.

Zahn, R. C., F. G. Hermann, et al. (2008). "Efficient entry inhibition of human and nonhuman primate immunodeficiency virus by cell surface-expressed gp41-derived peptides." Gene Ther 15(17): 1210-1222.

Zhang, L., U. Sankar, et al. (1998). "The Himar1 mariner transposase cloned in a recombinant adenovirus vector is functional in mammalian cells." Nucleic Acids Res 26(16): 3687-3693.

Zimmerman, P. A., A. Buckler-White, et al. (1997). "Inherited resistance to HIV-1 conferred by an inactivating mutation in CC chemokine receptor 5: studies in populations with contrasting clinical phenotypes, defined racial background, and quantified risk." Mol Med 3(1): 23-36.

Zufferey, R., T. Dull, et al. (1998). "Self-inactivating lentivirus vector for safe and efficient in vivo gene delivery." J Virol 72(12): 9873-9880.

21

Gene Therapy for HIV-1 Infection

Lisa Egerer, Dorothee von Laer and Janine Kimpel
Innsbruck Medical University, Department of Hygiene, Microbiology and Social Medicine, Division of Virology, Innsbruck Austria

1. Introduction

The introduction of the highly active antiretroviral therapy (HAART) for the treatment of HIV-1-infection has dramatically improved the quality of life and the survival of HIV-infected patients. HAART can effectively suppress virus replication and thereby helps to preserve immune functions. However, as HIV-1 persists in latently infected reservoirs (Finzi et al., 1997), complete eradication of the virus by antiretroviral drugs has never been achieved and life-long treatment is required. Moreover, emerging viral resistance and drug toxicity restrict long-term therapeutic efficacy (Brinkman et al., 1999; Vigouroux et al., 1999). As a consequence, HAART has not had a major impact on the global prevalence of HIV-infection and there is no vaccine in sight that could prevent further virus spread.

In addition to HAART and vaccines, gene therapy approaches for HIV-1 infection have been under investigation for more than two decades. Gene therapy could theoretically overcome the limitations of standard antiretroviral drug therapy and facilitate sustained suppression of virus replication after only few treatment cycles. Moreover, the choice of adequate genes or combinations of genes and expression systems could greatly reduce toxicity and prevent the generation of resistant virus strains. Although gene therapy is an expensive and technically challenging therapy today, future developments could simplify the procedures involved and bring down costs. Two basic gene therapeutic strategies for immune reconstitution of AIDS patients have been developed and the safety and efficacy of different approaches have been examined in preclinical and clinical studies. The first strategy aims to specifically kill HIV-infected cells by enhancing the antiviral host immune responses. The second approach, termed 'intracellular immunization', is based on the expression of antiviral genes that prevent HIV-1 replication in its target cells. Furthermore, therapeutic or prophylactic vaccination strategies that aim to enhance anti-HIV immunity and use DNA or viral vectors to express the viral antigens can formally be classified as gene therapy approaches. However, such vaccination strategies are not in the scope of this review.

2. Enhancing HIV-specific immunity: Adoptive transfer of $CD8^+$ T cells

The striking ability of HIV-1 to evade control by the host immune system is a fundamental problem in AIDS pathogenesis. Although most patients develop natural anti-HIV immune responses, the virus does not possess the immunogenicity to mount long-lasting responses strong enough to entirely suppress replication and to allow complete virus eradication from the body. In fact, most affected individuals initially develop immunodominant $CD8^+$ T cell (cytotoxic T lymphocyte, CTL) responses during the acute phase of HIV-1 infection, resulting in transient virus control and a decrease in plasma viremia (Borrow et al., 1994). The importance of CTLs was further confirmed in experiments with SIV-infected non-human primates, where acute infection could not be controlled in animals depleted of $CD8^+$ T lymphocytes (Schmitz et al., 1999). There is a strong negative correlation between emergence of virus-specific CTLs and the viral set point, as patients with strong early CTL responses show significantly lower viral set points and a slower disease progression (Streeck et al., 2009). However, later, during the chronic phase of HIV-1 infection generation of $CD8^+$ T cell responses seems to be impaired and dysfunctional CTLs fail to control virus replication in most patients. In contrast, long-term non-progressors - individuals which are HIV-1 seropositive, but do not progress to AIDS - retain high levels of virus-specific T cells, indicating that functional CTL responses are crucial for efficient virus control also in chronic infection (Rinaldo et al., 1995).

One reason for the failure of HIV-specific immunity during the chronic stage of infection may be the high variability of the virus resulting from a high replication rate and error-prone reverse transcription (Phillips et al., 1991). Moreover, HIV-1 attacks the immune system itself, the $CD4^+$ helper T cell being its major target cell. This results in the preferential infection and a massive loss of HIV-specific $CD4^+$ T cells already early upon infection, as the virus-specific helper cells migrate to the site of infection where they become activated thereby becoming more susceptible to HIV-1 infection (Demoustier et al., 2002; Douek et al., 2002). Yet, virus-specific $CD4^+$ T cells are urgently needed to help generating strong, durable immune responses and their absence impairs CTL activation and maturation (Kemball et al., 2007; Matloubian et al., 1994). In addition, progressive exhaustion of virus-specific $CD8^+$ T cells is a hallmark of the chronic immune activation during ongoing HIV-1 infection. Here, the constant antigen persistence prevents contraction of the effector T cell pool and development of long-lived memory cells. Instead, a stepwise exhaustion characterized by metabolic and transcriptional changes, reduced cytokine and chemokine secretion, loss of proliferation capacity and cytolytic activity is observed, resulting in impaired CTL effector functions and finally apoptosis (Shankar et al., 2000; Trimble & Lieberman, 1998).

Boosting of the natural CTL responses against HIV-1 by cell and gene therapeutic strategies may help to overcome these problems. For this purpose two different strategies have been developed; the adoptive transfer of autologous antigen-specific T cells after *ex vivo* selection and expansion, and the infusion of genetically armed $CD8^+$ T cells expressing HIV-specific T cell receptors (TCRs). A therapy combining these approaches with the protection of $CD4^+$ T cells to preserve important T-helper cell functions could potentially impact infection dynamics and ultimately facilitate clearance of the virus.

The adoptive transfer of autologous, antigen-specific $CD8^+$ T cell clones has been used successfully to treat persistent viral infections and cancer. The allogeneic organ transplantation from cytomegalovirus or Epstein-Barr virus seropositive donors, for instance, is associated with risks for the recipient, if untreated. Co-transplantation of virus-antigen-specific T cells isolated from the donor and expanded *in vitro*, enhanced T cell immunity to the viruses and prevented adverse effects in the immunosuppressed recipients (Heslop et al., 1996; Walter et al., 1995). For HIV-1, however, the transfer of *ex vivo* expanded virus-specific CTLs had only limited success in patients so far. In a study reported by Brodie et al. autologous Gag-specific CTLs were isolated and reinfused into HIV-positive individuals (Brodie et al., 1999). The CTLs engrafted in the patients and were found to migrate to the lymph nodes, which are the major sites of HIV-1 replication (Brodie et al.,

2000; Hufert et al., 1997). However, although the CTLs were capable of lysing HIV-1 infected cells *in vivo*, only a transient effect on virus replication was observed (Brodie et al., 1999; Brodie et al., 2000). A major problem of this therapeutic concept is that the CTLs isolated from patients with advanced disease are often exhausted and terminally differentiated and lack full effector functions. As *in vitro* expansion of these cells is accompanied with a further loss of function, the transferred cell numbers may be insufficient to induce long-term effects. Methods that allow generation of large numbers of fully functional CTLs therefore would be required to facilitate success of this promising therapy approach.

An alternative to the isolation and expansion of existing antigen-specific T cells from a patient, is the genetic modification of cells resulting in the expression of recombinant HIV-specific receptors. The cell types used for this genetic 'redirection' can be peripheral blood T cells, but also hematopoietic stem cells (HSC), which can afterwards differentiate into immune cells targeting HIV-1. As the isolation and manipulation of T cells is currently easier to perform compared to stem-cell modification, all studies that have been conducted so far used peripheral blood T cells. The receptors used to redirect the immune cells to target HIV-1 can either be natural T cell receptors or artificial chimeric antigen receptors (CARs). For the natural TCRs, CTL clones with high avidity TCRs specific for the target antigens are selected *in vitro*. The alpha and beta chains of these TCRs are then cloned and used to transduce patient T cells. This approach has been used successfully in the clinic to treat patients with melanoma, where in some cases tumor regression has been observed (Morgan et al., 2006). The isolation and cloning of high-avidity HIV-specific TCRs is also feasible. Joseph and colleagues constructed a lentiviral vector expressing a TCR specific for the HIV-1 Gag epitope SL9. Transduction of human primary T cells led to the conversion of peripheral blood $CD8^+$ T cells into HIV-specific CTLs (Joseph et al., 2008). These CTLs exerted anti-HIV activity *in vitro* and *in vivo* in a humanized mouse model. In a similar study, an SL9-specific TCR with enhanced affinity was shown to efficiently mediate control of HIV-1 *in vitro* (Varela-Rohena et al., 2008). Currently this approach is evaluated in a phase I clinical trial (www.ClinicalTrials.gov; identifier: NCT00991224). The use of natural TCRs to generate virus-specific CTLs is limited by the major histocompatibility complex (MHC)-restriction of the TCR. TCRs recognize peptides only if they are presented on a specific type of MHC. Therefore, T cells expressing a given TCR can only be used for treatment of MHC-matched patients. The clinical trial described above, for instance, can only include patients with the HLA-type A*02. For a broader application of this therapy concept a set of TCRs would be required that allows treatment of patients with various haplotypes. Besides, in gene modified CTLs, the genetically transferred TCR can mispair with the endogenous TCR, which may affect its function and lead to autoimmunity. Another drawback of the approach is the downregulation of MHC molecules in HIV-infected cells, which impedes the presentation of viral peptides and recognition by the CTLs (Sommermeyer et al., 2006).

CARs are chimeric antigen receptors composed of an extracellular antigen binding motive connected to an intracellular signal transduction domain via a flexible linker and a transmembrane domain. The antigen binding motive usually is an antigen-specific single-chain variable fragment derived from a monoclonal antibody, while the signal transduction part comes from the CD3 ζ-chain. CARs trigger an MHC-independent antigen recognition (Eshhar et al., 2001). Two CARs with HIV-1 specificity have been developed by Roberts and colleagues (Roberts et al., 1994). The antigen-binding part consists either of the gp120 binding domain from human CD4 or an antibody against gp41. T cells transduced with either of the receptors specifically recognized and killed HIV-infected cells *in vitro*. The receptor containing CD4 has been tested in three clinical trials. In these studies local effects on virus replication were observed, but unfortunately there was no overall change in viral load (Deeks et al., 2002; Mitsuyasu et al., 2000; Walker et al., 2000).

3. Intracellular immunization: Protection of $CD4^{+}$ T cells

The second gene therapeutic strategy for HIV-1 infection was termed 'intracellular immunization' (Baltimore, 1988) and involves the expression of an antiviral gene in cells susceptible to HIV-1 infection. The target cells for intracellular immunization strategies therefore are mainly peripheral T cells or hematopoietic stem cells. The gene product can either be a protein or an RNA that inhibits HIV-1 replication by interfering with crucial steps of the viral life cycle or by targeting a cellular factor required for virus replication. Efficient genetic protection of the HIV-1 target cell population, i.e. mainly $CD4^{+}$ T-helper cells, will deprive the virus of the possibility to produce progeny and is therefore expected to result in a drop of viral load and a regeneration of T cell counts. An additional antiviral effect can be achieved, if sufficient T-helper cell clones specific for HIV-1 antigens are protected against viral infection. These gene-protected $CD4^{+}$ T cells could support the immunologic control of viral replication, without risking infection facilitated by HIV-1 antigen activation. As mentioned above, previous studies have shown that HIV-specific T-helper cell clones, which are crucial for an effective immune control of HIV-1 replication, are preferentially infected by HIV and lost during the course of the disease (Douek et al., 2002).

3.1 Antiviral proteins

Various types of anti-HIV proteins have been developed over the past years. Dominant-negative forms of both, viral proteins and cellular proteins required for virus replication have been described. These dominant-negative mutant proteins antagonize the activity of their corresponding wild-type proteins and thus prevent viral replication. A transdominant form of the HIV-1 Rev protein, RevM10, has been extensively studied *in vitro* and *in vivo*. RevM10 prevents the export of genomic viral RNA from the nucleus and as a result inhibits production of progeny virus (Malim et al., 1989). In clinical trials genetic modification of $CD4^{+}$ T cells and $CD34^{+}$ hematopoietic stem cells with RevM10 has been shown to be safe and provide some selective survival advantage. However, no sustained absolute accumulation of gene-modified cells and accordingly no antiviral effect was observed (Morgan et al., 2005; Podsakoff et al., 2005; Ranga et al., 1998; Woffendin et al., 1996). Furthermore, transdominant mutants of HIV-1 Tat that prevent Tat transactiviation have been developed (Fraisier et al., 1998; Pearson et al., 1990), but were never tested in clinical trials. The same is true for transdominant forms of the HIV-1 proteins Gag (Trono et al., 1989) and Vif (Morgan et al., 1990; Vallanti et al., 2005).

Cellular proteins required for virus replication have also been targeted by dominant-negative mutants. Membrane expression of chemokine receptor 5 (CCR5), which acts as a co-receptor for HIV-1, has been blocked by transdominant negative CCR5 variants upon retroviral expression in human T cells (Luis Abad et al., 2003). Even though inhibition of virus replication was observed in the gene-modified cells, this concept was not pursued further. A truncated soluble form of the cell surface receptor CD4 (sCD4) has been described to protect T cells from entry of laboratory-adapted strains of HIV-1, however, inhibition was less efficient for primary virus isolates (Daar & Ho, 1991; Morgan et al., 1994; Morgan et al., 1990). In a clinical phase I study recombinant soluble CD4 was administered by continuous intravenous infusion to paediatric AIDS patients. Although the therapy was well tolerated, evidence of *in vivo* antiviral activity was not observed and consequently, sCD4 has never been investigated in gene therapy clinical trials (Husson et al., 1992).

Nevertheless, gene therapeutic strategies targeting early steps in the viral life cycle are expected to be the most promising therapeutics for HIV/AIDS, as discussed below. Protein-based inhibitors targeting the virus entry process are thought to be especially powerful tools as they can prevent infection of the cell. Our group has previously developed a membrane-anchored gp41-derived HIV-1 fusion inhibitor, maC46. This protein is expressed on the surface of T cells after transduction with retroviral or lentiviral vectors (Egelhofer et al., 2004; Hermann et al., 2009b; Perez et al., 2005). The protein binds to the HIV-1 gp41 heptad repeat 1 region thereby interfering with six-helix bundle formation during the viral and cellular membrane fusion process. MaC46 expressing T cells are almost completely protected from HIV-1 entry and have a strong selective survival advantage compared to unmodified cells *in vitro* and in mouse models of HIV-1 infection (Egelhofer et al., 2004; Hermann et al., 2009a; Kimpel et al., 2010). Likewise, maC46 has been shown to be one of the most potent anti-HIV gene products currently available (Kimpel et al., 2010). However, in a clinical trial with 10 HIV-1-infected patients with advanced disease and HAART failure, infusion of autologous $CD4^+$ T cells genetically modified to express maC46 did not achieve sustained success. Although a significant rise in overall $CD4^+$ T cell counts was observed in this study, the gene-protected cells did not accumulate over time and consequently, viral loads were not affected (van Lunzen et al., 2007). Recently, we described a secreted version of the fusion inhibitory C46 molecule. This '*in vivo* secreted antiviral entry inhibitor' (iSAVE) showed promising anti-HIV activity *in vitro* and has the potential to confer an overall antiviral effect *in vivo* despite low levels of gene marking (Egerer et al., 2011).

A different protein-based approach for HIV-1 gene therapy uses antibodies that bind and inactivate proteins and enzymes required for virus replication. Antibodies can be expressed within gene-modified cells as single-chain fragments (scFv), so-called intrabodies, or they can be secreted into the supernatant as neutralizing antibodies. Various intrabodies against HIV-1 proteins including Tat, Vif, Reverse Transcriptase and Integrase have been shown to inhibit virus replication in gene-modified cells *in vitro* (Goncalves et al., 2002; Kitamura et al., 1999; Levy-Mintz et al., 1996; Mhashilkar et al., 1995; Shaheen et al., 1996). Moreover, intrabodies against the viral co-receptors CXCR4 and CCR5 have been designed that retain these proteins in the ER (BouHamdan et al., 2001; Cordelier et al., 2004; Swan et al., 2006). Although these approaches efficiently inhibited HIV-1 replication in cell culture systems, intrabody techniques have not been further evaluated *in vivo*. The secreted version of the broadly neutralizing anti-gp41 monoclonal antibody 2F5 has been analyzed in a humanized mouse model of HIV-1 infection (Sanhadji et al., 2000). In this study, gene-modified cell lines expressing the antibody were implanted as neo-organs into immunodeficient mice repopulated with human $CD4^+$ T cells. The neo-organs engrafted in the peritoneum and permitted continuous secretion of the antibody. Upon infection of the mice with HIV-1, viral loads were greatly reduced compared to control animals. However, due to safety problems, the implantation of neo-organs is not an option for treatment of patients. Recently, Joseph and colleagues reported the secretion of therapeutic concentrations of the broadly neutralizing anti-gp120 antibody 2G12 in humanized mice. Here, immunodeficient mice were transplanted with human hematopoietic stem cells that had previously been modified with a lentiviral vector encoding 2G12. The transduced stem cells differentiated into human

progeny cells that secreted the functional antibody into the serum. This genetic immunization clearly reduced viral burden upon HIV-1 infection (Joseph et al., 2010).
Another strategy described by Sarkar et al. involves the expression of a modified version of the Cre recombinase (termed Tre) in HIV-1 infected cells. This recombinase has been engineered in a directed evolution approach to recombine a sequence present in the HIV-1 LTRs resulting in site-specific excision of the integrated provirus from an HIV-1 infected host cell genome (Sarkar et al., 2007). Even though proof-of-concept was provided *in vitro*, this approach is far from clinical application as the Tre recombinase is specific for one exclusive LTR sequence and does not recognize the LTRs of other virus strains.
Finally, zinc finger nucleases (ZFNs) are a novel tool in protein-based HIV-1 gene therapy. ZFNs are artificial fusion proteins composed of a DNA-binding and a DNA-cleavage domain. They can be engineered to bind any desired genome sequence and induce double-strand breaks in the targeted DNA. Repair of the damaged DNA is associated with the introduction of high-frequency deletions and insertions at the site of cleavage. Individuals with a naturally occurring 32 bp deletion mutant of the CCR5 receptor (CCR5Δ32) are perfectly healthy, but resistant to infection with R5-tropic strains of HIV-1 (Huang et al., 1996; Samson et al., 1996). Consequently, disruption of the CCR5 locus using ZFNs is not expected to alter immune functions, making it an ideal target for ZFN-based gene therapy. CCR5-specific ZFNs have been studied *in vitro* and in animal models and were shown to render the treated cells resistant to HIV-1 infection (Holt et al., 2010; Perez et al., 2008). Currently three clinical trials are recruiting patients to test this promising approach *in vivo* (www.ClinicalTrials.gov; identifier: NCT01044654, NCT01252641 and NCT00842634).

3.2 Antiviral RNAs

Antiviral RNAs for intracellular immunization can be grouped into four major categories: RNA interference (RNAi), ribozymes, anti-sense RNAs and RNA decoys. Several RNAi-based gene therapy regimens for treatment of HIV-1 infection have proven to be effective in blocking viral replication by selective degradation of either viral RNAs or mRNAs of host factors that are essential for HIV-1 replication. Basically all HIV-1 RNAs have been successfully downregulated by RNAi *in vitro* (Chang et al., 2005; Coburn & Cullen, 2002; Jacque et al., 2002; N. S. Lee et al., 2002; Novina et al., 2002). However, systemic delivery of siRNAs to the relevant cell types *in vivo* is difficult. Kumar and colleagues administered antiviral siRNAs conjugated to a T cell-specific single-chain antibody that undergoes internalization upon binding to T cell surface receptors to humanized mice. This approach allowed targeted delivery of the siRNAs to T cells, which resulted in effective virus inhibition and preserved $CD4^+$ T cell numbers (Kumar et al., 2008). An alternative to the regular injection of exogenous siRNAs is the expression of shRNAs directly in the HIV-1 target cells, but achieving stable transgene expression in the gene-modified cells is a challenge. Yet, constant endogenous expression would be required to obtain efficient suppression of HIV-1 replication and prevent viral escape mutants. At the same time, expression levels have to be tightly regulated in order to avoid cellular toxicity, as saturation of the cellular small RNA-processing pathway due to overexpression of shRNAs can lead to downregulation of cellular microRNAs (miRNAs) and cause severe toxicity (Grimm et al., 2006). Insertion of shRNAs into a natural miRNA backbone has been shown to reduce such toxic effects (McBride et al., 2008).
The high mutation rate of HIV-1 is an additional challenge in developing RNAi-based therapeutics, as a single point mutation within the targeted HIV-1 RNA sequence can

abolish function of small RNAs and escape mutants emerge rapidly (Boden et al., 2003; Das et al., 2004; Sabariegos et al., 2006). This problem can be partly overcome by using a combination of small RNAs targeting several conserved regions of the viral genome and ideally expressed from a single therapeutic vector (ter Brake et al., 2006). Alternatively, cellular genes required for virus replication can be targeted, including CD4, CXCR4, CCR5, nuclear factor κB, or LEDGF/p75, which all have been shown to be susceptible to RNAi silencing, thereby blocking viral entry or replication (Anderson & Akkina, 2005; Cordelier et al., 2003; Novina et al., 2002; Surabhi & Gaynor, 2002; Vandekerckhove et al., 2006). The CCR5 receptor is a particularly promising target, as disruption of the CCR5 gene does not alter immune functions (Huang et al., 1996; Samson et al., 1996). A highly potent and non-cytotoxic siRNA directed against CCR5 has been developed by the group of Irvin Chen. Stable long-term expression of the siRNA and silencing of the CCR5 gene was observed after transplantation of gene-modified $CD34^+$ hematopoietic progenitor cells in non-human primates. Gene-modified cells isolated from the animals were resistant to simian immunodeficiency virus infection *ex vivo* (An et al., 2007; Liang et al., 2010). The only RNAi approach that has been examined in patients so far is a tat/rev specific short hairpin RNA, which was tested in combination with a ribozyme targeting CCR5 and a TAR decoy in four patients receiving $CD34^+$ hematopoietic progenitor cell transplantation due to AIDS-related lymphoma. In this recently reported clinical trial, stable, but low-level expression of the antiviral RNAs from gene-modified cells was observed for up to 24 months; however, there were no major effects on viral load (DiGiusto et al., 2010).

Ribozymes are anti-sense RNA molecules with enzymatic activity that have been designed to target and site-specifically cleave essential viral RNAs or cellular mRNAs leading to gene silencing. Many ribozyme-based strategies for treatment of HIV-1 infection have been developed and show promising antiviral activity *in vitro* (Hotchkiss et al., 2004; Sarver et al., 1990; Zhou et al., 1994). Three ribozymes directed against HIV-1 tat/vrp (Amado et al., 2004; Macpherson et al., 2005; Mitsuyasu et al., 2009), HIV-1 rev/tat (Michienzi et al., 2003) and the viral U5 leader region (Wong-Staal et al., 1998) have already been tested in separate clinical trials. The gene transfer was proven to be safe in all studies, but none showed significant antiviral efficacy. As mentioned above, a CCR5-specific ribozyme has recently been analyzed in the clinic in combination with two other types of anti-HIV RNAs, but did not have a major influence on HIV-1 replication (DiGiusto et al., 2010).

Antisense RNAs are short or long single-stranded RNA molecules binding to complementary HIV-1 mRNAs resulting in the formation of non-functional duplexes. Antisense molecules directed against the HIV-1 trans-activation response element (TAR) and the viral envelope RNA have been developed (Humeau et al., 2004; Lu et al., 2004; Vickers et al., 1991). The conditionally replicating lentiviral vector VRX496™ encodes a long antisense gene against the HIV-1 envelope. In clinical trials patients received autologous $CD4^+$ T cells transduced with VRX496™. A stabilization of viral load and slightly increased $CD4^+$ T cell counts were observed, the significance of these results, however, remains unclear (Levine et al., 2006).

In contrast to the antiviral RNA molecules described above, RNA decoys do not attack the HIV-1 RNA. Instead, these small RNA fragments, which are derived from cis-acting elements in the viral genome, competitively bind and sequester viral proteins, thereby interfering with HIV-1 replication. Anti-HIV decoys are mainly based on the HIV-1 regulatory sequences TAR and Rev-responsive-element (RRE), which are bound by the two HIV-1 regulatory proteins Tat and Rev, respectively. The TAR element is a sequence contained in the 5′ region of all HIV-1 mRNAs, which forms a stable stem-loop structure (Baudin et al., 1993; Muesing et al., 1987). Binding of the HIV-1 Tat (trans-activator) protein to the TAR element mediates increased viral gene expression (Keen et al., 1996); moreover, the TAR region is required for initiation of reverse transcription (Harrich et al., 1996). Disruption of the Tat/TAR interaction by TAR decoy RNA was shown to effectively prevent HIV-1 replication *in vitro* (Sullenger et al., 1990, 1991). A combination of three antiviral RNAs including a TAR decoy was successfully tested in humanized mouse models of HIV-1 infection (Anderson et al., 2007) and, as mentioned above, was shown to be safe in a clinical trial, although only minor effects on HIV-1 infection could be observed (DiGiusto et al., 2010). Interaction of the viral Rev protein with the RRE is critically required for transport of the unspliced genomic viral mRNA to the cytoplasm (Olsen et al., 1990). RRE decoys provide strong inhibition of HIV-1 replication by blocking the nuclear export of genomic HIV-1 RNA (T. C. Lee et al., 1992; Michienzi et al., 2006). Genetic modification of CD34$^+$ hematopoietic stem cells by retroviral transfer of an RRE decoy gene followed by infusion of the gene-modified cells, was shown to be safe in a clinical trial with paediatric AIDS patients. However, transduction and engraftment levels were very low and no antiviral effect was observed (Kohn et al., 1999).

3.3 The mode of action: Classification of antiviral genes

The impact of gene-modified cells on systemic HIV-1 kinetics depends critically on the stage of the viral replication cycle at which the inhibition occurs. The antiviral genes can accordingly be grouped into three classes, depending on their effect on the viral life cycle (von Laer et al., 2006). Class I genes inhibit the first steps of the replication cycle prior to integration of the proviral DNA into the host cell genome and thus prevent infection of the cell. Hence, class I includes genes encoding entry inhibitors, as well as inhibitors of reverse transcription and integration. Class II genes have no effect on early steps of the viral replication cycle, but prevent the expression of viral RNA or proteins. Thus, they inhibit the production of infectious virus progeny and the viral cytopathic effect, however, integration of the proviral genome into the host cell chromosomes is not hindered. Cells expressing a class II gene and infected with HIV-1 resemble latently infected cells and according to computer simulations accumulate with time, counteracting the antiviral effect (von Laer et al., 2006). Furthermore, reverse transcription, which can give rise to resistant virus variants, is not inhibited by class II genes. Class III genes interfere with late steps in the viral life cycle such as virion assembly and budding. Consequently, they neither protect the infected cell from recognition by the immune system, as viral protein production is not inhibited, nor from the viral cytopathic effect. Therefore, class III genes alone are not expected to have an overall antiviral effect unless high percentages of cells are genetically modified.

Mathematical modelling predicts that only genes inhibiting early steps in the viral replication cycle provide a selective advantage strong enough to allow for the selection and accumulation of the gene modified cells (Lund et al., 1997; von Laer et al., 2006). Consequently, class I genes are the most promising candidates for successful intracellular immunization strategies. The group of Warner Greene recently found that in *ex vivo* cultures of human tonsils infected with HIV-1 the vast majority of CD4$^+$ T cells died due to non-productive abortive infection. In these non-permissive cells DNA reverse transcription intermediates elicited proapoptotic responses resulting in release of proinflammatory cytokines and caspase-mediated cell death (Doitsh et al., 2010). Inhibition of HIV-1 entry or early steps of reverse transcription could protect the cells from these fatal effects, indicating that very early inhibitors are even more favorable, as they can prevent the massive "bystander" killing observed in HIV-1 infection. However, combination of several antiviral genes, targeting different steps in the viral life cycle might synergize most efficiently and could be the only way to achieve sustained suppression of HIV-1 replication.

3.4 Selective survival advantage and bystander effect

The major drawback of intracellular immunization approaches is the huge number of HIV-1 target cells in the human body (> 10^{11}) that cannot be genetically modified with the available technologies. The frequencies of gene-modified $CD4^+$ T cells achieved *in vivo*, whether by T cell or stem cell targeting, have been disappointingly low, in the range of 0,01% to 1%, or less (Amado et al., 2004; Levine et al., 2006; Macpherson et al., 2005; Morgan et al., 2005; van Lunzen et al., 2007). A significant impact of these few genetically HIV-resistant cells is neither expected on overall HIV-1 infection dynamics nor on immune reconstitution. However, if the gene-protected cells are able to proliferate and preferentially survive compared with unmodified cells, they could accumulate with time and progressively repopulate the immune system (Lund et al., 1997; von Laer et al., 2006). A number of gene products that have been developed could theoretically mediate such a selective survival advantage of the transduced cells as they have been shown to efficiently suppress virus replication and protect the cells from the viral cytopathic effect *in vitro*. However, selective accumulation of gene-protected cells has never been observed in clinical trials so far. In a comparative study, we recently evaluated three intracellular immunization strategies that had previously been used in the clinic, with respect to antiviral activity and survival advantage (Kimpel et al., 2010): (1) the viral entry inhibitor maC46 (class I gene); (2) an HIV-1 tat/rev-specific small hairpin (sh) RNA (class II gene); and (3) an RNA antisense gene specific for the HIV-1 envelope (class II gene). We found robust inhibition of HIV-1 replication with the fusion inhibitor maC46 and the antisense envelope inhibitor. Interestingly, and importantly, a survival advantage was merely demonstrated for cells expressing the maC46 fusion inhibitor both *in vitro* and *in vivo* in a humanized xenotransplant mouse model (Kimpel et al., 2010). This finding confirms *in silico* predictions stating that only class I genes can confer a sufficient selective advantage to allow preferential survival and accumulation of gene-protected, non-infected cells *in vivo* (von Laer et al., 2006). However, even this highly active fusion inhibitor failed to show a clear accumulation of gene-protected cells to therapeutic levels in a previous clinical trial in 10 AIDS patients (van Lunzen et al., 2007). These data show that efficient engraftment and proliferation of the gene-protected cells remain a major challenge in gene therapy for HIV-1 infection.

Yet, such a strong selection and accumulation may not be required for a secreted antiviral gene product. Secreted antiviral proteins or peptides are expected to produce a bystander effect on unmodified neighboring cells, thereby suppressing virus replication and protecting the overall T cell pool even at low levels of gene modification. Such a bystander effect can only be conferred by antiviral proteins, but not by RNAs, as secretion is limited to proteins and peptides. However, the number of reports on secreted antiviral proteins in HIV-1 gene therapy is still very limited. Examples are neutralizing antibodies (Sanhadji et al., 2000), truncated soluble CD4 (Morgan et al., 1994; Morgan et al., 1990) and interferon β (Gay et al., 2004). We have recently reported the generation of an *in vivo* secreted antiviral entry inhibitor (iSAVE), which exerted a strong bystander effect in cell culture (Egerer et al., 2011). Lymphatic tissue is the major site of HIV-1 replication and thus T or B cells could be an ideal target cell for gene therapy approaches based on secreted gene products. Secretion of antiviral proteins directly in the lymphoid tissues is likely to lead to high and stable local peptide concentrations and to substantially suppress virus replication. On the other hand, secreted antiviral gene products no longer depend on expression in HIV-1 target cells, but instead several other cell types could serve as producer cells in the body. This facilitates the development of direct *in vivo* gene transfer approaches (e.g. by the use of AAV-vectors), making gene therapy less complex and practicable also for treatment of patients in the developing world. Furthermore, such strategies have the potential for application as a gene transfer vaccine in a prophylactic setting. In this regard, a secreted antiviral gene product could for instance be used as a genetic topical microbicide that aims at the prevention of HIV-1 mucosal transmission. High-level secretion of the antiviral molecules from gene-modified target cells in the vagina or rectum has the potential to confer local sterilizing immunity, thus preventing HIV-1 genital transmission.

3.5 Immunogenicity of the antiviral gene product

Gene therapeutic strategies based on the expression of antiviral proteins are limited by the potential immunogenicity of the antiviral gene product, which can severely impair survival of the transduced cells. Antiviral RNAs have an advantage here, as they generally lack immunogenicity. Also, natural or only slightly altered variants of human proteins are not expected to mount significant immune responses. However, many antiviral proteins are non-self and bear the risk of eliciting a cellular immune response. Thus, to prevent selective deletion of the gene-modified cells by transgene-specific CTLs, it is necessary to minimize or eliminate immunogenicity of the antiviral gene product. The fusion of a Glycine-Alanine repeat derived from the Epstein-Barr virus nuclear antigen 1 (EBNA-1) to immunogenic proteins, such as transdominant HIV-1 Gag, has been shown to significantly reduce immunogenicity and prolong survival of transduced cells *in vivo* (Hammer et al., 2008). The Glycine-Alanine repeat protects the fusion protein from proteasomal degradation and prevents subsequent presentation of potentially immunogenic peptides on MHC class I molecules (Levitskaya et al., 1997). This frustrates the induction of CTLs directed against the transgene product and conceals it from CTL-mediated immune attack.

Another possibility to facilitate immune-evasion, which is feasible for small antiviral peptides only, is the generation of peptides which are devoid of MHC class I epitopes. Our group recently developed antiviral C peptides with potentially reduced immunogenicity, by mutating *in silico*-predicted immunodominant CTL epitopes within the peptide sequence. The mutated peptides retained excellent anti-HIV activity, while no immune responses could be detected in ELIspot assays (unpublished data).

3.6 The target cell for intracellular immunization strategies

Target cells for intracellular immunization are usually cells that can become infected with HIV-1 (mainly CD4$^+$ T cells) or their progenitors (hematopoietic stem cells). For gene therapeutic approaches based on secreted antiviral molecules, the modification of non-HIV-target cells is also feasible. So far, mature T cells and hematopoietic stem cells have been used in clinical trials. Advantages and disadvantages of both cell types are summarized in Table 1. Both have in common that they are relatively easy to obtain, and there are protocols for efficient *ex vivo* cultivation and transduction available. Gene modification of HSC has greater therapeutic potential, as it could restore a normal T cell repertoire, allow regeneration of HIV-specific T-helper cells and also protect monocytes/macrophages. However, current stem-cell based therapies are associated with greater risks and toxicity.

Target cell	T cell	HSC
Easy to obtain	++	+
Conditioning required	-	+
Cell dose	>10^{10}	10^8-10^9
Regeneration of T cell repertoire	-	+
Protection of all HIV-1 target cells	-	+
Insertional mutagenesis	Limited	+

Table 1. The target cell: T cells versus hematopoietic stem cells (HSC).

4. Vector systems for gene transfer

The choice of the vector system may have a major impact on the efficacy of HIV-1 gene therapy approaches. There is no ideal vector suitable for all purposes, but the pros and cons have to be balanced for each application. Table 2 summarizes advantages and disadvantages of several vector systems commonly used for gene transfer.

Vector type	Application	Titer	Packaging capacity	Inte-gration	Immuno-genicity	Clinical trials
Adenoviral	*ex vivo* + *in vivo*	10^{13} VP/ml	up to 36 kb	-	++	+
AAV	*in vivo*	10^{13} VP/ml	3-5 kb	only with Rep	+	+
Gamma-retroviral	*ex vivo*	10^5-10^7 TU/ml	8-10 kb	+	-	+
Lentiviral	*ex vivo*	10^7 TU/ml (10^9-10^{10} TU/ml)*	up to 10 kb	+	-	+
SV-40	*ex vivo*	10^{12} VP/ml	up to 5 kb	+	-	-
Foamyviral	*ex vivo*	10^5-10^6 TU/ml (10^7 TU/ml)*	>9 kb	+	-	-

Table 2. Vector systems for gene transfer in HIV-1 gene therapy.
AAV, Adeno-Associated Virus; kb, kilo bases; SV-40, Simian Virus-40; TU, transducing units; VP, vector particles; * after concentration.

Basic questions to be asked are, whether *ex vivo* or *in vivo* gene transfer is preferred and if long-term expression of the gene product is required. To our knowledge, a vector system that allows efficient direct *in vivo* gene transfer specifically into $CD4^+$ T cells or HSC has not been developed so far. Therefore, approaches based on modification of these cell types (arming of T cells with TCRs or CARs, most intracellular immunizations) always rely on *ex vivo* gene transfer. In contrast, genes encoding secreted antiviral molecules may also be delivered to distinct production sites (e.g. liver, muscle) directly *in vivo* using adenovirus (Ad) or adeno-associated virus (AAV)-derived vectors. The second basic question deals with the long-term-expression of the transferred antiviral gene. Strategies involving arming of T cells with antigen-specific receptors and intracellular immunization require stable and long-lasting production of the antiviral molecules in proliferating cells (T cells or HSC). Consequently, for such approaches, integrating vectors are favorable. These include SV-40 vectors and vectors derived from retroviruses. Stable expression of secreted gene products from slowly dividing cells like liver or muscle cells may also be achieved using non-integrating vectors like adenoviral or AAV vectors.

4.1 Non-integrating viral vectors

The only vectors systems that currently allow direct *in vivo* gene transfer are non-integrating viral vectors. As their genome is not stably incorporated into the host cell chromosomes, these vectors have an improved safety profile compared to integrating vectors. For a direct *in vivo* application of integrating vectors, efficient systems for targeted vector delivery would be required, which are not yet available for use in man. Despite the lack of integration, non-integrating vector systems still allow sustained long-term transgene expression, if cells or tissues with a slow turnover are targeted, where the vector genome can stably persist. Moreover, non-integrating vectors can also be used to deliver zinc finger nucleases, which require only transient expression, to diving cells. A number of non-integrating viral vectors have been evaluated for gene transfer. Currently, adenoviral vectors and vectors derived from the adeno-associated virus are in the focus of interest. Accordingly, Ad vectors are currently used in the above mentioned clinical trials to deliver CCR5-specific zinc finger nucleases to T cells *ex vivo*.

Recombinant adenoviral vectors have been utilized as a gene transfer and vaccine platform for a long time. Ad vectors provide a huge packaging capacity (36 kb), allowing the transfer also of multiple therapeutic genes. Moreover, high-titer production is possible, facilitating direct *in vivo* application with high transduction efficacies. The major obstacle of adenoviral vectors is pre-existing immunity in the general human population. Vector-mediated immune responses cause rapid clearance of Ad vectors, moreover, severe side effects have been observed. This can be partly overcome by using engineered adenovirus serotypes (Dharmapuri et al., 2009). Moreover, production of Ad vectors is prone to contamination with replication competent adenovirus, which complicates clinical grade vector production.

AAV is a non-pathogenic virus that belongs to the family of Parvoviridae. AAV-derived vectors have recently gained particular interest as gene transfer vehicles due to their apathogenicity and very low immunogenicity. Moreover, they can be used for direct *in vivo* gene delivery to both dividing and non-dividing cells. AAV can infect a variety of cell types *in vivo* and different serotypes of AAV have been shown to have varying preferences in their target cell type of choice (Chao et al., 2000; Halbert et al., 2000). However, AAV variants with a preference for T cells or hematopoietic stem cells have not been described. In the absence of the viral Rep protein, AAV vectors do not integrate into the host cell genome, but are maintained in episomal form in the nucleus. This allows very stable transgene expression without causing genotoxicity. The major disadvantage of AAV vectors is their small packaging capacity. In addition, vector production used to be laborious in the past and large-scale manufacturing for clinical trials was complicated. However, novel production systems facilitate faster and simpler high-titer production of AAV vectors in scaleable processes (Clement et al., 2009; Lock et al., 2010).

4.2 Integrating viral vectors

Vectors derived from gamma-retroviruses (mostly murine leukaemia virus) and lentiviruses (HIV-1) have been used in numerous clinical trials, including *ex vivo* gene transfer trials for HIV-1 infection (DiGiusto et al., 2010; van Lunzen et al., 2007). Replication incompetent viral vectors are made from these viruses by deletion of all genes encoding enzymes and structural proteins (Gag, Pol, Env) from the viral genome. These genes have to be added *in trans* to produce infectious, but replication incompetent, vector particles. The tropism of the vector particles can be altered by modification of the envelope glycoprotein or by pseudotyping with the envelope protein from a different virus (Frecha et al., 2008; Funke et al., 2008). A major difference between gamma-retroviral and lentiviral vectors is that lentiviruses can infect dividing as well as non-dividing cells. In contrast, gamma-retroviruses can only transduce dividing cells, as they rely on the collapse of the nuclear membrane during mitosis to enter the nucleus (Roe et al., 1993). Lentiviral transduction protocols therefore usually require a shorter period of pre-activation of the cells. As prolonged *in vitro* culture is associated with differentiation and a loss of *in vivo* repopulation potential, especially for HSC, lentiviral vectors have an advantage here. However, large-scale production of lentiviral vectors is more difficult than gamma-retroviral vector production due to a lack of stable packaging cell lines.

Both, gamma-retroviral and lentiviral vectors integrate randomly into the host cell genome. While gamma-retroviruses usually integrate near transcriptional start sites, lentiviruses have a preference for transcribed regions (Mitchell et al., 2004). As a consequence, transduction with these vectors is always associated with a risk of transformation due to insertional mutagenesis. Indeed, severe side effects caused by vector integration have been reported in gene therapy clinical trials (Hacein-Bey-Abina et al., 2008; Howe et al., 2008). Experiments in animal models showed that vector genotoxicity is higher for transduction of hematopoietic stem cells than for mature T cells (Newrzela et al., 2008) and lower for self inactivating (SIN) vectors compared to conventional long terminal repeat (LTR)-driven vectors (Modlich et al., 2009). SIN vectors have deletions in the promotor and enhancer elements of the 3'LTR, thereby reducing the genotoxic risks, as transactivation of neighboring protooncogenes is less likely. In these vectors, expression of the transgene cassette is driven from an internal promoter.

Foamyviruses also belong to the family of retroviruses. Foamyviral vectors are generated by deleting enzymes and structural genes from the viral genome and adding these *in trans* during vector production (Rethwilm, 2007). Foamyvirus-derived vectors efficiently transduce resting cells, which makes them an ideal tool to transduce hematopoietic stem cells *ex vivo* (Hirata et al., 1996; Leurs et al., 2003). However, just like SV-40 vectors, foamyviral vectors have not yet been tested in clinical trials.

Simian virus-40 (SV-40) belongs to the family of Polyomaviridae. It has been one of the first viruses used as a gene transfer vehicle (Gething & Sambrook, 1981). For the construction of gene transfer vectors, all coding sequences except the origin of replication and the packaging signal can be deleted from wild type SV-40 (Strayer et al., 2002). The resulting vectors efficiently transduce hematopoietic stem cells and lymphocytes *in vitro*, but have never been tested in clinical trials (Strayer et al., 2005).

4.3 Targeted integration

Past clinical trials have shown that random integration of a transgene delivered by an integrating vector bears the risk of severe side effects due to insertional mutagenesis.

Targeted integration of transgenes into the host cell genome is therefore expected to massively increase safety. The CCR5 locus is considered to be a safe harbor for transgene integration, as a naturally occurring deletion of 32 bp in the coding sequence for CCR5 causes no clinical symptoms. Moreover, this deletion is associated with a reduced susceptibility for HIV-1 infection (Huang et al., 1996; Samson et al., 1996). Therefore, targeted integration of an anti-HIV transgene into the CCR5 locus could even provide an additional antiviral effect, due to disruption of the CCR5 gene. Zinc finger nucleases binding to CCR5 have been used *in vitro* and in animal models to destroy the CCR5 locus, rendering the treated cells resistant to HIV-1 infection (Holt et al., 2010; Perez et al., 2008). A combination of this approach with targeted integration of antiviral genes holds especially great promise. For such a strategy a donor DNA encoding the desired antiviral gene and containing sequences homologous to the target site has to be present in the cells during the repair of ZFN-induced double-strand breaks by cellular enzymes. This results in the incorporation of the foreign DNA into the targeted region of the host genome by non-homologous end joining mediated by the cellular DNA repair machinery (Cathomen & Joung, 2008). Such approaches require only transient expression of the zinc finger nuclease and the transgene to achieve stable integration into the host cell genome, which allows use of non-integrating vector systems for gene transfer.

As an alternative to zinc finger nucleases, AAV vectors that contain the viral Rep protein in *cis* or in *trans* can also be used for targeted integration, as in the presence of Rep, AAV vectors target their genome preferentially to a locus on the human chromosome 19, termed AAVS1, without causing any apparent adverse effects (Surosky et al., 1997). As the CCR5 locus, AAVS1 is thus considered a safe harbor for vector integration.

5. Conclusions

Gene therapeutic approaches for the treatment and possibly prevention of HIV-1 infection hold considerable promise. Although the final breakthrough has not yet been achieved in clinical trials, there has been substantial progress over the last years and future developments might leverage this technology. The major reason for the limited efficacy seen in all HIV-1 gene therapy clinical trials up to now has been the insufficient level of gene modification. It will therefore be particularly important to develop optimized therapeutic regimen and gene transfer technologies that allow therapeutically effective engraftment levels of functional, gene modified cells. Efficient protection of $CD4^+$ T cells could possibly be achieved by using a combination of antiviral genes targeting different steps of the viral life cycle, conferring a substantial *in vivo* selective survival advantage and ideally also a therapeutic bystander effect on unmodified cells. This review describes the potent gene therapeutic tools that have been developed in the past years and it will be exciting to see if these can be integrated into an effective treatment regimen in the near future.

6. References

Amado, R. G.; Mitsuyasu, R. T.; Rosenblatt, J. D.; Ngok, F. K.; Bakker, A.; Cole, S.; Chorn, N.; Lin, L. S.; Bristol, G.; Boyd, M. P.; MacPherson, J. L.; Fanning, G. C.; Todd, A. V.; Ely, J. A.; Zack, J. A. & Symonds, G. P. (2004). Anti-human immunodeficiency virus hematopoietic progenitor cell-delivered ribozyme in a phase I study: myeloid and lymphoid reconstitution in human immunodeficiency virus type-1-infected patients, *Hum Gene Ther*, Vol.15, No.3, pp. 251-262

An, D. S.; Donahue, R. E.; Kamata, M.; Poon, B.; Metzger, M.; Mao, S. H.; Bonifacino, A.; Krouse, A. E.; Darlix, J. L.; Baltimore, D.; Qin, F. X. & Chen, I. S. (2007). Stable reduction of CCR5 by RNAi through hematopoietic stem cell transplant in non-human primates, *Proc Natl Acad Sci U S A*, Vol.104, No.32, pp. 13110-13115

Anderson, J. & Akkina, R. (2005). CXCR4 and CCR5 shRNA transgenic CD34+ cell derived macrophages are functionally normal and resist HIV-1 infection, *Retrovirology*, Vol.2, pp. 53

Anderson, J.; Li, M. J.; Palmer, B.; Remling, L.; Li, S.; Yam, P.; Yee, J. K.; Rossi, J.; Zaia, J. & Akkina, R. (2007). Safety and efficacy of a lentiviral vector containing three anti-HIV genes--CCR5 ribozyme, tat-rev siRNA, and TAR decoy--in SCID-hu mouse-derived T cells, *Mol Ther*, Vol.15, No.6, pp. 1182-1188

Baltimore, D. (1988). Gene therapy. Intracellular immunization, *Nature*, Vol.335, No.6189, pp. 395-396

Baudin, F.; Marquet, R.; Isel, C.; Darlix, J. L.; Ehresmann, B. & Ehresmann, C. (1993). Functional sites in the 5' region of human immunodeficiency virus type 1 RNA form defined structural domains, *J Mol Biol*, Vol.229, No.2, pp. 382-397

Boden, D.; Pusch, O.; Lee, F.; Tucker, L. & Ramratnam, B. (2003). Human immunodeficiency virus type 1 escape from RNA interference, *J Virol*, Vol.77, No.21, pp. 11531-11535

Borrow, P.; Lewicki, H.; Hahn, B. H.; Shaw, G. M. & Oldstone, M. B. (1994). Virus-specific CD8+ cytotoxic T-lymphocyte activity associated with control of viremia in primary human immunodeficiency virus type 1 infection, *J Virol*, Vol.68, No.9, pp. 6103-6110

BouHamdan, M.; Strayer, D. S.; Wei, D.; Mukhtar, M.; Duan, L. X.; Hoxie, J. & Pomerantz, R. J. (2001). Inhibition of HIV-1 infection by down-regulation of the CXCR4 co-receptor using an intracellular single chain variable fragment against CXCR4, *Gene Ther*, Vol.8, No.5, pp. 408-418

Brinkman, K.; Smeitink, J. A.; Romijn, J. A. & Reiss, P. (1999). Mitochondrial toxicity induced by nucleoside-analogue reverse-transcriptase inhibitors is a key factor in the pathogenesis of antiretroviral-therapy-related lipodystrophy, *Lancet*, Vol.354, No.9184, pp. 1112-1115

Brodie, S. J.; Lewinsohn, D. A.; Patterson, B. K.; Jiyamapa, D.; Krieger, J.; Corey, L.; Greenberg, P. D. & Riddell, S. R. (1999). In vivo migration and function of transferred HIV-1-specific cytotoxic T cells, *Nat Med*, Vol.5, No.1, pp. 34-41

Brodie, S. J.; Patterson, B. K.; Lewinsohn, D. A.; Diem, K.; Spach, D.; Greenberg, P. D.; Riddell, S. R. & Corey, L. (2000). HIV-specific cytotoxic T lymphocytes traffic to lymph nodes and localize at sites of HIV replication and cell death, *J Clin Invest*, Vol.105, No.10, pp. 1407-1417

Cathomen, T. & Joung, J. K. (2008). Zinc-finger nucleases: the next generation emerges, *Mol Ther*, Vol.16, No.7, pp. 1200-1207

Chang, L. J.; Liu, X. & He, J. (2005). Lentiviral siRNAs targeting multiple highly conserved RNA sequences of human immunodeficiency virus type 1, *Gene Ther*, Vol.12, No.14, pp. 1133-1144

Chao, H.; Liu, Y.; Rabinowitz, J.; Li, C.; Samulski, R. J. & Walsh, C. E. (2000). Several log increase in therapeutic transgene delivery by distinct adeno-associated viral serotype vectors, *Mol Ther*, Vol.2, No.6, pp. 619-623

Clement, N.; Knop, D. R. & Byrne, B. J. (2009). Large-scale adeno-associated viral vector production using a herpesvirus-based system enables manufacturing for clinical studies, *Hum Gene Ther*, Vol.20, No.8, pp. 796-806

Coburn, G. A. & Cullen, B. R. (2002). Potent and specific inhibition of human immunodeficiency virus type 1 replication by RNA interference, *J Virol*, Vol.76, No.18, pp. 9225-9231

Cordelier, P.; Morse, B. & Strayer, D. S. (2003). Targeting CCR5 with siRNAs: using recombinant SV40-derived vectors to protect macrophages and microglia from R5-tropic HIV, *Oligonucleotides*, Vol.13, No.5, pp. 281-294

Cordelier, P.; Kulkowsky, J. W.; Ko, C.; Matskevitch, A. A.; McKee, H. J.; Rossi, J. J.; Bouhamdan, M.; Pomerantz, R. J.; Kari, G. & Strayer, D. S. (2004). Protecting from R5-tropic HIV: individual and combined effectiveness of a hammerhead ribozyme and a single-chain Fv antibody that targets CCR5, *Gene Ther*, Vol.11, No.22, pp. 1627-1637

Daar, E. S. & Ho, D. D. (1991). Relative resistance of primary HIV-1 isolates to neutralization by soluble CD4, *Am J Med*, Vol.90, No.4A, pp. 22S-26S

Das, A. T.; Brummelkamp, T. R.; Westerhout, E. M.; Vink, M.; Madiredjo, M.; Bernards, R. & Berkhout, B. (2004). Human immunodeficiency virus type 1 escapes from RNA interference-mediated inhibition, *J Virol*, Vol.78, No.5, pp. 2601-2605

Deeks, S. G.; Wagner, B.; Anton, P. A.; Mitsuyasu, R. T.; Scadden, D. T.; Huang, C.; Macken, C.; Richman, D. D.; Christopherson, C.; June, C. H.; Lazar, R.; Broad, D. F.; Jalali, S. & Hege, K. M. (2002). A phase II randomized study of HIV-specific T-cell gene therapy in subjects with undetectable plasma viremia on combination antiretroviral therapy, *Mol Ther*, Vol.5, No.6, pp. 788-797

Demoustier, A.; Gubler, B.; Lambotte, O.; de Goer, M. G.; Wallon, C.; Goujard, C.; Delfraissy, J. F. & Taoufik, Y. (2002). In patients on prolonged HAART, a significant pool of HIV infected CD4 T cells are HIV-specific, *Aids*, Vol.16, No.13, pp. 1749-1754

Dharmapuri, S.; Peruzzi, D. & Aurisicchio, L. (2009). Engineered adenovirus serotypes for overcoming anti-vector immunity, *Expert Opin Biol Ther*, Vol.9, No.10, pp. 1279-1287

DiGiusto, D. L.; Krishnan, A.; Li, L.; Li, H.; Li, S.; Rao, A.; Mi, S.; Yam, P.; Stinson, S.; Kalos, M.; Alvarnas, J.; Lacey, S. F.; Yee, J. K.; Li, M.; Couture, L.; Hsu, D.; Forman, S. J.; Rossi, J. J. & Zaia, J. A. (2010). RNA-based gene therapy for HIV with lentiviral vector-modified CD34(+) cells in patients undergoing transplantation for AIDS-related lymphoma, *Sci Transl Med*, Vol.2, No.36, pp. 36ra43

Doitsh, G.; Cavrois, M.; Lassen, K. G.; Zepeda, O.; Yang, Z.; Santiago, M. L.; Hebbeler, A. M. & Greene, W. C. (2010). Abortive HIV infection mediates CD4 T cell depletion and inflammation in human lymphoid tissue, *Cell*, Vol.143, No.5, pp. 789-801

Douek, D. C.; Brenchley, J. M.; Betts, M. R.; Ambrozak, D. R.; Hill, B. J.; Okamoto, Y.; Casazza, J. P.; Kuruppu, J.; Kunstman, K.; Wolinsky, S.; Grossman, Z.; Dybul, M.; Oxenius, A.; Price, D. A.; Connors, M. & Koup, R. A. (2002). HIV preferentially infects HIV-specific CD4+ T cells, *Nature*, Vol.417, No.6884, pp. 95-98

Egelhofer, M.; Brandenburg, G.; Martinius, H.; Schult-Dietrich, P.; Melikyan, G.; Kunert, R.; Baum, C.; Choi, I.; Alexandrov, A. & von Laer, D. (2004). Inhibition of human immunodeficiency virus type 1 entry in cells expressing gp41-derived peptides, *J Virol*, Vol.78, No.2, pp. 568-575

Egerer, L.; Volk, A.; Kahle, J.; Kimpel, J.; Brauer, F.; Hermann, F. G. & von Laer, D. (2011). Secreted Antiviral Entry Inhibitory (SAVE) Peptides for Gene Therapy of HIV Infection, *Mol Ther*, advance online publication, 01.03.2011 (doi: 10.1038/mt.2001.30)

Eshhar, Z.; Waks, T.; Bendavid, A. & Schindler, D. G. (2001). Functional expression of chimeric receptor genes in human T cells, *J Immunol Methods*, Vol.248, No.1-2, pp. 67-76

Finzi, D.; Hermankova, M.; Pierson, T.; Carruth, L. M.; Buck, C.; Chaisson, R. E.; Quinn, T. C.; Chadwick, K.; Margolick, J.; Brookmeyer, R.; Gallant, J.; Markowitz, M.; Ho, D. D.; Richman, D. D. & Siliciano, R. F. (1997). Identification of a reservoir for HIV-1 in patients on highly active antiretroviral therapy, *Science*, Vol.278, No.5341, pp. 1295-1300

Fraisier, C.; Abraham, D. A.; van Oijen, M.; Cunliffe, V.; Irvine, A.; Craig, R. & Dzierzak, E. A. (1998). Inhibition of Tat-mediated transactivation and HIV replication with Tat mutant and repressor domain fusion proteins, *Gene Ther*, Vol.5, No.7, pp. 946-954

Frecha, C.; Szecsi, J.; Cosset, F. L. & Verhoeyen, E. (2008). Strategies for targeting lentiviral vectors, *Curr Gene Ther*, Vol.8, No.6, pp. 449-460

Funke, S.; Maisner, A.; Muhlebach, M. D.; Koehl, U.; Grez, M.; Cattaneo, R.; Cichutek, K. & Buchholz, C. J. (2008). Targeted cell entry of lentiviral vectors, *Mol Ther*, Vol.16, No.8, pp. 1427-1436

Gay, W.; Lauret, E.; Boson, B.; Larghero, J.; Matheux, F.; Peyramaure, S.; Rousseau, V.; Dormont, D.; De Maeyer, E. & Le Grand, R. (2004). Low autocrine interferon beta production as a gene therapy approach for AIDS: Infusion of interferon beta-engineered lymphocytes in macaques chronically infected with SIVmac251, *Retrovirology*, Vol.1, pp. 29

Gething, M. J. & Sambrook, J. (1981). Cell-surface expression of influenza haemagglutinin from a cloned DNA copy of the RNA gene, *Nature*, Vol.293, No.5834, pp. 620-625

Goncalves, J.; Silva, F.; Freitas-Vieira, A.; Santa-Marta, M.; Malho, R.; Yang, X.; Gabuzda, D. & Barbas, C., 3rd (2002). Functional neutralization of HIV-1 Vif protein by intracellular immunization inhibits reverse transcription and viral replication, *J Biol Chem*, Vol.277, No.35, pp. 32036-32045

Grimm, D.; Streetz, K. L.; Jopling, C. L.; Storm, T. A.; Pandey, K.; Davis, C. R.; Marion, P.; Salazar, F. & Kay, M. A. (2006). Fatality in mice due to oversaturation of cellular microRNA/short hairpin RNA pathways, *Nature*, Vol.441, No.7092, pp. 537-541

Hacein-Bey-Abina, S.; Garrigue, A.; Wang, G. P.; Soulier, J.; Lim, A.; Morillon, E.; Clappier, E.; Caccavelli, L.; Delabesse, E.; Beldjord, K.; Asnafi, V.; MacIntyre, E.; Dal Cortivo, L.; Radford, I.; Brousse, N.; Sigaux, F.; Moshous, D.; Hauer, J.; Borkhardt, A.; Belohradsky, B. H.; Wintergerst, U.; Velez, M. C.; Leiva, L.; Sorensen, R.; Wulffraat, N.; Blanche, S.; Bushman, F. D.; Fischer, A. & Cavazzana-Calvo, M. (2008).

Insertional oncogenesis in 4 patients after retrovirus-mediated gene therapy of SCID-X1, *J Clin Invest*, Vol.118, No.9, pp. 3132-3142

Halbert, C. L.; Rutledge, E. A.; Allen, J. M.; Russell, D. W. & Miller, A. D. (2000). Repeat transduction in the mouse lung by using adeno-associated virus vectors with different serotypes, *J Virol*, Vol.74, No.3, pp. 1524-1532

Hammer, D.; Wild, J.; Ludwig, C.; Asbach, B.; Notka, F. & Wagner, R. (2008). Fusion of Epstein-Barr virus nuclear antigen-1-derived glycine-alanine repeat to trans-dominant HIV-1 Gag increases inhibitory activities and survival of transduced cells in vivo, *Hum Gene Ther*, Vol.19, No.6, pp. 622-634

Harrich, D.; Ulich, C. & Gaynor, R. B. (1996). A critical role for the TAR element in promoting efficient human immunodeficiency virus type 1 reverse transcription, *J Virol*, Vol.70, No.6, pp. 4017-4027

Hermann, F. G.; Egerer, L.; Brauer, F.; Gerum, C.; Schwalbe, H.; Dietrich, U. & von Laer, D. (2009a). Mutations in gp120 contribute to the resistance of human immunodeficiency virus type 1 to membrane-anchored C-peptide maC46, *J Virol*, Vol.83, No.10, pp. 4844-4853

Hermann, F. G.; Martinius, H.; Egelhofer, M.; Giroglou, T.; Tonn, T.; Roth, S. D.; Zahn, R.; Schult-Dietrich, P.; Alexandrov, A.; Dietrich, U.; Baum, C. & von Laer, D. (2009b). Protein scaffold and expression level determine antiviral activity of membrane-anchored antiviral peptides, *Hum Gene Ther*, Vol.20, No.4, pp. 325-336

Heslop, H. E.; Ng, C. Y.; Li, C.; Smith, C. A.; Loftin, S. K.; Krance, R. A.; Brenner, M. K. & Rooney, C. M. (1996). Long-term restoration of immunity against Epstein-Barr virus infection by adoptive transfer of gene-modified virus-specific T lymphocytes, *Nat Med*, Vol.2, No.5, pp. 551-555

Hirata, R. K.; Miller, A. D.; Andrews, R. G. & Russell, D. W. (1996). Transduction of hematopoietic cells by foamy virus vectors, *Blood*, Vol.88, No.9, pp. 3654-3661

Holt, N.; Wang, J.; Kim, K.; Friedman, G.; Wang, X.; Taupin, V.; Crooks, G. M.; Kohn, D. B.; Gregory, P. D.; Holmes, M. C. & Cannon, P. M. (2010). Human hematopoietic stem/progenitor cells modified by zinc-finger nucleases targeted to CCR5 control HIV-1 in vivo, *Nat Biotechnol*, Vol.28, No.8, pp. 839-847

Hotchkiss, G.; Maijgren-Steffensson, C. & Ahrlund-Richter, L. (2004). Efficacy and mode of action of hammerhead and hairpin ribozymes against various HIV-1 target sites, *Mol Ther*, Vol.10, No.1, pp. 172-180

Howe, S. J.; Mansour, M. R.; Schwarzwaelder, K.; Bartholomae, C.; Hubank, M.; Kempski, H.; Brugman, M. H.; Pike-Overzet, K.; Chatters, S. J.; de Ridder, D.; Gilmour, K. C.; Adams, S.; Thornhill, S. I.; Parsley, K. L.; Staal, F. J.; Gale, R. E.; Linch, D. C.; Bayford, J.; Brown, L.; Quaye, M.; Kinnon, C.; Ancliff, P.; Webb, D. K.; Schmidt, M.; von Kalle, C.; Gaspar, H. B. & Thrasher, A. J. (2008). Insertional mutagenesis combined with acquired somatic mutations causes leukemogenesis following gene therapy of SCID-X1 patients, *J Clin Invest*, Vol.118, No.9, pp. 3143-3150

Huang, Y.; Paxton, W. A.; Wolinsky, S. M.; Neumann, A. U.; Zhang, L.; He, T.; Kang, S.; Ceradini, D.; Jin, Z.; Yazdanbakhsh, K.; Kunstman, K.; Erickson, D.; Dragon, E.; Landau, N. R.; Phair, J.; Ho, D. D. & Koup, R. A. (1996). The role of a mutant CCR5 allele in HIV-1 transmission and disease progression, *Nat Med*, Vol.2, No.11, pp. 1240-1243

Hufert, F. T.; van Lunzen, J.; Janossy, G.; Bertram, S.; Schmitz, J.; Haller, O.; Racz, P. & von Laer, D. (1997). Germinal centre CD4+ T cells are an important site of HIV replication in vivo, *Aids*, Vol.11, No.7, pp. 849-857

Humeau, L. M.; Binder, G. K.; Lu, X.; Slepushkin, V.; Merling, R.; Echeagaray, P.; Pereira, M.; Slepushkina, T.; Barnett, S.; Dropulic, L. K.; Carroll, R.; Levine, B. L.; June, C. H. & Dropulic, B. (2004). Efficient lentiviral vector-mediated control of HIV-1 replication in CD4 lymphocytes from diverse HIV+ infected patients grouped according to CD4 count and viral load, *Mol Ther*, Vol.9, No.6, pp. 902-913

Husson, R. N.; Chung, Y.; Mordenti, J.; Butler, K. M.; Chen, S.; Duliege, A. M.; Brouwers, P.; Jarosinski, P.; Mueller, B. U.; Ammann, A. & et al. (1992). Phase I study of continuous-infusion soluble CD4 as a single agent and in combination with oral dideoxyinosine therapy in children with symptomatic human immunodeficiency virus infection, *J Pediatr*, Vol.121, No.4, pp. 627-633

Jacque, J. M.; Triques, K. & Stevenson, M. (2002). Modulation of HIV-1 replication by RNA interference, *Nature*, Vol.418, No.6896, pp. 435-438

Joseph, A.; Zheng, J. H.; Follenzi, A.; Dilorenzo, T.; Sango, K.; Hyman, J.; Chen, K.; Piechocka-Trocha, A.; Brander, C.; Hooijberg, E.; Vignali, D. A.; Walker, B. D. & Goldstein, H. (2008). Lentiviral vectors encoding human immunodeficiency virus type 1 (HIV-1)-specific T-cell receptor genes efficiently convert peripheral blood CD8 T lymphocytes into cytotoxic T lymphocytes with potent in vitro and in vivo HIV-1-specific inhibitory activity, *J Virol*, Vol.82, No.6, pp. 3078-3089

Joseph, A.; Zheng, J. H.; Chen, K.; Dutta, M.; Chen, C.; Stiegler, G.; Kunert, R.; Follenzi, A. & Goldstein, H. (2010). Inhibition of in vivo HIV infection in humanized mice by gene therapy of human hematopoietic stem cells with a lentiviral vector encoding a broadly neutralizing anti-HIV antibody, *J Virol*, Vol.84, No.13, pp. 6645-6653

Keen, N. J.; Gait, M. J. & Karn, J. (1996). Human immunodeficiency virus type-1 Tat is an integral component of the activated transcription-elongation complex, *Proc Natl Acad Sci U S A*, Vol.93, No.6, pp. 2505-2510

Kemball, C. C.; Pack, C. D.; Guay, H. M.; Li, Z. N.; Steinhauer, D. A.; Szomolanyi-Tsuda, E. & Lukacher, A. E. (2007). The antiviral CD8+ T cell response is differentially dependent on CD4+ T cell help over the course of persistent infection, *J Immunol*, Vol.179, No.2, pp. 1113-1121

Kimpel, J.; Braun, S. E.; Qiu, G.; Wong, F. E.; Conolle, M.; Schmitz, J. E.; Brendel, C.; Humeau, L. M.; Dropulic, B.; Rossi, J. J.; Berger, A.; von Laer, D. & Johnson, R. P. (2010). Survival of the fittest: positive selection of CD4+ T cells expressing a membrane-bound fusion inhibitor following HIV-1 infection, *PLoS One*, Vol.5, No.8, pp. e12357

Kitamura, Y.; Ishikawa, T.; Okui, N.; Kobayashi, N.; Kanda, T.; Shimada, T.; Miyake, K. & Yoshiike, K. (1999). Inhibition of replication of HIV-1 at both early and late stages of the viral life cycle by single-chain antibody against viral integrase, *J Acquir Immune Defic Syndr Hum Retrovirol*, Vol.20, No.2, pp. 105-114

Kohn, D. B.; Bauer, G.; Rice, C. R.; Rothschild, J. C.; Carbonaro, D. A.; Valdez, P.; Hao, Q.; Zhou, C.; Bahner, I.; Kearns, K.; Brody, K.; Fox, S.; Haden, E.; Wilson, K.; Salata, C.; Dolan, C.; Wetter, C.; Aguilar-Cordova, E. & Church, J. (1999). A clinical trial of retroviral-mediated transfer of a rev-responsive element decoy gene into CD34(+) cells from the bone marrow of human immunodeficiency virus-1-infected children, *Blood*, Vol.94, No.1, pp. 368-371

Kumar, P.; Ban, H. S.; Kim, S. S.; Wu, H.; Pearson, T.; Greiner, D. L.; Laouar, A.; Yao, J.; Haridas, V.; Habiro, K.; Yang, Y. G.; Jeong, J. H.; Lee, K. Y.; Kim, Y. H.; Kim, S. W.; Peipp, M.; Fey, G. H.; Manjunath, N.; Shultz, L. D.; Lee, S. K. & Shankar, P. (2008). T cell-specific siRNA delivery suppresses HIV-1 infection in humanized mice, *Cell*, Vol.134, No.4, pp. 577-586

Lee, N. S.; Dohjima, T.; Bauer, G.; Li, H.; Li, M. J.; Ehsani, A.; Salvaterra, P. & Rossi, J. (2002). Expression of small interfering RNAs targeted against HIV-1 rev transcripts in human cells, *Nat Biotechnol*, Vol.20, No.5, pp. 500-505

Lee, T. C.; Sullenger, B. A.; Gallardo, H. F.; Ungers, G. E. & Gilboa, E. (1992). Overexpression of RRE-derived sequences inhibits HIV-1 replication in CEM cells, *New Biol*, Vol.4, No.1, pp. 66-74

Leurs, C.; Jansen, M.; Pollok, K. E.; Heinkelein, M.; Schmidt, M.; Wissler, M.; Lindemann, D.; Von Kalle, C.; Rethwilm, A.; Williams, D. A. & Hanenberg, H. (2003). Comparison of three retroviral vector systems for transduction of nonobese diabetic/severe combined immunodeficiency mice repopulating human CD34+ cord blood cells, *Hum Gene Ther*, Vol.14, No.6, pp. 509-519

Levine, B. L.; Humeau, L. M.; Boyer, J.; MacGregor, R. R.; Rebello, T.; Lu, X.; Binder, G. K.; Slepushkin, V.; Lemiale, F.; Mascola, J. R.; Bushman, F. D.; Dropulic, B. & June, C. H. (2006). Gene transfer in humans using a conditionally replicating lentiviral vector, *Proc Natl Acad Sci U S A*, Vol.103, No.46, pp. 17372-17377

Levitskaya, J.; Sharipo, A.; Leonchiks, A.; Ciechanover, A. & Masucci, M. G. (1997). Inhibition of ubiquitin/proteasome-dependent protein degradation by the Gly-Ala repeat domain of the Epstein-Barr virus nuclear antigen 1, *Proc Natl Acad Sci U S A*, Vol.94, No.23, pp. 12616-12621

Levy-Mintz, P.; Duan, L.; Zhang, H.; Hu, B.; Dornadula, G.; Zhu, M.; Kulkosky, J.; Bizub-Bender, D.; Skalka, A. M. & Pomerantz, R. J. (1996). Intracellular expression of single-chain variable fragments to inhibit early stages of the viral life cycle by targeting human immunodeficiency virus type 1 integrase, *J Virol*, Vol.70, No.12, pp. 8821-8832

Liang, M.; Kamata, M.; Chen, K. N.; Pariente, N.; An, D. S. & Chen, I. S. (2010). Inhibition of HIV-1 infection by a unique short hairpin RNA to chemokine receptor 5 delivered into macrophages through hematopoietic progenitor cell transduction, *J Gene Med*, Vol.12, No.3, pp. 255-265

Lock, M.; Alvira, M.; Vandenberghe, L. H.; Samanta, A.; Toelen, J.; Debyser, Z. & Wilson, J. M. (2010). Rapid, simple, and versatile manufacturing of recombinant adeno-associated viral vectors at scale, *Hum Gene Ther*, Vol.21, No.10, pp. 1259-1271

Lu, X.; Yu, Q.; Binder, G. K.; Chen, Z.; Slepushkina, T.; Rossi, J. & Dropulic, B. (2004). Antisense-mediated inhibition of human immunodeficiency virus (HIV) replication by use of an HIV type 1-based vector results in severely attenuated mutants incapable of developing resistance, *J Virol*, Vol.78, No.13, pp. 7079-7088

Luis Abad, J.; Gonzalez, M. A.; del Real, G.; Mira, E.; Manes, S.; Serrano, F. & Bernad, A. (2003). Novel interfering bifunctional molecules against the CCR5 coreceptor are efficient inhibitors of HIV-1 infection, *Mol Ther*, Vol.8, No.3, pp. 475-484

Lund, O.; Lund, O. S.; Gram, G.; Nielsen, S. D.; Schonning, K.; Nielsen, J. O.; Hansen, J. E. & Mosekilde, E. (1997). Gene therapy of T helper cells in HIV infection: mathematical model of the criteria for clinical effect, *Bull Math Biol*, Vol.59, No.4, pp. 725-745

Macpherson, J. L.; Boyd, M. P.; Arndt, A. J.; Todd, A. V.; Fanning, G. C.; Ely, J. A.; Elliott, F.; Knop, A.; Raponi, M.; Murray, J.; Gerlach, W.; Sun, L. Q.; Penny, R.; Symonds, G. P.; Carr, A. & Cooper, D. A. (2005). Long-term survival and concomitant gene expression of ribozyme-transduced CD4+ T-lymphocytes in HIV-infected patients, *J Gene Med*, Vol.7, No.5, pp. 552-564

Malim, M. H.; Bohnlein, S.; Hauber, J. & Cullen, B. R. (1989). Functional dissection of the HIV-1 Rev trans-activator--derivation of a trans-dominant repressor of Rev function, *Cell*, Vol.58, No.1, pp. 205-214

Matloubian, M.; Concepcion, R. J. & Ahmed, R. (1994). CD4+ T cells are required to sustain CD8+ cytotoxic T-cell responses during chronic viral infection, *J Virol*, Vol.68, No.12, pp. 8056-8063

McBride, J. L.; Boudreau, R. L.; Harper, S. Q.; Staber, P. D.; Monteys, A. M.; Martins, I.; Gilmore, B. L.; Burstein, H.; Peluso, R. W.; Polisky, B.; Carter, B. J. & Davidson, B. L. (2008). Artificial miRNAs mitigate shRNA-mediated toxicity in the brain: implications for the therapeutic development of RNAi, *Proc Natl Acad Sci U S A*, Vol.105, No.15, pp. 5868-5873

Mhashilkar, A. M.; Bagley, J.; Chen, S. Y.; Szilvay, A. M.; Helland, D. G. & Marasco, W. A. (1995). Inhibition of HIV-1 Tat-mediated LTR transactivation and HIV-1 infection by anti-Tat single chain intrabodies, *Embo J*, Vol.14, No.7, pp. 1542-1551

Michienzi, A.; Castanotto, D.; Lee, N.; Li, S.; Zaia, J. A. & Rossi, J. J. (2003). RNA-mediated inhibition of HIV in a gene therapy setting, *Ann N Y Acad Sci*, Vol.1002, pp. 63-71

Michienzi, A.; De Angelis, F. G.; Bozzoni, I. & Rossi, J. J. (2006). A nucleolar localizing Rev binding element inhibits HIV replication, *AIDS Res Ther*, Vol.3, pp. 13

Mitchell, R. S.; Beitzel, B. F.; Schroder, A. R.; Shinn, P.; Chen, H.; Berry, C. C.; Ecker, J. R. & Bushman, F. D. (2004). Retroviral DNA integration: ASLV, HIV, and MLV show distinct target site preferences, *PLoS Biol*, Vol.2, No.8, pp. E234

Mitsuyasu, R. T.; Anton, P. A.; Deeks, S. G.; Scadden, D. T.; Connick, E.; Downs, M. T.; Bakker, A.; Roberts, M. R.; June, C. H.; Jalali, S.; Lin, A. A.; Pennathur-Das, R. & Hege, K. M. (2000). Prolonged survival and tissue trafficking following adoptive transfer of CD4zeta gene-modified autologous CD4(+) and CD8(+) T cells in human immunodeficiency virus-infected subjects, *Blood*, Vol.96, No.3, pp. 785-793

Mitsuyasu, R. T.; Merigan, T. C.; Carr, A.; Zack, J. A.; Winters, M. A.; Workman, C.; Bloch, M.; Lalezari, J.; Becker, S.; Thornton, L.; Akil, B.; Khanlou, H.; Finlayson, R.; McFarlane, R.; Smith, D. E.; Garsia, R.; Ma, D.; Law, M.; Murray, J. M.; von Kalle, C.; Ely, J. A.; Patino, S. M.; Knop, A. E.; Wong, P.; Todd, A. V.; Haughton, M.; Fuery, C.; Macpherson, J. L.; Symonds, G. P.; Evans, L. A.; Pond, S. M. & Cooper, D.

A. (2009). Phase 2 gene therapy trial of an anti-HIV ribozyme in autologous CD34+ cells, *Nat Med*, Vol.15, No.3, pp. 285-292

Modlich, U.; Navarro, S.; Zychlinski, D.; Maetzig, T.; Knoess, S.; Brugman, M. H.; Schambach, A.; Charrier, S.; Galy, A.; Thrasher, A. J.; Bueren, J. & Baum, C. (2009). Insertional transformation of hematopoietic cells by self-inactivating lentiviral and gammaretroviral vectors, *Mol Ther*, Vol.17, No.11, pp. 1919-1928

Morgan, R. A.; Looney, D. J.; Muenchau, D. D.; Wong-Staal, F.; Gallo, R. C. & Anderson, W. F. (1990). Retroviral vectors expressing soluble CD4: a potential gene therapy for AIDS, *AIDS Res Hum Retroviruses*, Vol.6, No.2, pp. 183-191

Morgan, R. A.; Baler-Bitterlich, G.; Ragheb, J. A.; Wong-Staal, F.; Gallo, R. C. & Anderson, W. F. (1994). Further evaluation of soluble CD4 as an anti-HIV type 1 gene therapy: demonstration of protection of primary human peripheral blood lymphocytes from infection by HIV type 1, *AIDS Res Hum Retroviruses*, Vol.10, No.11, pp. 1507-1515

Morgan, R. A.; Walker, R.; Carter, C. S.; Natarajan, V.; Tavel, J. A.; Bechtel, C.; Herpin, B.; Muul, L.; Zheng, Z.; Jagannatha, S.; Bunnell, B. A.; Fellowes, V.; Metcalf, J. A.; Stevens, R.; Baseler, M.; Leitman, S. F.; Read, E. J.; Blaese, R. M. & Lane, H. C. (2005). Preferential survival of CD4+ T lymphocytes engineered with anti-human immunodeficiency virus (HIV) genes in HIV-infected individuals, *Hum Gene Ther*, Vol.16, No.9, pp. 1065-1074

Morgan, R. A.; Dudley, M. E.; Wunderlich, J. R.; Hughes, M. S.; Yang, J. C.; Sherry, R. M.; Royal, R. E.; Topalian, S. L.; Kammula, U. S.; Restifo, N. P.; Zheng, Z.; Nahvi, A.; de Vries, C. R.; Rogers-Freezer, L. J.; Mavroukakis, S. A. & Rosenberg, S. A. (2006). Cancer regression in patients after transfer of genetically engineered lymphocytes, *Science*, Vol.314, No.5796, pp. 126-129

Muesing, M. A.; Smith, D. H. & Capon, D. J. (1987). Regulation of mRNA accumulation by a human immunodeficiency virus trans-activator protein, *Cell*, Vol.48, No.4, pp. 691-701

Newrzela, S.; Cornils, K.; Li, Z.; Baum, C.; Brugman, M. H.; Hartmann, M.; Meyer, J.; Hartmann, S.; Hansmann, M. L.; Fehse, B. & von Laer, D. (2008). Resistance of mature T cells to oncogene transformation, *Blood*, Vol.112, No.6, pp. 2278-2286

Novina, C. D.; Murray, M. F.; Dykxhoorn, D. M.; Beresford, P. J.; Riess, J.; Lee, S. K.; Collman, R. G.; Lieberman, J.; Shankar, P. & Sharp, P. A. (2002). siRNA-directed inhibition of HIV-1 infection, *Nat Med*, Vol.8, No.7, pp. 681-686

Olsen, H. S.; Nelbock, P.; Cochrane, A. W. & Rosen, C. A. (1990). Secondary structure is the major determinant for interaction of HIV rev protein with RNA, *Science*, Vol.247, No.4944, pp. 845-848

Pearson, L.; Garcia, J.; Wu, F.; Modesti, N.; Nelson, J. & Gaynor, R. (1990). A transdominant tat mutant that inhibits tat-induced gene expression from the human immunodeficiency virus long terminal repeat, *Proc Natl Acad Sci U S A*, Vol.87, No.13, pp. 5079-5083

Perez, E. E.; Riley, J. L.; Carroll, R. G.; von Laer, D. & June, C. H. (2005). Suppression of HIV-1 infection in primary CD4 T cells transduced with a self-inactivating lentiviral vector encoding a membrane expressed gp41-derived fusion inhibitor, *Clin Immunol*, Vol.115, No.1, pp. 26-32

Perez, E. E.; Wang, J.; Miller, J. C.; Jouvenot, Y.; Kim, K. A.; Liu, O.; Wang, N.; Lee, G.; Bartsevich, V. V.; Lee, Y. L.; Guschin, D. Y.; Rupniewski, I.; Waite, A. J.; Carpenito, C.; Carroll, R. G.; Orange, J. S.; Urnov, F. D.; Rebar, E. J.; Ando, D.; Gregory, P. D.; Riley, J. L.; Holmes, M. C. & June, C. H. (2008). Establishment of HIV-1 resistance in CD4+ T cells by genome editing using zinc-finger nucleases, *Nat Biotechnol*, Vol.26, No.7, pp. 808-816

Phillips, R. E.; Rowland-Jones, S.; Nixon, D. F.; Gotch, F. M.; Edwards, J. P.; Ogunlesi, A. O.; Elvin, J. G.; Rothbard, J. A.; Bangham, C. R.; Rizza, C. R. & et al. (1991). Human immunodeficiency virus genetic variation that can escape cytotoxic T cell recognition, *Nature*, Vol.354, No.6353, pp. 453-459

Podsakoff, G. M.; Engel, B. C.; Carbonaro, D. A.; Choi, C.; Smogorzewska, E. M.; Bauer, G.; Selander, D.; Csik, S.; Wilson, K.; Betts, M. R.; Koup, R. A.; Nabel, G. J.; Bishop, K.; King, S.; Schmidt, M.; von Kalle, C.; Church, J. A. & Kohn, D. B. (2005). Selective survival of peripheral blood lymphocytes in children with HIV-1 following delivery of an anti-HIV gene to bone marrow CD34(+) cells, *Mol Ther*, Vol.12, No.1, pp. 77-86

Ranga, U.; Woffendin, C.; Verma, S.; Xu, L.; June, C. H.; Bishop, D. K. & Nabel, G. J. (1998). Enhanced T cell engraftment after retroviral delivery of an antiviral gene in HIV-infected individuals, *Proc Natl Acad Sci U S A*, Vol.95, No.3, pp. 1201-1206

Rethwilm, A. (2007). Foamy virus vectors: an awaited alternative to gammaretro- and lentiviral vectors, *Curr Gene Ther*, Vol.7, No.4, pp. 261-271

Rinaldo, C.; Huang, X. L.; Fan, Z. F.; Ding, M.; Beltz, L.; Logar, A.; Panicali, D.; Mazzara, G.; Liebmann, J.; Cottrill, M. & et al. (1995). High levels of anti-human immunodeficiency virus type 1 (HIV-1) memory cytotoxic T-lymphocyte activity and low viral load are associated with lack of disease in HIV-1-infected long-term nonprogressors, *J Virol*, Vol.69, No.9, pp. 5838-5842

Roberts, M. R.; Qin, L.; Zhang, D.; Smith, D. H.; Tran, A. C.; Dull, T. J.; Groopman, J. E.; Capon, D. J.; Byrn, R. A. & Finer, M. H. (1994). Targeting of human immunodeficiency virus-infected cells by CD8+ T lymphocytes armed with universal T-cell receptors, *Blood*, Vol.84, No.9, pp. 2878-2889

Roe, T.; Reynolds, T. C.; Yu, G. & Brown, P. O. (1993). Integration of murine leukemia virus DNA depends on mitosis, *Embo J*, Vol.12, No.5, pp. 2099-2108

Sabariegos, R.; Gimenez-Barcons, M.; Tapia, N.; Clotet, B. & Martinez, M. A. (2006). Sequence homology required by human immunodeficiency virus type 1 to escape from short interfering RNAs, *J Virol*, Vol.80, No.2, pp. 571-577

Samson, M.; Libert, F.; Doranz, B. J.; Rucker, J.; Liesnard, C.; Farber, C. M.; Saragosti, S.; Lapoumeroulie, C.; Cognaux, J.; Forceille, C.; Muyldermans, G.; Verhofstede, C.; Burtonboy, G.; Georges, M.; Imai, T.; Rana, S.; Yi, Y.; Smyth, R. J.; Collman, R. G.; Doms, R. W.; Vassart, G. & Parmentier, M. (1996). Resistance to HIV-1 infection in caucasian individuals bearing mutant alleles of the CCR-5 chemokine receptor gene, *Nature*, Vol.382, No.6593, pp. 722-725

Sanhadji, K.; Grave, L.; Touraine, J. L.; Leissner, P.; Rouzioux, C.; Firouzi, R.; Kehrli, L.; Tardy, J. C. & Mehtali, M. (2000). Gene transfer of anti-gp41 antibody and CD4 immunoadhesin strongly reduces the HIV-1 load in humanized severe combined immunodeficient mice, *Aids*, Vol.14, No.18, pp. 2813-2822

Sarkar, I.; Hauber, I.; Hauber, J. & Buchholz, F. (2007). HIV-1 proviral DNA excision using an evolved recombinase, *Science*, Vol.316, No.5833, pp. 1912-1915

Sarver, N.; Cantin, E. M.; Chang, P. S.; Zaia, J. A.; Ladne, P. A.; Stephens, D. A. & Rossi, J. J. (1990). Ribozymes as potential anti-HIV-1 therapeutic agents, *Science*, Vol.247, No.4947, pp. 1222-1225

Schmitz, J. E.; Kuroda, M. J.; Santra, S.; Sasseville, V. G.; Simon, M. A.; Lifton, M. A.; Racz, P.; Tenner-Racz, K.; Dalesandro, M.; Scallon, B. J.; Ghrayeb, J.; Forman, M. A.; Montefiori, D. C.; Rieber, E. P.; Letvin, N. L. & Reimann, K. A. (1999). Control of viremia in simian immunodeficiency virus infection by CD8+ lymphocytes, *Science*, Vol.283, No.5403, pp. 857-860

Shaheen, F.; Duan, L.; Zhu, M.; Bagasra, O. & Pomerantz, R. J. (1996). Targeting human immunodeficiency virus type 1 reverse transcriptase by intracellular expression of single-chain variable fragments to inhibit early stages of the viral life cycle, *J Virol*, Vol.70, No.6, pp. 3392-3400

Shankar, P.; Russo, M.; Harnisch, B.; Patterson, M.; Skolnik, P. & Lieberman, J. (2000). Impaired function of circulating HIV-specific CD8(+) T cells in chronic human immunodeficiency virus infection, *Blood*, Vol.96, No.9, pp. 3094-3101

Sommermeyer, D.; Neudorfer, J.; Weinhold, M.; Leisegang, M.; Engels, B.; Noessner, E.; Heemskerk, M. H.; Charo, J.; Schendel, D. J.; Blankenstein, T.; Bernhard, H. & Uckert, W. (2006). Designer T cells by T cell receptor replacement, *Eur J Immunol*, Vol.36, No.11, pp. 3052-3059

Strayer, D. S.; Zern, M. A. & Chowdhury, J. R. (2002). What can SV40-derived vectors do for gene therapy?, *Curr Opin Mol Ther*, Vol.4, No.4, pp. 313-323

Strayer, D. S.; Akkina, R.; Bunnell, B. A.; Dropulic, B.; Planelles, V.; Pomerantz, R. J.; Rossi, J. J. & Zaia, J. A. (2005). Current status of gene therapy strategies to treat HIV/AIDS, *Mol Ther*, Vol.11, No.6, pp. 823-842

Streeck, H.; Jolin, J. S.; Qi, Y.; Yassine-Diab, B.; Johnson, R. C.; Kwon, D. S.; Addo, M. M.; Brumme, C.; Routy, J. P.; Little, S.; Jessen, H. K.; Kelleher, A. D.; Hecht, F. M.; Sekaly, R. P.; Rosenberg, E. S.; Walker, B. D.; Carrington, M. & Altfeld, M. (2009). Human immunodeficiency virus type 1-specific CD8+ T-cell responses during primary infection are major determinants of the viral set point and loss of CD4+ T cells, *J Virol*, Vol.83, No.15, pp. 7641-7648

Sullenger, B. A.; Gallardo, H. F.; Ungers, G. E. & Gilboa, E. (1990). Overexpression of TAR sequences renders cells resistant to human immunodeficiency virus replication, *Cell*, Vol.63, No.3, pp. 601-608

Sullenger, B. A.; Gallardo, H. F.; Ungers, G. E. & Gilboa, E. (1991). Analysis of trans-acting response decoy RNA-mediated inhibition of human immunodeficiency virus type 1 transactivation, *J Virol*, Vol.65, No.12, pp. 6811-6816

Surabhi, R. M. & Gaynor, R. B. (2002). RNA interference directed against viral and cellular targets inhibits human immunodeficiency Virus Type 1 replication, *J Virol*, Vol.76, No.24, pp. 12963-12973

Surosky, R. T.; Urabe, M.; Godwin, S. G.; McQuiston, S. A.; Kurtzman, G. J.; Ozawa, K. & Natsoulis, G. (1997). Adeno-associated virus Rep proteins target DNA sequences to a unique locus in the human genome, *J Virol*, Vol.71, No.10, pp. 7951-7959

Swan, C. H.; Buhler, B.; Steinberger, P.; Tschan, M. P.; Barbas, C. F., 3rd & Torbett, B. E. (2006). T-cell protection and enrichment through lentiviral CCR5 intrabody gene delivery, *Gene Ther*, Vol.13, No.20, pp. 1480-1492

ter Brake, O.; Konstantinova, P.; Ceylan, M. & Berkhout, B. (2006). Silencing of HIV-1 with RNA interference: a multiple shRNA approach, *Mol Ther*, Vol.14, No.6, pp. 883-892

Trimble, L. A. & Lieberman, J. (1998). Circulating CD8 T lymphocytes in human immunodeficiency virus-infected individuals have impaired function and downmodulate CD3 zeta, the signaling chain of the T-cell receptor complex, *Blood*, Vol.91, No.2, pp. 585-594

Trono, D.; Feinberg, M. B. & Baltimore, D. (1989). HIV-1 Gag mutants can dominantly interfere with the replication of the wild-type virus, *Cell*, Vol.59, No.1, pp. 113-120

Vallanti, G.; Lupo, R.; Federico, M.; Mavilio, F. & Bovolenta, C. (2005). T Lymphocytes transduced with a lentiviral vector expressing F12-Vif are protected from HIV-1 infection in an APOBEC3G-independent manner, *Mol Ther*, Vol.12, No.4, pp. 697-706

van Lunzen, J.; Glaunsinger, T.; Stahmer, I.; von Baehr, V.; Baum, C.; Schilz, A.; Kuehlcke, K.; Naundorf, S.; Martinius, H.; Hermann, F.; Giroglou, T.; Newrzela, S.; Muller, I.; Brauer, F.; Brandenburg, G.; Alexandrov, A. & von Laer, D. (2007). Transfer of autologous gene-modified T cells in HIV-infected patients with advanced immunodeficiency and drug-resistant virus, *Mol Ther*, Vol.15, No.5, pp. 1024-1033

Vandekerckhove, L.; Christ, F.; Van Maele, B.; De Rijck, J.; Gijsbers, R.; Van den Haute, C.; Witvrouw, M. & Debyser, Z. (2006). Transient and stable knockdown of the integrase cofactor LEDGF/p75 reveals its role in the replication cycle of human immunodeficiency virus, *J Virol*, Vol.80, No.4, pp. 1886-1896

Varela-Rohena, A.; Molloy, P. E.; Dunn, S. M.; Li, Y.; Suhoski, M. M.; Carroll, R. G.; Milicic, A.; Mahon, T.; Sutton, D. H.; Laugel, B.; Moysey, R.; Cameron, B. J.; Vuidepot, A.; Purbhoo, M. A.; Cole, D. K.; Phillips, R. E.; June, C. H.; Jakobsen, B. K.; Sewell, A. K. & Riley, J. L. (2008). Control of HIV-1 immune escape by CD8 T cells expressing enhanced T-cell receptor, *Nat Med*, Vol.14, No.12, pp. 1390-1395

Vickers, T.; Baker, B. F.; Cook, P. D.; Zounes, M.; Buckheit, R. W., Jr.; Germany, J. & Ecker, D. J. (1991). Inhibition of HIV-LTR gene expression by oligonucleotides targeted to the TAR element, *Nucleic Acids Res*, Vol.19, No.12, pp. 3359-3368

Vigouroux, C.; Gharakhanian, S.; Salhi, Y.; Nguyen, T. H.; Chevenne, D.; Capeau, J. & Rozenbaum, W. (1999). Diabetes, insulin resistance and dyslipidaemia in lipodystrophic HIV-infected patients on highly active antiretroviral therapy (HAART), *Diabetes Metab*, Vol.25, No.3, pp. 225-232

von Laer, D.; Hasselmann, S. & Hasselmann, K. (2006). Impact of gene-modified T cells on HIV infection dynamics, *J Theor Biol*, Vol.238, No.1, pp. 60-77

Walker, R. E.; Bechtel, C. M.; Natarajan, V.; Baseler, M.; Hege, K. M.; Metcalf, J. A.; Stevens, R.; Hazen, A.; Blaese, R. M.; Chen, C. C.; Leitman, S. F.; Palensky, J.; Wittes, J.; Davey, R. T., Jr.; Falloon, J.; Polis, M. A.; Kovacs, J. A.; Broad, D. F.; Levine, B. L.;

Roberts, M. R.; Masur, H. & Lane, H. C. (2000). Long-term in vivo survival of receptor-modified syngeneic T cells in patients with human immunodeficiency virus infection, *Blood*, Vol.96, No.2, pp. 467-474

Walter, E. A.; Greenberg, P. D.; Gilbert, M. J.; Finch, R. J.; Watanabe, K. S.; Thomas, E. D. & Riddell, S. R. (1995). Reconstitution of cellular immunity against cytomegalovirus in recipients of allogeneic bone marrow by transfer of T-cell clones from the donor, *N Engl J Med*, Vol.333, No.16, pp. 1038-1044

Woffendin, C.; Ranga, U.; Yang, Z.; Xu, L. & Nabel, G. J. (1996). Expression of a protective gene-prolongs survival of T cells in human immunodeficiency virus-infected patients, *Proc Natl Acad Sci U S A*, Vol.93, No.7, pp. 2889-2894

Wong-Staal, F.; Poeschla, E. M. & Looney, D. J. (1998). A controlled, Phase 1 clinical trial to evaluate the safety and effects in HIV-1 infected humans of autologous lymphocytes transduced with a ribozyme that cleaves HIV-1 RNA, *Hum Gene Ther*, Vol.9, No.16, pp. 2407-2425

Zhou, C.; Bahner, I. C.; Larson, G. P.; Zaia, J. A.; Rossi, J. J. & Kohn, E. B. (1994). Inhibition of HIV-1 in human T-lymphocytes by retrovirally transduced anti-tat and rev hammerhead ribozymes, *Gene*, Vol.149, No.1, pp. 33-39

22

HIV-Screening Strategies for the Discovery of Novel HIV-Inhibitors

María José Abad, Luis Miguel Bedoya and Paulina Bermejo
Department of Pharmacology, Faculty of Pharmacy, University Complutense, Ciudad Universitaria s/n, 28040, Madrid
Spain

1. Introduction

Since acquired immunodeficiency syndrome (AIDS) was recognized 27 years ago, 25 million people have died of human immunodeficiency virus (HIV)-related causes. On a global scale, although the HIV epidemic has stabilized since 2000, unacceptably high levels of new HIV infection and AIDS death still occur each year. In 2007, there were an estimated 33 million (30-36 million) people living with HIV, and 2 million (1.8-2.3 million) people died due to AIDS, compared with an estimated 1.7 million (1.5-2.3 million) in 2001.

There are two main types of HIV: type 1 (HIV-1) and type 2 (HIV-2) (Buonaguro et al., 2007). HIV-1 is the most prevalent in the worldwide pandemic. HIV-2 is present mainly in West Africa, where it was discovered in 1986, and infects about one million people worldwide. HIV-2 is slowly but continuously spreading throughout Europe, Asia and the Americas, and has reached a significant prevalence in countries such as Portugal and India. After more than 20 years of research, HIV remains a difficult target for a vaccine; thus the treatment of AIDS continues to focus on the search for chemical anti-HIV agents.

A working knowledge of the HIV replication cycle is essential for understanding the mechanism of action of antiviral drugs. The HIV is an enveloped virus that contains two copies of viral genomic RNA in its core. In addition to the copies of RNA, the viral core also contains the enzymes required for HIV replication. The first step in the HIV replication cycle is the interaction between the envelope proteins of the virus (gp120) and specific host-cell surface receptors (e.g. the T-cell receptor CD4 on the cellular membrane) of the host cell. In the second step, the virus binds to the chemokine coreceptors CXC-chemokine receptor 4 (CXCR4) and CC-chemokine receptor 5 (CCR5). This induces a conformational change in gp120 that opens up a high affinity binding site located within the third variable loop (V3) and surrounding surfaces for the chemokine coreceptors CXCR4 and CCR5. This gives rise to further conformational rearrangements of gp120 that expose the transmembrane glycoprotein gp41, and the heptad repeat (HR) regions of the three subunits of gp41, HR1 and HR2, fold into a six-helical bundle. This ultimately results in the "fusion" of the viral envelope and the cytoplasmic membrane. Fusion creates a pore through which the viral capsid enters the cells.

HIV encodes three enzymes required for replication: HIV-1 reverse transcriptase (RT), HIV-integrase (IN) and HIV-protease (PT). Following entry into the cell, the viral RT enzyme catalyzes the conversion of viral RNA into DNA. This viral DNA enters the nucleus and becomes inserted into the chromosomal DNA of the host cell (integration). This process is facilitated by the viral enzyme IN. Expression of the viral genes leads to production of precursor viral proteins. These proteins and viral RNA are assembled at the cell surface into new viral particles and leave the host cell by a process called budding. During the budding process, they acquire the outer layer and envelope. At this stage, the PT enzyme cleaves the precursor viral proteins into their mature products. If this final phase of the replication cycle does not take place, the released viral particles are non-infectious and not competent to initiate the replication cycle in other susceptible cells.

Once HIV has entered the cell, it must disarm and hijack the intracellular machinery for its own benefit. Normal cell functionality of viral hosts is altered by invading virus proteins to the benefit of the virus. Viral proteins are known to compete with the host proteins, thus disrupting the normal host protein-protein interaction network. HIV-1 encodes the regulatory proteins, Tat and Rev, and four accessory proteins: viral infectivity factor (Vif), viral protein R (Vpr), viral protein U (Vpu) and negative factor (Nef) (Romani & Engelbrecht, 2009, Romani et al., 2010). The regulatory proteins are essential for virus replication by controlling HIV gene expression in host cells. In contrast, accessory proteins are often dispensable for virus replication *in vitro*. The Vif directly binds to and inactivates cellular deoxycytidine deaminase APOBEC3G, a natural antiviral factor that promotes G- to A-hypermutation of viral DNA during reverse transcription. The Vpu has been shown to down-regulate the CD4 receptor, and is also required for effective release of newly formed viral particles.

Anti-HIV drugs are classified into different groups according to their activity on the replicative cycle of HIV. These are virus-cell adsorption, virus-cell fusion, uncoating, reverse transcription, integration, DNA replication, transcription, translation, budding (assembly/release) and maturation. There are currently 25 compounds approved for the treatment of HIV, and most of these are nucleoside reverse transcriptase inhibitors (NRTIs), non-nucleoside reverse transcriptase inhibitors (NNRTIs) or protease inhibitors (PIs) (Warnke & Barreto, 2007, Zhan et al., 2009) (Table 1). Highly active antiretroviral therapy (HAART), which combines several such drugs (typically three or four), has dramatically improved patients' lives. The therapeutic effects are limited, however, by adverse effects and toxicities caused by long-term use and the emergence of drug resistance.

GENERIC NAME	ADVERSE REACTIONS
Entry inhibitors	
Maraviroc (UK-427)	Upper respiratory tract infection, cough, pyrexia
Fusion inhibitors	
Enfuvirtide (T20)	Pruritus, pain, discomfort
Reverse transcriptase inhibitors	
Nucleoside inhibitors	
Abacavir (ABC)	Diarrhea, nausea, headache
Didanosine (ddl)	Rash, abdominal pain, peripheral neuropathy
Emtricitabine (FTC)	Hyperpigmentation of skin, rash, diarrhea
Stavudine (d4T)	Rash, nausea, lipoatrophy
Lamivudine (3TC)	Decrease in appetite, headache, fatigue
Tenofovir (DF)	Diarrhea, nausea osteopenia
Zalcitabine (ddC)	Hepatic steatosis, peripheral neuropathy

GENERIC NAME	ADVERSE REACTIONS
Zidovudine (AZT)	Headache, anorexia, leukopenia
Non-nucleoside inhibitors	
Delavirdine (DLV)	Rash
Efavirenz (EFV)	Dizziness, hallucinations, insomnio
Etravirine (THC125)	Rash
Nevirapine (NVP)	Rash, hepatotoxicity
Integrase inhibitors	
Raltegravir (MK-0518)	Diarrhea, injection-site reactions, headache
Protease inhibitors	
Amprenavir (AMP)	Stomach upset, diarrhea, nausea
Atazanavir (ATZ)	Rash, elevated bilirubin, depression
Darunavir (TMC-114)	Rash, hypertriglyceridemia, diarrhea
Fosamprenavir (GW-433908)	Stomach upset, diarrhea, nausea
Indinavir (IDV)	Kidney stones, vomiting, headache
Lopinavir (ABT-378)	Diarrhea, headache, fatigue
Nelfinavir (NFV)	Diarrhea, nausea, rash
Ritonavir (RTV)	Stomach upset, vomiting, taste disturbance
Saquinavir (SQV)	Stomach upset, headache, abdominal pain
Tripanavir (TPV)	Hypercholesterolemia, diarrhea, nausea

Table 1. Approved antiretroviral drugs for the treatment of HIV infection

The multiple steps of the HIV replication cycle present novel therapeutic targets other than the viral enzyme RT and PT for drug developement. Continued efforts have been made to discover new inhibitors that target not only RT and PT but also other viral targets, achievements that have been reviewed comprehensively in the literature. Several recent novel target inhibitors were discovered using virus-based screening approaches (Table 2). Alternatively, PIs, the next generation of NNRTIs, CCR5 antagonist and IN inhibitors were identified by structure-based drug design, receptor pharmacology and biochemical screening approaches (Westby et al., 2005, Menéndez-Arias & Tözser, 2008, Greene et al., 2008, Liang, 2008, Pang et al., 2009, Marchand et al., 2009, Tan et al., 2010). Historical precedent therefore suggests that diverse screening strategies should be employed for the discovery of new HIV-1 agents. In this review we present a brief overview of various HIV-1 screening strategies and highlight novel approaches and/or significant advances in HIV-1 screening technology.

2. HIV-1 Entry

As mentioned above, HIV cellular entry is a multistep process that requires the interaction of a viral envelope glycoprotein (gp120) and a host receptor (CD4), followed by binding to a coreceptor (CCR5 and CXCR4). The proteins involved in the entry process have become attractive targets for drug design, and HIV-1 replication screens have successfully identified compounds with antiviral activity that act at each of these three steps of HIV entry (Grande et al., 2008, Wang & Duan, 2009).

The chemokine receptors CCR5 and CXCR4, membrane proteins belonging to the G-protein coupled receptor super-family, have been identified as essential coreceptors for HIV entry into the cells, and molecules that inhibit HIV entry by targeting CCR5 and CXCR4 have been

Attachment inhibitors
CD4 binding peptides
Aminoglycoside-arginine conjugates
Poly-arginine aminoglycoside conjugates
Cyclotriazadisulfonamide
Sulfated polysaccharides
CCR5 antagonists
3-(4-benzylpiperidin-1-yl)-N-phenylpropylamine derivatives
1-(3,3-diphenylpropyl)-piperidinyl amides
Ureas
1,3,4-trisubstituted pyrrolidines
1-amino-2-phenyl-4-(piperidin-1-yl) butane analogs
Prostatin (12-deoxyphorbol ester)
CXCR4 inhibitors
Prostatin (12-deoxyphorbol ester)
Bicyclams
Non-cyclam polynitrogenated compounds
Cyclic penta- and tetrapeptides
Diketopiperazine mimetics
Tetrahydroquinolines
Thiazolylisothiourea derivatives
Benzodiazepines
Alkylamine analogs
Non-peptide derivatives
Fusion inhibitors
Fusion inhibitors peptides
Pyrrole derivatives
Reverse transcriptase inhibitors
Nevirapine analogs
Efavirenz analogs
Tetrahydroimidazo-[4,5,1-jk][1,4]-benzodiazepinone derivatives
Tetrazole thioacetinilide derivatives
Calanolide A
Integrase inhibitors
β-diketo acids
GS-9137
Chalcones
Protease inhibitors
Cyclic urea derivatives
Peptidomimetic protease inhibitors

Table 2. Selected novel target inhibitors with potential application for the treatment of HIV infection

in rapid development as antiviral agents. Additionally, the envelope glycoprotein gp120 exists in its native form as a homopolymeric trimer, held on the outer surface of the virion by non-covalent interactions with a fusion glycoprotein gp41 trimer. The crystal structure of gp120 core bound to CD4 reveals specific targets for developing anti-HIV drugs.

High-throughput screening technologies designed to identify compounds that inhibit binding of natural ligands to their cognate G-protein-coupled receptor have been used successfully by the pharmaceutical industry for many years. The disadvantage of this approach is the dependence upon a radiolabeled ligand, which involved a high cost and arouses significant environmental concern when screening large chemical libraries. It is therefore unlikely that radiolabeled ligand binding assays will be widely used in the future.

More recently, assays have been developed which identify compounds that inhibit receptor function rather than ligand binding (and thus avoid the need for radiolabeled chemokines). HIV is an enveloped virus, and its envelope proteins complex (Env) controls the key process of viral entry. Env is a complex composed of a transmembrane gp41 subunit and a noncovalently-associated surface gp120 subunit. Infection is initiated by the binding of the virion gp120 Env protein to the CD4 molecule present on some T-cells, macrophages and microglial cells. The interaction induces a conformational change that promotes secondary gp120 binding to the coreceptor CCR5 and CXCR4. Both coreceptors are members of the chemokine receptor family, but CCR5 is the coreceptor for HIV-1 strains that infect macrophages (M-tropic or R5 strains), while CXCR4 is the coreceptor for HIV-1 strains that infect T-cells (T-tropic or X4 strains). Ochsenbauer-Jambor et al. (2006) introduced a T-cell based receptor reporter cell line (JLTRG-RS) that expresses both HIV-1 coreceptors, CXCR4 and CCR5, and offers the convenience of using enhanced green fluorescent protein (EGFP) as a direct and quantitative marker. Unlike previous EGFP-based reporter cell lines, JLTRG-RS cells have an unusually high dynamic signal range, sufficient for plate reader detection using a 384-well format. Because EGFP can be directly and continuously quantified in cell culture, the reporter cell line requires no manipulation during assay preparation or analysis. These characteristics make the system extremely flexible, rapid and inexpensive. Due to its intrinsic flexibility, the JLTRG-RS cell-based reporter system provides a powerful tool which will considerably facilitate future screening for HIV inhibitors.

Immortalized cell lines, transfected with the HIV-1 Env gene, express gp120/gp41 on their surface and can fuse to cells co-expressing CD4 and either CCR5 and CXCR4. Screens based on this approach have been described by a number of laboratories. A cell-based enzyme-linked immunosorbent assay (ELISA) was developed using and anti-CXCR4 monoclonal antibody, 12G5, and cells expressing CD4 and CXCR5, the U373-MAGI-CXCR4 (CEM) cell line (Zhao et al., 2003). The assay was sensitive to the well-characterized CXCR4 antagonists, T22, T14012 (a downsized analog of T22) and AMD3100, which effectively inhibited 12G5 binding to CXCR4-expressing cells whereas HIV-1 entry inhibitors targeting CD4 and gp41 in addition to HIV-1 RT and PT inhibitors, did not block the binding of 12G5 to U373-MAGI-CXCR4 (CEM) cells. This suggests that the cell-based ELISA is specific, sensitive, convenient, rapid and economical.

More recently, two new T-cell-based reporter cell lines were established to measure HIV-1 infectivity (Chilba-Mizutani et al., 2007). One cell naturally expresses CD4 and CXCR4, making it susceptible to X4-tropic viruses, and the other cell line, in which a CCR5 expression vector was introduced, is susceptible to both X4- and R5-tropic viruses. Reporter cells were constructed by transfecting the human T-cell line HPB-Ma, which demonstrated high susceptibility to HIV-1, with genomes expressing two different luciferase reporters: HIV-1 long terminal repeat (LTR)-driven firefly luciferase and cytomegalovirus promoter-driven renilla luciferase. The cell lines were also beneficial for screening new antiretroviral agents, as false inhibition caused by the cytotoxicity of test compounds was easily detected by monitoring renilla luciferase activity.

3. HIV-1 enzyme targets

HIV-1 encodes three enzymes required for replication: HIV-1 RT, HIV-1 IN and HIV-1 PT. A number of assays have been developed for screening test compounds against thyese well-known targetrs fir drug discovery. Utilization in screening campaigns of RT or PT enzymes that contain drug resistant mutations is a common strategy for identifying next-generation HIV-1 inhibitors against these targets.

HIV-1 RT is a multifunctional enzyme involved in several essential activities for viral replication (Sarafianos et al., 2009, Herschhorn & Hiz, 2010). These activities include DNA- and RNA-dependent DNA polymerase, ribonuclease H (RNase H), strand transfer and strand displacement activities. RT has been the main target of current antiviral therapies against AIDS. NRTIs have been widely used in HAART, combined with PIs and/or NNRTIs. The high error rates characteristic of HIV-1 RT, however, are a presumed source of the viral hypermutability that contributes mainly to the emergence of resistant variants, although the significant toxicity associated with current anti-HIV drugs also results in treatment failure. These factors in combination drive pharmacologists to develop more potent and less toxic RT inhibitors against the native and drug-resistant variants, which will most certainly remain critical components of future drug regimens.

Although currently marketed agents inhibit the DNA polymerase activity of HIV-1 RT, inhibition of any of the step in the reverse transcription process would result in inhibition of viral replication. Therefore various assays suitable for testing compounds in a high-throughput screening format have been described for measuring the DNA polymerase, RNase H and DNA strand transfer activities of HIV-1 RT.

Examples of isotopic assays for measuring DNA polymerase activity include "microarray compound screening technology", and "scintillation proximity assay technology" (Xuei et al., 2003). Inhibition reverse transcription by targeting the RNase H activity of HIV-1 RT is another approach of interest, since mutations in the NNRTI allosteric domain or the RT active site are not expected to affect inhibitors that bind to the RNase H domain. Although RNase H-mediated cleavage of hybrid RNA/DNA duplex occurs either concurrently with DNA polymerization or independently, most RNase H assays target the latter. Parniak et al. (2003) described a homogeneous "fluorescence resonance energy transfer" (FRET) assay for measuring RNase H activity. The duplex substrate contains a fluorescein label on the 3′-end of the RNA, which is quenched by a Dabcyl label on the 5′-end of the DNA strand. When the substrate is cleaved by RNase H, the interaction between the fluorescein and Dabcyl is removed, resulting in an increase in the fluorescence signal.

A fluorescence polarization (FP) microplate assay for screening compounds against the RNase H activity of HIV-1 RT has also been developed (Nakayama et al., 2006). This homogeneous assay uses a hybrid 18-mer DNA/RNA duplex substrate composed of an RNA oligonucleotide labelled with 6-carboxytetramethyl rhodamine at the 3′-end, thast is annealed to a complementary unlabeled DNA strand substrate cleavage by RNase H to produce small RNA fragments (1-4 mer), resulting in a significant change in the measured FP value.

More recently, a 6-phenylpyrrolocytidine (PhpC)-based assay has been incorporated into high-throughput microplate assay format, and may form the basis for a new screen for inhibitors of HIV-1 RNase H (Wahba et al., 2010). The PhpC-containing RNA formed native-like duplex structures with complementary DNA or RNA. The PhpC-modification was found to act as a sensitive reporter group, and was non-disruptive to structure and the enzymatic activity of RNase H. A RNA/DNA hybrid possessing a single PhpC insert was an excellent substrate for

HIV-1 RT RNase, and rapidly reported cleavage of the RNA strand with a 14-fold increase in fluorescence intensity. The PhpC-based assay for RNase H was superior to the traditional molecular beacon approach in terms of responsiveness, speed and ease.

HIV-IN represents a potential target for the development of new anti-HIV chemotherapeutic agents. This viral enzyme is required for the integration of viral DNA into the host DNA, which catalyzes two reactions known as processing and strand transfer. The viral DNA is first cleaved by HIV IN at a CA dinucleotide at the 3′-end to leave the two-nucleotide overhanging. This step is known as processing. Then, the protein-DNA complex is transported into the nucleus. The host DNA is cleaved to leave a 5′ overhang of five bases, and the 3′-ends of the viral DNA are convalently linked to the 5′-end of the host DNA. Finally, the 5-bases gap between the 5′-end of the viral DNA and the 3′-end of the host DNA is filled in by host cell enzymes. Since IN-negative mutants of HIV do not produce infectious virus particles, and no cellular homologue of HIV IN has been described, IN is considered to be an attractive target. However, in contrast to RT and PT, not a single IN inhibitor has yet entered the anti-HIV drug market. However, using *in vitro* assay systems and the recombinant HIV-1 IN, a variety of HIN IN inhibitors have been identified.

Most currently used assays for HIV-1 IN target the strand transfer process and follow a similar premise. HIV IN is combined with donor dsDNA, which has been immobilized onto a solid support, to form an enzyme/DNA complex. The reaction is then initiated by the addition of target dsDNA labelled in some manner, and after an incubation period, the ligated product is quantified. John et al. (2005) reported a highly efficient and sensitive high-throughput screen, HIV IN Target SRI Assay for HIV-1 IN activity, using 5′ biotin-labelled DNA (5′ BIO donor) and 3′ digoxygenin-labelled DNA (3′ DIG target). Following 3′ processing of the 5′ BIO donor, strand transfer proceeds with integration of the 5′ BIO donor into the 3′ DIG target. The assay was used to screen drugs in a high-throughput format, and the assay was also adapted to study mechanistic questions regarding the integration process. For example, using variations of the assay format, it showed a high preference of the E strand of the LTR viral DNA as a target strand compared with its complementary A strand. Wang et al. (2005) described two homogeneous time-resolved FRET-based assays for the measurement of HIV-1 IN 3′-processing and strand transfer activities. These assays have also proven their utility for the identification of mechanistically interesting and biologically active inhibitors of HIV-1 IN that hold potential for further development into potential antiviral drugs.

In addition to recombinant enzyme screens, biochemical assays have been developed that measure HIV-1 IN activity in the context of the preintegration complex (PIC), which mediates the integration of the retroviral genome into host cell DNA. The HIV PIC is a large nucleoprotein complex containing the viral CDNA and IN as well as matrix Vpr, RT and a number of host proteins including histones and members of the non-homologous end joining pathway. It is possible that screening for PIC activity, analogous to that in a true infection, may offer an expanded set of targets and yield more biologically relevant compounds. A polymerase chain reaction-based assay for integration has been reported which employs HIV-1 PICs derived from cells infected with single-cycle HIV-1 reporter viruses.

4. HIV-1 protease

In a later stage of the HIV-1 life cycle, HIV PT hydrolyzes precursor polyproteins into functional proteins that are essential for viral assembly and subsequent activity. HIV-1 Gag and Pol polypeptide precursors are cleaved by the viral encoded aspartyl protease to form the mature structural and enzymatic gene products. During virus assembly, the viral Gag polyprotein must be effectively processed and transported to the cell membrane. Cofactors such as the phospholipid phosphatidylinositol (4,5) biphosphate, the ADP ribosylation factor binding proteins or tumour susceptibility gene 101, are required for the intracellular transport and budding of HIV particles. While these are just a few examples of virus-host cell interactions, each one represents a potential new target under rigorous research with their validation being actively pursued.

The functional structure of HIV-1 PT is a homodimer containing an active site created in the cleft between the monomers as part of a four-stranded β turn. The active site region is capped by two identical β-hairpin loops (the flaps, residues 45-55 in each monomer), which undergo significant conformational changes upon substrate binding. All PIs currently licensed for the treatment of HIV infections mimic the substrate and block the active site. Another strategy is to develop compounds that bind to the subunit interface and thus block dimerization. As a result, drug discovery efforts continue to focus on the identification of new inhibitors against this validated target that are active against HIV-1 variants which are resistant to the currently available HIV-1 PIs. In line with these efforts, the assays described here may be conducted with wild-type proteins or variants that contain mutations conferring resistance to current HIV-1 PIs.

FRET assays are more commonly used for HIV-1 PT. Synthetic peptide substrates typically consist of a cleavage sequence flanked with fluorescent donor and acceptor labels. The fluorescence signal is low in the intact peptide because the donor is quenched by the nearby acceptor. Once the substrate is cleaved by HIV-1 PT, the FRET interaction is removed, and the fluorescence increases. Hamilton et al. (2003) described a biochemical detection method for peptide products of enzymatic reactions, based on the formation of PSD95/Disc-large/ZO-1 (PDZ) domain* peptide ligand complexes. The product sensor involves using masked or cryptic PDZ domain peptide ligands as enzyme substrates. The practical applicability of this PDZ-based detection method is determined by the affinity of the PDZ* peptide ligand interaction, and the efficiency of the enzyme to process the masked peptide ligand. These results showed that the Na^+/H^+ exchanger regulatory factor, which binds to the consensus sequence Thr/Ser-X-Leu-COOH, can be used to extend the flexibility in the recognition of the carboxy-terminal amino acid of the ligand, and monitor the enzymatic activity of HIV PT.

In addition to enzyme assays, a number of cell-based assays have been reported for HIV-1 PT. A green fluorescent protein (GFP)-PT chimera was developed that can be expressed in mammalian cells, causing minimal toxicity until autocatalytic cleavage occurs (Lindsten et al., 2001). The precursor is activated *in vivo* by autocatalytic cleavage, resulting in rapid elimination of PT-expressing cells. Treatment with therapeutic doses of HIV-1 PIs results in a dose-dependent accumulation of the fluorescent precursor that can be easily detected and quantified by flow cytometric and fluorimetric assays. More recently, Majerova-Uhlikova et al. (2006) described a new assay that might serve as a non-infectious, rapid, cheap and reliable alternative to the currently used phenotypic assays. These investigations showed that in the GFP-PT reporter, the HIV wild-type PT can be replaced by a drug-resistant HIV PT mutant, yielding a simple and biologically relevant tool for the quantitative analysis of drug-resistant HIV PT mutant susceptibility to HIV PTs.

5. HIV-1 replication screens

Although biochemical high-throughput screening and structure-based drug design approaches are currently preferred over holistic approaches, HIV-1 replication screens have historically been used to identify antiviral compounds. HIV-1 replication assays offer the advantage of screening for multiple targets in the context of a natural infection.

As the methodology used in the determination of the antiviral activity and the interpretation of the results have been virtually specific to each laboratory and are thus not comparable to one another, simple procedures and guidelines for evaluating antiviral and/or virucidal activities of compounds are needed. Various cell culture-based assays are currently available and can be successfully applied for the antiviral or virucidal determination of substances. Antiviral agents interfere with one or more dynamic processes during virus biosynthesis, making them candidates for clinically useful antiviral drugs; whereas virucidal substances inactivate virus infectivity extracellularly and are therefore better candidates for antiseptics, exhibiting a broad spectrum of germicidal activities.

Cost, simplicity, accuracy and reproducibility are the key factors determining the selection of the assay system, but selectivity, specificity and sensitivity also need to be taken into account. The methods commonly used for evaluation of *in vitro* antiviral activities are based on the different abilities of viruses to replicate in cultured cells. Some viruses can cause cytopathic effect (CPE) or form plaques. Others are capable of producing specialized functions or cell transformation. Virus replications in cell culture may also be monitored by the detection of viral products such as viral DNA, RNA or polypeptides. Thus, the antiviral test selected may be based on inhibition of CPE, reduction or inhibition of plaque formation.

Several different HIV-1 replication assays have been described that could be adapted for medium-to-high-throughput screening. Such assays can generally be subdivided into one of three categories: reporter virus assays, reporter cell assays or cell protection assays.

In reporter virus assays, a reporter gene is introduced into the virus genome, usually in place of a viral gene not required for replication, in the target cells of interest. The concept of using HIV-1 reporter viruses to monitor HIV-1 replication was first introduced using a replication competent HIV-1 reporter virus containing the chloramphenicol acetyltransferase gene in place of HIV-1 Nef sequences. Cells are then infected with the recombinant reporter virus and virus replication is quantified by measuring the expression of the virally encoded reporter gene (Adelson et al., 2003; Dey & Berger, 2003).

For reporter cell assays, the target cells of interest are engineered to contain a reporter gene, which is activated upon viral infection. Virus replication is measured by monitoring induction of the reporter gene in the infected target cells. These assays have been used for some time to monitor HIV-1 infection and measure the activity of HIV-1 inhibitors. Kremb et al. (2010) presented a full HIV-replication system for the identification and analysis of HIV inhibitors. This technology is based on adherently growing HIV-susceptible cells, with a stable fluorescent reporter gene activated by HIV Tat and Rev. A fluorescence-based assay was designed to measure HIV infection through two parameters relating to the early and the late phases of HIV replication respectively. These results concluded that this technology is a versatile tool for the discovery and characterization of HIV inhibitors. Reporter cell assays have also been adapted to allow analysis of CCR5 as well as CXCR4 tropic HIV strains (Miyake et al., 2003).

In cell protection assays, CPE resulting from virus replication are measured by determining cell viability using a dye reduction method. These assays represent a more conventional approach to antiviral screening and have been used successfully to execute antiviral screens and identify new HIV-1 inhibitors. Although cell protection assay formats have been available for some time, they continue to be the cornerstone of many HIV-1 drug discovery programs.

6. Acknowledgements

The technical assistance of Ms. Brooke-Turner is gratefully acknowledged.

7. References

Adelson, M.E., Pacchia, A.L., Kaul, M., Rando, R.F., Ron, Y., Peltz, S.W., Dougherty, J.P. (2003). Toward the development of a virus-cell-based assay for the discovery of novel compounds against human immunodeficiency virus type 1. *Antimicrob. Agents Chemother.*, 47, 2, (February 2003), 501-508, ISSN 1098:6596

Buonaguro, L., Tornesello, M.L., Buonaguro, F.M. (2007). Human immunodeficiency virus type 1 subtype distribution in the Worlwide epidemic: pathogenetic and therapeutic implications. *J. Virol.*, 81, 19, (October 2007), 10209-10219, ISSN 0022-538X

Chilba-Mizutani, T., Mivra, H., Matsuda, M., Matsuda, Z., Yokomaku, Y., Miyauchi, K., Nishizawa, M., Yamamoto, N., Sigiura, W. (2007). Use of new T-cell-based cell lines expressing two luciferase reporters for accurately evaluating susceptibility to anti-human immunodeficiency virus type 1 drugs. *J. Clin. Microbiol.*, 45, 2, (February 2007), 477-487, ISSN 0095-1137

Dey, B., Berger, E.A. (2003). Current Protocols in Immunology, In: *Detection and Analysis of HIV*, Straber, W., 10, John Wiley & Sons, Inc., ISBN1934-368X, Sussex, England

Grande, F., Garofalo, A., Neamati, N. (2008). Small molecules anti-HIV therapeutics targeting CXCR4. *Curr. Pharm. Des.*, 14, 4, (April 2008), 385-404, ISSN 1381-6128

Greene, W.C., Debyser, Z., Ikeda, Y., Freed, E.O., Stephens, E., Yonemoto, W., Buckheit, R.W., Este, J.A., Cihlar, T. (2008). Novel targets for HIV therapy. *Antiviral Res.*, 80, 3, (December 2008), 251-265, ISSN 0166-3542

Hamilton, A.C., Inglese, J., Ferrer, M. (2003). A PDZ domain-based assay for measuring HIV protease activity: assay design considerarions. *Protein Sci.*, 12, 3, (March 2003), 458-467, ISSN 1469-896X

Herschhorn, A., Hiz, A. (2010). Retroviral reverse transcriptases. *Cell Mol. Life Sci.*, 67, 16, (August 2010), 2717-2747, ISSN 1420-682X

John, S., Fletcher, T.M., Jonsson, C.B. (2005). Development and application of a high-throughput screening assay for HIV-1 integrase enzyme activities. *J. Biomol. Screen.*, 10, 6, (September 2005), 606-614, ISSN 1087-0571

Kremb, S., Helfer, M., Heller, W., Hoffmann, D., Wolff, H., Kleinschmidt, A., Cepok, S., Hemmer, B., Durner, J., Brack-Werner, R. (2010). EASY-HIT: HIV full-replication technology for broad discovery of multiple classes of HIV inhibitors. *Antimicrob. Agents Chemother.*, 54, 12, (December 2010), 5257-5268, ISSN 1098:6596

Liang, X. (2008). CXCR4 inhibitors and mechanism of action. *Chem. Biol. Drug Des.*, 72, 2, (August 2008), 97-110, ISSN 1747-0285

Lindsten, K., Uhlikova, T., Konvalinka, J., Masucci, M.G., Dantuna, N.P. (2001). Cell-based fluorescence assay for human immunodeficiency virus type 1 protease activity. *Antimicrob. Agents Chemother.*, 45, 9, (September 2001), 2616-2622, ISSN 1098:6596

Majerova-Uhlikova, T., Dantuma, N.P., Lindstein, K., Masucci, M.G., Konvalinka, J. (2006). Non-infectious fluorimetric assay for phenotyping of drug-resistant HIV proteinase mutants. *J. Clin. Virol.*, 36, 1, (May 2006), 50-59, ISSN 1386-6532

Marchand, C., Maddali, K., Metifiot, M., Pammier, Y. (2009). HIV-1 IN inhibitors 2010 update and perspectives. *Curr. Top. Med. Chem.*, 9, 11, (November 2009), 1016-1037, ISSN 1568-0266

Menéndez-Arias, L., Tözser, J. (2008). HIV-1 protease inhibitors: effects on HIV-2 replication and resistance. *Trends Pharmacol. Sci.*, 29, 1, (January 2008), 42-49, ISSN 0165-6147

Miyake, H., Iizawa, Y., Baba, M. (2003). Novel reporter T-cell line highly susceptible to both CCR5- and CXCR4-using human immunodeficiency virus type 1 and its application to drug susceptibility tests. *J. Clin. Microbiol.*, 41, 6, (June 2003), 2515-2521, ISSN 0095-1137

Nakayama, G.R., Binghom, P., Tan, D., Maegley, K.A. (2006). A fluorescence polarization assay for screening inhibitors against the ribonuclease H activity of HIV-1 reverse transcriptase. *Anal. Biochem.*, 351, 2, (April 2006), 260-265, ISSN 0003-2697

Ochsenbauer-Jambor, C., Jones, J., Heil, M., Zammit, K.P., Kutsch, O. (2006). T-cell line for HIV drug screening using EGFP as a quantitative marker of HIV-1 replication. *Bio Techniques*, 40, 1, (January 2006), 91-100, ISSN 0736-6205

Pang, W., Tam, S.C., Zheng, Y.T. (2009). Current peptide HIV type-1 fusion inhibitors. *Antivir. Chem. Chemother.*, 20, 1, (January 2009), 1-18, ISSN 0956-3202

Parniak, M.A., Min, K.L., Budihas, S.R., Le Grice, S.F.J., Beutle, J.A. (2003). A fluorescence based high throughput screening assay for inhibitors of human immunodeficiency virus-1 reverse transcriptase-associated ribonuclease H activity. *Anal. Biochem.*, 322, 1, (November 2003), 33-39, ISSN 0003-2697

Romani, B., Engelbrecht, S. (2009). Human immunodeficiency virus type 1 Vpr: functions and molecular interactions. *J. Gen. Virol.*, 90, 8, (August 2009), 1795-1805, ISSN 0022-1317

Romani, B., Engelbrecht, S., Glashoff, R.H. (2010). Functions of Tat: the versatile protein of human immunodeficiency virus type 1. *J. Gen. Virol.*, 91, 1, (January 2010), 1-12, ISSN 0022-1317

Sarafianos, S.G., Marchand, B., Das, K., Himmel, D.M., Parniak, M.A., Hughes, S.H., Arnold, E. (2009). Structure and function of HIV-reverse transcriptase: molecular mechanism of polymerization and inhibition. *J. Mol. Biol.*, 385, 3, (January 2009), 693-713, ISSN 0022-2836

Tan, J.J., Cong, X.J., Hu, L.M., Wang, C.X., Jia, L., Liang, X.J. (2010). Therapeutic strategies underpinning the development of novel techniques for the treatment of HIV infection. *Drug Discover. Today*, 15, 5/6, (March 2010), 186-197, ISSN 1359-6446

Wahba, A.S., Esmaeili, A., Damha, M.J., Hudson, R.M. (2010). A single-label phenylpyrrolocytidine provides a molecular beacon-like response reporting HIV-1 RT RNase H activity. *Nucleic Acid Res.*, 38, 3, (January 2010), 1048-1056, ISSN 0305-1048

Wang, Y., Klock, H., Yin, H., Wolff, K., Bieza, K., Niswonger, K., Matzen, J., Gunderson, D., Hale, J., Lesley, S., Kuhen, K., Caldwell, J., Brinker, A. (2005). Homogeneous high-throughput screening assays for HIV-1 integrase 3β-processing and strand transfer activities. *J. Biomol. Screen.*, 10, 5, (August 2005), 456-462, ISSN 1087-0571

Wang, T., Duan, Y. (2009). HIV co-receptor CCR5: structure and interactions with inhibitors. *Infect. Disord. Drug Targets*, 9, 3, (March 2009), 279-288, ISSN 1871-5265

Warnke, D., Barreto, J. (2007). Antiretroviral drugs. *J. Clin. Pharmacol.*, 47, 12, (December 2007), 1570-1579, ISSN 0091-2700

Westby, M., Nakayama, G.R., Butler, S.L., Blair, W.S. (2005). Cell-based and biochemical screening approaches for the discovery of novel HIV-1 inhibitors. *Antiviral Res.*, 67, 3, (September 2005), 121-140, ISSN 0166-3542

Xuei, X., David, C.A., Middleton, T.R., Lim, B., Pithawalla, R., Chen, C.M., Tripathi, R.L., Burns, D.J., Warrior, V. (2003). Use of SAM2® biotin capture membrane in microarrayed compound screening (μARCS) format for nucleic acid polymerization assays. *J. Biomol. Screen.*, 8, 3, (June 2003), 273-282, ISSN 1087-0571

Zhan, P., Lia, X., Li, Z. (2009). Recent advances in the discovery and development of novel HIV-1 NNRTI platforms: 2006-2008 update. *Curr. Med. Chem.*, 16, 22, (July 2009), 2876-2889, ISSN 0929-8673

Zhao, Q., Lu, H., Schols, D., De Clercq, E., Jiang, S. (2003). Development of a cell-based enzyme-linked immunosorbent assay for high-throughput screening of HIV type entry inhibitors targeting the coreceptor CXCR4. *AIDS Res. Hum. Retroviruses*, 19, 11, (November 2003), 947-955, ISSN 0889-2229

Part 8

Vaccine Development

23

HIV Vaccine

Alexandre de Almeida, Telma Miyuki Oshiro,
Alessandra Pontillo and Alberto José da Silva Duarte
University of São Paulo
Brazil

1. Introduction

More than three decades after the discovery of Human Immunodeficiency Virus (HIV) as the causative agent of Acquired Immunodeficiency Syndrome (AIDS), a vaccine is still considered as the best hope for controlling the epidemic. In fact the history of medicine shows that no viral disease have ever been controlled without a vaccine.

Remarkable success in the AIDS treatment has been achieved with the development of antiretroviral drugs that, by interfering with various aspects of the HIV life cycle, allowed an impressive control of infection (Fischl et al., 1987; Egger et al., 1997). The use of these drugs, however, was accompanied by new challenges related to side effects, high cost and resistance development (Carr, 2000; Hawkins, 2010; Menéndez-Arias, 2010; www.hivresourcetracking.org/treatments/vaccines).

Antiretroviral treatment cannot prevent early infection events, such as transmission to sexual partners during the post-infection peak of viremia (Wawer et al., 1999) and the massive destruction of intestinal CD4+T cells during the first weeks of infection (Brenchley et al., 2004). Furthermore drugs delivery to poor and endemic areas is often hard due to practical limitations. In resource-limited countries only 1 out 4 HIV-positive individuals has access to antiretroviral medications, and for each person who begins the therapy, there are about 6 new infections (www.who.int/entity/hiv/mediacentre/universal_access_progress_report_en.pdf). These factors made difficult to control the pandemic through antiretroviral therapy.

Others approaches could be taken in account to reduce HIV-1 infection in subjects at risk of exposure, including public health involvement (i.e.: screening of donor blood products), educational effort (i.e.: risk reduction counselling), or social imprinting (i.e.: male circumcision and behaviour modifications such as condom usage). In high seropositive communities, pre-exposure or post-exposure antiretroviral prophylaxis may reduce susceptibility to HIV infection, as well as the vertical HIV transmission from mother to child.

The creation of an HIV-1 vaccine represents an unprecedented scientific challenge and it's an absolute priority in field of HIV prevention. We must remember that vaccines are one of the most effective public health interventions ever known, but unfortunately, in HIV infection, the current perspective is that we will not have a product, even moderately effective, in the coming years.

The truth is that often in the history of vaccinology it takes a long time since the discovery of infectious agents to the licensing of an effective vaccine (Heyward et al., 1998). This is due in part to the fact that even today no one knows for sure how the immune system protects us against infections and, consequently, how to handle it for this to occur. In HIV/AIDS, the stimulation of a specific immune response is unlikely to immunize against HIV: there are no established immune correlates of protection (i.e.: humoral or cellular response), no documented cases of spontaneous recovery from AIDS or HIV infection, and no animal model that faithfully predicts HIV disease or vaccine responses in humans beyond the variability of the virus. Moreover HIV entries predominantly through mucosal surfaces, targets preferentially CD4+T cells, and rapidly establishes a persistent reservoir of latently infected cells, making difficult the study of the host/virus interaction as well as the development of an interventional strategy.

Novel approaches for an HIV vaccination need a rational vaccine design, including a better integration of emerging scientific concepts and knowledge derived from vaccinology research fields.

Models of natural resistance to HIV infection, including individuals able to control the infection (elite controllers) and some species of non-human primates, show that some level of control can be achieved (Dunham et al., 2006; Sumpter et al., 2007; Walker, 2007; Lederman et al., 2010; Poropatich & Sullivan, 2011).

The creation of an effective HIV vaccine will require continued scientific research and cooperation between academic community and biotechnology industry with the contributions of brightest scientists, long-term commitments of stable and flexible funding, trials and vaccines accessibility for developing countries. In coming years, the prospect is that several area of scientific community will be involved seeking to combine the knowledge necessary to develop new strategies, new candidates and evaluating these products.

This chapter will describe some aspects of the development of HIV vaccines, with emphasis on scientific efforts and challenges made to producing a safe and effective vaccine, strategies and methods used in the development of anti-HIV vaccines, current outlook and perspectives in this area.

2. Major challenges to get an HIV vaccine

Primary in prevention and control of infectious diseases, vaccines are a highly effective way to stimulate the immune system to fight pathogens. In the case of HIV infection, it has not yet been possible to obtain a vaccine to control infection, despite the efforts of the scientific community, the large financial investment and scientific and technological progress achieved.

Considering the natural history of infection, an HIV vaccine has the principal aim to prevent the integration of HIV genetic material into the genome of the host cell in order to prevent systemic infection and the establishment of viral reservoirs. This occurs within a few days after exposure, when HIV rapidly replicates in the lymphoid tissues, so the window of opportunity to prevent the establishment of a persistent infection is very brief. Therefore an effective HIV vaccine should be able to activate the immune system against the virus very early after the infection.

The complexity and diversity of HIV, its high capacity to evade the immune system and the missing gap in effective host immune response against the virus represent some major challenges to design an optimal vaccine. Moreover the absence of an experimental model able to mimic human infection represents another limit for pre-clinical studies.

2.1 HIV heterogeneity and cell targets

HIV presents a genome of about 10,000 base pairs, composed of three structural genes (*gag*, *pol* and *env*) beyond the six accessory genes (*vif,vpr*, *rev*, *tat,vpu* and *nef*). The *gag* gene encodes the viral core protein as the capsid, matrix and nucleocapsid, *pol* encodes the viral enzymes (reverse transcriptase, protease, ribonuclease and integrase) and *env* gene encodes the envelope glycoproteins. Some products of these genes are targets of choice for the study of vaccines.

The great genetic diversity of HIV represents a major obstacle to developing an effective vaccine. Such diversity is the result of a highly HIV replicative rate (new 10^{10} viral particles/day) and of its prone to errors retrotranscriptase (1 new nucleotide substitution/replication for a genome of approximately 10 000 bp).

The highest degree of HIV diversity is found in the envelope glycoproteins. The amino acid sequences of Env may differ by about 15% between isolates of the same clade and in more than 35% between envelopes of different clades (Gaschen et al 2002).

As a consequence of this high degree of mutational rate, HIV can counteract the selective pressure imposed by the host immune response, and it soon become able to evade an effective response. This aspect makes it difficult to identify potential HIV targets against which the immune system could be directed.

Another important point is that an effective vaccine may protect against various HIV subtypes and clades prevalent in every region of the world. HIV is classified into two types: HIV-1 and HIV-2 that have a genetic homology around 40-50%. While HIV-2 is less pathogenic and its incidence is confined to Africa, HIV-1 is the causative agent of a worldwide pandemic. HIV-1 is divided into three groups M, O and N. The groups O and N are restricted to Central Africa, while group M is responsible for the AIDS pandemic.

Within group M, HIV-1 isolates are divided into six subtypes and clades (A, B, C, D, E and G) and have distinct geographic distributions. While subtype B is prevalent in the Americas and Europe, subtype C, which accounts for more than 50% of AIDS cases worldwide, is prevalent in Southeast Asia and Africa. The difference between the amino acid sequences among viral clades differs by 20% and the variation within clades can reach over 10% in amino acid sequence. Furthermore, different subtypes may be associated with generating circulating recombinant forms (CRFs), further increasing the viral diversity.

Another major challenge that hinders the design of an effective vaccine is the HIV tropism for immune cells. HIV uses the CD4 molecule as a receptor for cell entry. This molecule, in turn, is expressed mainly by T helper lymphocytes and to a lesser degree by dendritic cells, macrophages and monocytes. Since these are strategic cells within the immune system, the immune response in HIV-infected individuals is compromised (Figure1).

Belonging to retroviruses, HIV integrates its genetic material into host cell genome. Days after infection the virus begins its haematogenous spreading from mucosal to lymphoid sites, particularly gut-associated lymphoid tissue (GALT) where a lot of CD4+ CCR5+ T memory lymphocytes are destructed (Matapallil et al., 2005).

The massive loss of CD4+ T cells compromises the host immune response during the infection. Moreover, since the HIV genome is integrated latently until cells become activated, establishing viral reservoirs that hinder the complete elimination of infection.

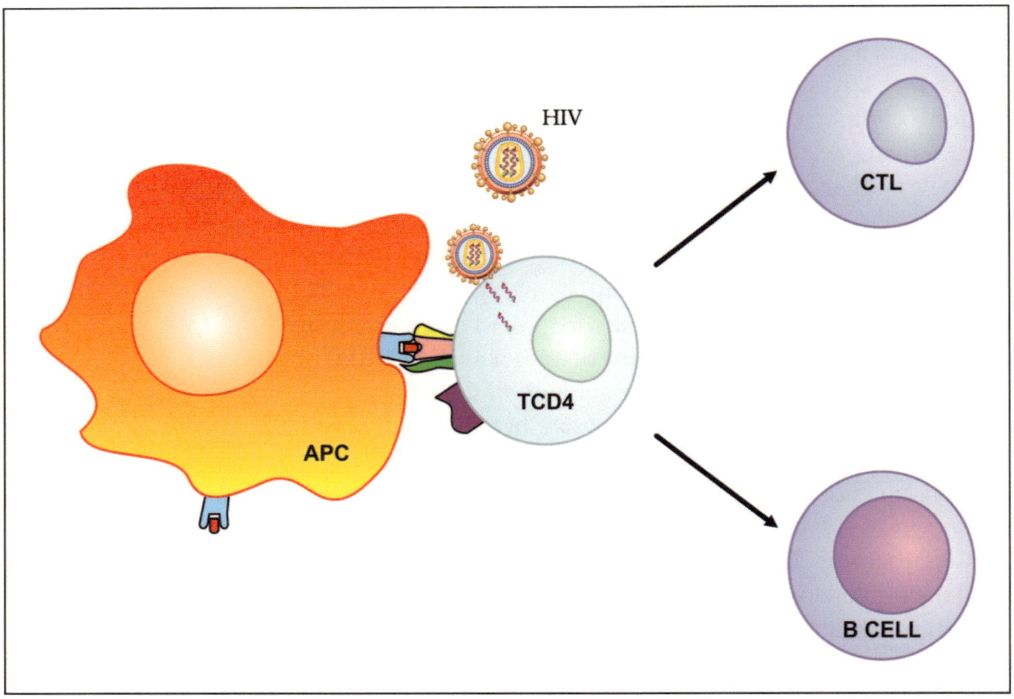

Fig. 1. HIV cell target. HIV predominantly infects CD4+ lymphocytes, which play a fundamental role in the induction of specific immune response.
APC: Antigen-presenting cell
CTL: Cytotoxic T lymphocyte

2.2 Host/virus interaction

A key feature of the immune system is to "remember" and respond to antigens with which they've previously met. This property, called immunological memory, is the basis of the vaccination process. To play its role, a vaccine must therefore deliver the antigen to the immune system in order to stimulate it and to enable the development of memory.
In this sense, a basic problem in developing an HIV vaccine is the lack of definition of the correlates of immune protection in HIV infection, so that is not completely clear what types of immune response should ideally be stimulated by vaccination and consequently what measure and criteria should be used to evaluate the effectiveness of the vaccine.
Initially the first strategies implied to obtain an HIV vaccine were focused on inducing neutralizing antibodies against the viral envelope proteins (Dolin, 1995) and from mid-1990, studies began to focus on the activation of a cellular immune response.
Stimulation of neutralizing antibodies with broad specificity for all HIV variants would be definitely interesting for a vaccine strategy. Evidence in nonhuman primates suggest that a protection could be afforded if neutralizing antibodies could be present in high concentration both in blood and mucosa at the time of first infection (Parren et al., 2001). However, the induction of neutralizing antibodies against HIV is hampered by some specific characteristics of the virus, such as

a. The high epitopes mutation rate, which causes loss of recognition capacity by antibodies;

b. The large number of subtypes of HIV that exhibit little cross-reactivity;
c. The high rate of glycosylation on the viral envelope
d. The existence of hidden CD4/receptor binding sites which difficult the access of the antibodies. (Figure 2)

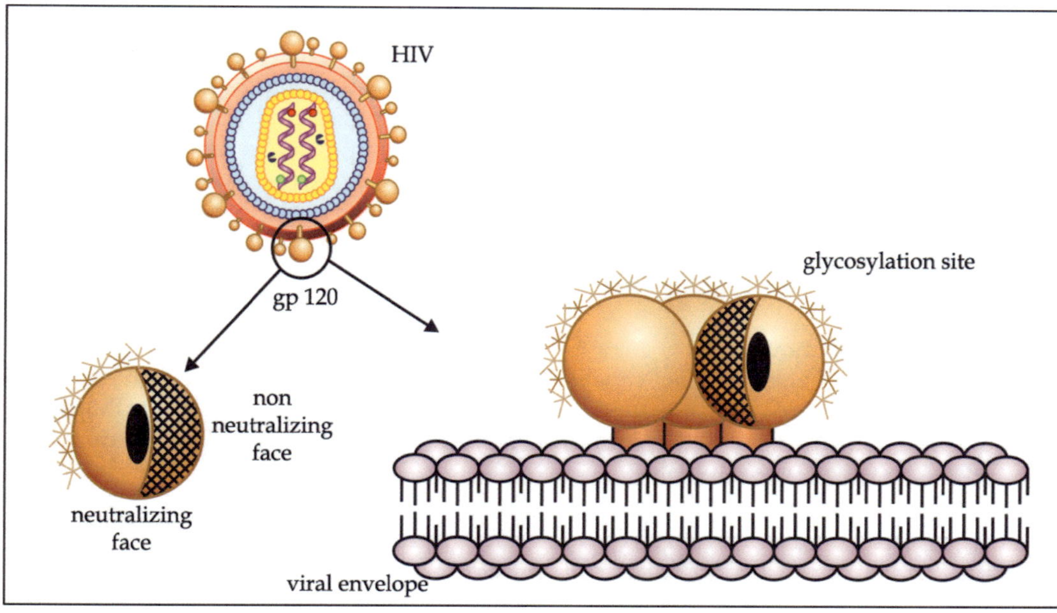

Fig. 2. Sites of antibody binding to gp120. Neutralizing and non-neutralizing sites of gp120. The sites of glycosylation of the molecule are also shown.

Considering that HIV infects CD4+ T cells, the stimulation of a cellular response is important for the destruction of infected cells by cytotoxic T lymphocytes (CTLs) before the release of new viral particles. Thus, in a context of an anti-HIV vaccine CD4+ T cells should be rapidly expanded to stimulate the right cytotoxic response against infected cells and drive memory cells to sites potentially susceptible to infection such as mucosal and lymph nodes.
Although many studies provide strong evidence that a cellular response can effectively suppress HIV (Rowland-Jones et al., 1998; Hladik et al., 2003), it remains unclear how this viral suppression occurs and how a vaccine could stimulate it. Peculiar characteristics of the virus and the nature of infection hinder the development of an appropriate cellular response, for example,

a. The reduction of the expression of MHC class I molecules mediated by the HIV Nef protein;
b. The establishment and maintenance of latent viral reservoirs in cells
c. The massive destruction of T cells specific or not for HIV, caused mainly by activation-induced apoptosis. (Cadogan & Dalgleish, 2008).

In this context, even though there are not clear evidences regarding the type of immune response to be induced by an HIV vaccine, it is reasonable to assume that elements of the immune response important to ensure a real effectiveness of an HIV vaccine may depend on both neutralizing antibody and specific cellular immunity, and besides, also on innate immunity. In a simplified view, neutralizing antibodies prevent the entry of virus into the

cell by blocking the transmission and infection, while the cellular response would act destroying HIV-infected cells before the release of new viral particles in order to control an yet established infection.
Another interesting tips is that being mucosal the primary site of natural HIV infection (Kozlowski & Neutra, 2003) an effective vaccine must induce anti-HIV-1 neutralizing antibodies at mucosal surfaces to prevent the infection and cytotoxic T lymphocytes (CTLs) in sub-mucosal areas to kill virus-infected cells, or a combination of both. Unfortunately, the immune response within the mucosa may be associated with a high viral replication and dissemination: HIV activates and recruits a lot of target cells and the virus uptake by dendritic cells allow its dissemination to draining lymph nodes avoiding antibody recognition. The challenge to an effective vaccine is to activate mucosal immunity at the right time. Moreover, all mucosal vaccines have to overcome tolerance, which is related with regulatory cells and depend on the nature of the antigen, the dosage, the method of delivery and on whether or not adjuvant is used.

2.3 Lack of animal models

Actually there is no animal model capable of to mimic the human HIV infection and AIDS development. The use of animal models could help the investigation of disease pathogenesis and provide information about toxicity and efficacy of drugs and vaccines to reduce risk, duration and cost of a clinical trial.
Despite its relatively low cost and ease of maintenance in animal houses, the use of small rodents as experimental models for HIV infection is not appropriate since HIV is unable to sustain infection in murine cells. More recently it has been demonstrated the use of humanized mice models (Van Duyne et al., 2009).
Studies in non-human primates (NHP; i.e.: *Macaca rhesus*), when allowed, even if expensive, gave some good results and have the advantage of sharing a high genetic background with humans. NHP are the natural host of a retrovirus of the same HIV family, SIV (Simian Immunodeficiency Virus) which has a very low mutational rate compared to HIV. In some studies the SHIV, a hybrid virus composed of parts of the genome of HIV and SIV, has been implied to create the infection model (Stapransan et al, 2010).
Although providing crucial information about viral immunobiology and vaccine design, it must be taken in account that important differences in the viral infection exist between humans and NHP. Data from NHP models should be critically evaluated for their predictive value in human trials (Shedlock et al., 2009).

3. Strategies and methods used in the development of anti-HIV vaccines

Like most vaccines, candidates for HIV vaccine contained weakened or killed forms of the virus or viral components which resembling original HIV and could be able to stimulate the immune system to develop an appropriate response. Taking in account all these considerations, in the past decades several aspects related to the vaccine composition, route of immunization and vaccine strategy have been tested in the effort to develop an effective HIV vaccine.

3.1 Vaccine composition

3.1.1 Immunogen production

Many techniques have been employed in order to produce relevant immunogenic HIV antigens, such as:

- chemical (eg. alcohols) or heat inactivated virus particles;
- viral proteins or peptides artificially synthesized (mimetopos) or produced by the insertion of relevant genes in biological vectors (recombinants);
- proteins expressed in the form of virus like particles (VLP), consisting of structurally preserved viral epitopes (i.e.: parts of the virus surface proteins), without the viral genetic material, thus preventing their replication.
- HIV genetic material to insert directly into cells that will express their products. Usually this material is inserted in the form of plasmids, which are molecules of extra-chromosomal circular DNA, with independent replication. The insertion of genetic material in the body can be made directly (eg. electroporation or gene guns using compressed gas) or through biological vectors.

Live attenuated virus vaccines have not been investigated in anti-HIV vaccines due to the risk of development of virulence, as evidenced in a model of NHP (Whatmore et al., 1995).

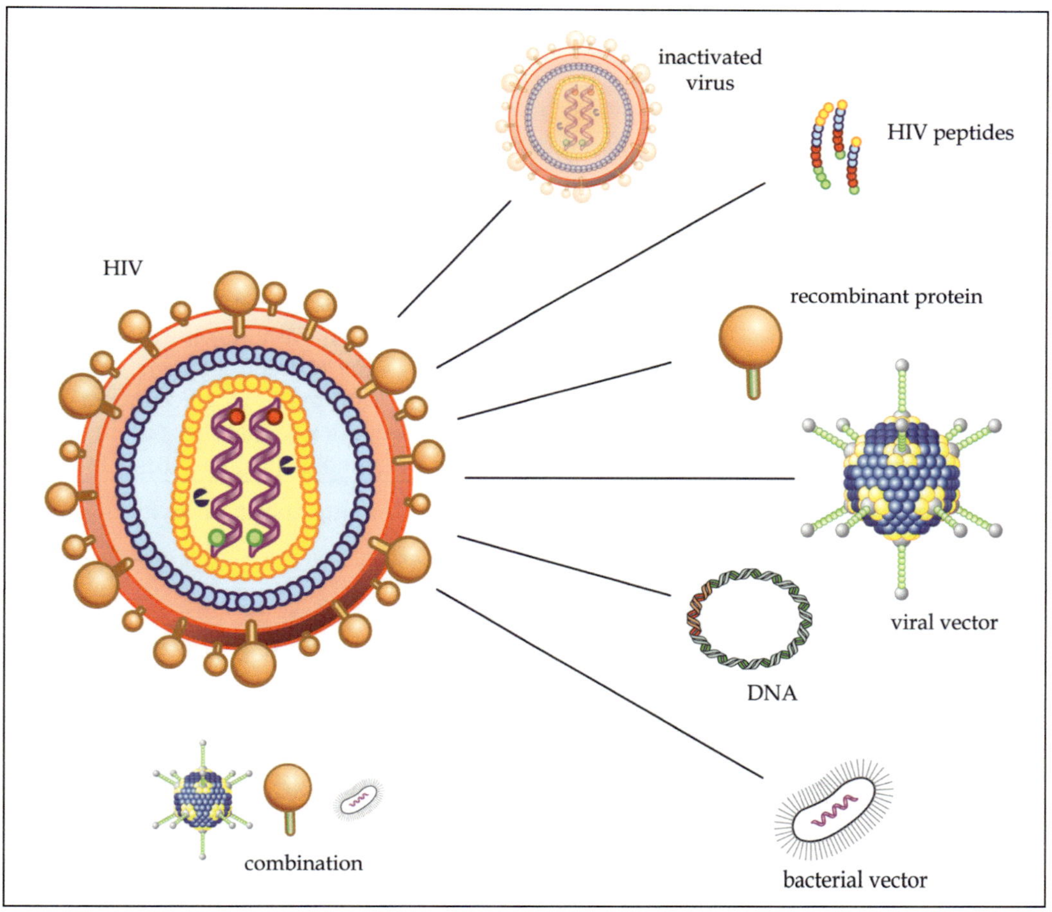

Fig. 3. Immunogens used in the composition of HIV vaccines. There are three types of immunogens: whole vital particle, peptides or recombinant proteins and genetic material of the virus, which may or may not be inserted within vectors. Sometimes the combination of different immunogens can be used (prime-boost strategy).

The advantages and disadvantages of some types of immunogens used in the development of HIV vaccines are summarized in Table 1.

PRODUCT	ADVANTAGE	DISADVANTAGE
Inactivated virus	- whole virus is included in the vaccine	-risk that the preparation contains active virus - difficult to produce in large scale -the response induced by chance is directed only to the type of virus
Peptide	-production relatively simple and inexpensive -safe	-un representative in terms of immunogenic epitopes
Recombinant proteins	-production relatively simple -safe	-low immunogenic
DNA	-production relatively simple and inexpensive	-there are gaps of knowledge about the integration of DNA in the human genome -low immunogenic
Vaccines based on biological vectors	-safe -it is possible to control the type and amount of HIV protein	- limited ability to incorporate HIV genes (in the case of viral vectors) - limited immunogenicity by the existence of prior immunity to the vector - production platforms more complex (viral vectors)

Table 1. Advantages and disadvantages of some types of immunogens used in the development of HIV vaccines

3.1.2 Adjuvants

A vaccine adjuvant is a component that potentiates the immune responses to an antigen and/or modulates it towards the desired immune responses (i.e.: with respect to immunoglobulin classes and induction of cytotoxic or helper T lymphocyte responses). In addition, certain adjuvants can be used to promote antibody responses at mucosal surfaces.
Activation of innate immune system and in particular of dendritic cells (DCs) is a crucial mechanism by which adjuvants stimulate protective adaptive immunity against the vaccine antigen.
As immune response is typically initiated by activation of antigen presenting cells (APCs), notably dendritic cells (DCs). There has been significant interest in improving APC-stimulating adjuvants as a key step in constructing better vaccines
Adjuvants have several forms, ranging from mineral salts such as alum to oil-based emulsions. Moreover molecular adjuvants such as proteins, lipids, nucleic acids, carbohydrates, or chemical compounds have a known receptor in DCs (i.e.: Toll Like

receptors - TLRs) and result in an improvement in the quantity or quality of the ensuing immune response (Kornbluth & Stone, 2006).

CLASS	EXAMPLE
CD40 agonists	CD40L or its derivates, Agonistic anti-CD40 antibodies, Heat shock protein (Hsp70)
NKT cell ligand	CD1d-binding NKT
TLRs agonists	poly(I:C), LPS, and imidazoquinolines act on TLR3, TLR4, and TLR7 (mDCs) imidazoquinolines and CpG ODP act on TLR7 and TLR9 (pDCs) flagellin act on TLR5 (Vassilieva et al., 2011)
NLRs agonists	MDP act on NOD2 and NALP3, extracellular ATP and pathogen RNA act on NALP3
Chemokines	MIP-1a, CCL19/EBI1-ligand and CCL21/SLC

Table 2. Molecular adjuvants for HIV vaccine strategy.

Many adjuvants have been developed in the past, but were never accepted for routine vaccination because of safety concerns (e.g. acute toxicity and the possibility of delayed side effects).

3.2 Route of administration

Vaccine delivery systems are the sum of pharmacologic technologies (including drug preparation, route of administration, site targeting, metabolism and toxicity) and have the principal aim to make the vaccine preparation faster and easier available to immune system. In its broadest sense, the concept of vaccine delivery systems can be expanded to include a diverse range of devices and physical delivery systems that are designed to improve the potency of vaccines or to allow immunization using novel, non-invasive routes (eg. gene-gun approach, devices designed to fire powdered vaccines into the skin through the use of helium gas and vaccine patches). Delivery systems may function to improve antigen access to lymph nodes in a number of ways:

a. increase antigens presenting cells (APCs), generally dendritic cells (DC), infiltration into the injection site;
b. promote the uptake of antigen in APCs through activating phagocytosis;
c. deliver antigen from the injection site to the local lymph node trough into the lymphatic system

Various routes of HIV vaccine administration have been used starting from the most common (eg. subcutaneous, intramuscular) to more specific such as mucosal with different outcomes. HIV transmission occurs through mucosal (specially of the genital tract) and many efforts have been done to better characterize the mucosal associated lymphoid tissue (MALT) and its involvement in early HIV infection, with the final purpose to use the mucosal route of immunization. For vaccine design, the choice of mucosal inductive site is critical in determining the distal effector site to which induced memory cells will home. In

HIV vaccine research, many mucosal sites were chosen to administer the immunogen: nasal mucosal (Vajdy & Singh, 2006), intratracheal/aerosol vaccination (Corbett et al., 2008), oral vaccination (Stahl-Hennig et al., 2007, N. Cuburu et al., 2007), rectal/colonic vaccination (Belyakov et al., 2006), intravaginal vaccination- (Pialoux et al., 2008).

3.3 Vaccination strategies

The vaccination strategy comprehends the combination of diverse types of vaccine (immunogen, adjuvant, route of immunization) with different schedules to increasing the vaccine potential immunogenic effect. In HIV vaccine several combinations of immunogens (inactivated virus, viral proteins, recombinant viral DNA), routes and schedules have been tested to augment the delivery of HIV antigens to the immune system.

For example, viral vectors are efficient to place HIV relevant epitopes within the target cells and, due to their composition, to stimulate the innate response, promoting an adjuvant effect, although it has been observed that the immunogenicity of these vectors could be affected by the competition between HIV and vector epitopes in the context of antigen presentation. For these reason it was developed the strategy to combined this type of vaccine with a vaccine based on HIV proteins or peptides in a such called prime-boost regimen.

Prime-boost strategy was first time used in 1992 in NHP studies (Hu et al., 1992). Briefly, it consists in the administration of one type of vaccine, such as a live-vector vaccine, followed by or together with a second type of vaccine, such as a recombinant subunit vaccine. The intent of this combination regimen is to induce different types of immune responses and enhance the overall immune response, a result that may not occur if only one type of vaccine were to be given for all doses (Ranasinghe et al., 2009).

3.4 Steps of vaccine development

The development of a vaccine is a process that requires several steps aiming to answer specific questions and to test concepts through experimental practice. Scientific knowledge generated from the execution of each stage or phase will give useful data for planning the next step.

The development of an effective vaccine against HIV infection, due to its unique aspects, will be an unprecedented challenge, and scientific rigor and discipline, statistical principles and bioethics should be required to achieve success.

The preliminary step is to generate more ideas. Established scientists in universities, research institutes and industry use the existing scientific knowledge and technology to develop ideas of how a vaccine might work.

From there, preclinical studies should be performed before human trials to assess whether a novel product has scientific merit to be a candidate vaccine. Such pre-clinical studies involve *in vitro* experiments and *in vivo* tests in available animal models to obtain information regarding the efficacy, toxicity and pharmacokinetics, using varying doses of the product being tested.

The transformation process of a candidate product in a vaccine logarithmic increases the cost and complexity of the research, as it moves from laboratory to clinical application. It is also important to emphasize that only a small percentage of the candidate products being studied in preclinical development is considered safe and promising enough to be evaluated in humans (clinical phase).

Once proven its potential as a vaccine candidate, the clinical phase of the study will start to evaluate safety, immunogenicity and efficacy of the product. Phases I-III are required for licensing the product. In the process of vaccine development, clinical trials may last for many years and the number of volunteers is increasing at every step. The goals set for each stage involves pharmacological and clinical issues, evaluated in a progressive manner throughout the process (www.ich.org - General Considerations for Clinical Trials).

The clinical trial itself begins in Phase I: the candidate vaccine is first evaluated in a small group of human volunteers in order to evaluate its safety, tolerability, pharmacokinetics and pharmacodynamics and identify possible side effects.

In Phase I trial it is also possible to evaluate efficacy markers (e.g.: the generation of antibodies and/or cytotoxic T response), allowing a preliminary assessment of the ability of the vaccine to generate an immune response. Once the safety of the candidate product has been checked, the research could proceed to the next step (Phase II).

The objective of Phase II is to test the candidate vaccine in a larger number of volunteers with two principal purposes: identify side effects related to the product use (within the perspective of future safety analysis, i.e.: toxicity) and collect preliminary indications of product potential effectiveness (efficacy).

Sometimes these aims are studied in different moments and the Phase II trials are divided into:

a. Phase IIa: designed to determine the optimal dose of vaccine (dose-response studies).
b. Phase IIb: designed to study the vaccine efficacy.

The Phase III trials are the last stage before possible licensing of the vaccine for marketing. They are randomized controlled trials, often multi-centric, involving large numbers of patients. The primary objective of this step is to evaluate the effectiveness of the product. Achieving a high level of effectiveness at this stage, however, does not necessarily guarantee that the product is effective in the general population, which will be evaluated in phase IV.

Phase IV trials, also called post-evaluation of efficacy, are pharmacovigilance studies performed after licensing the product and that aim to measure the effect of the product in a population. The importance of this phase is to assess the real impact of a vaccine in the epidemic.

The conduct of clinical trials involving prophylactic and therapeutic vaccines for HIV remains a challenge. In terms of design and implementing Phase I and early Phase II are relatively easy to do, although studies involving analysis of effectiveness show a higher degree of complexity. For prophylactic vaccines, the statistical requirements to demonstrate a real prevention of infection require a very large number of patients and they are sometimes prohibitive. Clinical trials for HIV vaccines require the appropriate preclinical studies and the development of better laboratory markers of efficacy.

The role of society is essential for the success of all the program to develop HIV vaccines and the establishment of a genuine dialogue with the community facilitates clinical research with HIV vaccines.

4. Current outlook

Obtaining an HIV vaccine has been one of the biggest challenges of this century. To date numerous clinical trials have been conducted to test candidate products as prophylactic vaccine.

Most initial approaches have focused on the gp120 HIV envelope protein. At least thirteen different gp120 candidates have been evaluated in Phase I trials in the USA predominantly through the AIDS Vaccine Evaluation Group, showing to be safe and immunogenic in diverse populations. They have induced neutralizing antibody, but rarely induced CD8+ cytotoxic T lymphocytes (CTL). Moreover it was very difficult to induce and maintain the high anti-gp120 antibody titers necessary to have any hope of neutralizing an HIV exposure. The availability of several recombinant vectors (adenovirus, canarypox) carrying HIV gens (gag, pol, nef or env) has provided interesting results characterized principally by a poly-functional CTL responses.

Currently, about 20 clinical trials are underway, most protocols for Phase I.

PROTOCOL	SPONSOR	PRODUCT	N	TRIAL SITE	fase
HVTN 082	NIAID, HVTN	VRC-HIVDNA016-00-VP; VRC-HIVADV014-00-VP		USA	I
PedVacc001 & PedVacc002	Medical Research Council	MVA.HIVA	48	Kenya	I
HVTN 078	NIAID, EuroVacc, HVTN	NYVAC-B; VRC-HIVADV038-00-VP	80	Switer zland	I/II
HVTN 505	NIAID, HVTN	VRC-HIVDNA016-00-VP; VRC-HIVADV014-00-VP	1,350	US	II
B001	IAVI, University of Rochester Medical Center	Prime: VRC-HIVDNA016-00-VP Adenovirus serotype 35 vector. Ad35-GRIN/ENV consists of two vectors: Ad35-GRIN vector with *gag*, reverse transcriptase, integrase, and *nef*Ad35-ENV vector with gp140 *env*	42	USA	I
HIVIS 05	Swedish Institute for Infectious disease Control	MVA-CMDR	24	Swede n	I
P001	IAVI, Indian Council of Medical Research, Tuberculosis Research Centre, Chennai; National AIDS Research Institute, Pune	Prime: ADVAX (DNA vaccine containing env, gag, pol, nef and tat) Boost: TBC-M4 (MVA vector with env, gag, RT, rev, tat and nef)	32	India	I
Tiantianvaccinia HIV Vaccine	Chinese Center for Disease Control and Prevention, National Vaccine and SerumInstitute, Peking Union Medical College	HIV-1 CN54 gag, pol and env genes with DNA and rTV vectors	80	China	I
Ad5HVR48.ENVA.01	NIAID, Brigham and Women's Hospital	Recombinant Adenovirus HIV-1 Vaccine, Ad5HVR48.ENVA.01	48	USA	I
HVTN205	GeoVax, HVTN	Prime: DNA vaccine containing gag, pol, env, rat,rev, vpu Boost: MVA vaccine containing gag, pol, env	225	USA, Peru	II
HVTN 073	HVTN, SAAVI, Brigham and Women's Hospital CRS, Fenway Community Health, Clinical Research Boston,	Prime: SAAVI DNA-C2 Boost: SAAVI MVA-C; DNA plasmid vaccine with *gag, RT, tat, nef, env*	48	USA, South Africa	I

PROTOCOL	SPONSOR	PRODUCT	N	TRIAL SITE	fase
	Crossroads, Chris Hani BaragwanathHospita				
VRC 015 (08-1-0171)	NIAID, VRC, NIH Clinical Center	Multiclade Recombinant HIV-1 Adenoviral Vector Vaccine, VRCHIVADV014-00-VP	40	USA	I
Ad26.ENVA.01	NIAID, IPCAVD, Brigham and Women's Hospital, Beth Israel Deaconess Medical Center, Crucell	Recombinant adenovirus serotype 26 (rAd26) vaccine	48	USA	I
NCHECR-AE1	NCHECR, University of New South Wales, Thai Red Cross AIDS Research Centre	A candidate prophylactic DNA prime-rFPV boost HIV vaccination strategy (rFPV-HIV-AE;pHIS-HIV-AE)	8	Thaila nd	I/II
VRC 012	NIAID, VRC	HIV-1 adenovirus vector vaccine VRC-HIVADV027-00VP: dose escalation and prime-boost with an HIV-1 adenovirus vector vaccine, VRC-HIVADV038-00-VP	35	USA	I
HVTN 077	NIAID, HVTN, Alabama Vaccine, San Francisco Vaccine and Prevention, Hope Clinic of the Emory Vaccine Center, NY Blood Ctr./Union Square, NY Blood Ctr./Bronx, University of Rochester HVTN	Recombinant Adenoviral Subtype 35 (rAd35) and Subtype 5 (rAd5) HIV-1 Vaccines When Given as a Heterologous Prime-Boost Regimen or as Boosts to a Recombinant DNA Vaccine in Healthy, Ad5-Naïve and Ad5-Exposed (VRC-HIVDNA044-00-VP;VRC-HIVADV027-00-VP;VRC-HIVADV038-00-VP)	192	USA	I
HPTN 027	HVTN, International Maternal Pediatric Adolescent AIDS Clinical Trials Group,Makerere University, Johns Hopkins University, Mulago Hospital, Sanofi-Pasteur	Canarypox viral vector with *env*and*gag-pol*	50	Ugand a	I
HVRF-380-131004	Moscow Institute of Immunology, FederalMedical and Biological Agency, Russian Federation Ministry of Education and Science	VICHREPOL with polyoxidonium adjuvant	15	Russia	I
RV 138; B011	Walter Reed Army Institute of Research, US Military HIV	Sanofi Pasteur Live Recombinant ALVAC-HIV (vCP205, HIV-1 Env/Gag/Pol) subcutaneously, intradermally, or intramuscularly	36	USA	I
EnvDNA	St. Jude's Children's Research Hospital	Recombinant HIV-1 multi-envelope DNA plasmid vaccine with *env*	6	USA	I
RV 156A	NIAID, HVTN, VRC, MHRP, Makerere U.	VRC-HIVADV014-00-VP alone or as a boost to VRCHIVDNA009-00-VP	30	Ugand a	I

Table 3. Ongoing clinical trials (www.avac.org/ht/a/GetDocumentAction/i/3436).

The results of Phase II and Phase III major prophylactic trials are summarized above.

4.1 VAX 004 trial (Phase III, USA 1998-2002)

The phase III VAX 004 trial enrolled 5,403 USA participants between 1998 and 1999. Volunteers received 7 injections of either vaccine or placebo (ratio, 2:1) over 30 months.

The study vaccine contained 2 rgp120 HIV-1 envelope antigens (300 mg each of two recombinant proteins rgp120/HIV-1 MN and GNE8) (AIDSVAX B/B; VaxGen) that had been derived from 2 different subtype B strains and that were adsorbed onto 600 mg of alum. GNE8 gp120 was cloned directly from peripheral-blood mononuclear cells and had the CCR5 phenotype; the GNE8 gp120 DNA sequence was deposited in GenBank.

The vaccine did not prevent HIV-1 acquisition and there was no overall protective effect (Flynn et al., 2005).

4.2 STEP trial (Phase II, USA, 2004-2007)

On December 13, 2004, the HIV Vaccine Trials Network (HVTN) began recruiting for the STEP study, a 3,000-participant phase II clinical trial of a novel HIV vaccine, at sites in North America, South America, the Caribbean and Australia.

The trial was co-funded by the National Institute of Allergy and Infectious Diseases (NIAID/NIH, USA), and the pharmaceutical company Merck & Co. Merck developed the experimental vaccine called V520 which contains a adenoviral vector rAd5 carrying three subtype B HIV genes (gag/pol/nef). The vaccine was administered in prime-boost regimen at 0, 1 and 6 months. The follow up of vaccinated subjects showed the lack of efficacy of this vaccine, as well as an increment in HIV-1 infection in individuals with prior immunity to adenovirus. Adenovirus vectors and many other viral vectors currently used in HIV vaccines, will induce a rapid memory immune response against the vector. This results in an impediment to the development of a T cell response against the inserted antigen.

For this reason the phase II trial was closed in September 2007 and other vaccine protocols in progress including the same vector vaccine such as the HVTN503 (Phambili) were cancelled or modificated (Barouch & Korber, 2010).

While the final results of STEP have been disappointing, this study has raised its contribution to redefine the priorities in HIV vaccines research field, demonstrating the need to focus on basic research, preclinical and clinical studies.

4.3 RV144 trial (Phase III, Thailand, 2003-2009)

The phase III HIV vaccine RV144 involved more than 16,000 young Thailandese adults at variable risk for infection between October 2003 and September 2009. Ever six months, volunteers received a prime-boost vaccination including six injections of a vaccine called ALVAC-HIV (vCP1521, Sanofi Pasteur) with the last two of the six injections being a combination of that vaccine and another one called AIDSVAX B/E (gp120, Genentech).

ALVACHIV consists of a viral vector containing genetically engineered versions of three HIV genes (env, gag and pro).The ALVAC vector is an inert form of canarypox, a bird virus which cannot cause disease or replicate in humans. AIDSVAX B/E is composed of genetically engineered gp120. The RV 144 protocol was sponsored by the Surgeon General of the United States Army and conducted by the Thailand Ministry of Public Health with support from the United States Army Medical Research and Materiel Command and the NIAD/NIH.

The rate of HIV infection among volunteers who received the experimental vaccine being tested in the trial was 31% lower than the rate of HIV infection among volunteers who received placebo (Rerks-Ngarm et al., 2009).

Although showing only a modest benefit, this work has renewed optimism in this field of research. However, criticisms related primarily to the study design and statistical method employed to analyse data generated debate about the results (Cohen, 2009; Letvin, 2009).

4.4 Dendritic cell based immunotreatment

In addition to trials aimed at obtaining prophylactic HIV vaccine, has been also developed protocols for therapeutic vaccination using dendritic cells (DC) for the treatment of individuals already infected with HIV.

DCs are potent antigen presenting cells that act as controllers and regulators of the immune system and are the only cells capable of fully activate naive CD4 lymphocytes and thus initiate a specific response (Banchereau & Steinman, 1998). In the context of an HIV vaccine

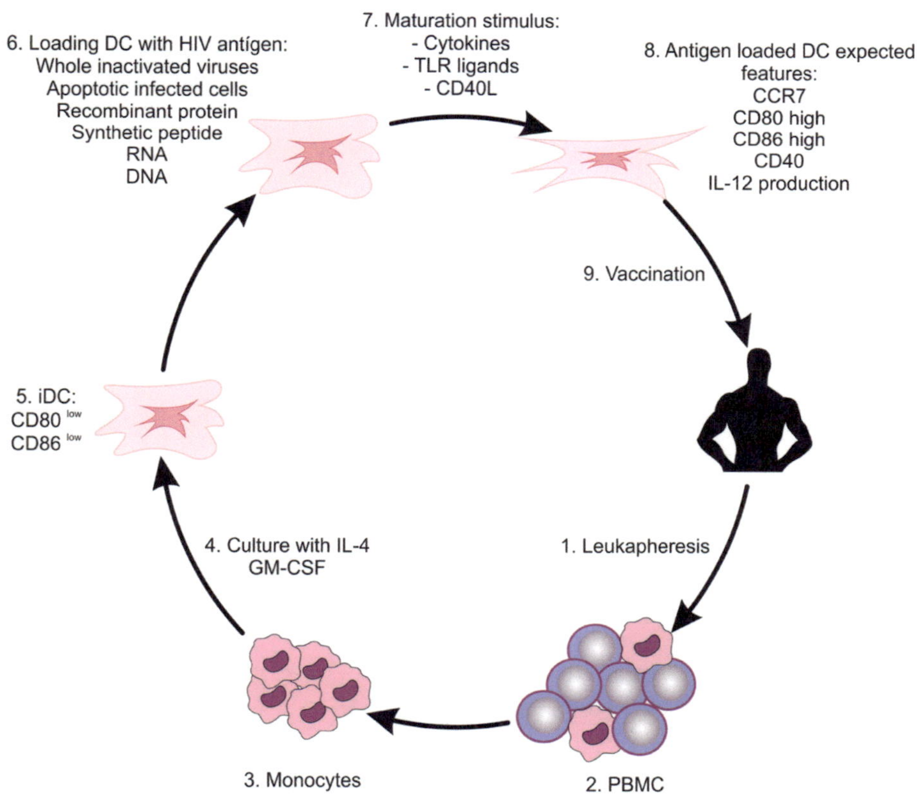

Fig. 4. Treatment of HIV infected patients with monocyte-derived DCs. Peripheral blood mononuclear cells (PBMC) are obtained by leukapheresis and monocytes are separated and cultured in the presence of IL-4 and GM-CSF to obtain immature DCs (iDCs). iDCs are loaded with the antigen of interest and are activated by different stimuli for maturation. Mature DCs (MDCs), potentially able to migrate and to present antigens, are reinoculate into the patient.

AUTHORS	n	TYPE OF ANTIGEN	IMMUNOGENICITY ASSESSMENT
Kundu et al., 1998	6	Recombinant HIV-1 MN gp160 or HLA-A2-restricted synthetic peptides of envelope, Gag, and Pol	Envelope-specific CTL- and lymphocyte-proliferative responses, IFN-gamma and IL-2 production, peptide-specific lymphocyte-proliferative responses
Lu W et al., 2004	18	Chemically inactivated autologous HIV-1	Serum neutralizingantibodytiters, HIV-1-specific interferon-γ (IFN-γ) expressing CD4+ T and CD8+ cells, HIV-1-specific IL-2- expressing CD4+ T cells, HIV-1 gag–specific CD8+ T cells, HIV-1 gag–specific CD8+ T cells expressing perforin
Garcia F et al.,2005	12	Heat-inactivated autologous human immunodeficiency virus type 1 (HIV-1)	Lymphoproliferation, Th1 cell levels, cytotoxic T lymphocyte [CTL] levels, serum neutralizingantibodytiters and changes in lymphoid tissue
Ide F et al., 2006	4	HIV-1-derived cytotoxic T lymphocytes (CTL) peptides	IFN-g production in CD8 lymphocytes
Connolly NC et al., 2008	18	Gag, Env, and Pol peptides	Gamma interferon (IFN-γ)-producing cells (PBMC)
Ghandhi RT et al., 2009	29	Viral vector (canarypox) expressing HIV-1 envandgag and a synthetic polypeptide encompassing epitopes from nefandpol	Gamma interferon (IFN-γ)-producing cells (PBMC), lymphocyte-proliferative responses
Garcia F et al, 2011	24	Heat-inactivated autologous human immunodeficiency virus type 1 (HIV-1)	Lymphoproliferation, serum neutralizing antibody titers, ELISPOT

Table 4. Parameters used in the post-vaccine immune response assessment
HLA= **Human Leukocyte Antigen.** IL-2= **Interleukin-2** . PBMCs=Peripheral Blood Mononuclear Cells.

becomes desirable to induce a specific and effective activation of the immune system against the viral chronic infection.

Protocols of immunotherapy with DCs began in the late 1990 and since then a growing number of studies evaluating this strategy. Because it is an individualized protocol, the number of individuals in the tests is always limited, never exceeding a few tens of individuals.

It is a strategy that involves the collection of mononuclear cells from HIV-infected individual, separation of monocytes and stimulation of these cells with cytokines to differentiate into immature dendritic cells. Dendritic cells are then sensitized (pulsed or loaded) with the antigen of interest, activated and reinoculated into the individuals (Figure 4). The objective of this strategy is to stimulate the immune response by enhancing antigen presentation mediated by dendritic cells.

An overview of the works conducted so far (Table 4) shows although that the products are always safe and the results are quite heterogeneous (Kundu et al., 1998; García et al., 2005, 2011; Ide at al., 2006; Connolly et al., 2008, Lu et al., 2004, Ghandhi, 2009)

Considering the difficulty to obtain an HIV prophylactic vaccine, the immunotherapy offers a unique opportunity to study the mechanisms of immune response against the virus and contribute to the definition of correlates of protection in HIV infection. Knowledge generated from studies of DC-based immunotherapy may contribute also to the development of prophylactic vaccines.

5. Conclusions

Despite numerous difficulties and great scientific challenges that must be overcome to obtain an HIV vaccine, the extraordinary advance in biomedical research and the remarkable progress achieved show clear reasons for optimism.

Knowledge has been accumulated on the biology and diversity of HIV; new methods have been used for the production of immunologically relevant antigens; the study of immune response in exposed not-infected individuals and in elite controllers has generated important information regarding the type of effective immune response against HIV. Furthermore, immunotherapy protocols in infected individuals provide a unique opportunity to studying immune mechanisms against the virus.

Lessons from the failure of the previous protocols can effectively guide the design and refinement of the next generation of candidate vaccines. In this scenario, the perspective is that knowledge of the various interdisciplinary areas of science can provide an environment leading to overcome these scientific challenges.

6. References

Banchereau, J., Steinman, R.M. (1998). Dendritic cells and the control of immunity. *Nature* , Vol 392, No. 6673, (Mar 1998), pp. 245-252, ISSN 0028-0836.

Barouch, D.H., Korber B. (2010). HIV-1 vaccine development after STEP. Annu Rev Med, Vol. 61, (Feb 2010), pp.153-167, ISSN 0066-4219.

Belyakov, I.M., Kuznetsov, V.A., Kelsall, B., Klinman, D., Moniuszko, M., Lemon, M., Markham, P.D., Pal, R., Clements, J.D., Lewis, M.G., Strober, W., Franchini, G. and Berzofsky J.A. (2006). Impact of vaccine-induced mucosal high-avidity CD8+ CTLs in delay of AIDS viral dissemination from mucosa. Blood, Vol. 107, pp. 3258–3264, ISSN 1528-0020.

Brenchley, J.M., Schacker, T.W., Ruff, L.E., Price, D.A., Taylor, J.H., Beilman G.J., Nguyen P.L., Khoruts, A., Larson M., Haase, A.T., Douek, D.C. (2004). CD4+ T cell depletion during all stages of HIV disease occurs predominantly in the gastrointestinal tract. *J Exp Med*, Vol. 200, No. 6, (Sep 2004), pp. 749-759, ISSN 0022-1007.

Cadogan, M., Dalgleish, A.G. (2008). HIV immunopathogenesis and strategies for intervention. *Lancet Infect Dis*, Vol. 8, No. 11, pp:675-684. ISSN 1473-3099.

Carr, A. (2000). HIV protease inhibitor-related lipodystrophy syndrome. *Clin Infect Dis*, Vol 30, Suppl 2, pp.S135-42, ISSN 1537-6591

Cohen, J. (2009). HIV/AIDS research. Beyond Thailand: making sense of a qualified AIDS vaccine "success". *Science*, Vol. 326, No. 5953, pp. 652-653, ISSN 1095-9203.

Connolly, N.C., Whiteside, T.L., Wilson, C., Kondragunta, V., Rinaldo, C.R., Riddler, S.A. (2008). Therapeutic immunization with human immunodeficiency virus type 1 (HIV-1) peptide-loaded dendritic cells is safe and induces immunogenicity in HIV-1-infected individuals. *Clin. Vac. Immunol.* Vol. 15, No 2, pp. 284-92, ISSN 1556-679X.

Corbett M., Bogers, W.M., Heeney, J.L., Gerber, S., Genin, C., Didierlaurent, A., Oostermeijer, H., Dubbes, R., Braskamp, G., Lerondel, S., Gomez, C.E., Esteban, M., Wagner, R., Kondova, I., Mooij, P., Balla-Jhagjhoorsingh, S., Beenhakker, N., Koopman, G., van der Burg, S., Kraehenbuhl, J.P. and Le Pape, A. (2008). Aerosol immunization with NYVAC and MVA vectored vaccines is safe, simple, and immunogenic. *Proc Natl Acad Sci USA*, Vol. 105, pp. 2046–2051, ISSN 1091-6490.

Cuburu, N., Kweon. M.N., Song, J.H., Hervouet, C., Luci, C., Sun, J.B., Hofman, P., Holmgren, J., Anjuere, F. and Czerkinsky, C. (2007). Sublingual immunization induces broad-based systemic and mucosal immune responses in mice. *Vaccine* Vol. 25, pp. 8598–8610, ISSN 0264-410X.

Dolin, R. (1995). Human studies in the development of human immunodeficiency virus vaccines. *J Infect Dis*. Vol. 172, No. 5, pp.1175-1183,ISSN 1537-6613.

Dunham, R., Pagliardini, P., Gordon, S., Sumpter, B., Engram, J., Moanna, A., Paiardini, M., Mandl, J.N., Lawson, B., Garg, S., McClure, H.M., Xu, Y.X., Ibegbu, C., Easley, K., Katz, N., Pandrea, I., Apetrei, C., Sodora, D.L., Staprans, S.I., Feinberg, M.B., Silvestri, G. (2006). The AIDS resistence of naturally SIVinfected sooty mangabeys is independent of cellular immunity to the virus. *Blood*, Vol. 108, No 1, pp. 209-217, ISSN 1528-0020.

Egger, M., Hirschel, B., Francioli, P., Sudre, P., Wirz, M., Flepp, M., Rickenbach, M., Malinverni, R., Vernazza, P., Battegay, M.(1997). Impact of new antiretroviral combination therapies in HIV infected patients in Switzerland: prospective multicentre study. Swiss HIV Cohort Study. *BMJ*, Vol. 315, pp. 1194-1199, ISSN 09598138.

Fischl, M.A., Richman, D.D., Grieco, M.H., Gottlieb, M.S., Volberding, P.A., Laskin, O.L., Leedom, J.M., Groopman, J.E., Mildvan, D. Schooley, R.T et al. (1987). The efficacy of azidothymidine (AZT) in the treatment of patients with AIDS and AIDS-related complex. A double-blind, placebo-controlled trial. *N Engl J Med,* Vol.317, pp. 185-191, ISSN 1533-4406.

Flynn, N.M., Forthal, D.N., Harro, C.D., Judson, F.N., Mayer, K..H., Para ,M.F.; rgp120 HIV Vaccine Study Group. (2005). Placebo-ControlledPhase 3 Trial of a RecombinantGlycoprotein 120 Vaccine to Prevent HIV-1 Infection. J Infect Dis, Vol. 91, pp. 654–65, ISSN ISSN 1537-6613.

García, F., Lejeune, M., Climent, N., Gil, C., Alcamí, J., Morente, V., Alós, L., Ruiz, A., Setoain, J., Fumero, E., Castro, P., López, A., Cruceta, A., Piera, C., Florence, E., Pereira, A., Libois, A., González, N., Guilá, M., Caballero, M., Lomeña, F., Joseph, J., Miró, J.M., Pumarola, T., Plana, M., Gatell, J.M., Gallart, T. (2005). Therapeutic Immunization with dendritic cells loaded with heat-inactivated autologous HIV-1 in patients with chronic HIV-1 Infection. *J. Infect. Dis.* Vol. 191, pp. 1680-1685, ISSN 1537-6613.

García, F., Climent, N., Assoumou, L., Gil, C., González, N., Alcamí, J., León, A., Romeu,. J., Dalmau J., Martínez-Picado, J., Lifson, J., Autran, B., Costagliola, D., Clotet, B., Gatell, J.M., Plana, M., Gallart, T. DCV2/MANON07- AIDS Vaccine Research Objective Study Group. (2011). A therapeutic dendritic cell-based vaccine for HIV-1 infection. J Infect Dis, Vol 203, No. 4, pp. 473-478, ISSN 1537-6613.

Gaschen, B., Taylor, J., Yusim, K., Foley, B., Gao, F., Lang, D., Novitsky, V., Haynes, B., Hahn, B.H., Bhattacharya, T., Korber, B. (2002) Diversity considerations in HIV-1 vaccine selection. *Science,* Vol. 296, No 5577, pp. 2354–2360, ISSN 1095-9203.

Gandhi RT, O'Neill D, Bosch RJ, Chan ES, Bucy RP, Shopis J, Baglyos L, Adams E, Fox L, Purdue L, Marshak A, Flynn T, Masih R, Schock B, Mildvan D, Schlesinger SJ, Marovich MA, Bhardwaj N, Jacobson JM; AIDS Clinical Trials Group A5130 team. (2009). A randomized therapeutic vaccine trial of canarypox-HIV-pulsed dendritic cells vs. canarypox-HIV alone in HIV-1-infected patients on antiretroviral therapy. Vaccine, Vol 27, No. 43, pp. 6088-6094, ISSN 0264-410X.

Hawkins, T. (2010). Understanding and managing the adverse effects of antiretroviral therapy. *Antiviral Res,* Vol 85, No 1, pp. 201-209, ISSN 0166-3542.

Heyward, W.L., MacQueen, K.M., Goldenthal, K.L. (1998). HIV vaccine development and evaluation: realistic expectations. AIDS Res&Hum Retroviruses, Vol. 14, Suppl 3:S205-10, ISSN 1931-8405.

Hladik, F., Desbien, A., Lang, J., Wang, L., Ding, Y., Holte, S., Wilson, A., Xu, Y., Moerbe, M., Schmechel, S., McElrath, M.J. (2003). Most highly exposed seronegative men lack HIV-1-specific, IFN-gamma-secreting T cells. *J Immunol,* Vol. 171, No 5, pp. 2671-83, ISSN 1550-6606.

Hu, S.L., Abrams, K., Barber, G.N., Moran, P., Zarling, J.M., Langlois, A.J., Kuller, L., Morton, W.R., Benveniste, R.E. (1992). Protection of macaques against SIV infection by subunit vaccines of SIV envelope glycoprotein gp160. *Science,* Vol. 255, No. 5043, pp. 456-459, ISSN 1095-9203.

Ide, F., Nakamura, T., Tomizawa, M., Kawana-Tachikawa, A., Odawara, T., Hosoya, N. and Iwamoto, A. (2006). Peptide-loaded dendritic-cell vaccination followed by treatment interruption for chronic HIV-1 infection: a phase 1 trial. *J. Med. Virol,* Vol. 78, No. 6, pp. 711-718, ISSN 1096-9071.

Kornbluth, R.S., Stone, G.W. (2006). Immunostimulatory combinations: designing the next generation of vaccine adjuvants. J Leukoc Biol, Vol. 80, No. 5, pp.1084-1102, ISSN 0741-5400.

Kozlowski, P.A., Neutra, M.R. (2003). The role of mucosal immunity in prevention of HIV transmission. *Curr Mol Med*, Vol. 3, No 3, pp. 217-228, ISSN 1566-5240.

Kundu, S.K., Engleman, E., Benike, C., Shapero, M.H., Dupuis, M., van Schooten, W.C., Eibl, M., Merigan, T.C. (1998). A pilot clinical trial of HIV antigen-pulsed allogeneic and autologous dendritic cell therapy in HIVinfected patients. *AIDS Res. Hum. Retrovir.* Vol. 14, pp. 551–560, ISSN 1931-8405.

Lederman, M.M., Alter, G., Daskalakis, D.C., Rodriguez, B., Sieg, S.F., Hardy, G., Cho, M., Anthony, D., Harding, C., Weinberg, A., Silverman, R.H., Douek, D.C., Margolis, L., Goldstein, D.B., Carrington, M., Goedert, J.J. (2010). Determinants of protection among HIV-exposed seronegative persons: an overview. *J Infect Dis*, Vol. 202, Suppl 3:S333-8, ISSN 1537-6613.

Letvin, N.L. (2009). Virology. Moving forward in HIV vaccine development. *Science*, Vol. 26, No 5957, pp. 1196-8, ISSN 1095-9203.

Lu, W., Arraes, L.C., Ferreira, W.T., Andrieu, J.M. (2004). Therapeutic dendritic-cell vaccine for chronic HIV-1 infection. *Nat. Med, Vol,* 10, pp. 1359–65, ISSN 1078-8956.

Mattapallil, J.J., Douek, D.C., Hill, B., Nishimura, Y., Martin ,M., Roederer, M. (2005). Massive infection and loss of memory CD4+ Tcells in multiple tissues during acute SIV infection. *Nature*, Vol. 434, pp. 1093–1097, ISSN 0028-0836.

Menéndez-Arias L. (2010). Molecular basis of human immunodeficiency virus drug resistance: an update. *Antiviral Res.* Vol. 85, No. 1, pp. 210-231, ISSN 0166-3542.

Parren, P.W., Marx, P.A., Hessell, A.J., Luckay, A., Harouse, J., Cheng-Mayer, C., Moore, J.P. and Burton, D.R. (2001). Antibody protects macaques against vaginal challenge with a pathogenic R5 simian/human immunodeficiency virus at serum levels giving complete neutralization in vitro. *J Virol*, Vol. 75, No. 17, pp. 8340-8347, ISSN 1098-5514.

Pialoux, G., Hocini, H., Perusat, S., Silberman, B., Salmon-Ceron, D., Slama, L., Journot, V., Mathieu, E., Gaillard, C., Petitprez, K., Launay, O. and Chene, G. (2008). Phase I study of a candidate vaccine based on recombinant HIV-1 gp160 (MN/LAI) administered by the mucosal route to HIV-seronegative volunteers: The ANRS VAC14 study. *Vaccine*, Vol. 26, pp. 2657–2666, ISSN 0264-410X.

Poropatich, K., Sullivan, D.J.Jr. (2011). Human immunodeficiency virus type 1 long-term non-progressors: the viral, genetic and immunological basis for disease non-progression. *J Gen Virol*, Vol. 92 Pt 2, pp. 247-68, ISSN 1465-2099.

Ranasinghe, C., Ramshaw, I.A. (2009). Genetic heterologous prime–boost vaccination strategies for improved systemic and mucosal immunity. *Expert Rev Vaccines* , Vol. 8, pp. 1171–1181, ISSN 1476-0584.

Rerks-Ngarm, S., Pitisuttithum, P., Nitayaphan, S., Kaewkungwal, J., Chiu, J., Paris, R., Premsri, N., Namwat, C., de Souza, M., Adams, E., Benenson, M., Gurunathan, S., Tartaglia, J., McNeil, J.G., Francis, D.P., Stablein, D., Birx, D.L., Chunsuttiwat, S., Khamboonruang, C., Thongcharoen, P., Robb, M.L., Michael, N.L., Kunasol, P., Kim, J.H. and MOPH-TAVEG Investigators. (2009). Vaccination with ALVAC and

AIDSVAX to prevent HIV-1 infection in Thailand. , Vol. 361, No. 23, pp. 2209-2220, ISSN 1533-4406.

Rowland-Jones, S.L., Dong, T., Fowke, K.R., Kimani, J., Krausa, P., Newell, H., Blanchard, T., Ariyoshi, K., Oyugi, J., Ngugi, E., Bwayo, J., MacDonald, K.S., McMichael, A.J. and Plummer, F.A. (1998). Cytotoxic T cell responses to multiple conserved HIV epitopes in HIV-resistant prostitutes in Nairobi. *J Clin Invest*, Vol. 102, No. 9, pp. 1758-1765, ISSN 1558-8238.

Shedlock, D.J., Silvestri, G., Weiner, D.B. (2009). Monkeying around with HIV vaccines: using rhesus macaques to define 'gatekeepers' for clinical trials. *Nat Rev Immunol*, Vol. 9, No. 10, pp. 717-728, ISSN 1474-1733.

Stahl-Hennig, C., Kuate, S., Franz M., Suh, Y.S., Stoiber, H., Sauermann, U., Tenner-Racz, K., Norley, S., Park, K.S., Sung, Y.C., Steinman, R., Racz, P., and Uberla, K. (2007) Atraumatic oral spray immunization with replication-deficient viral vector vaccines. *J Virol*, Vol. 81, pp.13180–13190, ISSN 1098-5514.

Stapransa, S.I., Feinberga, M.B., Shiverb, J.W. and Casimiro, D.R. (2010). Role of nonhuman primates in the evaluation of candidate AIDS vaccines: an industry perspective. Current Opinion in HIV and AIDS, Vol. 5, No. 5, pp. 377–385, ISSN 1746-6318.

Sumpter, B., Dunham, R., Gordon, S., Engram, J., Hennessy, M., Kinter, A., Paiardini, M., Cervasi, B., Klatt, N., McClure, H., Milush, J.M., Staprans, S., Sodora, D.L. and Silvestri, G. (2007). Correlates of preserved CD4(+) T cell homeostasis during natural, non-pathogenic simian immunodeficiency virus infection of sooty mangabeys: implications for AIDS pathogenesis. *J. Immunol*, Vol. 178, No. 3, pp. 1680-1691, ISSN 1550-6606.

Vajdy, M. and Singh M. (2006). Intranasal delivery of vaccines against HIV. *Expert OpinDrug Deliv*, Vol. 3, pp. 247–259, ISSN 1742-5247.

Van Duyne, R., Pedati, C., Guendel, I., Carpio, L., Kehn-Hall, K., Saifuddin, M., Kashanchi, F. (2009). The utilization of humanized mouse models for the study of human retroviral infections. *Retrovirology*, Vol. 6, pp. 76, ISSN 1742-4690.

Vassilieva, E.V., Wang, B.Z., Vzorov, A.N., Wang, L., Wang, Y.C., Bozja, J., Xu, R., Compans, R.W. (2011). Enhanced Mucosal Immune Responses to HIV Virus-Like Particles Containing a Membrane-Anchored Adjuvant. *MBio*, Vol. 2, No. 1, ISSN 2150-7511.

Walker, B.D. (2007). Elite control of HIV Infection: implications for vaccines and treatment. *Top HIV Med*, Vol. 15, No. 4, pp. 134-136, ISSN 1542-8826.

Wawer, M.J., Sewankambo, N.K., Serwadda, D., Quinn, T.C., Paxton, L.A., Kiwanuka, N., Wabwire-Mangen, F., Li , C., Lutalo, T., Nalugoda, F., Gaydos, C.A., Moulton, L.H., Meehan, M.O., Ahmed, S., Gray, R.H. (1999). Control of sexually transmitted diseases for AIDS prevention in Uganda: a randomized community trial. Rakai Project Study Group. *Lancet*, Vol 353, pp. 525-535, ISSN 0140-6736.

Whatmore, A.M., Cook, N., Hall, G.A., Sharpe, S., Rud, E.W., Cranage, M.P. (1995). Repair and evolution of nef in vivo modulates simian immunodeficiency virus virulence. *J. Virol*, Vol. 69, pp.5117–5123, ISSN 1098-5514.

Towards Universal Acess: Scaling up priority HIV/AIDS Interventions in the health sector. WHO, UNAIDS, UNICEF, 2007. www.who.int/entity/hiv/mediacentre/universal_access_progress_report_en.pdf
www.ich.org - General Considerations for Clinical Trials
www.hivresourcetracking.org/treatments/vaccines
www.avac.org/ht/a/GetDocumentAction/i/3436

24

Towards a Functional Cure for HIV Infection: The Potential Contribution of Therapeutic Vaccination

Maja A. Sommerfelt
Bionor Pharma ASA
Norway

1. Introduction

Human immunodeficiency virus (HIV-1) currently infects 33.3 million people globally. In 2009, 1.8 million people died from acquired immunodeficiency syndrome (AIDS) marking a decline in AIDS deaths by 19% since 1999, the estimated peak of the pandemic. This is largely due to the introduction of combination antiretroviral therapy (ART) in 1996 and its expanding access in recent years. However, despite continued efforts to improve ART availability worldwide, only 5 of the estimated 15 million people living with HIV-1 in low- and middle-income countries have access (UNAIDS, 2010). Furthermore, the number of new infections continues to outpace the number of people being put on ART each day. ART is costly, and places a formidable financial burden on healthcare services. This in turn compromises efforts for universal access.

Combination ART has made a significant impact on HIV-1 morbidity and mortality (Vittinghoff et al., 1999, Palella et al., 2006) and represents the 'gold standard' for HIV-1 treatment. Despite early optimism that combination ART could potentially eradicate infection (Perelson et al., 1996, Ho, 1997), it has since become clear that virus invariably returns if ART is stopped. As a result, ART remains a daily lifelong treatment requiring a high level of compliance to avoid the development of (multi) drug resistance.

Where ART is available, the diagnosis 'AIDS' becomes less frequent, and HIV-1 infection may no longer be considered a irrevocable terminal disease but rather a chronic manageable infection. However, recent studies have observed that ART does not restore life expectancy completely (Neuhaus et al., 2010a; The Antiretroviral Therapy Cohort, 2008). Furthermore, as those living with HIV-1 do become older, age-related toxicities emerge (Powderly, 2007, 2010) as well as other ART co-morbidities such as increased risk of cardiovascular disease, metabolic disorders, neurocognitive abnormalities, liver and renal disease, bone disorders, malignancy and frailty (Deeks & Phillips, 2009).

Untreated HIV-1 infection is characterised by a substantial depletion of CD4+ T-cells in the mucosa as well as a gradual progressive decline of CD4+ T-cells in peripheral blood. When CD4+ T-cell levels in peripheral blood fall below 200 cells/mm^3, immune competence is reduced leading to susceptibility to opportunistic infections and conditions that characterise AIDS as well as significant increases in viral load (Levy, 2007). It is primarily the level of CD4+ T-cells in peripheral blood that determines the requirement for ART (Panel on Antiretroviral Guidelines for Adults and Adolescents, 2011).

In recent years it has become apparent that disease progression in HIV-1 infection is not simply due to a loss of CD4+ T-cells as a result of chronic cytopathic viral infection. Instead, HIV-1 infection is accompanied by a progressive generalised immune activation (Neuhaus et al., 2010b; Kuller et al., 2008). Indeed, expression of the activation marker CD38 particularly on CD8+ T-cells has been found to be more predictive of disease progression than viral load (Giorgi et al., 1993; Hazenberg et al., 2003). Although immune activation may be reduced on effective ART, it is not completely absent but remains higher than in uninfected individuals. This may in part explain the loss and/or lack of optimal gain in CD4+ T-cell counts despite effective viral suppression below the level of detection (Hunt et al., 2003). It is intriguing that a similar immune activation is also observed in rhesus macaques infected with simian immunodeficiency virus (SIVsmm or SIVagm) but not in the natural host for these viruses, the sooty mangabey and African green monkey respectively, despite high viral loads (Silvestri et al., 2003). Furthermore, HIV-2 in contrast to HIV-1, is associated with slower disease progression and lower levels of immune activation (Sousa et al., 2002).

The underlying causes of the generalised immune activation associated with HIV-1 infection are presently not fully understood, but are probably associated with multiple mechanisms. These may include reactivation of latent viruses during HIV-1 infection, such as cytomegalovirus (CMV) or Epstein-Barr virus (EBV). The most widely considered mechanism is based on the significant depletion of CD4+ T-cells in the mucosa leading to a disruption of the gut lining and translocation of microbial flora to the systemic immune system (Brenchley et al., 2006). HIV-1 is known to incorporate host human leukocyte antigens (HLA) into its envelope during budding, that may play a role in immune activation. Furthermore, the conserved C5 region of gp120 may also be involved in immune activation (Cadogan & Dalgleish, 2008) by virtue of similarity with the peptide binding domains of HLA molecules. This region of gp120 has been shown to bind peptide and promote activation of antigen-specific T-cell clones (Sheikh et al., 2000).

A small percent (<5%) of individuals have been found to control HIV-1 infection for long periods in the absence of ART. Virus levels, although very low - are never eliminated in these individuals (Hunt et al., 2011). These elite and viraemic controllers (that have a low viral load) have been shown to have narrow cell-mediated immune responses preferentially targeting Gag, and lower immune activation (Rosenberg et al., 1997; Zuniga et al., 2006; Walker, 2007; Saez-Cirion et al., 2007; Binley et al., 1997; Kiepiela et al., 2007). The fact that some individuals can control HIV-1 viraemia suggests that long-term immunological control of HIV-1 infection is possible. This therefore provides credence to the concept of therapeutic vaccination as a means to confer relevant immune stimulation that can ultimately lead to a sustained virological response, emulating a long-term nonprogressor status where the risk of virus transmission is reduced. As a result, more focus will need to be directed to understanding the mechanism(s) behind the control of HIV-1 in elite and viraemic controllers (Autran et al., 2011).

Long-term control of HIV-1 infection in the absence of ART forms the basis for the term 'functional cure' where virus and immune activation levels become equivalent to that found in elite controllers or natural virus suppressors (Jeffries, 2010). In contrast, a 'sterilising cure' relates to HIV-1 eradication, that is, the permanent removal of the HIV-1 by the complete elimination of viral reservoirs. The eradication concept has been inspired by 'The Berlin Patient' who received a bone marrow transplant from a donor that had the CCR5 Δ32 mutation rendering the cells resistant to virus strains using this co-receptor for infection (Hütter et al., 2009). The Berlin patient has remained virus-free for four years to date (Allers et al., 2011).

Therapeutic vaccines have the advantage of being able to penetrate sanctuary sites less well accessed by ART such as lymphoid tissue (Pantaleo et al., 1991; Fox et al., 1991) and the central nervous system (Alexaki et al., 2008), that represent regions for viral persistence. This relates to therapeutic interventions targeting both the virus itself as well as HIV-associated immune activation. This chapter will discuss the potential contribution of therapeutic vaccination to achieve a functional cure for HIV-1 infection.

2. HIV-1 persistence in reservoirs

The failure of ART to eradicate HIV-1 infection lies in the observation that HIV-1 remains quiescent in latent reservoirs. Latently infected resting CD4+ cells (either naive or long lived memory cells) carry transcriptionally silent HIV-1 and represent the predominant reservoir of HIV-1 infection. Other cells may also act as reservoirs (Reviewed in Alexaki et al., 2008) such as macrophages, dendritic cells and astrocytes (where HIV-1 infection occurs via a CD4-independent mechanism). It is these latent reservoirs that represent the major challenge to eradication of HIV-1 infection. More than 80% of individuals on suppressive ART have persistent viraemia below the level of detection (Maldarelli et al., 2007). This low level viraemia is not reduced further despite ART intensification (Dinoso et al., 2009) supporting the concept that HIV-1 rebounds on ART cessation from the rapid reactivation of virus from latently infected cells rather than from continuous ongoing low level replication (Joos et al., 2008). Long lived memory cells comprise approximately 1 cell per million with an extremely low decay rate explaining why 73 years is required to eliminate HIV-1 from infected individuals (Finzi et al., 1999, Siliciano, 2010).

It is clear that to achieve a functional cure, therapeutic vaccination will need to induce not only effective antigen-specific immune responses but also combat the generalised immune activation induced by HIV-1.

3. The concept of a functional cure

The ultimate aim of a functional cure for HIV-1 infection is to induce long-term remission by depleting virus reservoirs to such an extent that a 'controller' status is achieved. In this way virus is maintained at low levels for long periods of time in the absence of ART, equivalent to that observed in known HIV-1 controllers (Lambotte et al., 2005) natural virus suppressors (Sajadi et al., 2007) and elite controllers (Deeks & Walker, 2007). This concept can be compared to achieving a sustained virological response for hepatitis C virus (HCV) infection following interferon/ribavirin treatment. If a sustained virological response is observed for HCV (undetectable virus for at least 6 months), the patient is considered cured. The potential for curing HCV infection is theoretically greater than for HIV-1 since HCV, a separate genus *Hepacivirus* within the virus family Flaviviridae, replicates solely in the cytoplasm of infected cells. As such, on cell division, the virus may remain in only one of the daughter cells. In contrast, HIV-1 is a retrovirus that integrates into the host genome and as such, on cell division will be automatically present in both daughter cells.

A sustained virological response for HIV-1 could be envisaged as either:

a. Indefinite virus control below the limits of detection (<50 copies HIV-1 RNA/ml) (equivalent to a sterilising cure/eradication).
b. Long-term low level virus replication, as for a natural virus suppressor or long-term non progressor, with concomitant low levels of immune activation (equivalent to a functional cure).

Approaches towards eradication include attempts to purge reservoirs by selective activation of latently infected cells (such as memory cells) in the presence of ART such that released virus may not infect and replicate in neighbouring cells (Richman et al., 2009). Agents include histone deacetylase inhibitors, cytokines, such as IL-2 and IL-7, as well as bryostatin, the protein kinase C activator (Kovochich et al., 2011). However, such interventions may also be associated with side effects, resistance and high cost.

Maintaining HIV-1-infected cells in a continuously latent (transcriptionally silent) state, akin to true latency characteristic of herpesviruses, represents the opposite extreme that has received less attention. HIV-1 is produced from activated CD4+ T-cells. At present it is not clear how HIV-1 can be maintained transcriptionally silent whilst still allowing for the CD4+ T-cell activation required to mount an immune response.

3.1 Functional cure and treatment interruption

In order to demonstrate a sustained virological response (functional cure) for patients that are well controlled on ART, treatment will ultimately need to be stopped in order to show that virus levels remain controlled (low/undetectable).

Treatment interruption has been intensely investigated in the past as a means to overcome the limitations of lifelong ART which include side effects, drug resistance and high cost. Today, treatment interruption *per se,* is viewed with scepticism due to safety concerns arising from the SMART study, the largest treatment interruption study to date (El-Sadr et al., 2006). In the SMART study and numerous previous smaller studies, ART was interrupted without any additional immunological support. Treatment interruption in the SMART study was CD4-guided, where ART was discontinued when CD4 levels rose above 350 cells/mm^3 and resumed if CD4 counts fell below 250 cells/mm^3. However, the study was prematurely halted since patients in the treatment conservation group (treatment interruption) experienced greater side effects and adverse events than those in the continuous ART arm. The SMART study therefore concluded that treatment interruption was not safe and that ART should remain a continuous life-long treatment. These safety concerns have affected the design of all treatment interruption trials including those for therapeutic vaccines. Interestingly, a more recent large study of the Swiss Cohort, has suggested that treatment interruption of up to six months can be safely tolerated particularly if patients are well monitored (Kauffman et al., 2011).

Earlier clinical studies have shown that upon cessation of ART, and in the absence of therapeutic immunisation, CD4+ T-cell counts and virus load rebound to preART levels (i.e. the preART set point) (Oxenius et al., 2002a; Wit et al., 2005; Oxenius et al., 2002b; Mata et al., 2005). However, not all patients have available preART viral load information and therefore efforts have been made to identify alternate markers that may predict where the viral load may settle on treatment interruption in the absence of any other intervention. This is necessary in order to determine whether an intervention has lowered the viral load set point in a subject. Proviral DNA levels at baseline have been shown to correlate with the preART viral load, (Yerly et al., 2005), however, this approach will require further validation before it can be taken in to routine use. Until alternative markers are available, preART RNA values will remain the best predictor of the viral load set point that may be obtained on treatment interruption in the absence of therapeutic immunisation. Consequently, the effect of different therapeutic interventions on the viral load will therefore be compared to the preART values.

CD4+ T-cell counts represent the major parameter that determines the need for ART initiation. For this reason, earlier efforts within therapeutic vaccination aimed to improve CD4+ T-cell counts in order to slow disease progression. However, in light of the SILCAAT and ESPRIT studies that focused on improving CD4+ T-cell counts using IL-2 (which provides nonspecific immune stimulation unlike a therapeutic vaccine that is antigen-specific), the conclusion was that improving CD4 counts *per se* was not associated with clinical benefit (INSIGHT-ESPRIT and SILCAAT Study groups, 2009). Consequently, reducing viral load now represents the unequivocal major endpoint for any therapeutic vaccine or intervention aimed at effecting a functional cure or ultimately eradication.

The current scepticism regarding treatment interruption means that inclusion criteria for patients in such studies will take in to consideration both preART and nadir (lowest ever) CD4+ T-cell counts since this has been shown to be a critical parameter in determining the outcome of treatment interruption (Willberg & Nixon, 2007). In subjects with low CD4+ T-cells nadir (200-250 cells/mm^3), CD4+ T-cell levels fall rapidly on treatment interruption requiring earlier re-initiation of ART (Toulson et al., 2005). Patients selected may therefore be relatively newly infected and have robust preART CD4+ T-cell levels and less well established viral reservoirs.

3.1.1 Functional cure scenario 1: Long lasting remission on ART interruption

One approach towards a functional cure could involve therapeutic vaccination in combination with ART followed by treatment interruption with the aim of providing long lasting sustained virological suppression. The advantage of immunising individuals in the presence of ART is that patients have usually regained CD4+ T-cell counts, including naive CD4+ T-cells that can be stimulated to target HIV-1. Furthermore, virus replication is controlled allowing for immunisation in the absence of circulating virus. The immunisation itself will provide some immune activation as CD4+ T-cells harbouring virus become activated leading to a virus burst which would nevertheless be contained by ART. It would therefore be important to allow for vaccine-induced immune activation to subside before stopping ART. Antigen-specific therapeutic vaccines inducing cell-mediated immune responses against gene products from multiply spliced RNA such as Tat may function in the presence of ART and remove infected cells. This is because these early gene products are not targeted by current antiretroviral therapy. Furthermore, Tat expression is not dependent on the activation state of the infected cell and is therefore also synthesized in quiescent T-cells in the absence of virus replication (Wu & Marsh, 2001). In contrast, for therapeutic vaccines targeting products requiring the expression of structural genes such as Gag and Env, ART would need to be stopped in order for the immune system to identify HIV-1 infected cells expressing these antigens.

Therapeutic vaccination using antigen-specific immune stimulation could be combined with other interventions to provide a long-lasting reduction of HIV-1-associated generalised immune activation and consequently reduce the level of viral rebound even further. The aim would be that when patients are removed from ART, CD4+ T-cell counts would remain sustained and a virus set point would be established at a level compatible with a long-term non-progressor, or elite controller for a significant period of time (Figure 1). The therapeutic vaccine may also attenuate the height of the initial peak rebound so that it does not necessarily overshoot the preART value. This scenario may be most beneficial for newly infected subjects that have robust CD4 T-cell counts.

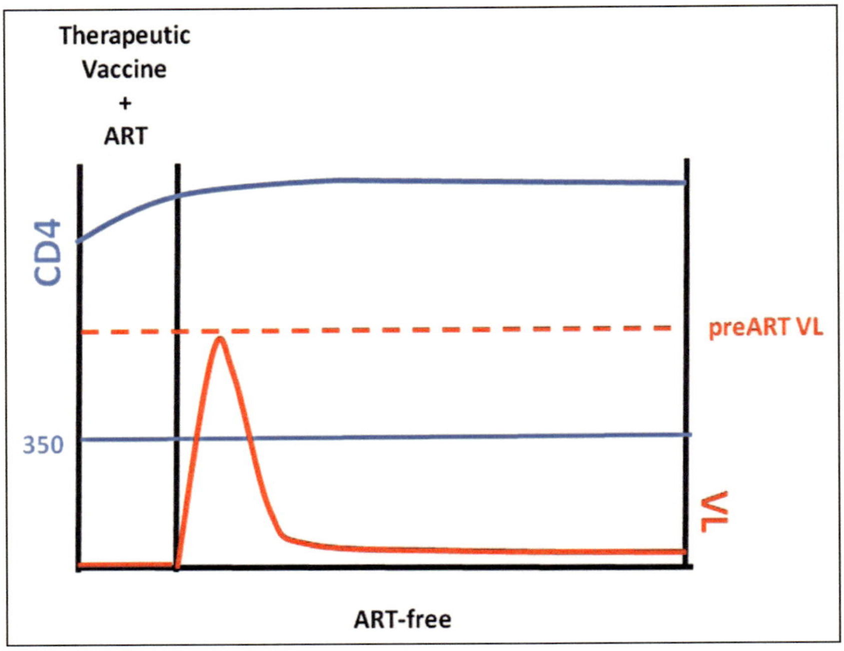

Stippled line at 350 indicates CD4 count below which ART should be initiated. Thick solid line: CD4 count. Thin line: viral load (VL). Dashed line: PreART viral load

Fig. 1. Scenario 1: Therapeutic vaccination in combination with ART leading to sustained virological response (long-lasting remission). Viral rebound may not necessarily overshoot the preART viral load. CD4+ T-cell levels would remain above the level of 350 cells/mm^3 that necessitates a return to ART according to current guidelines

3.1.2 Functional cure scenario 2: Remission following intermittent ART

It is possible that on treatment interruption as in scenario 1, viral load levels may stabilize at a lower set point, but not sufficiently low to be compatible with an HIV controller. This may be the case for individuals that started ART later on in disease course, where the number of viral reservoirs is greater, and the CD4+ T-cell nadir lower. To address this, therapeutic vaccination may be used to allow ART to become safely intermittent and where the viral set point may be sequentially reduced following multiple cycles of ART and booster immunisations with the therapeutic vaccine (Figure 2). In such a scenario, due to the safety concerns, the duration of the ART-free period should not exceed the 6 month time period shown to be safe in the Swiss cohort study (Kauffman et al., 2011). This approach of intermittent ART in combination with therapeutic immunisation and booster immunisations has not been investigated to date and may be viewed with scepticism due to the safety concerns arising from the SMART study. However, the underlying basis for the SMART study, i.e. a need to combat ART side effects, drug resistance and high cost remain relevant issues that need to be resolved.

Similarly to scenario 1, therapeutic vaccination may also attenuate the size of the initial peak of rebound during the first treatment interruption allowing the set point to establish below the preART level. Following subsequent booster immunisations on ART in this scenario, as the viral load set point is lowered, CD4+ T-cell decline would also become less marked and would ultimately stabilise above the level necessitating ART (350 cells/mm^3).

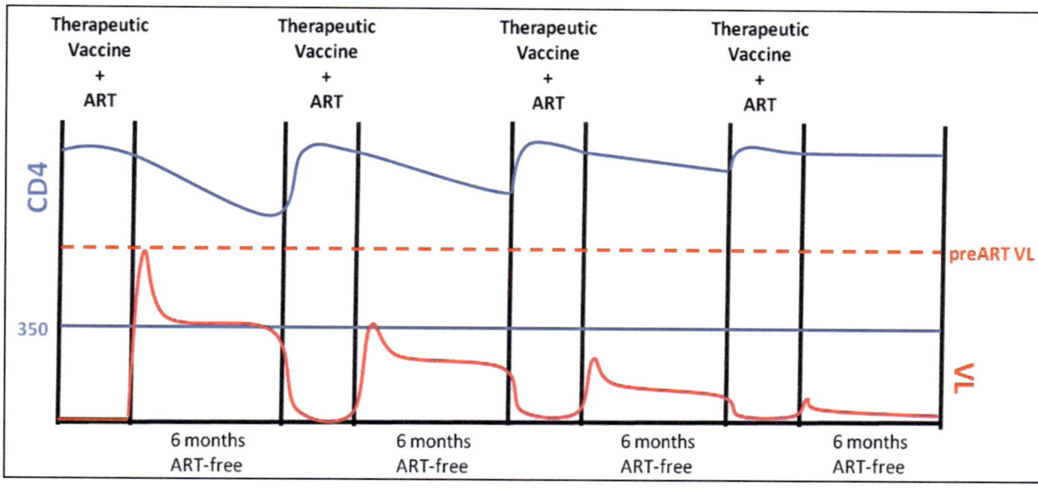

Stippled line at 350 indicates CD4 count below which ART should be initiated. Thick solid line: CD4 count. Thin line: viral load (VL). Dashed line: PreART viral load

Fig. 2. Scenario 2: Functional cure over time: intermittent ART supported by therapeutic vaccination, where viral rebound achieves a lower set point for each successive treatment interruption with a concomitant slower CD4+ T-cell decline over time

Any therapeutic vaccination approach involving treatment interruption involves concerns that viral reservoirs would become repopulated. It is interesting to note that viral reservoirs are also repopulated in elite controller patients since they never manage to eliminate their virus despite maintaining a viral set point below the level of detection (Hunt et al., 2011).

3.1.3 Functional cure scenario 3: On continuous ART

Although potentially applicable to all patient categories, this third scenario for achieving a functional cure on continuous ART may be particularly suited for subjects where treatment interruption is not considered a viable option due to poor CD4+ T-cell reconstitution on ART, low CD4+ T-cell nadir or a very high preART viral load set point. This approach could involve combining continuous ART with therapeutic vaccination and reservoir purging agents (Figure 3).

In this scenario, subjects would be maintained on continuous ART. Therapeutic vaccination would be carried out in the presence of ART as in scenarios 1 and 2 with the aim of generating more effective responses to HIV-1. However, instead of removing patients from ART as in scenarios 1 and 2, reservoir purging agents would be used to reverse latency and allow for the expression of viral genes. Viral replication and spread would be hindered due to the presence of ART. Expression of viral genes would render infected cells 'visible' to the immune system allowing for their removal as a consequence of the improved immune responses resulting from therapeutic immunisation. However, to show ultimately that viral reservoirs have been reduced significantly or even fully depleted, subjects will need to be removed from ART.

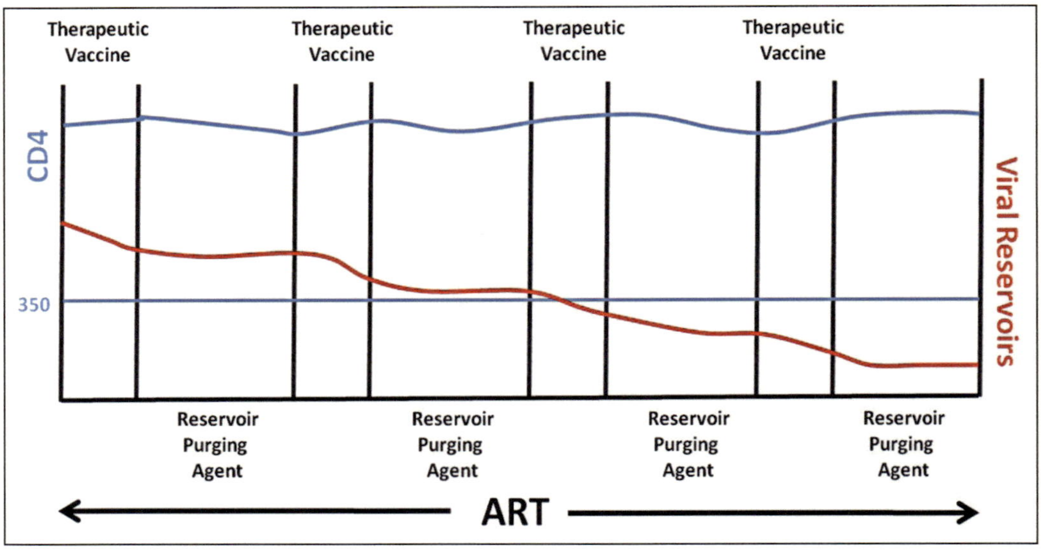

Stippled line at 350 indicates CD4 count below which ART should be initiated. Thick solid line: CD4 count. Thin line: viral reservoirs

Fig. 3. Scenario 3: Subjects remain on continuous ART. Therapeutic vaccination takes place in the presence of ART and the immune responses generated can remove infected cells that release virus following the use of reservoir purging agents. This procedure may need to be repeated to gradually remove virus reservoirs over time

3.2 Functional cure and treatment naive patients

Therapeutic vaccination of individuals that are treatment naive would be an attractive proposition in regions where ART availability is incomplete and where the financial burden to sustain life long treatment is greatest. In this case, subjects would be immunised in the presence of circulating virus to improve and direct immune responses to important epitopes such that viral load is decreased, CD4+ T-cell numbers have the potential to increase and the initiation of treatment delayed. However, therapeutic vaccination itself may result in a transient immune activation that could result in the seeding of further reservoirs with functional and 'fit' (replication competent) virus.

Treatment naive individuals currently represent a study population where the effects of therapeutic vaccination on viral load and CD4+ T-cell counts can be readily observed. However, clinical trials involving treatment naive subjects will likely involve enrolment of patients that are early in disease course and where ART is not yet indicated. Such patients would likely have robust CD4+ T-cell counts and viral loads below 100 000 copies/ml. It is likely that viral reservoirs in these patients would be less well established. The more robust the CD4+ T-cell count, the more likely that the patient may provide an immunological response to the therapeutic vaccine.

4. Approaches to therapeutic vaccination in clinical development

A number of different approaches to HIV-1 therapeutic vaccination are currently in clinical development, although not necessarily at this point in time directly aiming to achieve a functional cure (Tables 1-3). The majority of products aim to induce T-cell immunity whereas a minority aim to induce antibody responses to specific viral antigens.

The viral antigens used as therapeutic vaccine candidates include peptides, polypeptides, fusion proteins, recombinant proteins, DNA, RNA either alone or with viral vectors such as poxviruses or adenoviruses, as well as inactivated autologous virus. These antigens can be injected directly or via *ex vivo* bombardment of autologous dendritic cells that are re-infused into the patient. The overall objective of therapeutic vaccine candidates is to reduce viral load, although some also aim to concurrently sustain CD4+ T-cell counts upon ART interruption.

The potency of *ex vivo* stimulation of dendritic cells with inactivated autologous virus was first appreciated following the original studies by Lu et al., (2004) and Garcia et al., (2005) where subjects experienced a significant although transient reduction of viral load. Such approaches require access to autologous virus prior to ART initiation either for purification and inactivation or use as the basis for amplification of viral genes. This approach requires access to advanced technology and may require intermittent boosting to maintain the effect.

Therapeutic vaccines are also being developed that aim to target dendritic cells *in situ*. This usually involves intradermal administration. Since intradermal injection requires trained personnel, alternative approaches are being developed to target dendritic cells such as topical patches/plasters.

Company	**Product**	**Clinical phase**	**Technology**
Argos Therapeutics	AGS-004	II n=34 NCT00672191	Autologous DCs co-electroporated with amplified *in vitro* transcribed RNA encoding CD40L and autologous HIV-1 antigens derived from the patient's own plasma taken immediately prior to the initiation of ART.
Baylor University/ ANRS	DC Vaccine	I n=19 NCT00796770	DALIA study: *Ex vivo* administration of Lipopeptides to Nef, Gag and Env to DCs followed by reinfusion to patient
Bionor Pharma	Vacc-4x	IIb n=137 NCT00659789	Peptides to conserved domains of HIV p24 injected intradermally with GM-CSF.
Genetic Immunity	LC002	II n=16 NCT00918840	Clade B DNA in nanoparticles and delivered to DCs in a patch (Dermavir).
NIAID/ Profectus Biosciences	MRK Ad5 HIV-1 gag	II n=120 NCT00080106	Replication defective adenovirus vector carrying HIV-1 gag.

Table 1. Therapeutic vaccine candidates immunising subjects on ART with a treatment interruption phase in the study. DC:dendritic cell, TI: treatment interruption. NCT provides the clinical trial identifier for trials listed on www.clinicaltrials.gov

Viral vectors derived from adenoviruses or poxviruses have also been extensively used to deliver DNA-based vaccines most often in a prime boost strategy. For such approaches it will likely be necessary to determine the serological status of vaccine recipients to the viruses that have been used as a basis for these vectors since prior immunity may negatively affect vaccine efficacy. Similarly, maintenance of vaccine effect may require boosting using a heterologous virus vector, to avoid inhibitory effects of prior vaccine-induced immunity to the original vector.

Although the induction of neutralising antibodies remains the major goal for an effective preventative vaccine, therapeutic vaccines aim to induce antibody responses to other viral antigens such as the HIV-1 Tat protein. Earlier studies have shown that loss of antibody responses to Tat correlated with disease progression (van Baalen et al., 1997; Rezza et al., 2005). Such a vaccine may also address pathogenic effects of Tat released from infected cells (Ensoli et al., 1993).

Company	Product	Clinical phase	Technology
Imperial College	GTU-MultiHIV-B (FIT06)	I n=30 NCT01130376	DNA plasmid. Intradermal injections in combination with GM-CSF and IL-2 as well as a growth hormone.
Univ. Oxford Med Research Council.	MVA.HIVconsv	I n=20 NCT01024842	MVA vector encoding a DNA that carries conserved domains in Gag, Vif, Pol, Env.
University Pennsylvania / Drexel University	PENNVAX B,GENEVAX IL-12-4532, pIL15EAM	I n=38 NCT00775424	PENNVAX-B is a DNA vaccine encodes synthetic HIV-1 envelope protein, Gag and Pol. GENEVAX and pIL15 are DNA adjuvants (IL-12 and IL-15)
Massachusetts General Hospital	DNA	I n=21 NCT00833781	Dendritic cells transfected with vectors encoding consensus (clade B) HIV Gag and Nef mRNA.
NIAID	HIV Antigens & IL-12	I n=60 NCT01266616	Plasmid DNA with IL-12 to enhance the response.

Table 2. Therapeutic vaccine candidates in clinical development where therapeutic vaccination occurs in the presence of continuous ART. DC: dendritic cell. NCT provides the clinical trial identifier for trials listed on www.clinicaltrials.gov

5. The challenges facing therapeutic vaccination

No preventative vaccine has yet been developed for HIV-1 infection. This is despite intense efforts since the virus was first isolated in 1983 (Barre-Sinoussi et al., 1983). The challenges faced by preventative and therapeutic vaccines are similar in that HIV-1 shows extensive genetic variation and a propensity for immune escape. Furthermore, human populations are also varied and this is characterised by a variety of human leukocyte antigens (HLA). HLA function to present HIV-1 epitopes at the surface of infected cells to allow for recognition and removal by cytotoxic T-lymphocytes. The association of certain HLA with virus control (e.g. HLA-B57) and disease progression (e.g. B35) has recently been highlighted

(International HIV Controllers Study Study, 2010). However these HLA alleles are not present in a large proportion of individuals. It has been suggested that patients in clinical studies should be HLA tested to help explain and understand the results (Li et al., 2011).
One salient difference between the preventative and therapeutic vaccines lies in their objectives. At present it is considered remote that a vaccine can be developed that will yield sterilising immunity and complete protection from HIV-1 infection. For this reason, the objective of a preventative vaccine is now to prevent infection as far as is possible, and should infection occur the immune system will be sufficiently primed to ensure that the disease course is milder (Johnston & Fauci, 2007). This was the aim of the STEP trial, which used an adenovirus vector. However, unexpectedly, prior exposure to adenovirus infection resulted in greater susceptibility to HIV-1 infection in study participants (Buchbinder et al., 2008).

Company	Product	Clinical phase	Technology
Genetic Immunity	LC002	II n=36 NCT00711230	Clade B DNA incorporated into nanoparticles and delivered to DCs in a patch (Dermavir).
SEEK (previously PepTcell)	HIV-v	I n=55 NCT01071031	Mixture of polypeptide T-cell epitope sequences to conserved domains of HIV (internal proteins). Single subcutaneous injection
Statens seruminstitutt, DK, EU clinical trials partnership	AFO-18	I n=20 NCT01141205	Peptides representing 3 CD4 and 17 CD8 minimal HIV epitopes. Adjuvant CAF01.
Thymon	TUTI-16	I/II n=24 NCT00848211	Tat Lipopeptide. Subcutaneous injection, acts as own adjuvant.
FIT Biotech	FIT06 (GTU-MultiHIV-B)	II n=60	DNA plasmid using GTU® Technology patented by FIT Biotech (Gene Transport Unit). Gag, Rev, Nef, Tat. Clade B.
Hospital Clinic of Barcelona	DCV2	I/II n=60 NCT00402142	Autologous dendritic cell pulsed *ex vivo* with patient's own virus.
Istituto Superiore di Sanita	ISS T003	II n= 160 NCT01029548	Inactivated Tat protein injected intradermally (i.d.) to induce antibodies to Tat. This study is an observational cohort.

Table 3. Therapeutic vaccine candidates in clinical development immunising subjects that are treatment naive.

6. Conclusion

The complexity of HIV-1 infection represents a challenge to achieving a functional cure or ultimately eradication of infection. A number of scenarios have been suggested in this chapter where therapeutic vaccination is combined with ART and also potentially with virus purging agents. At present it is unlikely that any one scenario will suit all purposes, indeed, the choice of approach will likely depend upon the availability of ART, how far advanced the infection is on diagnosis and when during the disease course ART was initiated since these considerations will influence the size of viral reservoir.

It is unlikely that there will ever be a single product that will either prevent HIV-1 infection completely or eradicate HIV-1 infection. Therefore, combinations may be more appropriate. Harnessing the immune system is a rational approach to combine with ART bearing in mind that the immune system may penetrate regions of the body not reached by current therapy. Combination ART has been more successful than monotherapy. Similarly combining ART with therapeutic vaccination and/or virus purging agents will likely be more effective than any of these interventions on their own. The recent Thai study provides is an example where two preventative vaccine candidates that had not shown effect earlier, provided an improved response leading to a marginally significant effect when combined (Reks-Ngarm et al., 2009).

Ultimately a therapeutic vaccine will need to confer effective immune responses in all individuals regardless whether they possess HLA compatible with virus control or not. It is therefore important that therapeutic vaccine candidates take into consideration genetic variation in both human and viral populations in order to be able to elicit the most effective responses leading to control of infection. Strictly, the term 'functional cure' can be considered misleading since virus is not completely removed from the body, but rather the patient experiences remission from symptoms. The term 'functional control' would therefore be more appropriate.

Eradication approaches will require much research and development, where both novel and known compounds will be tested in new ways to determine a potential effect on eradication without incurring too many side effects. It may therefore take significant time before such products are available on the market. In contrast, a functional cure may be achievable in the shorter term and represent a more realistic goal since virus reduction has been shown for a number of therapeutic vaccine candidates. Approaches that aim to successfully combat HIV-1 infection will need to address both the virus (virus-specific approaches including ART and therapeutic vaccines) as well as the generalized immune activation that drives the infection. It is likely that to achieve a functional cure, a combination of different interventions may ultimately be required.

7. Acknowledgments

This work has been partly supported by a grant from the Research Council of Norway GLOBVAC programme. Many thanks to Birger Sørensen, Ingebjørg Baksaas, Vidar Wendel-Hansen and Giuseppe Pantaleo for reading and commenting the manuscript.

8. References

Alexaki, A.; Liu, Y. & Wigdahl B. (2008). Cellular reservoirs of HIV-1 and their role in viral persistence. *Curr. HIV Res.* 6:388-400.

Allers, K.; Hütter, G.; Hofmann, J.; Loddenkemper, C.; Rieger, K.; Thiel, E.; Schneider, T. (2009). Evidence for the cure of HIV infection by CCR5Δ32/Δ32 stem cell transplantation. *Blood* 117:2791-99.

Autran, B.; Descours, B.; Avettand-Fenoel, V. & Rouzioux, C. (2011). Elite controllers as a model of functional cure. *Curr. Opin. HIV and AIDS* 6:181-187.

Barré-Sinoussi, F., Chermann, J.C., Rey, F., Nugeyre, M.T., Chamaret, S., Gruest, J., Dauguet, C., Axler-Blin, C., Vézinet-Brun, F., Rouziousx, C., Rosenbaum, W., Montagnier, L. (1983). Isolation of a T-lymphotropic retrovirus from a patient at risk for acquired immunodeficiency syndrome AIDS. *Science* 220:868-71.

Binley, J.M.; Klasse, P.J., Cao, Y.; Jones, I.; Markowitz, M.; Ho, D.D. & Moore, J.P.(1997). Differential regulation of the antibody responses to Gag and Env proteins of human immunodeficiency virus type 1. *J. Virol.* 71:2799-2809

Brenchley, J.M. Price, D.A.; Schacker, T.W.; Asher, T.E.; Silvestri, G.; Rao, S.; Kazzaz, Z.; Bornstein, E.; Lambotte, O.; Altmann, D.; Blazar, B.R.; Rodriguez, B.; Teixeira-Johnson, L.; Landay, A.; Martin, J.N.; Hecht, F.M.; Picker, L.J.; Lederman, M.M.; Deeks, S.G. & Douek, D.C. (2006). Microbial translocation is a cause of systemic immune activation in chronic HIV infection. *Nat. Med.* 12:1365-71

Buchbinder, S.P.; Mehrotra, D.V.; Duerr, A.; Fitzgerald, D.A.; Mogg, R.; Li, D. Gilbert, P.B.; Lama, J.R.; Marmor, M.; del Rio, C.; McElrath, J.; Casimiro, D.R.; Gottesdiener, K.M.; Chodakewitz, J.A.; Corey, L. & Robertson, M.N. The Step Study Protocol Team (2008). *Lancet* 372:1881–93

Cadogan, M. & Dalgleish, A.G. (2008). Pathogenesis of HIV: non-specific immune hyperactivity and its implications for vaccines. *Clinical Medicine* 8:267-71.

Deeks, S.G. & Phillips, A.N. (2009). HIV infection, antiretroviral treatment, ageing and non-AIDS-related morbidity. *BMJ* 338:a3172.

Deeks, S.G. & Walker, B.D. (2007). Human immunodeficiency virus controllers: mechanisms of durable virus control in the absence of therapy. *Immunity* 27:406-416.

Dinoso, J.B.; Kim, S.Y.; Wiegand, A.M.; Palmer, S.E.; Gange, S.J.; Cranmer, L.; O'Shea, A.; Callender, M.; Spivak, A., Brennan, T.; Kearney, M.F.; Proschan, M.A.; Mican, J.M.; Rehm, C.A.; Coffin, J.M.; Mellors, J.W.; Siliciano, R.F. & Maldarelli, F. (2009). Treatment intensification does not reduce residual HIV-1 viraemia in patients in highly active antiretroviral therapy. *Proc. Nat. Acad. Sci. USA* 106:9403-08.

El-Sadr, W.M., Lundgren, J.D.; Neaton, J.D.; Gordin, F.; Abrams, D.; Arduino, R.C.; Babiker, A.; Burman, W.; Clumeck, N.; Cohen, C.J., Cohn, D.; Cooper, D.; Darbyshire, J.; Emery, S.; Fätkenheuer, G.; Gazzard, B.; Grund, B.; Hoy, J.; Klingman, K.; Losso, M.; Markowitz, N.; Neuhaus, J.; Phillips, A.; Rappoport, C. & the SMART Study Group. CD4+ count-guided interruption of antiretroviral treatment. *N. Engl. J. Med.* 2006; 355:2283-96

Ensoli, B.; Buonaguro, L.; Barillari, G.; Fiorelli, V.; Gendelman, R.; Morgan, R.A.; Wingfield, P. & Gallo, R.C. (1993) Release, uptake, and effects of extracellular human immunodeficiency virus type 1 Tat protein on cell growth and viral transactivation. *J. Virol* 67:277–87.

Finzi, D.; Blankson, J.; Siliciano, J.D.; Margolick, J.B.; Chadwick, K.; Pierson, T.; Smith, K.; Lisziewicz, J.; Lori, F.; Flexner, C.; Quinn, T.C.; Chaisson, R.E.; Rosenberg, E.; Walker, B.; Gange, S.; Gallant, J. & Siliciano, R.F. (1999). Latent infection of CD4+ T cells provides a mechanism for lifelong persistence of HIV-1, even in patients on effective combination therapy. *Nat. Med.* 5:512–517.

Fox, C.H.; Tenner-Racz, K.; Firpo, A.; Pizzo, P.A. & Fauci, A.S. (1991) Lymphoid germinal centers are reservoirs of human immunodeficiency virus type 1 RNA. *J. Infect. Dis.* 164:1051–57.

Garcia, F.; García, F.; Lejeune, M.; Climent, N.; Gil, C.; Alcamí, J.; Morente, V.; Alós, L.; Ruiz, A.; Setoain, J.; Fumero, E.; Castro, P.; López, A.; Cruceta, A.; Piera, C.; Florence, E.; Pereira, A.; Libois, A.; González, N.; Guilá, M.; Caballero, M.; Lomeña, F.; Joseph, J.; Miró, J.M.; Pumarola, T.; Plana, M.; Gatell, J.M. & Gallart, T. (2005). Therapeutic immunization with dendritic cells loaded with heat-inactivated autologous HIV-1 in patients with chronic HIV-1 infection. *J. Infect. Dis.* 191:1680-5

Giorgi, J.V.; Liu, Z.; Hultin, L.E.; Cumberland, W.G.; Hennessey, K. & Detels, R. (1993). Elevated levels of CD38+CD8+ T cells in HIV infection add to the prognostic value of low CD4+ T-cell levels: Results of 6 years follow-up. The Los Angeles Center, Multicenter AIDS Cohort Study. *J. Acquir. Immune Def. Syndr.* 6:904-12.

Hazenberg, M.D.; Otto, S.A.; van Benthem, B.H.; Roos, M.T.; Coutinho, R.A.; Lange, J.M.; Hamann, D.; Prins, M. & Miedema, F. (2003). Persistent immune activation in HIV-1 infection is associated with progression to AIDS. *AIDS* 17:1881-8.

Ho, D.D. (1997). How far can you knock down HIV? An interview with David D. Ho, MD. Interview by Mark Mascolini. *J. Int. Assoc. Physicians AIDS Care.* 3:40-4.

Hunt, P.W.; Martin, J.N.; Sinclair, E.; Bredt, B.; Hagos, E.; Lampiris, H. & Deeks, S.G. (2003). T cell activation is associated with lower CD4+ T-cell gains in human immunodeficiency virus-infected patients with sustained viral suppression during antiretroviral therapy. *J. Infect. Dis.* 187:1534-43.

Hunt, PW.; Hatano, H.; Sinclair, E.; Lee, T-H.; Busch, MP.; Martib, JN.; McCune, JM. & Deeks, SG. (2011). HIV-specific CD4+ T cells may contribute to viral persistence in HIV controllers. *Clin. Infec. Dis.* 52:681-7.

Hütter, G.; Nowak, D.; Mossner, M.; Ganepola, S.; Musig, A.; Allers, K.; Schneider, T.; Hofmann, J.; Kucherer, C.; Blau, O.; Blau, IW.; Hofmann, WK. & Thiel, E. (2009). Long-Term Control of HIV by CCR5 Delta32/Delta32 Stem-Cell Transplantation. *N. Engl. J. Med.* 360:692-8.

INSIGHT-ESPRIT and SILCCAT study Groups. (2009). Interleukin-2 therapy in patients with HIV infection. *N. Engl. J. Med.* 361:1548-59.

International HIV Controllers Study. (2010). The major genetic determinants of HIV-1 control affect HLA class I peptide presentation. *Science* 330:1551-7

Jeffries, RJ. (2010). Workshop report: Towards a cure: HIV reservoirs and strategies to control them. Journal of the International AIDS Society 13(Suppl. 3):I1. (http://www.jiasociety.org/content/13/S3/I1)[Accessed 11th July 2011]

Johnston, M. & Fauci, A. (2007). An HIV Vaccine – Evolving concepts. *N. Engl. J. Med.* 356:2073-81

Joos, B.; Fischer, M.; Kuster, H.; Pillai, S.K.; Wong, J.K.; Böni, J.; Hirscheld, B.; Webera, R.; Trkolaa, A.; Günthard, H.F.; & The Swiss HIV Cohort Study (2008). HIV rebounds from latently infected cells, rather than from continuing low-level replication. *Proc. Natl. Acad. Sci. USA* 105:16725-30.

Kaufmann, GR.; Elzi, L.; Weber, R.; Furrer, H.; Giulieri, S.; Vernazza, P.; Bernasconi, E.; Hirschel, B. & Battegay, M.; the Swiss HIV Cohort Study (2011). Interruptions of cART limits CD4 T-cell recovery and increases the risk of opportunistic complications and death. *AIDS* 25:441-451.

Kiepiela, P.; Ngumbela, K.; Thobakgale, C.; Ramduth, D.; Honeyborne, I.; Moodley, E.; Reddy, S.; de Pierres, C.; Mncube, Z.; Mkhwanazi, N.; Bishop, K.; van der Stok, M.; Nair, K.; Khan, N.; Crawford, H.; Payne, R.; Leslie, A.; Prado, J.; Prendergast, A.; Frater, J.; McCarthy, N.; Brander, C.; Learn, G.H.; Nickle, D.; Rousseau, C.; Coovadia, H.; Mullins, J.I.; Heckerman, D.; Walker, B.D.; Goulder, P. (2007). CD8+ T-cell responses to different HIV proteins have discordant associations with viral load. *Nat. Med.* 13:46-53.

Kovochich, M.; Marsden, M.D. & Zack, J. (2011). Activation of latent HIV using drug-loaded nanoparticles. *PLoS ONE* 6 (4):e18270.

Kuller, L.H.; Tracy, R.; Belloso, W.; De Wit, S.; Drummond, F.; Lane, H.C.; Ledergerber, B.; Lundgren, J.; Neuhaus, J.; Nixon, D.; Paton, N.I. & Neaton, J.D. INSIGHT SMART Study Group (2008) Inflammatory and Coagulation Biomarkers and Mortality in Patients with HIV Infection. *Plos Med.* Oct 21;5(10):e203.

Lambotte, O.; Boufassa, F.; Madec, Y.; Nguyen, A.; Goujard, C.; Meyer, L.; Rouzioux, C.; Venet, A. & Delfraissy, J.F. SEROCO-HEMOCO Study Group (2005). HIV controllers: a homogeneous group of HIV-1 infected patients with spontaneous control of viral replication. *Clin. Infect. Dis.* 41:1053-1056.

Levy J. (2007). Overall features of HIV pathogenesis: prognosis for long-term survival. In: *HIV and the Pathogenesis of AIDS* 3rd Edition pp317-357. ASM Press. ISBN-13 978-1-55581-393-2.

Li, J.Z.; Brumme, Z.L.. Brumme,, C.J.; Wang, H.; Spritzler, J.; Robertson, M.N.; Lederman, M.M.; Carrington, M.;Walker, B.D.; Schooley,R.T.; & Kuritzkes, D.R. for the AIDS Clinical Trials Group A5197 Study Team (2011). Factors associated with viral Rebound in HIV-1-infected individuals enrolled in a therapeutic HIV-1 gag vaccine trial. *J. Infect. Dis.* 203:976–83

Lu, W.; Arraes, L.C.; Ferreira, W.T. & Andrieu, J. M. (2004). Therapeutic dendritic cell vaccine for chronic HIV-1 infection. *Nat. Med.* 10:1359-65

Maldarelli, F.; Palmer, S.; King, M.S.; Wiegand, A.; Polis, M.A.; Mican, J.; Kovacs, J.A.; Davey, R.T.; Rock-Kress, D.; Dewar, R.; Liu, S.; Metcalf, J.A.; Rehm, C.; Brun, S.C.; Hanna, G.J.; Kempf, D.J.; Coffin, J.M. & Mellors, J.W. (2007). ART suppresses plasma HIV-1 RNA to a stable set point predicted by pretherapy viremia. *PLOS Pathog.* 13:e46

Mata, R.C.; Viciana, P.; de Alarcon, A.; Lopez-Cortes, L.F.; Gomez-Vera, J.; Trastoy, M. & Cisneros, J.M. (2005). Discontinuation of antiretroviral therapy in patients with chronic HIV infection: Clinical, virologic, and immunologic consequences. *AIDS Patient Care STDS* 19:550–562.

Neuhaus, J.; Angus, B.; Kowalska, J.D.; La Rosa, A.; Sampson, J.; Wentworth, D. & Mocroft, A. INSIGHT SMART and ESPRIT study groups. (2010a). Risk of all-cause mortality associated with nonfatal AIDS and serious non-AIDS events among adults infected with HIV. *AIDS* 24: 697-706.

Neuhaus, J.; Jacobs, D.R. Jr.; Baker, J.V.; Calmy, A.; Duprez, D.; La Rosa, A.; Kuller, L.H.; Pett, S.L.; Ristola, M.; Ross, M.J.; Shlipak, M.G.; Tracy, R. & Neaton, J.D. (2010b)

Markers of inflammation, coagulation and renal function are elevated in adults with HIV infection. *J. Infect. Dis.* 201:1788-1795.

Oxenius, A.; Price, D.A.; Dawson, S.J.; Günthard, H.F.; Fischer, M.; Perrin, L.; Ramirez, E.; Fagard, C.; Hirschel, B.; Scullard, G.; Weber, J.N.; McLean, A.R. & Phillips RE; Swiss HIV cohort study (2002a). Residual HIV-specific CD4 and CD8 T cell frequencies after prolonged antiretroviral therapy reflect pretreatment plasma virus load. *AIDS* 16:2317-22.

Oxenius, A.; Price, D.A.; Günthard, H.F.; Dawson, S.J.; Fagard, C.; Perrin, L.; Fischer, M.; Weber, R.; Plana, M.; García, F.; Hirschel, B.; McLean, A. & Phillips, R.E. (2002b). Stimulation of HIV-specific cellular immunity by structured treatment interruption fails to enhance viral control in chronic HIV infection. *Proc. Natl. Acad. Sci. USA* 99:13747-13752.

Palella, FJ, Jr., Baker, R.K.; Moorman, A.C.; Chmiel, J.S.; Wood, K.C.; Brooks, J.T. & Holmberg, S.D. HIV Outpatient Study Investigators (2006). Mortality in the Highly Active Antiretroviral Therapy Era. Changing Causes of Death and Disease in the HIV Outpatient Study. *J. Acquir. Immune Def. Syndr.* 43:27-34

Panel on Antiretroviral Guidelines for Adults and Adolescents. Guidelines for the use of antiretroviral agents in HIV-1-infected adults and adolescents. Department of Health and Human Services. January 10, 2011; 1–166. Available at http://www.aidsinfo.nih.gov/ContentFiles/AdultandAdolescentGL.pdf [Accessed 7th May 2011]

Pantaleo, G.; Graziosi, C. & Butini, L. (1991). Lymphoid organs function as major reservoirs for human immunodeficiency virus. *Proc. Natl. Acad. Sci. USA* 88:9838–42.

Perelson, AS.; Neumann, AU.; Markowitz, M.; Leonard, J.M. & Ho, D.D. (1996). HIV-1 dynamic in vivo: Infected cell lifespan, and viral generation time. *Science* 271:1582-86.

Powderly, W. (2007). The three ages of antiretroviral therapy - its evolution and the emergence of long-term safety concerns. *European Infectious Disease* 1:19-25.

Powderly, W. (2010). Growing old with HIV-dealing with co-morbidities. *Journal of the International AIDS Society* 13(Suppl 4):025.

Rerks-Ngarm, S.; Pitisuttithum, P.; Nitayaphan, S.; Kaewkungwal, J.; Chiu, J.; Paris, R.; Premsri, N.; Namwat, C.; de Souza, M.; Adams, E.; Benenson, M.; Gurunathan, S.; Tartaglia, J.; McNeil, J.G.; Francis, D.P.; Stablein, D.; Birx, D.L.; Chunsuttiwat, S.; Khamboonruang, C.; Thongcharoen, P.; Robb, M.L.; Michael, N.L., Kunasol, P. & Kim, J.H. MOPH-TAVEG Investigators (2009). Vaccination with ALVAC and AIDSVAX to Prevent HIV-1 Infection in Thailand. *N. Engl. J. Med.* 361:2209-20.

Rezza, G.; Fiorelli, V.; Dorrucci, M.; Ciccozzi, M.; Tripiciano, A.; Scoglio, A.; Collacchi, B.; Ruiz-Alvarez, M.; Giannetto, C.; Caputo, A.; Tomasoni, L.; Castelli, F.; Sciandra, M.; Sinicco, A.; Ensoli, F.; Buttò, S. & Ensoli, B. (2005). The presence of anti-Tat antibodies is predictive of long-term nonprogression to AIDS or severe immunodeficiency: findings in a cohort of HIV-1 seroconverters. *J. Infect. Dis.* 191:1321-4.

Richman, DD.; Margolis, DM.; Delaney, M.; Greene, WC.; Hazuda, D. & Pomerantz RJ. (2009). The challenge of finding a cure for HIV infection. *Science* 323:1304-1307.

Rosenberg, E.S.; Billingsley, J.M.; Caliendo, A.M.; Boswell, S.L.; Sax, P.E.; Kalams, S.A. & Walker, B.D.(1997). Vigorous HIV-1-specific CD4+ T cell responses associated with control of viremia. *Science* 278:1447 -50.

Sáez-Cirión, A.; Lacabaratz, C.; Lambotte, O.; Versmisse, P.; Urrutia, A.; Boufassa, F.; Barré-Sinoussi, F.; Delfraissy, J.F.; Sinet, M.; Pancino, G. & Venet, A. Agence Nationale de Recherches sur le Sida EP36 HIV Controllers Study Group (2007). HIV controllers exhibit potent CD8 T cell capacity to suppress HIV infection *ex vivo* and peculiar cytotoxic T lymphocyte activation phenotype. *Proc. Natl. Acad. Sci. USA* 104:6776-81.

Sajadi, M.M.; Heredia, A.; Le, N.; Constantine, N.T. & Redfield, R.R. (2007). Natural virus suppressors: Control of viral replication in the absence of therapy. *AIDS* 19:517-9.

Schooley, R.T.; Spritzler, J.; Wang, H.; Lederman, M.M.; Havlir, D.; Kuritzkes, D.R.; Pollard, R.; Battaglia, C.; Robertson, M.; Mehrotra, D.; Casimiro, D.; Cox, K. & Schock, B.; AIDS Clinical Trials Group 5197 Study Team (2010). AIDS clinical trials group 5197: A placebo-controlled trial of immunization of HIV-1 infected persons with replication deficient adenovirus type 5 vaccine expressing HIV-1 core protein. *J. Inf. Dis.* 202:705-16.

Sheikh, J.; Souberbielle B.; Westby, M.; Austen, B. & Dalgleish, A.G. (2000). HIV gp120 plus specific peptides are recognized in a similar way to specific HLA plus peptide by HLA restricted antigen specific cell lines. *Viral Immunol.* 13:9-17.

Siliciano, RF. (2010). Prospects of curing HIV infection. *Top. HIV Med.* 18:104-8.

Silvestri G.; Sodora D.L.; Koup, R.A.; Silvestri, G.; Sodora, D.L.; Koup, R.A.; Paiardini, M.; O'Neil, S.P.; McClure, H.M.; Staprans, S.I. & Feinberg, M.B. (2003). Nonpathogenic SIV infection of sooty managebeys is characterised by limited bystander immunopathology despite chronic high level viremia. *Immunity* 18:441-52.

Sousa, A.E.; Carneiro, J.; Meier-Schellersheim, M.; Grossman, Z. & Victorino, R.M. (2002). CD4 T-cell depletion is linked directly to immune activation in the pathogenesis of HIV-1 and HIV-2 but only indirectly to viral load. *J. Immunol.* 169:3400-6.

The Antiretroviral Therapy Cohort Collaboration (2008). Life expectancy of individuals on combination antiretroviral therapy in high-income countries: a collaborative analysis of 14 cohort studies. *Lancet* 372:293-9

Toulson, A.R.; Harrigan, R.; Heath, K.; Yip, B.; Brumme, Z.L.; Harris, M.; Hogg, R.S. & Montaner, J.S. (2005). Treatment interruption of highly active antiretroviral therapy in patients with nadir CD4 cell counts >200 Cells/mm^3. *J. Infect. Dis.* 192:1787–93.

UNAIDS Report on the Global AIDS Epidemic (2010). ISBN 978-92-9173-871-7. Available at http://www.unaids.org [Accessed 11th July 2011]

van Baalen, C.A.; Pontesilli, O.; Huisman, R.C.; Geretti, A.M.; Klein, M.R.; de Wolf, F.; Miedema, F.; Gruters, R.A.; & Osterhaus, A.D. (1997). Human immunodeficiency virus type 1 Rev- and Tat-specific cytotoxic T lymphocyte frequencies inversely correlate with rapid progression to AIDS. *J. Gen. Virol.* 78:1913–18.

Vittinghoff, E.; Scheer, S., O'Malley, P.; Colfax, G.; Holmberg, S.D. & Buchbinder, S.P. (1999). Combination antiretroviral therapy and recent declines in AIDS incidence and mortality. *J. Infect. Dis.* 179:717-20.

Walker B. (2007). Elite control of HIV infection: Implications for vaccines and treatments. *Top. HIV Med.* 15:134-6.

Willberg, C.B. & Nixon, D.F. (2007). Treatment interruption in chronic HIV-1 infection: does it deliver? *Curr. Opin. HIV AIDS* 2:26-30.

Wit, F.W.; Blanckenberg, D.H.; Brinkman, K.; Prins, J.M.; van der Ende, M.E.; Schneider, M.M.; Mulder, J.W.; de Wolf, F. & Lange, J.M. ATHENA Study Group.(2005). Safety of long-term interruption of successful anti-retroviral therapy: the ATHENA cohort study. *AIDS* 19:345-48.

Wong, J.K.; Hezareh, M.; Günthard, H.F.; Havlir, D.V.; Ignacio, C.C.; Spina, C.A. & Richman, D.D. (1997). Recovery of replication competent HIV despite prolonged suppression of plasma viraemia. *Science* 278:1291-5.

Wu, Y. & Marsh, J.W. (2001). Selective transcription and modulation of resting T cell activity by preintegrated HIV DNA. *Science* 293:1503-6.

Yerly, S.; Günthard, H.F.; Fagard, C.; Joos, B.; Perneger, T.V.; Hirschel, B.; & Perrin, L. Swiss HIV Cohort Study. (2004). Proviral HIV-DNA predicts viral rebound and viral setpoint after structured treatment interruptions *AIDS*. 24;18:1951-3.

Zuñiga, R.; Lucchetti, A.; Galvan, P.; Sanchez, S.; Sanchez, C.; Hernandez, A.; Sanchez, H.; Frahm, N.; Linde, C.H.; Hewitt, H.S.; Hildebrand, W.; Altfeld, M.; Allen, T.M.; Walker, B.D.; Korber, B.T.; Leitner, T.; Sanchez, J. & Brander, C. (2006). Relative dominance of Gag p24-specific cytotoxic T-lymphocytes is associated with human immunodeficiency virus control. *J. Virol.* 80:3122-5.

Part 9

Beyond Conventional

25

Micronutrient Synergy in the Control of HIV Infection and AIDS

Raxit J. Jariwalla, Aleksandra Niedzwiecki and Matthias Rath
Dr. Rath Research Institute, Santa Clara, CA
USA

1. Introduction

Acquired immune deficiency syndrome (AIDS) has become a global health pandemic and the most common cause of death among young adults aged 20-24 years (Patton et al., 2009). According to the UN/AIDS Global Report published in November 2010 (UNAIDS 2010), about 1.8 million persons died from AIDS-related causes in the year 2009 alone. At the end of that year, the epidemic had left behind totally 16.6 million orphans, defined as those under 18 who had lost one or both parents to AIDS. Since the beginning of the epidemic, nearly 30 million people have died from AIDS-related causes.

At the end of 2009, an estimated 30.8 million adults and 2.8 million children were living with HIV, the human immunodeficiency virus linked to AIDS; with women accounting for just over one-half of all adults living with HIV worldwide. During the same year, about 2.6 million persons became newly infected with HIV, including 370,000 children. Of all people living with HIV, about 68% reside in Sub-Saharan Africa (UNAIDS 2010).

Despite these gruesome statistics, there is no cure in sight. Current treatment is based on the use of antiretroviral (ARV) drugs targeted against HIV at various steps in viral replication (Sleaseman and Goodenow 2003). Although ARV drugs can reduce viral load in the bloodstream, they neither cure HIV infection nor restore the immune system to combat AIDS (Roederer 1998, Pakker et al., 1998). Virus is known to persist indefinitely in reservoirs of latently-infected cells and emergence of drug-resistant strains is common. Furthermore, the effectiveness of ARVs in having any clinical benefits at all depends upon a number of factors, particularly the CD4 count and the nutritional status of patients at the point at which ARV treatment is commenced (Hong et al., 2001, Paton et al., 2006). Additionally, drugs are higly toxic and are often associated with adverse side effects to various organs of the body, including the bone marrow and liver, (Fischl et al., 1987, Richman et al., 1987, Costello et al., 1988, Abrescia et al., 2008), cellular mitochondria (Carr et al., 2001), and with lipodystrophy and dyslipidemia (Carr et al., 1998).

Consequently, there is need for safe and effective, nontoxic therapy that can not only restore the immune system and keep virus multiplication/spread in check but also block AIDS progression without harming cells of the host. This review will focus on the relationship of nutrition to infection and immunity and evidence from experimental and clinical studies on the potential value of micronutrients and their combinations in controlling HIV infection and reducing symptoms associated with AIDS.

2. Nutritional deficiencies in HIV and AIDS

The relationship between nutrition, infection and immunity is well established since the early 1940's (Scrimshaw 2003, Webb and Villamor 2007). It is for instance well recognized that nutritional deficiency can lower immunity and predispose individuals to microbial infection. Conversely, nutritional supplementation can improve immune function and prevent/confer resistance to infection.

As the latent period between HIV infection and AIDS manifestation has been estimated at 8-10 years (Morgan et al 2002), nutritional cofactors, besides HIV, have been implicated in AIDS development (Beach et al., 1992, Baum et al., 1995, Jariwalla et al., 2008a, 2009). Furthermore, nutrient supplementation in asymptomatic HIV-infected individuals was shown to delay the onset of AIDS (Abrams et al., 1993, Tang et al., 1993), supporting involvement of nutritional status as a contributory factor in AIDS development.

It is universally known since the emergence of the AIDS epidemic in the early 1980's that nutritional deficiencies are prevalent in persons with HIV infection and AIDS (Gray 1984, Beach et al., 1992, Jariwalla 1995; see also Table 1). These deficits include: (i) specific micronutrient abnormalities such as reduced blood levels of the common ACE vitamins, minerals, trace elements including selenium, amino acids such as cysteine, and the tri-peptide glutathione, which displays a global systemic deficiency; (ii) macronutrient abnormalities such as protein calorie malnutrition, which has been linked to a wasting disease, characteristic of AIDS. Malnutrition has also been linked to the spread of AIDS and TB in developing countries and with reduced survival (Paton et al., 2006, Turchenko et al., 2008)

MICRONUTRIENT ABNORMALITIES	
Vitamins	**Trace Elements**
Vitamin A	Selenium
Vitamin B12	Zinc
Vitamin B6	
Vitamin C	**Amino Acids**
Vitamin E	Cysteine
	Peptides
	Glutathione

MACRONUTRIENT DEFECITS
Protein Calorie Malnutrition
Abnormal Lipids (Dyslipidemia)

Table 1. Commonly occurring nutritional deficiencies in HIV infection and AIDS

3. Impact of nutritional deficiencies

Micronutrient deficiencies in particular vitamin and mineral deficiencies can promote and strengthen microbial growth by weakening the immune system of the host, making it prone to acquiring new infections (Scrimshaw 2003, Webb and Villamor 2007; see Fig 1).

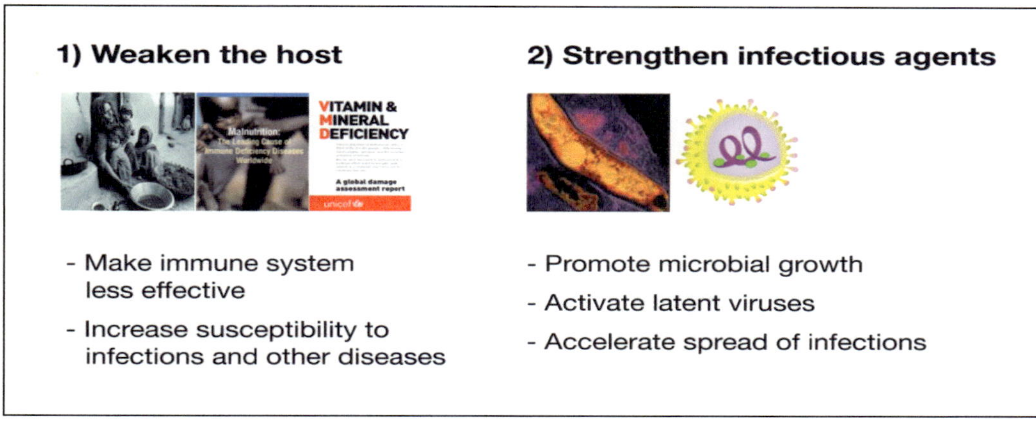

Fig. 1. Impact of micronutrient deficiencies on infectious diseases

4. Essential role of micronutrients in cell physiology and immunity

Micronutrients are essential for sustaining all cellular functions including metabolic reactions in the cytosol and biochemical functions within cellular organelles (Fig 2). Vitamins and minerals are needed in smaller amounts than proteins, fats and sugars but without them, cells cannot convert food into biological energy and build different body structures.

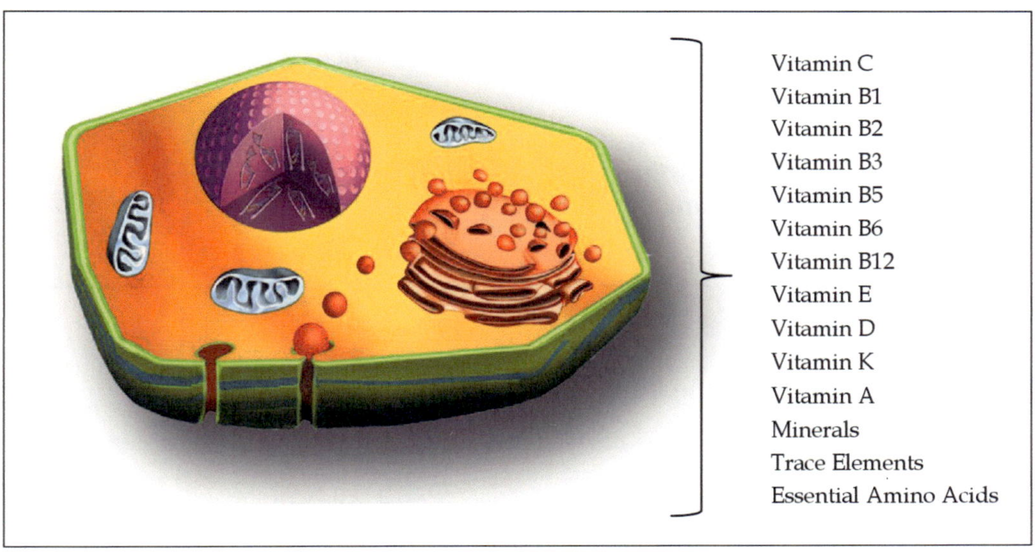

Fig. 2. Micronutrients are essential for sustaining all cellular functions

Micronutrients are also critical for optimum functioning of the immune system including cell-mediated immunity, antibody production (humoral immunity) and optimum thymus function (Fig. 3).

The pathological basis of AIDS is a dysfunctional immune system clinically indicated by abnormally low levels of white blood cells. Micronutrients are essential for blood formation, including white blood cells. Of particular importance are: vitamin B-3, vitamin B-5, vitamin B-6, vitamin B-12, vitamin C, folic acid and iron. Any textbook of biology or biochemistry documents these scientific facts. Moreover, no less than nine Nobel Prizes in Medicine have been awarded to date on the discovery of the health benefits of vitamins, relevant to their role in cellular physiology and impact on the immune system (Nobel Prize Committee website, Nobelprize.org).

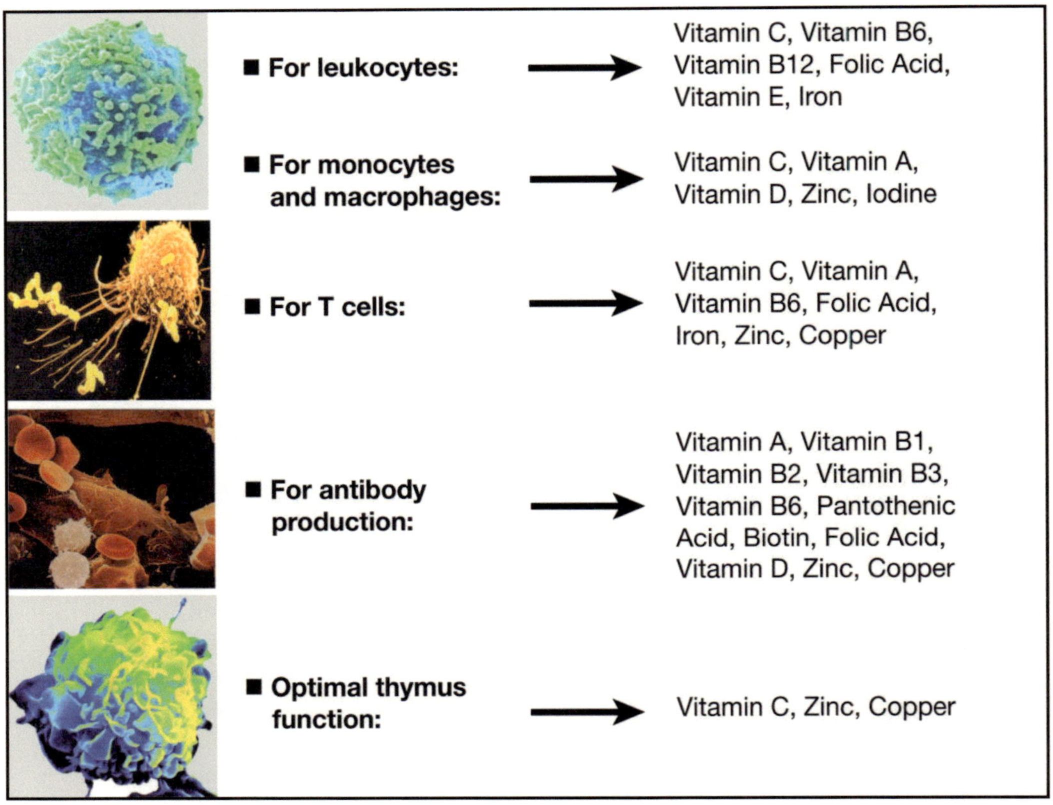

Fig. 3. Nutrients are critical for optimum immune defense of a host

5. Role of micronutrients in suppression of virus infection

Additionally, experimental studies have shown that specific micronutrients can suppress virus infection at various steps in the viral life cycle that include blocking (a) virus entry, (b) virus multiplication, (c) virus activation in latently infected cells and (d) virus spread (Fig 4).
Prevent viral entry into cells (Vitamin C, EGCG)
Stop viral multiplication (Vitamin C, N-Acetylcysteine)
Prevent activation of "silent" viruses (Vitamin C)
Limit spread of infections (Lysine, Vitamin C)
In the case of HIV, micronutrients have been shown to block virus expression at all stages of virus-host interactions, which include acute infection, chronic expression and activation from latently infected cells (Fig 5). The specific micronutrients demonstrated to affect different phases of virus infection are listed in Table 2. Most of them are reducing agents

with antioxidant properties. They include: vitamins C and E, amino acid thiols such as cysteine or its derivative N-acetyl cysteine (NAC), disulfides such as alpha-lipoic acid, tripeptides such as glutathione and its derivative glutathione monoester, polyphenols such as epigallo-catecheine gallate (EGCG from green tea) and the trace element selenium. Among them, ascorbic acid (vitamin C or ascorbate) is the most versatile, capable of blocking HIV replication in all phases of HIV infection namely, acute, chronic and latent infection (Harakeh et al., 1990; Harakeh and Jariwalla, 1991, 1995). Cysteine and glutathione monoester inhibit chronic HIV expression (Mihm et al., 1991; Kalebic et al., 1991) whereas NAC and selenium are effective in inhibiting HIV activation in latently-infected cells (Roederer et al., 1990, Harakeh and Jariwalla 1991; Sappey et al., 1994). It has been reported that alpha-lipoic acid can block acute infection (Bauer et al., 1991) and flavonoids including the polyphenol EGCG inhibit HIV at an early stage, blocking interaction of the virus with

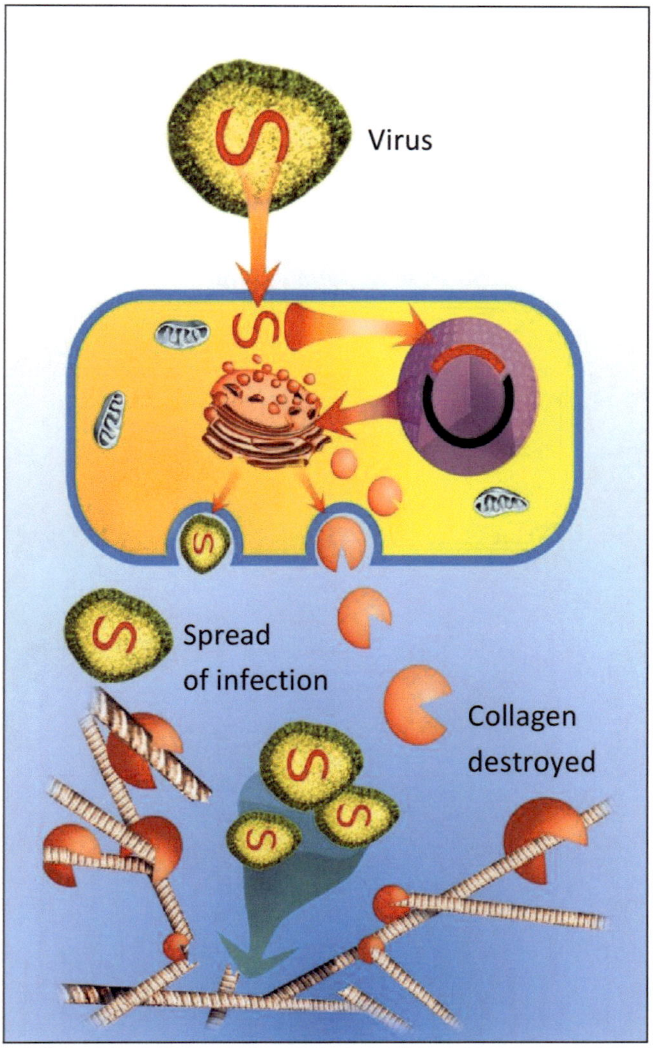

Fig. 4. Nutrients can directly suppress viral infections

host-cells receptor (Mahmood et al., 1993, Fassina et al., 2002). More recently, green tea extract enriched in such polyphenols (80% by weight) was shown to suppress HIV production in chronically and latently infected cells (Jariwalla et al., 2010).

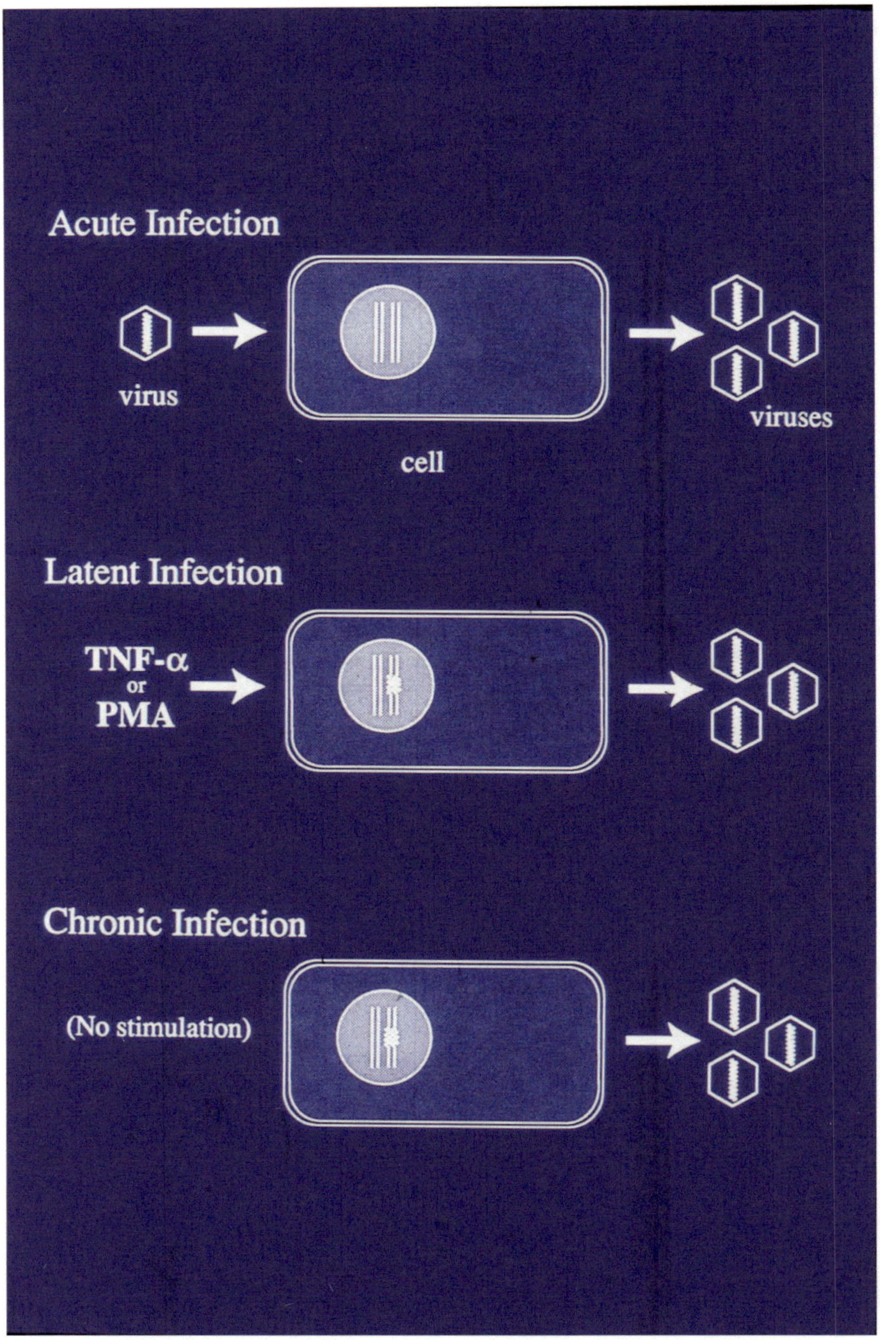

Fig. 5. Micronutrients can target different stages in HIV-host cell interaction

Nutrient	Inhibitory Effect Targeted at	Reference
Vitamin E	Latent infection	Suzuki *et al* 1993
Vitamin C	Acute, chronic and latent infection	Harakeh and Jariwalla (1991, 1995)
Cysteine, alpha-lipoic acid	Chronic and acute infection	Mihm *et al* 1991, Baur *et al* 1991
NAC, Selenium	Chronic and latent infection	Roederer *et al* 1990, Harakeh & Jariwalla 1991, Sappey *et al* 1994.
Glutathione monoester	Chronic infection	Kalebic *et al* 1991
Flavonoids, EGCG, green tea extract	Acute infection	Mahmood et al 1993, Fassina *et al* 2002, Jariwalla et al 2010
Nutrient mixture (NM)*	Synergistic HIV suppression in chronic and latent infection	Jariwalla *et al* 2010

Table 2. Action of micronutrients on phases of HIV infection
* containing (vitamin C, green tea extract, lysine, proline, arginine, NAC, selenium)

6. Our approach to controlling virus infection with nutrient synergy

Although specific, single nutrients have been shown to suppress HIV in previous studies, little attention has been directed at blocking virus expression with nutrient combinations. To investigate this, we have utilized the principle of nutrient synergy i.e. use of nutrients in combination at low to moderate (physiological) levels for prevention and control of disease (Rath and Niedzwiecki 1996, Rath et al., 2005, Jariwalla et al., 2008a, 2009). The principle underlying nutrient synergy is that nutrients work in the body in harmonious synergy, not isolation, and they allow for maximal benefits when used in combination at physiological doses. In nutrient synergy 1 + 1 is more than 2 (Fig 6). We have applied this principle to both experimental studies of HIV infection as well as the in vivo evaluation of a defined multi-micronutrient supplement in AIDS patients in a community wide setting.

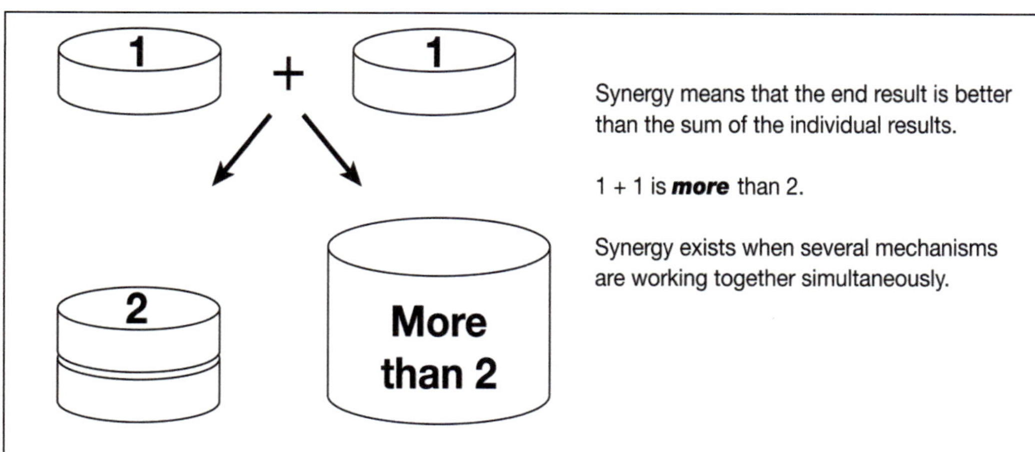

Fig. 6. The benefits of nutrient synergy

All nutrients work in our bodies in harmonious synergy, not in isolation.
Nutrient Synergy allows for achieving maximum health benefits and keeping cellular processes in balance using smaller quantities of nutrients. Use of single vitamins in very high-doses or a randomly selected nutrient combination is not recommended as an optimal approach to health.

7. Experimental studies in HIV infection

Studies conducted by us of micronutrient combinations in laboratory cultures of HIV infected cells have provided further support for nutritional efficacy in viral immunodeficiency disease (Jariwalla et al., 2010). In these studies, we compared the ability of micronutrient combinations to single nutrients in the suppression of HIV replication in both chronically and latently infected cells. H9-HTLV IIIB is a model, chronically-infected T lymphocytic cell line that constitutively produces HIV cytopathic virus in the cell culture supernatant (Popovic et al., 1984, Gallo et al., 1984, Harakeh et al., 1990, Harakeh and Jariwalla 1991). Exposure of these cells to low/moderate concentrations of single micronutrients such as ascorbic acid, green tea extract and the amino acids such lysine produced only small inhibitory effects on virus production. In contrast, exposure of cells to combinations of micronutrients conferred significantly greater HIV suppression compared to single nutrients, indicating a synergistic effect. A nutritional mixture (NM), consisting of vitamin C, green tea extract, amino acids (lysine, proline, arginine), NAC and selenium also gave enhanced suppression of HIV production in this cell line compared to single nutrients (Jariwalla et al., 2010; see also Table 2). A similar inhibitory effect on cytokine-stimulated virus expression was obtained in latently infected T cells, indicating that micronutrients cooperate to suppress virus expression in both chronically and latently-stimulated cells (Jariwalla et al., 2010; Table 2).

8. Clinical nutrition studies in AIDS patients

Based on the above scientific evidence of micronutrient effectiveness in laboratory cultures of virally-infected cells, we have incorporated the use of micronutrients in natural control of HIV infection. Our studies conducted in persons with AIDS symptoms have provided further support for micronutrient efficacy in viral immunodeficiency disease (Jariwalla et al., 2008a, 2009). This in vivo confirmation of micronutrient efficacy was demonstrated in AIDS patients in a community wide program conducted in South Africa between 2005 and 2008. In this community program, the Dr. Rath Foundation donated a micronutrient supplement to the South African National Civic Organization (SANCO) who distributed it among people affected by AIDS in various townships in South Africa.
The micronutrient supplement contained vitamins and trace elements (except iron) that are known to modulate the immune system (listed in Fig. 3) plus selenium, essential minerals and other important nutrients such as amino acids, green tea extract, bioflavonoids, N-acetyl cysteine, inositol and coenzyme Q10. This supplement was given to subjects to be taken 3 times a day with meals. The characteristics of participants, patient selection, informed consent, administration of questionnaire grading AIDS-defining symptoms and the evaluation methodology were reported previously (Jariwalla et al., 2008a, 2009).
The first township where a pilot nutritional program was evaluated was Khayelitsha, a township near Cape Town (Jariwalla et al., 2008a). In this pilot protocol, 56 AIDS patients completed all 3 examinations and their completed questionnaires were evaluated for

changes in severity of symptoms seen after the first 3 visits (8-12) weeks from the beginning of micronutrient supplementation. Table 3 lists the AIDS-defining symptoms for Africa, other physical symptoms, pain symptoms and symptoms of well-being. Tables 4-6 show a summary of the impact on these symptoms from micronutrient supplementation. The results showed that within 10-12 weeks, the micronutrient supplement statistically significantly suppressed all AIDS-defining symptoms compared to baseline. The supplement also significantly suppressed other physical symptoms frequently seen in AIDS patients including state of well-being (Jariwalla et al., 2008a).

AIDS-Defining Symptoms	**Symptoms of Well Being**
Fever	Appetite
Diarrhoea	Energy
Cough	Enjoyment of life
Weight loss	Fear of future
TB	Concentration
Oppurtunistic infections	Anxiety
	Depression
Other Physical Symptoms	Insomnia
Swollen glands	Fatigue
Colds, flu	
Rashes	
Wounds, sores, ulcers	
Headache	
Bloating, gas	
Other physical symptoms	

Table 3. AIDS-Related Symptoms, Conditions and Diseases Monitored in Community Wide Micronutrient Program

The micronutrient supplement evaluated in Khayelitsha was also rolled out in KwaZulu Natal district (near Durban) where a very large group (522 patients) completed all 3 exams and questionnaires. Similar to Khayelitsha, the same trend in reduction of AIDS-defining symptoms, other physical AIDS-associated symptoms and pain symptoms was seen (Tables 4-6). The results were also confirmed in two other townships (Western Cape and Free State), for a total of 813 participants from all 4 townships (Tables 4-6).

Site	**Total no of patients**	**% decrease in AIDS-defining symptoms from baseline after 3 visits ***
Khayelitsha	50	33-61%
Kwazulu-Natal (KZN)	473	37-48%
Western Cape	153	51-78%
Free State	82	23-26%

Table 4. Impact of micronutrient supplementation on AIDS defining symptom in a community wide program
*8-12 weeks except Free State (= 40 weeks)

Site	Total no of patients	% decrease in other physical symptoms from baseline after 3 visits *
Khayelitsha	45	37-60%
Kwazulu-Natal (KZN)	522	17-54%
Western Cape	153	44-83%
Free State	78	17-47%

Table 5. Impact of micronutrient supplementation on other physical symptoms in AIDS patients in community wide program
* 8-12 weeks except Free State (= 40 weeks)

Site	Total no of patients	% decrease in pain symptoms from baseline after 3 visits *
Khayelitsha	44	38-49%
Kwazulu-Natal (KZN)	511	32-50%
Western Cape	149	43-64%
Free State	79	24-35%

Table 6. Impact of micronutrient supplementation on pain symptoms in AIDS patients in community wide program
* 8-12 weeks except Free State (= 40 weeks)

9. Conclusion

The results we have seen are not in isolation. Beneficial effects of micronutrients and their combinations have been seen in clinical studies conducted by other researchers as summarized in Table 7. These studies have evaluated nutrients in combination and reported beneficial effects on various outcomes including improvement in viral and immune parameters, antioxidant protection from cellular damage, slowing of disease progression, reduction of AIDS-related symptoms and improvement of birth outcomes in pregnant women. The impact of nutritional support and vitamin and micronutrient supplementation in the treatment of HIV and AIDS is a seriously under-investigated area. Repeated calls have been made for more studies in this area by international health agencies. Although micronutrients are not a cure for AIDS, in the absence of an effective cure or vaccine and in the face of the toxicity and limited efficacy of ARVs, they are a safe, effective and affordable way to halt progression towards and even reduce the symptoms of the AIDS disease and to improve the quality of life of AIDS patients.

The implications of micronutrient supplementation results for public health and control of infectious and immunodeficiency disease are enormous. If properly evaluated, micronutrients have the potential of being incorporated into strategies for fighting viral pandemics on a global scale. Implementation of the above positive findings could save millions of lives.

Micronutrient Supplement	Clinical change	Reference
Multivitamin Supplement	Delayed onset of AIDS in HIV positive asymptomatic persons	Abrams *et al* 1993, Tang *et al* 1993
N-acetylcysteine (NAC)	Increased survival compared to placebo	Herzenberg *et al* 1997
Vitamin C plus E	1) Reduced oxidative stress, viral load 2) Prevention of AZT-induced miochondrial damage	Allard *et al* 1998, de la Asuncion *et al* 1998
NAC plus vitamin C	Enhanced immune responses and reduced viral load in advanced AIDS	Muller *et al* 2000
Multivitamin Supplement	Reduced fetal death among HIV-infected Tanzanian women	Fawzi *et al* 1998, 2004
Multi-micronutrient Supplement	Increased survival among HIV-infected persons in Bangkok	Jiamton *et al* 2003
Micronutrient Supplement	Improved CD4 count	Kaiser *et al* 2006
Nutritional Supplements	Delayed AIDS progression in HIV-infected persons	Namulemia *et al* 2007
Alpha-lipoic acid	Enhanced blood glutathione and improved lymphocyte function	Jariwalla *et al* 2008b
Micronutrient Supplement (see text, page 8)	Reduced AIDS related and pain symptoms; improved state of well being	Jariwalla *et al* 2008a; 2009

Table 7. Clinical improvements seen upon micronutrient supplementation in HIV and AIDS patients, in peer-reviewed published studies.

10. Acknowledgement

We would like to thank Lisa Smith for help with formatting/presentation of the graphics and Anupriya Pandit for tabulating data and organizing references.

11. References

Abrams B, Duncan D & Hertz-Picciotto I. (1993). A prospective study of dietary intake and acquired immune deficiency syndrome in HIV-seropositive homosexual men. *J Acquir Immune Defic Syndr.*, Vol. 6, No. 8, pp. 949-58.

Abrescia N, D'Abbraccio M, Figoni M, Busto A, Maddaloni A & De Marco M. (2005). Hepatotoxicity of antiretroviral drugs. *Current Pharmaceutical Design,* Vol. 11, pp. 3697-3710.

Allard JP, Aghdassi E, Chau J, Tam C, Kovacs CM, Salit IE & Walmsley SL. (1998). Effects of vitamin E and C supplementation on oxidative stress and viral load in HIV-infected subjects. *AIDS*, Vol. 12, No. 13, (September 10), pp. 1653-9.

de la Asunción JG, del Olmo ML, Sastre J, Millán A, Pellín A, Pallardó FV & Viña J. (1998). AZT treatment induces molecular and ultrastructural oxidative damage to muscle mitochondria. Prevention by antioxidant vitamins. *J Clin Invest.*, Vol.102, No. 1, (July 1), pp. 4-9.

Bauer A, Harrer T, Peukert M, Jahn G, Kalden JR & Fleckenstein B. (1991). Alpha-lipoic acid is an effective inhibitor of human immuno-deficiency virus (HIV-1) replication. *Klin Wochenscher,* Vol. 69, No. 15, (October 2), pp. 722-724.

Baum MK, Shor-Posner G, Lu Y, Rosner B, Sauberlich HE, Fletcher MA, Szapocznik J, Eisdorfr C, Buring JE & Hennekens CH. (1995). Micronurients and HIV-1 disease progression. *AIDS*, Vol. 9, No. 9, pp. 1051-1056.

Beach RS, Mantero-Atienza E, Shor-Posner G, Javier JJ, Szapocznik J, Morgan R, Sauberlich HE, Cornwell PE, Eisdorfer C & Baum MK. (1992). Specific nutrient abnormalities in asymptomatic HIV-1 infection. *AIDS*, Vol. 6, No. 7, pp. 701-8.

Carr A, Samaras K, Chisholm DJ & Cooper DA. (1998). Pathogenesis of HIV-1-protease inhibitor-associated peripheral lipodystrophy, hyperlipidaemia, and insulin resistance. *Lancet*, Vol. 351, No. 9119, (June 20), pp. 1881-3.

Carr A, Morey A, Mallon P, Williams D & Throburn DR. (2001). Fatal portalhypertension, liver failure, and mitochondrial dysfunction after HIV-1 nucleoside analogue-induced hepatitis and lactic acidaemia. *Lancet*, Vol. 357, No. 9266, (May 5), pp. 1412-4.

Costello C. (1988). Haematological abnormalities in human immunodeficiency virus (HIV) disease. *Journal of clinical pathology*, Vol. 41, pp. 711-715.

Fassina G, Buffa A, Benelli R, Varnier OE, Noonan DM & Albini A. (2002). Polyphenolic antioxidant (-)-epigallocatechin-3-gallate from green tea as a candidate anti-HIV agent. *AIDS*, Vol. 16, No. 6, (April 12), pp. 939-41.

Fawzi WW, Msamanga GI, Spiegelman D, Urassa EJ, McGrath N, Mwakagile D, Antelman G, Mbise R, Herrera G, Kapiga S, Willett W & Hunter DJ. (1998). Randomised trial of effects of vitamin supplements on pregnancy outcomes and T cell counts in HIV-1-infected women in Tanzania. *Lancet*, Vol. 351, No. 9114, (May 16), pp. 1477-82.

Fawzi W, Msamanga G, Antelman G, Xu C, Hertzmark E, Spiegelman D, Hunter D & Anderson D. (2004). Effect of prenatal vitamin supplementation on lower-genital levels of HIV type 1 and interleukin type 1 beta at 36 weeks of gestation. *Clin Infect Dis.*, Vol. 38, No. 5, (Mar 1), pp. 716-22.

Fischl MA, Richman DD, Grieco MH, Gottlieb MS, Volberding PA, Laskin OL, Leedom JM, Groopman JE, Mildvn D, Schooley RT *et al.* (1987). The efficacy of azidothymidine (AZT) in the treatment of patients with AIDS and AIDS-related complex. A double-blind, placebo-controlled trial. *N Engl J Med*, Vol. 317, No. 4, (July 23), pp. 185-91.

Gallo RC, Salahuddin SZ, Popovic M, Shearer GM, Kaplan M, Haynes BF, Palker TJ, Redfield R, Oleske J, Safai B, et al. (1984). Frequent detection and isolation of cytopathic retroviruses (HTLV-III) from patients with AIDS and at risk for AIDS. , Vol. 224, No. 4648, (May 4), pp. 500-3.

Gray RH. (1984). Similarities between AIDS and PCM. *AM J Public Health*, Vol. 73, No. 11, pp. 1332.

Harakeh S, Jariwalla RJ & Pauling L. (1990). Suppression of human immunodeficiency virus replication by ascorbate in chronically and acutely infected cells. *Proc. Natl. Acad. Sci USA*, Vol. 87, No. 18, pp. 7245-49.

Harakeh S & Jariwalla RJ. (1991). Comparative study of the anti-HIV activities of ascorbate and thiol-containing reducing agents in chronically HIV-infected cells. *Am J Clin. Nutr.*, Vol. 54, No. 6S, pp. 1231S-1235S.

Herzenberg LA, De Rosa SC, Dubs JG, Roederer M, Anderson MT, Ela SW & Deresinski SC. (1997). Glutathione deficiency is associated with impaired survival in HIV disease. *Proc Natl Acad Sci U S A*, Vol. 94, No. 5, (March 4), pp. 1967-72.

Hogg RS, Yip B, Chan KJ, Wood E, Craib KJ, O'Shaughnessy MV & Montaner JS. (2001). Rates of disease progression by baseline CD4 cell count and viral load after initiating triple-drug therapy. *JAMA*, Vol. 286, No. 20, (November 28), pp. 2568-77.

Jariwalla RJ. (1995). Micronutrient imbalance in HIV infection and AIDS: Relevance to pathogenesis and therapy. *J Nutr Environ Med*, Vol. 5, pp. 297-306.

Jariwalla RJ, Niedzwiecki A, & Rath M. (2008a). Micronutrients and nutrient synergy in immunodeficiency and infectious disease. In: *Botanical Medicine in Clinical Practice* (R. R. Watson & V. R. Preedy, Eds), pp 203-12. CAB International, London, UK.

Jariwalla RJ, Lalezari J, Cenko D, Mansour SE, Kumar A, Gangapurkar B & Nakamura D. (2008b). Restoration of blood total glutathione status and lymphocyte function following alpha-lipoic acid supplementation in patients with HIV infection. *J Altern Complement Med.*, Vol. 14, No. 2, pp. 139-46.

Jariwalla RJ, Niedzwiecki A, & Rath M. (2009). The essentiality of nutritional supplementation in HIV infection and AIDS: Review of clinical Studies and results from a community helath micronutrient program. In: Bioactive Foods in Promoting Health: Fruits and Vegetables (R. R. Watson & V. R. Preedy, Eds), pp 323-342. Oxford: Academic Press, ISBN: 978-0-12-374628-3.

Jariwalla RJ, Gangapurkar B, Pandit A, Kalinovsky T, Niedzwiecki A & Rath M. (2010). Micronutrient cooperation in the suppression of HIV production in chronically and latently infected cells. *Mol Med Report,* Vol. 3, No. 3, pp. 377-85.

Jiamton S, Pepin J, Suttent R, Filteau S, Mahakkanukrauh B, Hanshaoworakul W, Chaisilwattana P, Suthipinittharm P, Shetty P & Jaffar S. (2003). A randomized trial of the impact of multiple micronutrient supplementation on mortality among HIV-infected individuals living in Bangkok. *AIDS,* Vol. 17, No. 17, (November 21), pp. 2461-9.

Kaiser JD, Campa AM, Ondercin JP, Leoung GS, Pless RF & Baum MK. (2006). Micronutrient supplementation increases CD4 count in HIV-infected individuals on highly active antiretroviral therapy: a prospective, double-blinded, placebo-controlled trial. *J Acquir Immune Defic Syndr.*, Vol. 42, No. 5, (August 15), pp. 523-8.

Kalebic T, Kinter A, Poli G, Anderson ME, Meister A & Fauci AS. (1991). Suppression of human immunodeficiency virus expression in chronically infected monocytic cells by glutathione, glutathione ester, and N-acetylcysteine. *Proc Natl Acad Sci USA,* Vol. 88, No. 3, (February 1), pp. 986-90.

Mahmood N, Pizza C, Aquino R, De Tommasi N, Piacente S, Colman S, Burke A & Hay AJ. (1993). Inhibition of HIV infection by flavonoids. *Antiviral Res.*, Vol. 22, No. 2-3, pp. 189-99.

Mihm S, Ennen J, Pessara U, Kurth R & Droge W. (1991). Inhibition of HIV-1 replication and NF-κB by cysteine and cysteine derivatives. *AIDS,* Vol. 5, No. 5, pp. 497-503.

Morgan D, Mahe C, Mayanja B, Okongo, Lubega R & Whitworth JA. (2002). HIV-1 infection in rural Africa: Is there a difference in median time to AIDS & survival compared with that in industrialized countries. *AIDS,* Vol. 16, No. 4, (March 8), pp. 597-603.

Müller F, Svardal AM, Nordoy I, Berge RK, Aukrust P & Frøland SS. (2000).Virological and immunological effects of antioxidant treatment in patients with HIV infection. *Eur J Clin Invest.*, Vol. 30, No. 10, pp. 905-14.

Namulemia E, Sparling J & Foster HD. (2007). Nutritional supplements can delay the progression of AIDS in HIV-infected patients: results from a double-blinded, clinical trial at Mengo hospital, Kampala, Uganda. *Journal of orthomolecular Medicine,* Vol. 22, pp. 129-136.

Nobelprize.org (1929-1964). The nobel prize and the discovery of vitamins (by K.J. Carpenter), Retrieved from http://nobelprize.org/nobel_prizes/medicine/articles/carpenter

Pakker NG, Notermans DW, de Boer RJ, Roos MT, de Wolf F, Hill A, Leonard JM, Danner SA, Miedema F & Schellekens PT. (1998). Biphasic kinetics of peripheral blood T cells after triple combination therapy in HIV-1 infection: a composite of redistribution and proliferation. *Nat Med.*, Vol. 4, No. 2, pp. 208-14.

Paton NI, Sangeetha S, Earnest A & Bellamy R. (2006). The impact of malnutrition on survival and the CD4 count response in HIV-infected patients starting antiretroviral therapy. *HIV Med.*, Vol. 7, No. 5, pp. 323-30.

Patton GC, Coffey C, Sawyer SM, Viner RM, Haller DM, Bose K, Vos T,Ferguson J & Mathers CD. (2009). Global patterns of mortality in young people: a systematic analysis of population health data. *Lancet*, Vol. 374, No. 9693, (September 12), pp. 881-92.

Popovic M, Sarngadharan MG, Read E & Gallo RC. (1984). Detection, isolation, and continuous production of cytopathic retroviruses (HTLV-III) from patients with AIDS and pre-AIDS. *Science*, Vol. 224, No. 4648, (May 4), pp. 497-500.

Rath M & Niedzwiecki A. (1996). Nutritional supplement program halts progression of early coronary atherosclerosis documented by ultrafast computed tomography. *Journal of Applied Nutrition*, Vol. 48, pp. 67-78.

Rath M, Kalinovsky T & Niedzwiecki A. (2005). Reduction in the frequency of arrhythmic episodes in patients with paroxysmal atrial arrhythmia with a vitamin/essential nutrient program. *JANA*, Vol. 8, pp. 21-25.

Richman DD, Fischl MA, Grieco MH, Gottlieb MS, Volberding PA, Laskin OL, Leedom JM, Groopman JE, Mildvan D, Hirsch MS, Jackson GG, Durack DT & Nusinoff-Lehrman S. The AZT collaborative working group. (1987). The toxicity of azidothymidine (AZT) in the treatment of patients with AIDS and AIDS related complex. A double-blind, placebo-controlled trial. *New England Journal of Medicine*, Vol. 317, pp. 192-197.

Roederer M. (1998). Getting to the HAART of T cell dynamics. *Nat Med.*, Vol. 4, pp. 145-6.

Roederer M, Staal FJ, Raju PA, Ela SW & Herzenberg LA. (1990). Cytokine-stimulated human immunodeficiency virus replication is inhibited by N-acetyl-L-cysteine. *Proc. Natl. Sci USA*, Vol. 87, No. 12, pp. 4884-8.

Sappey C, Legrand-Poels S, Best Belpomme M, Favier A, Rentier B & Piette J. (1994). Stimulation of glutathione peroxidase activity decreases HIV type 1 activation after oxidative stress. *AIDS Res. Hum. Retroviruses*, Vol. 10, No. 11, pp. 1451-61.

Scrimshaw NS. (2003). Historical concepts of interactions, synergism and antagonism between nutrition and infection. *Journal of Nutrition*, Vol. 133, No. 1, pp. 316S-321S.

Sleaseman JW and Goodenow MM. (2003). HIV-1 infection. *J Allergy Clin Immunol.*, Vol. 111, No. 2 suppl, pp. S582-S592.

Suzuki YJ & Packer L. (1993). Inhibition of NF-κB activation by vitamin E derivatives. *Biochem. Biophys. Res. Commun.*, Vol. 193, No. 1, (May 28), pp. 277-83.

Tang AM, Graham NM, Kirby AJ, McCall LD, Willett WC & Saah AJ. (1993). Dietary micronutrient intake and risk of progression to acquired immunodeficiency syndrome (AIDS) in human immunodeficiency virus type 1 (HIV-1)-infected homosexual men. *Am J Epidemiol.*, Vol. 138, No. 11, (December 1), pp. 937-51.

Turchenko LV, Voloshchuk EO, Ivanov V, Kalinovsky T, Niedzwiecki A & Rath M. (2008). Clinical improvement of active tuberculosis patients with complex treatment and nutritional supplementation. *The Open Natural Products Journal*, Vol. 1, pp. 20-26.

UNAIDS (2010). UNAIDS Report on the Global AIDS Epidemic, Retrieved from http://www.unaids.org/globalreport/

Webb AL & Villamor E. (2007). Update: effects of antioxidant and non-antioxidant vitamin supplementation on immune function. *Nutr Rev.*, Vol. 65, No. 5, pp. 181-217.

26

Substance Abuse Treatment Utilizing Medication Assisted Treatment as HIV Prevention

Thomas F Kresina, Robert Lubran and Laura W. Cheever
Centre for Substance Abuse Treatment, Substance Abuse and Mental Health Services Administration and HIV/AIDS Bureau, Health Resources and Services Administration
USA

1. Introduction

International guidelines have been developed for the use of medications in the treatment of substance use disorders (WHO, 2008; WHO, 2009). Medications used in the detoxification from drug abuse and dependence provide symptomatic relief of drug and alcohol withdrawal. For long term treatment or medical maintenance treatment, medications eliminate the physiological effects of drug use by blocking drug-receptor binding in the brain and are an important part of the recovery process. The use of medication assistant treatment (MAT) is part of a comprehensive treatment plan for drug and alcohol dependence that addresses the medical, social, and psychological needs of the patient (SAMHSA, 2005; SAMHSA, 2009). An effective long term treatment paradigm for the successful treatment of alcohol or opioid dependence is the concomitant use of medications that block the effects of drug use in concert with behavior change counseling and psychotherapy. Medications which have demonstrated effectiveness in the long term treatment of opioid dependence are methadone, buprenorphine (subutex®, suboxone®), and naltrexone (Revia®, Depade®) or extended release injectable naltrexone (vivitrol®). Pharmacotherapies used in the treatment of alcohol dependence include acamprosate (Campral®), disulfiram (antabuse®, antabus®) and naltrexone (Revia®, Depade®) or extended release injectable naltrexone (vivitrol®).

Time in treatment is a reliable indicator for successful treatment of drug dependence. Patients remain in treatment for longer periods of time when they perceive that their health care environment is supportive and non-stigmatizing, have a good patient-provider relationship, and feel that their needs are identified and met. Access to community-based substance abuse treatment that includes MAT is fundamental to achieving broad service coverage. Given that substance abuse treatment is Human Immunodeficiency Virus (HIV) prevention and the frequent co-morbidity of substance abuse and HIV infection, the provision of prevention, care and treatment for both need to be addressed in a coordinated manner for ideal patient outcomes. There are several models to achieve excellent patient outcomes for both HIV infection and the treatment of substance abuse (Proeschold-Bell et al 2010; Weiss et al, 2011). The highest level of coordinated care model has MAT and HIV services fully integrated with both the same medical record and health providers for both services. Alternatively, MAT and HIV services can be separately managed but co-located to allow convenient utilization of both MAT and HIV services in another form of "one stop shopping". A third approach is coordinated care and treatment where MAT and HIV services are provided at distinct locations, and case managers, peer facilitators, or others promote coordination of referrals. This third model can pose significant barriers to substance users who are heavily stigmatized and medically disenfranchised and who have multiple competing medical, psychological and social needs that limit access to care. MAT programs that offer comprehensive services and care options can best contribute to improving the health of these individuals thereby reducing HIV infection in the community.

2. Drug and alcohol use and their linkage to HIV infection

Exposure to the HIV can result in a patent viral infection. HIV infection can occur via two transmission routes: direct injection of the virus through the use of injection equipment infected with HIV and through sexual contact with an infected individual. There is a direct linkage between these disparate behaviours and drug and alcohol use.

For people who inject drugs, there is a risk of HIV infection when the injection equipment is reused and not sterilized after use or when there is direct sharing of the injection equipment with individuals who may be infected with HIV. Drug users who are under the influence of drugs may engage in risk behaviours for HIV that they would not while sober. In addition, for drug users who develop dependence, withdrawal induced drug cravings may result in the exchange of sex for money or drugs or other behaviours that increase risk of HIV acquisition. Similarly, alcohol consumption increases sexual risk-taking including high risk behaviors (Figure 1). That includes sexual acts without the use of condoms and an increased number of sexual partners. Concurrent sexual partnerships are a significant risk factor for the transmission of HIV (Epstein & Morris, 2011). Alcohol can also be an important contributor in the progression of HIV infection to acquired immune deficiency syndrome (AIDS) (Hahn & Samet , 2010). Alcohol consumption is an important consideration in the medical management of patients with HIV infection, particularly those co-infected with the hepatitis C virus (HCV) (Edlin et al 2001). Studies have also shown that alcohol consumption can modify drug metabolism in the liver, and thereby potentially influence the effectiveness of HIV antiretroviral therapy. Alcohol-induced cirrhosis can result in changes in drug metabolism in the liver through compromised liver function. Research has shown that alcohol consumption greater than 50 g/day (4–5 drinks) is a risk factor for disease progression for patients with HIV/HCV co-infection.

All substance abuse, whether the use of opioids, stimulants, or excessive alcohol, can negatively influence the course of HIV disease progression when the use results in low antiretroviral adherence or facilitates missed medical appointments. Substance abuse has been associated with less access to antiretroviral medications, lower medication adherence, and increased mortality among HIV infected patients.

2.1 Alcohol abuse, medication assisted treatment and HIV infection

Alcohol abuse and dependence are global problems of major medical importance with high societal impact (WHO, 2010). In determining the global burden of disease, the World Health Organization (WHO) has noted that a leading cause of disability is alcohol and drug use disorders. Alcohol consumption is estimated to cause 4% of the total of Disability-Adjusted

Life Years and 3.2% of deaths, globally. The WHO estimates that about 2 billion individuals worldwide consume alcoholic beverages.

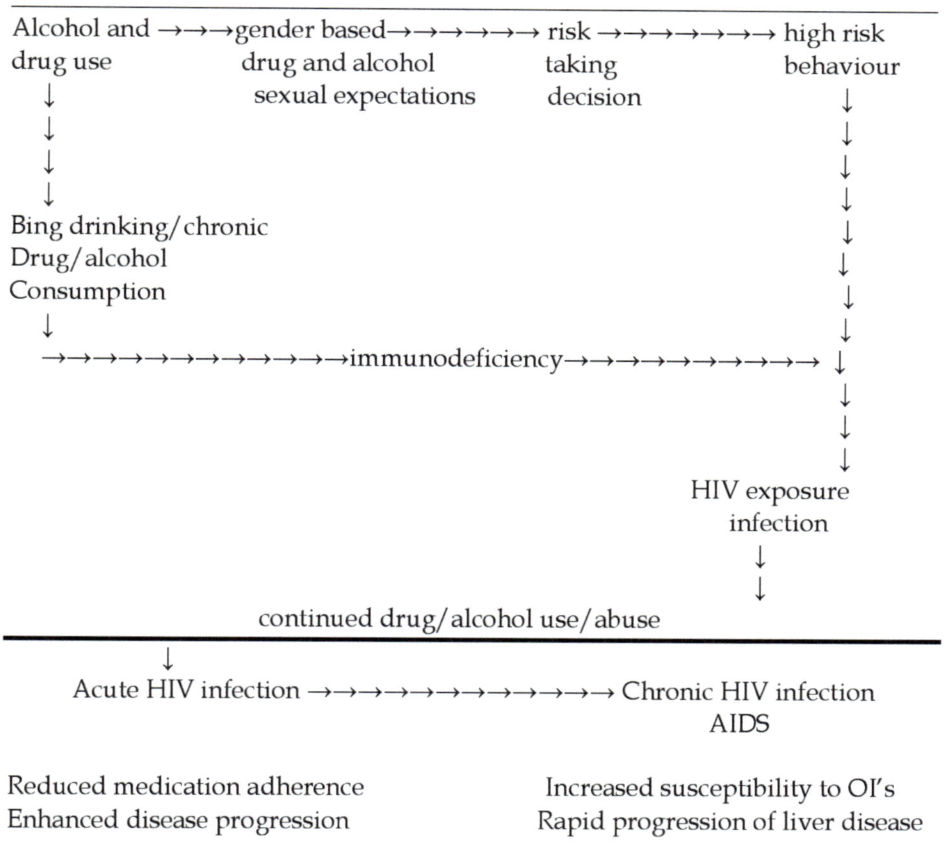

Fig. 1. Interactions and linkages between drug and alcohol use and abuse in the course of HIV infection and AIDS.

Alcoholic beverage consumption can be described based on quantity. Abstainers or light/occasional drinkers comprise roughly 40% of a general population while moderate drinkers comprise about 35% of the general population. Both groups comprise approximately 55–75% of a general medical practice. At-risk drinkers, those with hazardous drinking patterns or quantities, and alcohol abusers, those with harmful drinking (meeting the required clinical criteria) comprise approximately 20% of the population and 20–35% of a general medical practice. At-risk drinkers are males who drink more than two drinks a day or greater than four drinks per occasion. For females and individuals over the age of 65, at-risk drinkers are those who drink greater than one drink per day or greater than three drinks per occasion. These individuals consume alcohol at levels that place them at-risk for alcohol-related social and/or medical problems (Dufour, 1999). These at-risk individuals are best managed through the use of brief interventions that can be provided by primary care physicians, health care providers or specialists, upon training. Usually these brief interventions are outpatient interventions that include some form of counseling.

Approximately 76.3 million individuals have a diagnosable alcohol use disorder. Alcohol and drug use disorders are defined clinically as alcohol/drug abuse or dependence (WHO, 2004). Diagnostic and Statistical Manual of Mental Disorders-4th edition (DSM-IV) definitions of abuse and dependence are maladaptive patterns of alcohol or drug use that result in clinically significant impairment or distress as well as significant behavior modifications. Individuals with alcohol dependence comprise approximately 5% of the population and around 5–10% of a general medical practice. Alcohol abusers and alcohol-dependent individuals exhibit a varying degree of social and/or medical dysfunction. These individuals require intensive treatment, including structured counseling and/or pharmacotherapy (Fiellin et al., 2000). Severely involved dependent patients have been traditionally thought of requiring treatment in a specialty setting. However, studies (Fiellin et al., 2000a) have shown that primary care physicians may also have an important role in providing treatment to these individuals.

Pharmacotherapy for alcohol dependence is an important adjunct to behavioral therapies to reduce the risk of relapse to drinking after an initial period of abstinence (SAMHSA, 2009). Pharmacotherapy for alcohol consumption is also important for patients with co-occurring conditions such as patients with HIV and/or HCV infection(s) where alcohol consumption can augment disease progression. For these patients alcohol dependence treatment has been reported with either acamprosate, naltrexone, vivitrol or disulfiram (Collins et al, 2006). Acamprosate and naltrexone have different mechanisms of action and modify different behavioral aspects of alcohol dependence. Acamprosate is a long acting compound that prolongs periods of abstinence by normalizing glutamateric neurotransmission. Glutamateric neurotransmission in the brain is dysregulated during chronic alcohol consumption and withdrawal. Naltrexone is a fast acting opioid receptor antagonist that reduces heavy drinking through a decrease of the reward effects of ethanol. An evidence-based risk -benefits assessment can be used to inform health care providers on medication choice (Mason, 2003). However, the safety and efficacy of treatment using both medications for alcohol dependence has been shown in double blind studies (Kiefer & Wiedemann, 2004). Disulfiram, another pharmacotherpy option, blocks the oxidation of alcohol at the acetaldehyde stage of its metabolism. The increase in the levels of acetaldehyde resulting in a series of unpleasant symptoms (e.g., flushing, headache, and vomiting). Although disulfiram is widely used, particulalry is the setting of opioid dependence, superior data of studies support the use of naltrexone and acamprosate as pharmacologic treatments of alcoholism (Kiefer et al 2005). For resource limited settings, a series of factors acting synergistically may be creating the "perfect storm" promoting alcohol availability, alcohol consumption, and reducing alcohol control policies, thereby increasing the need for public health efforts (Table 1) to reduce alcohol consumption the beyond the use of medication-assisted treatment for alcohol abuse and dependence (Caetano & Laranjeira, 2006).

Use of alcohol may impact the care and course of HIV infection for an individual patient (Baum et al, 2010; Hahn & Samet, 2010). Optimal management of HIV infected patients with alcohol problems requires recognition of the impact of alcohol on a number of issues: patient's linkage to medical care; adherence to anti-retroviral treatment, impact on co-morbid conditions (such as HCV infection), liver function, and the stage of HIV disease. Due to its many ramifications, the clinical approach to the HIV infected patient with alcohol problems takes on a high priority, yet it is similar in many ways to the standard optimal approach to any medical patient (Bogart et al., 2000). It requires the effective screening for

Public Health Educational Efforts to Prevent HIV Transmssion in the Context of Aclohol Consumption :

- Public education to inform youth and adults of the harms associated with at-risk alcohol consumption
- Education of women of the gender related issues regarding alcohol use and abuse
- Public education on changing societal norms for heavy drinking, and awareness of HIV related risk, including condom use
- Beverage industry collaboration to promote responsible drinking.

Integration of targeted alcohol information, education and interventions in HIV/AIDS prevention programs for persons at high risk for HIV/AIDS:

- Women of child-bearing age
- HIV-positive persons and their partners
- Anti-retroviral treatment patients
- Sex trade workers and truckers
- Injection drug users
- MSM

Brief Interventions. Screening, brief advice & motivational interventions for at-risk drinkers

- By HIV healthcare workers
- By HIV peer outreach workers
- By VCT and anti-retroviral professionals

Detoxification

- Community-based detoxification for acute stabilization prior to outpatient or residential treatment
- Hospital detoxificaion - as medically required

Specialty treatment for alcohol abusers and dependent persons

- Inpatient or residential treatment
- Therapeutic Community Model
- Outpatient treatment and Aftercare- Community drop-in centers for alcohol-free activities and outreach, peer support
- Supportive Residential- Half-way or similar residential support post-discharge
- Treatment approaches- Motivational Interviewing, Cognitive Behavioral, and 12-step based treatmen, Relapse Prevention, and Peer Support
- Medications (Naltrexone, Acamprosate, Disulfiram, Vivitrol)

Peer Recovery Community Support

Table 1. Approaches to Alcohol Use and Abuse in HIV/AIDS

the prevalent condition of alcohol abuse, assessment of the severity of the alcohol problem, and skills to intervene effectively to reduce the harm associated with alcohol use/abuse. New strategies to target alcohol use/ abuse in HIV populations need to be implemented in the context of existing recommended HIV clinical approaches. Addressing alcohol problems in HIV-infected persons has the potential to improve the overall management of HIV disease in a substantial proportion of the population

2.2 Illicit opioid abuse, medication assisted treatment and HIV infection

Based on the 2010 World Drug Report (UNODC, 2010) from the United Nations Office on Drugs and Crime (UNODC), it is estimated that between 175- 250 million people from almost every country, or 5 percent of the global population age 15-64, have used illicit drugs at least once in the last 12 months. Cannabis is by far the most widely used drug, followed by stimulants, such as amphetamines and ecstasy, then cocaine use and then opioids. While most individuals occasionally use or have casually tried illicit drugs, UNODC estimates that there are between 18-38 million problem drug users. These individuals consume most of the drugs and likely fulfill the criteria for a diagnosis of drug abuse or dependence.

These medical co-occurring conditions are specifically prevalent in injection drug users (IDU). Estimates for IDU's are available for at least 130 countries with approximately 78% of the 13.2 million IDU's living in developing or transitional countries (Aceijas et al 2004). Forty-one countries have reported a high prevalence (>5%) of HIV infection in this high-risk population. Globally, IDU's now account for at least 10% of all new HIV infections which are estimated at 5 million per year (IHRDP, 2006). In chronic HIV infection, AIDS has been reported as the leading cause of death in IDUs (Chin, 2007). Epidemiological data of HIV infection show that generalized HIV epidemics can result from diffusion transmission of HIV from high risk groups, such as IDUs. Thus, it is important for countries and regions to undertake surveillance studies to identify current alcohol and drug use patterns and develop best practices for the treatment of individuals who use and abuse alcohol and illicit drugs.

Drug dependence is a chronic, relapsing neurophysiological disease resulting from the prolonged effects of drug(s) on the brain. The neurochemical abnormalities resulting from chronic use are the underlying cause of many of the observed physical and behavioral aspects of abuse and dependence. The brain abnormalities associated with addiction are wide ranging, complex, and long lasting (Chana et al 2006; Goodkin et al 1998; Langford et al 2003). They can involve abnormal brain signaling pathways, psychological conditioning or stress and social factors that result in cravings leading to a predisposition to relapse even months or years after drug(s) use cessation. Thus, substance abuse/dependence can be most effectively addressed in a multifaceted medical-based paradigm that comprises a comprehensive program of interventions that are delivered through the course of long term treatment. Such comprehensive treatment programs include behavioral, social rehabilitative components, as well as biological (pharmacological) components Table 2. Behavioral therapy interventions have been extensively researched and are critical components of the treatment of all drug addictions. Social rehabilitative components are also important and may prove suited to certain treatment environments.

In the United States, opioid abuse/dependence can be treated in two differing medical paradigms. In the highly regulated and structured environment, methadone is dispensed daily at Opioid Treatment Programs (OTPs). These OTPs are increasingly providing "wrap-around" services to address important patient needs, enhance time in treatment, and promote recovery. Alternatively, buprenorphine can be prescribed in a primary care health care setting similar to other illnesses to reduce the stigma/discrimination of drug dependence. Both medical paradigms need to address the reduced quality of life, physical and mental functioning, compared to the general population that is associated with drug abuse/dependence (Millson et al. 2006). In addition, multiple comorbidities are associated with substance abuse and dependence that also contribute to the lower quality of life

Drug Use, Abuse and Dependence
(1)PREVENTION OF DRUG INITIATION Individual targeted interventions through the life span Family targeted interventions Community interventions
(2)IDENTIFICATION OF SUBSTANE USE CONDITIONS Screening for drug use Case finding Assessment & Diagnosis
(3)INITIATION AND ENGAGEMENT IN DRUG TREATMENT Brief intervention Promoting Engagement, case management/ care navagators Detoxification/ Withdrawal Management Assessment of social, co-morbid medical conditions and co-occurring disorders
(4) LONG TERM TREATMENT OF SUBSTANCE USE ILLNESS Psychosocial Pharmacotherapy Treatment of co-morbid medical conditions and co-occurring disorders Promotion of treatment engagement & social stability through legal, social, educational, financial support
(5) PRIMARY CARE AND POST TREATMENT MANAGEMENT OF PATIENT Recovery Relapse prevention Rehabilitation Medical Home

Table 2. Elements of the Continuum of Care in the Treatment of Opioid Abuse/Dependence

experienced and documented by opioid dependent individuals. Life priorities of opioid users have been reported as concern about HIV and treatment of infection with HIV, housing, money, and protection from violence (Mizuno et al, 2003).

Substance abuse is a complex medical disorder composed of multiple physiologic, social and behavioral problems often interrelated with psychological illness. Health care providers need to screen substance misusing patients for psychological illness (Schuckit, 2006). Although it can be difficult to ascertain whether substance abuse, psychological illness, or infectious comorbidities should be addressed first, an initial focus on the medical treatment of drug abuse is often necessary to create sufficient patient stability from which other treatments can begin. Stability is further increased with both mental health services and substance abuse treatment, subsequently enhancing the medical outcomes of treatment for comorbidities.

In the United States, multiple pharmacological treatments, including both agonists and antagonists have been developed and approved by the Food and Drug Administration for specific drug dependence. Currently, medications and evidence-based treatment paridigms utilizing these pharmacotherapies are available for the treatment of nicotine, alcohol, and opioid substance use disorders. Although none are available for stimulants, such as cocaine and methamphetamine, many potential medications are now being developed for these drugs of abuse and are expected to be available over the next few years. An effective treatment strategy for drug abuse and dependence is to match a comprehensive treatment plan to the individual's particular substance abuse problems and needs. Desired treatment outcomes should: a) reduce dependence on drugs of abuse, b) reduce morbidity and mortality of and associated with drugs of abuse, and c) maximize the patients' abilities to access services and achieve social integration.

2.2.1 Medication assited treatment utilizing methadone

In most countries that utilize MAT for the treatment of opioid dependence, methadone is the pharmacotherapy of choice. Methadone is usually the least expensive medication and when used in evidence-based treatment paridigms is cost effective and can result in abstenence from illicit drug use over time and the achievement of recovery (Connock et al 2007; Skinner et al 2011). Methadone is a synthetic μ-opioid receptor agonist with pharmacological properties qualitatively similar to morphine and was originally used to treat the painful symptoms of withdrawal from heroin and other opioids (Gowing et al 2006; Payte & Zweben , 1998). Administered daily as an oral dose for the treatment of opioid dependence, an individual therapeutic dosage is determined to maintain an asymptomatic state and stabilize a patient, without episodes of opioid overmedication or withdrawal. The therapeutic dosage for a patient is a function of many factors including: absorption, metabolism, drug-drug interactions, physiology, diet and the use of alternative medications. Minimum retention time in treatment varies for residential and outpatient methadone treatment programs. The National Institutes of Health consensus panel on opioid-addiction treatment (NIH, 1997) concluded that individuals treated for fewer than three months with methadone do not show substantial medical gain. As time in treatment progresses, study outcomes have reported partial reductions of illicit opioid use progressing to abstinence. Relapse to opioid use is common when methadone is discontinued without further support or behavioral treatment. In the United States, OTPs or methadone maintenance treatment programs, MMTP, under the certification of the Substance Abuse and Mental Health Services Administration (SAMHSA), dispense methadone and can provide a comprehensive therapeutic milieu comprised of primary medical care, psychosocial counseling, vocational rehabilitation, HIV testing and counseling, hepatitis C education and testing and other vital medical and social services. Methadone treatment is effective as both primary and secondary HIV prevention (Kerr et al 2004) and cost-effective to society (Barnett et al 2001; Doran et al 2003). In addition to improving health outcomes, methadone treatment also substantially improves the quality of life of patients over the course of methadone treatment (Giacomuzzi et al 2005).

Barriers to retention in methadone treatment include the severity of drug, medical and social problems at initiation of treatment, as well as patient readiness for treatment and motivation. Integrating multiple components of the drug treatment program is fundamental to successful treatment outcomes. Treatment programs that offer a broader array of "wrap-around" services and a greater frequency of services have reported improved retention in treatment and treatment outcomes (Fiellin et al 2003). Programs responsive to the severity of drug abuse during initial stages of drug treatment have been shown to produce positive treatment outcomes based on greater retention time in treatment and patient satisfaction with treatment services. Maximum retention time in methadone treatment is associated with comprehensive treatment, provision of frequent health service, as well as appropriate methadone dosing (Litwin et al 2001).

2.2.2 Medication assited treatment utilizing buprenorphine

In the United States and globally, primary care physicians can expand the accessibility of substance abuse treatment while mitigating the stigma associated with drug use and treatment through an outpatient treatment setting in primary care and the use of buprenorphine. However, in the United States, buprenorphine-only OTPs have been recently developed where buprenorphine is provided to opioid dependent patents under the highly regulated rules and regulations that apply to methadone. Buprenorphine, a partial mu-receptor opiate agonist (Ling & Smith 2002), differs significantly from full agonists. Most significantly, buprenorphine has a plateau of its agonist properties at higher doses. This results in an improved safety profile compared with a full agonist. Specifically, buprenorphine has a favorable 'ceiling effect' on respiratory depression precluding overdose potential (Walsh et al 1994). However, the abuse of other substances that may enhance respiratory depression (e.g., benzodiazepines) remains a contraindication with buprenorphine as with methadone. Improved safety and thrice weekly flexible dosing promotes patient acceptance. In addition, buprenorphine has two features that decrease street diversion. Buprenorphine can precipitate opiate withdrawal when buprenorphine is taken by an opiate dependent patient (Schuh et al. 1996) and buprenorphine can be marketed both alone (Subutex®) and in combination with naloxone (Suboxone®). In the latter formulation, if it is crushed and injected, acute opiate withdrawal symptoms will ocuur which are a potent disincentive for prescription opioid abuse (Yokell et al. 2011).

2.2.3 Medication assited treatment utilizing naltrexone

Naltrexone is a non-narcotic long-acting, opioid antagonist that blocks the euphoric effects of opioids binding the mu opioid receptor. Unlike methadone, there is no negative reinforcement (opioid withdrawal) upon discontinuation. Due to naltrexone's opioid antagonism, patients must abstain from opioids for a minimum of seven days prior to starting treatment to avoid the precipitation of opioid withdrawal. The effectiveness of naltrexone treatment depends upon patient motivation and social support system (Greenstein et al 1983). Thus, in cultures where there is strong family or social support for the patient in care, oral naltrexone has been shown to be effective in the prevention of relapse to heroin use (Krupitsky et al 2010). Because of a lack of positive reinforcing effects with naltrexone and low motivation on the part of many patients, as well as, poor clinician acceptability, it is not widely prescribed for the treatment of opioid dependence in the United States.

Vivitrol is an injectable extended-release formulation of naltrexone that has recently been approved for the treatment of opioid abuse and dependence. Vivitrol addresses the concern of medication adherence as a monthly injectable formulation and has been shown to be more effective than oral naltrexone (Krupitskya & Blokhina, 2010). This was also shown in a recent Phase 3 clinical trial that confirmed vivitrol's safety and efficacy in the prevention of relapse to heroin use in a cohort of injection drug users. A higher retention in care and higher rates of opioid-free urine screens were observed along with a significant reduction in opioid craving compared to placebo. Currently, studies are underway to determine the most efficacious service model(s) for the use of vivitrol in the treatment of relapse prevention to heroin use.

3. Medication assisted treatment: Stages of treatment and recovery

The stages or phase of MAT are shown in Table 3. The patient travels through these three stages of treatment, sometimes linearly and sometimes with oscillations between phases. The ultimate goal upon entering MAT is a good clinical outcome which includes the

- Induction
  - Medication is chosen based on clinical and patient circumstances
  - MAT initiation where initial dosing of medication is observed and dosing titration is performed by a clinician
  - Dosing and dose titration is based on expression and control of withdrawal symptoms and is a critical period in terms of risk of opioid overdose in treatment
  - procedures for patient observation during and after dose titration are incorporated into the clinic setting
  - Induction can last 7-10 days with the goal of obtaining a therapeutic dose of opioid medication
- Stabilization
  - stabilization phase occurs when the patient no longer exhibits drug seeking behavior or craving
  - The correct dosage of medication is critical (overdosing versus underdosing) as well as successful participation of the patient in behavioral therapies and rehabilitation services
  - MAT provider determines stabilization based on patient symptoms, not on opioid free urine samples
  - Individual patient health (e.g. pregnancy, liver disease, etc.), other medical treatments including HAART and TB treatments, and other drug use or alcohol consumption affects stabilization
- Maintenance
  - Maintenance pharmacotherapy occurs when the patient is responding optimally to medication treatment and routine dose adjustments are not needed.
  - Patients at this stage have stopped using illicit opioid and resumed productive lifestyles away from the local drug culture.
  - It is also at this stage that patients should have minimal or normal medical needs and can move away from intensive drug treatment settings and receive their medications in a primary care/community setting.
  - Typically take home medication of controlled medications is allowed for patients
  - If maintenance phase cannot be reached, other drug dependence treatment approaches should be explored to complement MAT

Table 3. Stages or Phases of MAT

recovery from opioid abuse and dependence and social reintegration back into society. The individual in recovery is a functioning member of the community and contributes to the social fiber and health of the community. Thus, a foundation of MAT is the obtainment of Recovery from opioid abuse and dependence (Davidson & White , 2007).

The recovery process is the individual way in which a person actively manages their substance use disorder with efforts to reclaim full functional and meaningful lives in the community. Recovery is personal process of growth and change which embraces hope, autonomy and the elements that result in establishing a satisfying and productive life. MAT is a recovery oriented system of care when integrated with other medical, social and rehabilitative services in support of the individual's and family's long term efforts to reclaim full and meaningful lives in the community. Important in recovery is the provision of comprehensive services in the context of MAT but also a supportive, enabling environment that fosters individual responsibility over one's health and empowerment to change to a healthy lifestyle (Sowers, 2005).

MAT, as a recovery orientated system of care, has four phases as shown in Table 4, along with a set of recovery oriented goals, strategies, and services (White & Mojer-Torres, 2010). An important consideration in phase four, long term sustained recovery, is the personal decision to continue with medical maintenance of pharmacotherapy or to taper the medication. In either case, the home or living environment is critical to the prevention of relapse to opioid use. To prevent relapse of opioid use the individual in recovery needs a drug free environment. While significant gains have been made through national prevention programs such as "Drug Free Communities", it remains a Herculean task to keep a community entirely free of illicit drug use. Thus, for long term recovery the home or living environment is where recovery is nucleated (Ashcraft et al, 2008). Local peer recovery programs as well as recovery oriented systems of care that link to or provide individualized, quality long term supportive care are critical (Jason & Ferrari, 2010). These settings provide a network of people to support abstinence as well as a low risk environment to support recovery. Receiving abstinence support, guidance and information from a recovery home, that is committed to long term sobriety, reduces the risk of relapse to illicit opioid use. These homes need to be considered as a fundamental component in the development and maintenance of the public health of communities.

4. Service models for medication assisted treatment

Health service programs deliver MAT in a regulatory environment where both the federal government and state/local government provide a regulatory framework for the access to and delivery of medications that are controlled by international convention (Kresina et al, 2009). In the United States, state and local regulation can enhance the federal regulations but they can not negate the federal regulations. The MAT federal regulations can be found in the Code of Federal Regulations (CFR, 2002) and establish procedures to determine if a health practitioner is qualified to dispense methadone in the treatment of opioid abuse and dependence in opioid treatment programs, as well as, the quantity of methadone that can be provided for unsupervised use by patients. Thus, the federal regulations address the balance needed in the use of controlled medications for treatment versus the restrictions to limit diversion of the controlled medication (Yokell et al 2011).

The MAT federal regulations do not regulate the health service models that can be use to maximize access to MAT as well as time in treatment. These are two important

- *Recovery initiation and stabilization*
  - Major goal- eliminate use of illicit opioid use for at least twenty-four hours as well as other drug of abuse
    - Educate the patient about the risk and benefits of pharmacotherapy
    - Provide a choice of alternate/supplemental therapeutic approaches
    - Identify patient's treatment needs and engage early
    - Minimize sedative and side effects of medication
    - Asses safety and adequacy of each dose after administration
    - Discourage self medication of withdrawal symptoms
    - Assess and initially address medical, social, legal, family and other problems
    - Develop initial coping and craving strategies
- *Early recovery and rehabilitation*
  - Major goal- empower individuals to cope with life problems, medical needs co-occurring disorders vocational and educational needs, family problems, legal issues and develop long term goals for education, employment and family reconciliation
    - Insure medication dose promotes daily comfort
    - Link patient to family and peer-recovery support
    - Develop recovery plan
    - Assess and initially address personal strengths and needs
- *Recovery Maintenance*
  - Major goal- patient assumes primary responsibility for their life
    - Patient receives needed integrated services
    - Patient is active in community recovery support programs
    - Patient receives take home medication from an OTP
    - Decision on medical maintenance or tapering of pharmacotherapy
- *Long-term Sustained Recovery*
  - Major goal- continued primary responsibility for life
    - Taper from pharmacotherapy- quarterly or biannual check-up from substance abuse treatment program
    - Continuing pharmacotherapy- continued regular check-up with substance abuse treatment provider
    - Continued engagement with peer-based recovery support program
    - Patient becomes a recovery support for other patients

Table 4. Phases and Goals of MAT Recovery Oriented Systems of Care

characteristics to maximize as one designs model MAT programs to ensure good clinical and public health outcomes. Barrier free access to MAT is important for obtaining maximal public health impact and reaching all opioid abusing individuals seeking treatment. Research studies have shown that the more time in MAT the better the treatment outcome. Thus, MAT programs providing comprehensive services as part of the continuum of care (see Table 2) in an enabling environment result in quality and effective substance abuse treatment services that promote individual well-being and improved community health.

4.1 Integrated models of medication assisted treatment

Health service models for MAT that provide comprehensive services interface substance abuse treatment services with primary medical care and social/rehabilitation services. That interface can be comprehensive through the integration of substance abuse treatment services, primary medical care, infectious disease prevention, care and treatment and social/rehabilitation services. An integrated care and treatment model, where MAT services are provided within primary care using a single medical record, minimizes the sigma and discrimination associated with drug treatment services while improving overall health outcomes in a cost-effective manner (Collins et al 2010).

For OTPs dispensing methadone, primary medical care and social/rehabilitation services are integrated on-site in the structured environment where methadone is dispensed (Freidman et al 1999; Kresina et al 2008). Based on patient needs, various types of health services can be integrated into OTP MAT services including primary care, mental health, and infectious diseases. Specific limiting factors for the integration of services have been shown to be the organizational structure of the OTP and cost.

Buprenorphine, a less regulated opioid agonist medication, is approved in the United States for office based opioid treatment. An office based setting provides enhanced treatment access to MAT using buprenorphine in a less stigmatized environment enabling integrated medical care of infectious diseases and co-morbid conditions (Gunderson & Fiellin , 2008). Multiple models have been piloted for the integration of MAT using buprenorphine within HIV primary care (Sullivan et al 2006). These include an on-site combination of addiction treatment/HIV specialist treatment; a HIV primary care physician prescribing buprenorphine; a non-physician health care provider integrating medical care and substance abuse treatment services using buprenorphine; and a community outreach model where buprenorphine is provided along with medical services in a mobile van. These pilot projects have uncovered barriers to integrating MAT using buprenorphine within HIV primary care that are both financial and regulatory. Regulatory challenges include licensing and training restrictions imposed by the Drug Addiction Treatment Act of 2000 and confidentiality regulations for alcohol and drug treatment records (Schackman et al 2006). A recent study has shown that in a primary care setting that used buprenorphine, prescription opioid dependent patients showed better clinical outcomes compared to patients who were dependent on heroin (Moore et al, 2007).

Naltrexone is a non-narcotic and therefore non-controlled medication for the treatment of opioid abuse as well as alcohol abuse. Naltrexone integrated with mental health services, particularly psychosocial treatment has been shown to be an effective maintenance treatment for reducing heroin use after detoxification (Minozzi et al. 2006). In addition, using clonidine and naltrexone together has been shown to be successfully integrated into a primary care setting (O'Connor et al. 1997). In this study retention in care and successful detoxification from opioid abuse was observed with MAT using either naltrexone or buprenorphine. In other care settings, treatment of alcohol use disorders using naltrexone has been successfully integrated into the treatment of patients who have tuberculosis (Greenfield et al. 2010). Current efforts are determining the optimum conditions to integrate vivitrol (extended release naltrexone) into HIV primary care programs. Additionally, how to integrate vivitrol into an OTP setting and in primary medical care as a relapse prevention intervention for patients following their completion of maintenance treatment with either methadone or buprenorphine, is currently moving forward.

4.2 Coordinated care models of medication assisted treament

Health service models for MAT that provide comprehensive services can connect substance abuse treatment services with primary medical care and social/rehabilitation services in a non-integrated but coordinated fashion. Here, MAT services coordinate with primary medical care and social/rehabilitation services to promote good patient outcomes and enhance community health. MAT, health services and social/rehabilitation services can be separately managed with a different network of health care providers but co-located to allow convenient utilization of primary care, MAT and other services. An additional coordinated approach provides primary care, MAT and other services at distinct locations through a differing network of health care providers. As shown in a recent study where twice as many patients retained in MAT when the MAT services were provided at single location compared to referral of MAT to a distant location (Lucas et al 2010), providing needed health services at distinct locations is less than optimal. However, coordinated programs can be effective when case managers, peer facilitators, care navigators or others promote or support service utilization at the various locations. For example, a referral system intervention was modeled with linkages to treatment services for substance use, mental health and social services for HIV+ patients receiving HIV primary care (Zaller et al. 2007). Patients receiving the intervention were referred to MAT either at an OTP or in an office based setting that prescribed buprenorphine. An alternative model provided highly stable OTP patients with 28 days of methadone doses and required monthly check-ins. Successful patients were noted to have increased family and social activities and failed patients were provided stepped treatment intensification (King et al. 2006). Community -wide health service delivery programs also provide an alternative to integration through enhanced access to networked drug treatment and co-morbidity health services (Neufeld et al 2010).

Unique to buprenorphine is the model that a substance abuse treatment specialist provides the initial treatment (induction) with buprenorphine until the patient is stabilized. Then the patient is transferred/referred to a primary care physician who can then provide maintenance buprenorphine treatment and medical primary care. This so called 'wheel and spoke model' allows for substance abuse treatment specialists to manage the more difficult portion of buprenorphine treatment (early treatment -or induction phase) while the primary care medical program manages the long term maintenance phase of buprenorphine treatment (BBI, 2008). This model is important in the United States since the Drug Addiction Treatment Act of 2000 limits the number of patients a qualified buprenorphine treatment provider can manage in their practice (DATA, 2000). This model has been adapted to HIV+ patients where the buprenorphine induction is performed by the substance abuse treatment specialist and then the patient is transferred/ referred to the HIV primary care physician (Basu et al. 2006).

Coordinated MAT for patients seeking relapse prevention interventions after detoxification from opioid use can be provided by naltrexone or the recently approved vivitrol. As noted earlier, naltrexone it is not widely prescribed for the treatment of opioid dependence in the United States, but is provided as an office based treatment for opioid dependence after detoxification. In addition, studies have shown that the extended release formulations are effective in reducing opioid use and retaining patients in care after detoxification (Comer et al 2006; Kunoe et al. 2010). Fishman et al 2010 has shown good clinical outcomes (retention in care and reduced opioid use) for adolescents receiving vivitrol over a four month period. This study is important because of the limted use of controlled pharmacotherapies in adolescent populations as part of national regulatory frameworks.

5. Preventing HIV infection by integration of medication assisted treatment into HIV prevention services

Important HIV prevention interventions for people who inject drugs are the provision of clean needles and syringe through syringe service programs and associated HIV testing and counseling programs. These HIV prevention interventions, when integrated into MAT programs, maximize the enrollment in treatment programs for opioid and alcohol abuse, and thereby maximize HIV prevention efforts (Kidorf et al 2009; Lloyd et all 2005). Maximizing HIV prevention efforts targeting peple who use drugs and those dependent on opioids and alcohol are critcial to prevent HIV infection in these most-at -risk populations.

Integrating drug abuse treatment and early HIV prevention interventions, particulaly HIV testing and counseling, are important as components of the newly emerging Seek,Test, Treat and Retain" strategy (Crawford & Vlahov, 2010; Taege, 2011). This is an engagement and retention strategy that outreach workers can employ with injection drug users to reduce their risk for HIV infection. By utilizing outreach workers to seek out most-at-risk people who inject drugs, establish their HIV status through HIV testing, followed by sexual risk reduction councelling, HIV risk behaviors can be addressed with subsequent emphasis on treatment for their substance use disorder.

Unfortuately, there is not signifcant integration of HIV testing and counseling in OTPs. In the US, while approaximely 90% of opioid treatment programs provide some form of federally mandated HIV/AIDS education, only 74% of opiod treatment progams offered HIV testing (Kresina et al 2005). These services appear underutilized in that approximately one-in-three persons receiveving subtance abuse treatment also received HIV testing and counselling (Pollack & D'Aunno, 2010). Globally, although subtantial efforts are being made to increase the availability of HIV testing, most-at-risk populations remain underserved with regard to HIV prevention service utilization. It is estimated that only 10% of persons at-risk for HIV infection receive HIV testing. Thus, strategies such as opt-out testing, home-based testing, dor-to-door testing as well as providing dedicated HIV testings counselors at point-of-service locations are being utilized to enhance the uptake of HIV testing for people who use alcohol and inject drugs. Studies have shown that most-at-risk populations prefer point-of-service HIV testing, however, this intervention requires additional measures to support HIV positive individuals entering into HIV care and treatment (Keller et al 2011).

6. Preventing HIV transmission by integration of medication assisted treatment into HIV care and treatment

A significant factor in not reducing the global HIV epidemic is the lack of entrance into HIV care and treatment by most-at-risk populations. These populations, which include illicit

drug users and alcohol abusers, encounter numerous barriers in accessing HIV care and treatment. In addition, once in treatment these individuals often suffer stigma and discrimination as they receive their needed medical care. The result is an increase in the prevalence of medical and psychiatric co-morbidities as well as social issues and high risk behaviors, in addition to worse clinical outcomes with a higher mortality rate compared to the non-drug and non-alcohol using populations infected with HIV (Altice et al 2010).
The increased mortally rate noted in people who inject drugs is related to their late presentation for HIV care. Patients who present late for care and treatment of HIV/AIDS are at a higher risk of significant clinical complications and are thus more difficult to clinically manage. Late presentation for treatment of HIV/AIDS is a common scenario leading to death (Moreno et al 2010). A recent study has documented a highly lethal neurological syndrome found in HIV-infected drug abusers (Newsome et al 2011). Although rare, the newly described syndrome is highly lethal with a mean survival time of 21 days after diagnosis. The authors suggest that access and initiation of antiretroviral therapy may provide a better outcome for these patients. In addition, substance abuse treatment, particularly MAT, which has been shown to enhance the health status, reduce mortality and quality of life of injection drug users, would be an important adjunct to anti-retroviral treatment for these patients. Thus, as noted earlier integrating both MAT with anti-retroviral treatment in a HIV primary care setting is a paradigm to optimize health outcomes and the health status of HIV-infected injection drug users.
How MAT is integrated in HIV primary care programs depends on the country's regulatory framework. In the United States, all medications accept methadone, can be prescribes to patients in a HIV primary care or outpatient HIV clinical care setting. The federal regulations in the United States require methadone to be dispenses in OTPs. However, in this setting studies have shown that HIV care and anti-retroviral treatment can be effectively prescribed either as directly observed therapy or as routine care. Other countries, such as Australia, have less stringent federal regulations for prescribing controlled medications and all medications comprising MAT can be provided in a primary care setting. In either case, the important aspect of providing integrated MAT and HIV primary care is the single location/clinic. In that case, the patient can receive all the needed services to support their recovery from drug/alcohol dependence as well as care and treatment for HIV infection.

7. Essential health interventions for the prevention of HIV infection in people who inject opioids

The WHO, UNODC and UNAIDS has approved and advocates for a package of essential interventions for the prevention, treatment and care of HIV for people who inject drugs (WHO, 2009a). These evidence based intervention, shown in Table 6, need three important characteristics in their implementation to maximize effectiveness. These interventions need to be part of a public health policy that is human rights based, gender responsive, and community owned.
As noted earlier, no single intervention alone will prevent or reverse to growing national HIV epidemics due to injection drug use and abuse. However, the greatest impact will be obtained when the interventions are provided through an integrated services platform in a comprehensive fashion. And in order to reach all of those seeking HIV prevention, care and treatment services, health service platforms need to provide an enabling environment that establishes confidentiality. In addition, they also need to develop patient –provider trusting

relationships. Both community outreach and peer -to-peer services can promote full service utilization. The national Ministries of Health need to embrace and support these health services and interventions through a supportive legal and policy framework validating their place in the public health area and in society as they improve community health.

Prevention, Care and Treatment for People Who Inject Drugs
1. Needle and Syringe Programmes (NSP)/Syringe Service Programs (SSP)
2. Drug dependence treatment including Medication Assisted Treatment (MAT) and Opioid Substitution Treatment (OST)
3. HIV Testing and Counselling
4. Antiretroviral Therapy (ART)
5. Prevention and Treatment of Sexually Transmitted Infection (STI)
6. Condom distribution programs for People Who Inject Drugs and their sex partners
7. Targeted information, education and communication (IEC) for People Who Inject Drugs and their sex partners
8. Vaccination, diagnosis and treatment of viral hepatitis infection
9. Prevention, diagnosis and treatment of tuberculosis

Table 5. Listing of Internationally Accepted Essential Interventions for HIV

8. Conclusion

Substance abuse treatment is HIV prevention. The use of medication assisted treatment as a component of a comprehensive treatment plan for those individuals who abuse opioids and/or alcohol is an effective, evidence-based treatment paradigm that results in good medical outcomes including a reduction in HIV transmission as well as a reduction of incident infections in opioid and alcohol abusing populations.

9. References

Aceijas, C., Stimson, G.V., Hickman, M., & Rhodes, T. (2004) Global overview of injecting drug use and HIV infection among injection drug users. *Acquir Immun Defic Syndr* vol 18 no 17 pp 2295-2303.

Altice, FL., Kamarulzaman, A., Soriano, V., Schechter, M., & Friedland, GH. (2010) Treatment of medical, psychiatric and substance use comorbidities in people infected with HIV who use drugs. *The Lancet* vol 376 no 9738 pp367-387.

Ashcraft, L., Anthony, W.A,&, Martin C. (2008) Home is where recovery begins. *Behav Health* vol 28 no 5 pp 13-15.

Barnett, P.G., Zaric, G.S.& Brandeau, M..L.(2001) The cost-effectiveness of buprenorphine maintenance therapy for opiate addiction in the United States. *Addiction.* vol 96 no 9 pp1267-78.

Basu, S., Smith-Rohrberg, D., Bruce, R.D.& Altice, F.L. (2006) Models for integrating buprenorphine therapy into the primary HIV care setting. Clin Infect Dis vol 42 no 5 pp 716-721

Baum, MK., Rafie, C., Lai, S., Sales, S., Page, JB., & Campa, A. (2010) Alcohol use accelerates HIV disease progression. *AIDS Res Hum Retroviruses* vol 26 no 5 pp 511-518.

BBI (2008) *Baltimore Buprenorphine Initiative Newsletter*. Baltimore Buprenorphine Initiative Updates. October 2008.Retreived from: http://www.bsasinc.org/media/doc/Baltimore%20buprenorphine%20initiativenewsletteroctober200

Bogart, LM., Kelly, JA., Catz, SL., & Sosman. (2000) Impact of medical and nonmedical factors on physician decision making for HIV/AIDS antiretroviral treatment. *J Acquir Immune Defic Syndr* vol 23 no 5 pp 396-404.

Caetano, R. & Laranjeira, R. A. (2006) A 'perfect storm' in developing countries: economic growth and the alcohol industry. *Addict* vol 101 no 2 pp149-52.

CFR (2002) Part 8 Certification of Opioid Treatment Programs. *Code of Federal Regulations.* Title 42. Public Health. Chapter 1 Public Health Service, Department of Health and Human Services.. retrieved from: http://www.access.gpo.gov/nara/cfr/waisidx_02/42cfr8_02.html

Chana, G., Everall, I.P., Crews, L., Langford, D., Adame, A., Grant, I., Cherner, M., Lazzaretto, D., Heaton, R., Ellis, R., Masliah, E. & HNRC Group (2006). Cognitive deficits and degeneration of interneurons in HIV+ methamphetamine users. *Neurology* vol 67 no 8 pp 1486-1489.

Chin, J. (2007). *The AIDS Pandemic: the collision of epidemiology with political correctness.* Oxford: Radcliffe Publishing. ISBN-13: 978-1846191183

Collins, C., Hewson, D.L., Munger, R. & Wade, T.(2010) Evolving models of behavioral health integration in primary care. *Milbank Memorial Fund Report*, New York available at: http://www.milbank.org/reports/10430EvolvingCare/EvolvingCare.pdf

Collins, G.B., McAllister, M.S. & Adury, K. (2006) Drug adjuncts for treating alcohol dependence. *Cleve Clin J Med.* vol 73 no 7 pp 641-644

Comer, S.D., Sullivan, M.A., Yu, E., Rothenberg, J.L., Kleber, H.D., Kampman, K., Dackis, C.& O'Brain, C.P.(2006) Injectable, sustained-release naltrexone for the treatment of opioid dependence. A randomized, placebo controlled trial. *Arch Gen Psychiatry*. vol 63 no 2 pp 210-218.

Connock, M., Juarez-Garcia, A., Jowett, S., Fre, E., Liu, Z., Taylor, R.J., Fry-Smith, A., Day, E., Lintzeris, N., Roberts, T., Burls, A. & Taylor , R.S.(2007) Methadone and buprenorphine for the management of opioid dependence: a systematic review and economic evaluation. *Health Technol Aassess* vol 11 no 9 pp 1-171.

Crawford, N.D. & Vlahov, D. (2010) Progress in HIV reduction and prevention among injection and noninjection drug users. *J Acquir Immune Defic Syndr* vol 55 suppl 2 ppS84-87.

DATA (2000). *Drug Addiction Treatment Act of 2000.* Public Law 106-310 106th Congress Retrieved from: http://www.naabt.org/documents/DATA2000LAWTEXT.pdf

Davidson, L.& White, W. (2007) The concept of recovery as an organizing principle for integrating mental health and addiction services. *J Behave Health Ser Res* vol 34 no 2 pp 109-120.

Doran, C.M., Shanahan, M., Mattick, R.., Ali, R., White, J.& Bell, J.(2003) Buprenorphine versus methadone maintenance: a cost-effectiveness analysis. *Drug Alcohol Depend.* vol 71no 3 pp295-302.

DSM-IV (1999), Substance Related Disorders. In *DSM-IV™ Diagnostic and Statistical Manual of Mental Disorders- 4th edition.* American Psychiatric Association Publishers, ISBN 0-89042-062-9, Washington, DC pp175-272.

Dufour, M. (1999). What is moderate drinking? Defining « drinks » and drinking levels. *Alcohol Res Health* vol 23 no 1 pp5-14.

Edlin, B.R., Seal, K.H., Lorvick, J., Kral, A.H., Ciccarone D.H. & Moore ,L.D. (2001) Is it justifiable to withhold treatment for hepatitis C from illicit-drug users?, *New England Journal of Medicine* vol 345 no 3 pp. 211–214.

Epstein, H., & Morris, M. (2011) Concurrent partnerships and HIV : An inconvenient truth. *J Int AIDS Soc* vol 14 no 1 pp13-23.

Fiellin, DA., Reid, MC., & O'Connor PG. (2000) New therapies for alcohol problems: application to primary care. *Am J Med* vol 108 no 3 pp227-237.

Fiellin, DA., Reid, MC., & O'Connor PG. (2000a). Screening for alcohol problems in primary care : a systematic review. *Arch Intern Med* vol 160 no 13 pp1977-1989.

Fiellin, D.A., Rosenheck, R.A. & Kosten, T.R..(2003) Coordination of medical care and opioid dependence treatment in primary care: A case report. *Substance Abuse* vol 24 no 1 pp 43-46.

Fishman, M.J., Winstanley, E.L., Curran, E., Garrett, S. & Subramanian, G. (2010) Treatment of opioid dependence in adolescents and young adults with extended release naltrexone: preliminary case-series and feasibility. *Addiction* vol 105 no 9 pp1669-1676.

Freidmann, P.D. Alexander, J.A., Jin, L. & D'Aunno, T.A. (1999) On-site primary care and mental health services in outpatient drug abuse treatment units. *J Behav Health Ser Res* vol 26 no 1 pp 80-94.

Giacomuzzi, S.M., Ertl, M., Kemmler, G., Riemer, Y. & Vigl, A. (2005) Sublingual buprenorphine and methadone maintenance treatment: a three year follow-up of quality of life assessment. *Scientific World* J vol 5 pp 452-68

Goodkin, K., Shapshak, P., Metsch, L.R., McCoy, C.B., Crandall, K.A., Kumar, M., Fujimura, R.K., McCoy, V., Zhang, B.T., Reyblat, S., Xin, K.Q. & Kumar, A.M. (1998). Cocaine abuse and HIV-1 infection: epidemiology and neuropathogenesis. *J Neuroimmunol.* vol 83 no 1-2 pp 88-101

Gowing, L., Ali, R. & White, J. (2006) Opioid antagonists under heavy sedation or anaesthesia for opioid withdrawal. *Cochrane Database Syst Rev* April 19, 2006, no 2 CD002022.

Greenfield, S.F., Shields, A., Connery, H.S., Livchits, V., Yanov, S.A., Lastimoso, C.S., Strelis, A.K., Mishustin, S.P., Fitzmaurice, G., Mathew, T.A., Shin, S. (2010) Integrated management of physician-delivered alcohol care for tuberculosis patients: Design and implementation. *Alcohol Clin Exp Res* vol 34 no 2 pp 317-330

Greenstein, R.A., Evan, B.D., McLellan, A.T. & O'Brien, C.P. (1983) Predictors of favorable outcome following naltrexone treatment. *Drug Alcohol Depend* vol 12 no 2 pp 173-180.

Gunderson, E.W. & Fiellin D.A..(2008) Office-based maintenance treatment of opioid dependence: how does it compare with traditional approaches? *CNS Drugs* vol 22 no 2 pp 99-111

Hahn, JA., & Samet, JH. (2010) Alcohol and HIV disease progression: weighing the evidence. *Curr HIV/AIDS Rep* vol 7 no 4 pp226-233.

IHRDP (International Harm Reduction Development Program). (2006). Harm reduction developments 2005: countries with injection-driven HIV epidemics. New York: Open Society Institute. Retrieved from: http://www.soros.org/initiatives/health/focus/ihrd/articles_publications/publications/ihrdreport_20060417/ihrd_ar.pdf

Jason, L.A. & Ferrari J.R. (2010) Oxford House recovery homes: characteristics and effectiveness. *Psychol Serv* vol 7 no 2 pp 92-102.

Kerr, T., Wodak, A., Elliott, R., Montane,r .JS.& Wood, E. (2004)Opioid substitution and HIV/AIDS treatment and prevention. *Lancet*. vol 364 no 9449 pp1918-9

Keller, S., Jones, J., & Erbelding, E. (2011) Choice of Rapid HIV testing and entrance into care in Baltimore City sexually transmitted infection clinics. *AIDS Patient Care* STD vol 24 no 4 pp237-243..

Kidorf, M., King, V.L., Neufeld, K., Peirce, J., Kolodner, K. & brooner, R.K. (2009) Improving substance abuse treatment enrollment in community syringe exchangers. *Addiction* vol 104 no 5 pp786-795.

Kiefer, F., Helwig, H., Tarnaske, T., Otte, C., Jahn, H. & Wiedermann, K (2005). Pharmacological relapse prevention of alcoholism: clinical predictors of outcome. *Eur Addict Res vol* 11 no 2 pp 83-91.

Kiefer, F. & Wiedemann, K. (2004) Combined therapy: what does acamprosate and naltrexone combination tell us? *Alcohol Alcohol* vol 39 no 6 pp 542-547.

King, V.L., Kidorf, M.S., Stoller, K.B., Schwartz, R., Kolodner, K.& Brooner, R.K.(2006) A 12 month controlled trial of medical methadone maintenance integrated into an adaptive treatment model. *J Sub Abuse Treat* vol 31 no4 pp 385-393.

Kresina, T.F., Bruce, R.D., Lubran, R. & Clark, H.W. (2008) Integration of viral hepatitis services into opioid treatment programs. *J Opiod Manag* vol 4 no 6 pp 369-381.

Kresina, T.F., Litwin, A., Marion, I., Lubran, R. & Clark, H.W. (2009) Federal government oversight and regulation of medication assisted treatment for the treatment of opioid dependence. *J Drug Policy Anal* vol 2 no 1 pp 1-23.

Kresina, T.F., Maxwell, C., Parrino, M.W. & Lubran, R. (2005). Testing and Counseling for Hepatitis B, Hepatitis C, and HIV Infections in Opioid Treatment Programs (OTP's). Summary results from two surveys. Abstract presented at the *2005 CDC HCV Prevention Conference*. Washington, DC

Krupitsky, E., Zvartau, E. & Woody, G. (2010). Use of naltrexone to treat opioid addiction in a country in which methadone and buprenorphine are not available. *Curr Psychiatry Rep* vol 12 no 5 pp 448-453.

Krupitskya, E.M. & Blokhina, E.A. (2010) Long-acting depot formulations of naltrexone for heroin dependence: a review. *Curr Opin Psychiatry* vol 23 pp 210–214

Kunoe, N., Lobmaier, P., Vederhus, J.K., Hjerkinn, B., Hegstad, S., Gosso,p M, Kristensen, O. & Waal, H. (2010) Retention in naltrexone implant treatment for opioid dependance. Drug Alcohol Depend vol 111 no 1-2 pp 166-169

Langford, D., Adame, A., Grigorian, A., Grant, I., McCutchan, J.A., Ellis, R.J., Marcotte, T.D. & Masliah, E. (2003). HIV Neurobehavioral Research Center Group. Patterns of selective neuronal damage in methamphetamine-user AIDS patients. *J Acquir Immun Defic Syndr*. vol 34: no 5 pp 467-474

Ling, W. &. Smith, D. (2002) Buprenorphine: blending practice and research. *J Sub Abuse Treat*. vol 23 no 2 pp 87-92

Litwin, A.H., Soloway, I.& Gourevitch, M.N. (2005) Integrating services for injection drug users infected with hepatitis C virus with methadone maintenance treatment: challenges and opportunities. *Clin Infect Dis* vol 40: Suppl 5 pp S339-3345

Lloyd, J.J., Ricketts, E.P., Strathdee, S.A., Cornelius, L.J., Bishai, D., Heuttner, S., Havens, J.R. & Latkin, C. (2005) Social contextual factors associated with entry into opiate agonist treatment among injection drug users. *Am J DrugAlcohol Abuse* vol 31 no 4 pp 555-570.

Lucas, G.M., Chaudhry, A., Hsu, J., Woodso, T., Lau, B., Olse, Y., Keruly, J.C., Fiellin, D.A., Finkelstein, R., Barditch-Crovo, P., Cook, K.& Moore, R.D. (2010) Clinic-based treatment of opioid –dependent HIV-infected patients versus referral to an opioid treatment program: a randomized trial. *Ann Intern Med* vol 152 no 11 pp 704-711

Mason BJ. (2003). Acamprosate and naltrexone treatment for alcohol dependence: an evidence based risk -benefits assessment. *Eur Neuropsychopharm* vol 13 no 6 pp 469-475.

Millson, P., Challacombe, L., Villeneuve, P.J, Strike, C.J., Fischer, B., Myers, T., Shore, R.& Hopkins, S. (2006). Determinants of health-related quality of life of opiate users at entry to low-threshold methadone programs. *Eur Addict Res* vol 12 no 2 pp 74-82.

Minozzi, S., Amato, L., Vecchi, S., Davoli, M., Kirchmayer, U. & Verster, A. (2006) Oral naltrexone maintenance treatment for opioid dependence. *Cochrane Database of Systematic Reviews* CD001333DOI:101002/14651858.CD001333.pub2

Moore, B.A., Fiellin, D.A., Barry, D.T., Sullivan, L.E., Chawarski, M.C.,O'Connor, P.G.& Shottenfeld, R.S. (2007) Primary care office-based buprenorphine treatment: comparison of heroin and prescription opioid dependent patients. *J Gen Intern Med* vol 22 no 4 pp 527-530

Moreno, S., Mocroft, A., & Monforte, A. (2010) Medical and social consequences of late presentation. *Antivir Ther* vol 12 Suppl 1 pp9-15.

Neufeld, K., Kidorf, M., King, V., Stoller, K., Clark, M., Peirce, J., & Brooner, R.K. (2010) Using enhanced and integrated services to improve response to standard methadone treatment : changing the clinical infrastructure of treatment networks. *J Subst Abuse Treat* vol 38 no 3 pp170-177.

Newsome, SD., Johnson, E., Pardo, C., McArthur, JC., & Nath, A. (2011) Fulminent encephalopathy with basal ganglia hyperintensities in HIV-infected drug users. *Neurology* vol 76 no 9 pp787-794.

NIH (National Institutes of Health). (1997) Effective Medical Treatment of Opiate Addiction. *NIH Consensus Statement*. Bethesda, MD: National Institutes of Health. no 15 pp:1-38.

O'Connor, P.G., Carroll, K.M., Shi J.M., Schottenfeld, R.S,. Kosten, T.R.& Rounsaville B.J. (1997). Three methods of opioid detoxification in a primary care setting. A randomized trial. *Ann Intern Med* vol 127 no 7 pp526-530

Payte, J.T & Zweben, J.E. (1998) Opioid maintenance therapies. In: *Principles of Addiction Medicine*. 2nd ed. Chevy Chase, MD: American Society of Addiction Medicine, Inc publisher pp 557-570

Pollack, H.A. & D'Aunno, T. (2010) HIV testing and counseling in the nation's outpatient subtance absue treatment system, 1995-205. *J Subst Abuse Treat* vol 38 no 4 pp307-316.

Proeschold-bell, R.J., Heine, A., Pence, B.W., McAdam, K & Quinlivan, E.B. (2010) A cross-site, comparitive effectivenss study of an integreated Hiv and subtance use treatment program. *AIDS Patient Care STDS* vol 24 no 10 pp 651-658.

SAMHSA (Substance Abuse and Mental Health Services Administation) (2005). Medication Assisted Treatment for Opioid Addiction in Opioid Treatment Programs. *A Treatment Improvement Protocol, TIP 43* Department of Health and Human Services Publication (SMA)-05-4048.

SAMHSA (Substance Abuse and Mental Health Services Administation) (2009).Incorporating Alcohol Pharmacotherapies into Medical Practice. *A Treatment Improvement Protocol, TIP 43* Department of Health and Human Services Publication (SMA)-09-4380.

Schackman, B.R., Merrill, J.O., McCarty, D., Lev,i J.& Lubinsk,i C. (2006) Overcoming policy and financing barriers to integrated buprenorphine and HIV primary care. *Clin Infect Dis* vol 43 Suppl 4 pp S247-253

Schuckit, M.A. (2006) Comorbidity between substance use disorders and psychiatric conditions. *Addiction* vol 101: suppl 1 pp 76-88.

Schuh, K.J., Walsh, S.L., Bigelow, G.E., Preston, K.L. & Stitzer, M.L. (1996) Buprenorphine, morphine and naloxone effects during ascending morphine maintenance in humans. *J Pharm Exp Therap.* vol 278 no 2 pp 836-846.

Sinner, M.L., Haggarty, K.P., Fleming, C.B., Catalano, R.F. & Gainey, R.R. (2011) Opiate-addicted parents in methadone treatment: long term recovery, health and family relationship. *J Addict Dis* vol 30 no 1 pp 17-26.

Sowers W. (2005) Transforming systems of care: The American Association of Community Psychiatrists guidelines for recovery oriented services. *Community Mental Health J* vol 41 no 6 pp 757-774

Sullivan, L.E., Bruce, R.D., Haltiwanger, D., Lucas, G.M., Eldred, L., Finkelstein, R. & Fiellin, D.A..(2006) Initial strategies for integrating buprenorphine into HIV care settings in the United States. *Clin Infect Dis* vol 43 Suppl 4 pp S191-196

Taege,A. (2011) Seek and treat : HIV update 2011. *Cleve Clin J Med* vol 78 no 2 pp 95-100.

UNODC (2010). Executive Summary. *The World Drug report 2010.* United Nations Office on Drugs and Crime Publishers. ISBN 97-92-1-148256-0 Geneva. pp15-20.

Walsh, S.L., Preston, K.L., Stitzer, M.L., Cone, E.J. & Bigelow, G.E (1994). Clinical pharmacology of buprenorphine: ceiling effects at high doses. *Clin Pharm Therap.* vol 55 no 5 pp 569-580.

Weiss, L. Netherland, J., Egan, J.E., Flanigan, T.P., Finkelstein, R., Altice, F.L., & BHIVES Collaborative (2011). Integreationof buprenorphine/naloxone treatment into HIV clinical care: lessons from the BHIVES collaborative *J Acquir Immune Defic Syndr* vol 56 suppl 1 pp S68-75.

White W.L.& Mojer-Torres L (2010). *Recovery-oriented Methadone Maintenance.* Published by the Great Lakes Addiction Technology Transfer Center, the Philadelphia Department of Behavioral Health and Mental Retardation Services, and the NortheastAddiction Technology Transfer Center 2010. Retrieved from: http://www.ireta.org/resources/romm-exsum.pdf

WHO (World Health Organization) (2004). Alcohol consumption and beverage preferences. *Global Status Report on Alcohol 2004.* Department of Mental Health and Substance Abuse. World Health Organization Publishers. ISBN 92 4 156272 2 Geneva pp9-15.

WHO (World Health Organization) (2008). *Guidelines for the Psychosocially assisted pharmacological treatment of opioid dependence.* World Health Organization, WHO Press ISBN 978 92 4 154754 3 0 Geneva, Switzerland

WHO (World Health Organization) (2009). *Scaling up care for mental, neurological and substance use disorders.* mhGAP Mental Health Gap Action Programme. World Health Organization, WHO Press ISBN 978 92 4 159620 6 Geneva, Switzerland

WHO (World Health Organization) (2009a). *WHO,UNODC, UNAIDS Technical guide for countries to set targets for universal access to HIV prevention, treatment and care for injection drug users.* World Health Organization, WHO Press ISBN 978 92 4 159776 0 Geneva, Switzerland

WHO (World Health Organization) (2010). *Global strategy to reduce the harmfull use of alcohol.* WHO Press. ISBN 978 92 4 159993 1. Geneva, Switzerland

Yokell, M.A., Zaller, N.D., Green, T.C. & Rich, J.D. (2011) Buprenorphine and buprenorphine/naloxone diversion, misue and illicit use: An international review. *Curr Drug Abuse Rev* April 5 [Epub ahead of print]

Zaller, N., Gillani, F.S.& Rich, J.D.(2007) A model of integrated primary care for HIV-positve patients with underlying substance use and metal illness. *AIDS Care* vol 19 no 9 pp 1128-1133.

The Pertinence of Applying Qualitative Investigation Strategies in the Design and Evaluation of HIV Prevention Policies

Carmen Rodríguez, Teresa Blasco, Antonio Vargas and Agustín Benito
National Centre for Tropical Medicine, Health Institute Carlos III
Spain

1. Introduction

"We think that there still exists a vast sector of science in which we are no further than in taylorian stages of intellectual work rationalization and which can do nothing but contribute to scientific rigor. Rigor when reasoning is more important that rigor when calculating. Questions is more important than rigor than questionnaires."
Edgar Morin [1]

In the last decade, the incidence of HIV has globally diminished by 19% (Joint United Nations Programme on HIV/Aids, [Unaids], 2010). Likewise, new cases of children infected by HIV have diminished due to the spread of vertical mother-child prevention among pregnant women. The percentage of people who received anti-retroviral treatment increased by 30% due to improvements in the accessibility of therapeutic treatment. Also, the annual percentage of death caused by Aids has decreased (Unaids, 2010). Nevertheless, in spite of this progress, HIV/Aids pandemic continues to be one of the main threats to global health.

On a world scale, pandemic epidemiological data shows alarming numbers: there are more than 33 million people around the world living with HIV. Approximately, 7,000 new cases of infection arise every day. Every year, an average of 1,800,000 people die as a consequence of Aids. It is estimated that 12 million children have been orphaned (Unaids, 2010).

However, such numbers are distributed in unequal proportions throughout the world. Thus, since not every country presents the same level of prevalence, big differences can be found. Currently, most of the countries suffering from HIV pandemic are developing countries. Also, these countries show low or medium levels of human development. The Table 1 shows the relation between Human Development Index in some countries with a higher pandemic level.

As seen on table 1, the distribution of the pandemic tendency throughout these countries reveals a clear correlation: The less socio-economically developed a country is, the higher the HIV prevalence is. This being so, it is hardly surprising that sub-Saharan African or Asian countries present widespread epidemic HIV levels. On a world scale, these countries hold the highest Multidimensional Poverty Index (United Nations Development Programme, [Unpd], 2010). For instance, the worst Human Development Index in the world belongs to

[1] Morin, Eder. (2006). *The method* (ed. Cátedra).

Countries	2009 HIV estimates in Adults and children	HDI 2010
Nigeria	3,300,000	0.432
India	2,400,0000	0.59
United Republic Of Tanzania	140,000	0.398
Zimbawe	120,000	0.140
Uganda	120,000	0.422
Malawi	920,000	0.385
Zambia	98,000	0.395

Table 1. Relation between HIV and HDI prevalence
Self-made

belongs to Zimbabwe (0.291) and, at the same time, the highest levels of HIV prevalence can be found there - around 20% and 25%-, (UNPD, 2010). With the one before, in countries like Sweden, where the Human Development Index is very high, (0.773) such prevalence varies between 1% and 5% (UNPD, 2010).

Therefore, the highest number of cases are to be found in lesser developed countries, bearing almost 90% of the whole HIV prevalence worldwide. In these countries, the HIV epidemic is one of the largest National Health problems faced by their Governments. As a consequence, strategic plans of prevention, together with the provision of welfare coverage in the treatment of HIV, are given top priority by the National policies. Nonetheless, HIV epidemic does not only mean a challenge at political level, it also entails a menace to entails a menace to democracy and governability in these countries' political systems. Regarding this last statement, the South African Institute for Democracy has published a report highlighting the negative effect of HIV/Aids in the electoral processes of these countries.

HIV epidemic in these countries does not only mean a medical and sanitary problem, it also constitutes one of the main obstacles for their socio-economic development. Given the huge percentage of adults who die as a consequence of Aids, these countries lose their young people, those who could help with their economic development to a higher degree. In addition, economic productivity also decreases due to the fact that the number of people infected by Aids or those who take care of them must quit their jobs. Besides, their educational systems are affected due to the percentage of teachers who die as a consequence of Aids. This situation brings about an important loss of highly educated inhabitants. Likewise, medical expenses generated out of the provision of health services to people who live with HIV (PLHIV) and Aids, involve budgetary restrictions in the investment of public expenses in other sectors, with the aim of promoting the economic and social development of these countries. In connection with this, the UNPD estimates that in Bostwana the State Revenue dropped by 20% in 2010 as a direct result of HIV/Aids (PNUD, 2010).

Regarding families, the consequences of this epidemic in the domestic economy of these countries are also devastating. When they lose the "head of the family" -the one who has to meet the economic needs of the family- they lose their income, their nutrition worsens, agricultural production falls, medical expenses increase, savings turn into debts, funeral expenses multiply, children leave schools, people's health deteriorates, and so on. In fact, a survey carried out in Zambia shows that two thirds of urban homes which have lost the head of the family as a consequence of Aids have seen their income drop by 80%. The same survey revealed that 61% of these families moved to cheaper places to live, 39% lost their access to drinking water and also 21% of girls and 17% of boys gave up their school studies (PUND, 2001).

Finally, the spread of the epidemic in these countries is increasing, deepening existing poverty and social inequality, and reversing the trend towards their level of human development. Hence, HIV/Aids epidemic has become one of the main key aspects in national policies of Poverty Reduction Strategies (PRS) (PNUD, 2002) Such strategies are becoming the main national planning instrument in many countries. That is why HIV/Aids plays a central role in the processes of national development planning and in the budgetary allocation of these States. This contributes to the creation of adequate policies and providing the necessary resources, in order to give a wide multisectorial response to the HIV problem.

Generally, a higher prevalence of the pandemic in countries with low human development index increases social injustice and emphasizes the north-south divide. So that the fight against HIV/Aids together with the fight poverty has become two parts of the same parts of the same battle. Therefore, regarding poverty in certain countries, there will be no possibility to achieve the Millenium Development Goals (MDGs) unless HIV/Aids is efficiently treated. That is why the fight against HIV/Aids has been chosen as the sixth MDG (United Nations, [Nu], 2000).

2. The importance of prevention in the response to the epidemic

After three decades fighting against the epidemic, in the field of public health there is no doubt that the intervention from prevention policies is the most efficient weapon in order to eliminate and combat the epidemic (World Health Organization, [Who], 2010). In this sense, competent international organizations struggle more and more to make governments and other institutions aware of the importance of implementing efficient actions in order to prevent HIV. So, the last UNAIDS world report has included measurement indexes for different aspects of prevention processes carried out in different countries as evaluative indicators of the current state of the epidemic (Unaids, 2010).

All over the world, the high number of new cases of HIV in 2010 corroborate the pressing need for intervention in order to stop the development of the epidemic. There again, a higher incidence of HIV cases in developing countries has established prevention as a priority in the national policies of these countries. In connection with this, it is worth knowing that 97% of the new infections produced every day are to be found in people who live in countries with medium or low human development index (Unaids, 2010). Specifically, it is in the African context where the cases of incidence occur more frequently.

As for the development of HIV prevention policies, experience reveals that there are no universal formulae for success that might be applied to all countries. Therefore, certain strategies of prevention proved to be successful in a given country may not constitute any guarantee in another, due to the multiple factors that interfere in the development of the different policies. For instance, each context presents a set of specific needs which must be taken into account for the design and implementation of such policies. Among other things, exclusive qualities of the social and cultural elements also play a part when defining the context in which the intervention is going to take place. That is why it is advised to take into account all of these aspects and adapt the design of HIV prevention policies to the context in which they will be implemented.

Currently, there is a big concern about how to adapt prevention policies to African countries. On the one hand, it is due to the urgent need to change the development of the epidemic considering its magnitude and, on the other hand, to the ineffectiveness shown by prevention policies to date, considering the high rates of incidence. As a consequence, the epidemic stabilization has not yet been reached in some countries.

2.1 Prevention policies in the African context

HIV prevention actions developed in Africa are key to slow down the great development of this disease. Besides, prevention actions have an added value since either they must be linked to or they must incorporate values, such as justice, fairness and the promotion of dignity. At the same time, it constitutes basic principles which help to improve the African context.

Now, some of the international recommendations on public health as well as some of the existing evidence on HIV prevention in the African context to date are described.

Prevention actions must be aware of the main HIV routes of transmission in the continent. In Africa, the HIV epidemic spreads mainly through sexual intercourse. The percentage of people who became infected by this disease through routes other than the sexual intercourse is low. Nevertheless, mother-to-child transmission and hemoderivatives transfusion are the other two relevant aspects when assessing prevention measures in countries where, like in the African context, the investment in public health is not enough.

It is advisable to develop HIV prevention policies that interact with the different levels of prevention. According to the World Organization of Family Doctors (Wonca), there are four grades of prevention. Primary prevention is the one that involves action before the disease appears and, among these actions are the ones in charge of promoting health, those focused on environmental hygiene or those like vaccination or chemical prophylaxis. Secondary prevention deals with actions aimed at identifying ill patients within the population, implementing strategies of population sifting, enabling the early detection of diseases. Through implemented actions, tertiary prevention involves easing or avoiding the effects of the disease once it has been contracted. Finally, in 1986 Marc Jamoulle defined quaternary prevention as *"those actions designed to restrict unnecessary damage produced as a consequence of health-care activity"*.

Within the current priority of international recommendations on health-HIV, five guidelines for intervention have been developed. These guidelines are especially relevant in countries with higher prevalence, as in most of the African countries (Who, 2009). They mainly include preventive actions in the three first levels:

1. Strengthening actions in primary prevention of the disease from the health sector.
2. Making it possible for the population to know its serological status.
3. Accelerating the spread of the treatment as well as the HIV/Aids care.
4. Strengthening health systems capacities.
5. Increasing knowledge in order to improve response.

In general, as a maxim of intervention in public health, the development of HIV-related actions, including all actions and not only preventive ones, should be adapted to each and every context in three determining factors. Firstly, they should adapt to the specific characteristics of the epidemic in question, like the particular context of each country as well as that of its community. Secondly, they should pay attention to the cultural context and, thirdly, to the level of provision of services and resources set aside for health. Related to this last aspect and in order to strengthen the adaptation of international frameworks at local level, actions developed to prevent HIV are considered to be complex interventions as regards their evaluation processes (Campbell et al., 2000). In order to do so, it is advisable to take into account the adaptation of the process to the local circumstances before being implemented once it has been completely standardized. Therefore, for an optimal implementation, it is currently considered as necessary to have the adequate knowledge to orientate this process of adaptability of the standard theoretical framework.

In the African context, a low specific applicability of these criteria can be found. That is why a low level of key targets for prevention has been achieved. It is worth mentioning that only 32% of the African population knows their serological status. Likewise, only 45% of pregnant women receive proper care in order to prevent their children from contracting the disease. (Who, 2010).

As regards the type of epidemic, actions carried out in the African context must have plenty of characteristics unique to the generalized epidemic. This is the most common epidemiological situation in most countries of the continent. The fact of presenting generalized epidemic levels determines the monitoring of intervention priorities within the prevention area:

- Using strategies that would cover all risk behaviour of contracting the disease. Besides, these strategies must be as accessible as possible to the population in need of help.
- Decentralizing the provision of services by incorporating primary care actions as well as community actions.
- Integrating prevention services together with treatment and care services into primary care services.
- Giving priority to actions aimed at tertiary prevention making it possible to interrupt the epidemiological chain of the disease, diminishing the appearance of new cases.
- Recommending the diagnostic sifting of every person who makes use of health care services and to all pregnant women or those in a lactation period.

The existence of a whole multiplicity of cultural components characteristic of every area and unique to every social group is something that, for the time being, has not been sufficiently reflected in the adaptation of the general frameworks to each context. The recommendation that second generation epidemiological vigilance (Grulich & Kaldor, 2002) (Who, 2000) should be integrated into the tracking and monitoring processes of the disease makes it possible to count on a broader knowledge of people's attitudes and practices. Moreover, adaptation to strategies has improved. The use of qualitative methodologies in order to generate this knowledge is still very recent and, in some contexts, almost nonexistent. This is shown as a tool that supplies key elements, having a deeper impact on health when adapting actions to contexts.

Weakness in health systems which implement actions and policies is a very common factor all around Africa. Such weakness does not always derive from the low budget allocated to its development. In the last years, poor systems and limited resources, together with important obstacles that eliminate the possibility to improve these systems, demand the need to search for evidence-based knowledge in order to determine which actions are the most cost-effective in HIV. This knowledge would help to establish criteria that could improve the management of the intervention.

Out of all this generated knowledge, taking into account the target context of the chapter as well as efficiency criteria previously mentioned, we wanted to pay special attention to the value of implementing associated measures of secondary and tertiary prevention, like diagnosis and treatment, respectively.

The initial intervention model in the fight against HIV implemented only tertiary prevention measures, in spite of its low efficiency when trying to reduce the progression of the disease.

The target was to reduce the high rate of mortality caused by this disease at that time. Nowadays, the antiretroviral treatment has evolved and it is considered to be highly active (HAART). Cohort studies in serodiscordant couples and pregnant women living with HIV have proved that patients who receive good treatment and have an undetectable viral load are less likely to transmit the disease (Quinn et al., 2000). This ART has proved to be a very good method to reduce the transmission of this disease and that is the reason why, currently, on a global scale, all countries are advised to reach universal coverage (Granich et al, 2009) of the treatment. The reason is not only that the rate of mortality decreases but also its effect on the transmission chain.

There is a great variability when it comes to value the cost-effectiveness of HIV strategies depending, above all, on the country where the action is implemented (Andrew, 2002). Following this criteria, actions of prevention that cause a deeper impact and those enjoying a better cost-effectiveness criteria are meant to limit mother-to-child transmission of the disease.

Regarding the diagnosis of the disease in the population, the HIV strategies meet the requirements defined by Frame and Carslon (Frame & Carslon, 1975) in order to be able to carry out actions of secondary prevention and, therefore, make quite an impact both on the health of the patient and on the health of the whole population. The necessary criteria for this applicability are the following:

1. The disease must be an important health problem, having a clear effect on the quality of life and life expectancy.
2. The disease must develop through an asymptomatic initial stage and its natural history must be known.
3. There must be an effective treatment accepted by the population in the case that the disease is detected in its initial state.
4. There must be a sifting test which has to be quick, safe, easy-to-do, highly sensitive, highly specific, of high positive predictive value and well accepted by doctors and patients.
5. The sifting test must keep a good cost-effectiveness balance.
6. The early detection of the disease and its treatment during the asymptomatic period must diminish morbidity as well as global or each of them separately.

In the last years, the scientific community issued an appeal for the innovation of developed prevention strategies (Piot,2008). Current recommendations in order to cause a greater impact on health in the African context suggest that actions of secondary prevention, such as diagnosis, and actions of tertiary prevention, such as ARV treatment, are joined (Dood, 2010). It is important to bear in mind that without diagnosis there is no treatment and, as seen before, preventing this disease from being transmitted becomes a limited task.

3. Application of qualitative methodologies in HIV prevention

"Aids has proved that epidemics take place at different levels: biological event, social perception, collective response and individual phenomenon, both existential and moral [...].Each disease, as social phenomenon, is a unique configuration of events and responses both in the biological sphere and in the social sphere"(Mariano Bronfman[2]).

In the scientific field, HIV epidemic has traditionally been investigated by clinical epidemiology. For this reason, the predominant theoretical development has been the

[2] Mariano Bronfman: Social Sciences and Aids. Magazine of Public Health and Mexico 1999;Vol.41(2):83-84.

biomedical model. Concerning this subject, most of the investigations to be found on scientific literature are prevalence and/or ecological studies. In this sense and in general terms, knowledge based on data that mainly describe the way this epidemic is distributed throughout the population according to certain factors predominate (Caitlin et al., 2010).

However, the relevance and significance that HIV epidemic has gained in the social sphere nowadays constitute evidence. This fact can be clearly seen, for instance, when paying attention to the social stigma generated around HIV (Skinner & Mfecane, 2004). That is why most of the interventions being carried out in the field of HIV take into account the social dimension of the problem. In this sense, epidemic research beyond simple observation of how it is distributed throughout a given population is required.

Currently, the HIV epidemic represents a social phenomenon that mainly affects the area of public health. The HIV epidemic as a social phenomenon acquires different meanings depending on the kind of society in which it is found, since cultural and social contexts play an important role in all countries. For example, although HIV is seen as a cronical disease in the collective unconscious of most developed countries, this virus is considered to be fatal and lethal in the developing countries (Conde, 1997). There again, as HIV is meddled in social constructs like life, health, dead and disease, it is also steeped in specific connotations that every culture attributes to these social values.

So that HIV acquires meanings, representations, perceptions, values and erelated to social and cultural contexts. Such contexts give meaning and guide people's behaviour and actions to confront HIV. These distinctive values, meanings and so forth, will have an effect on preventive actions that are being taken in order to face the HIV phenomenon. As can be seen, qualitative aspects that are also important to know in order to prevent and eliminate the epidemic mark the HIV phenomenon.

By applying the methodologies which have developed the traditional approaches to HIV study, the knowledge of HIV qualitative aspects is difficult to achieve. Nowadays, with the aim of setting out a deeper and more holistic HIV knowledge, other perspectives and theoretic approaches belonging to disciplines other than health are applied. For instance, approaches to the epidemic phenomenon have been carried out by different sciences -like hermeneutics, phenomenology or ethnography- in which their theoretical frameworks from disciplines like Anthropology or Sociology (Arachu & Pau, 2003). The efforts made by UNESCO in order to develop and promote a cultural approach to the HIV epidemic are especially worthy of notice (United Nations Educational, Scientific and Cultural Organozation, [Unicef], 2003).

Theoretical approaches in the field of social sciences have incorporated HIV study methodologies different from the quantitative, which is traditionally applied by clinic epidemiology. Among these methodologies, the use of qualitative methodology prevails. Therefore, qualitative methodology is no longer a method exclusively used in disciplines connected to the social sphere. In this sense, it appears more and more frequently in health related studies, whose scientific expansion displays as much on publications and seminars as on medicine and public health related conferences.

On an international level, different authors have placed particular emphasis on the necessity and in the advantages of using this methodology in the field of public health (Bryman, 1984). Also, its relevance to social epidemiology has been highlighted. For instance, it has been pointed out its importance when used in order to evaluate peoples' health care from a more dynamic and comprehensive perspective. It has also been stated the necessity to know both the adaptation of qualitative methodology for its study and the socio-cultural background together with people's values as health determining factors.

As compared to other diseases or to other health related subjects, qualitative methodology has been widely used in the study of the HIV. However, qualitative investigations performed in this field are still few. But there are still fewer qualitative research aimed at putting into practice the necessary knowledge in order to evaluate and design HIV prevention policies.

Nevertheless, the results of the studies carried out show the adaptation and benefits of this methodology to the understanding and comprehension of the different factors that intervene in the HIV epidemic phenomenon. So that the adaptation of qualitative strategies to the study of the HIV phenomenon constitutes a potential instrument of support to design effective preventive strategies and, therefore, carry out effective and efficient policies in the intervention of this epidemic.

4. Application of a case: Equatorial Guinea

4.1 Epidemiological context

The HIV/Aids epidemic is also severely affecting Guinean people's health. On the basis of parameters established by the WHO, Equatorial Guinea suffers from generalized epidemic (Unaids, 2010 b). The HIV prevalence among people between 15 and 49 years of age is 3.2% (IC 95% 2.0 -4.4%). Likewise, Aids represents the main cause of individual mortality (Who, 2008).

In a context of generalized epidemic, competent international organizations warn of the urgent need for these countries to set appropriate measures in motion in order to reverse the epidemic curve. They also emphasize the importance of carrying out prevention policies with the aim of diminishing and eliminating the magnitude of the epidemic. At the same time, they urge the governments of these countries to establish and coordinate effective strategic plans for the prevention of the HIV. In this regard, one of the preventive measures recommended by the WHO is to spread the HIV diagnosis tests throughout the whole population, regardless whether there is clinical suspicion or not, and suggests having the test done at least once a year (Who, 2007) given the positive results that this action would carry with it in both individual level and community level. On an individual level: it initiates and holds preventive behaviour towards the HIV acquisition and transmission, immediate access to care, treatment and support of people living with HIV, major efficacy on interventions in order to prevent mother-to-child transmission, better planning to improve the future life. On community level: it diminishes denial, stigma and discrimination associated to the HIV and demands aid for an adequate answer. However, evidence suggests that, in terms of cost-effectiveness, everyone having the test done becomes profitable on the long term, regardless whether they take part in high risk behaviour or not. (Patiel, 2005).

As for HIV preventive measures carried out by the Guinean population, there is almost no information that describes and explains this aspect due to the lack of research in this field of study. Nevertheless, there is some data extracted from a transversal study conducted by ISCIII in collaboration with MINSABS. In this study, people aged between 15 and 50 were given a questionnaire - the CAP survey[3] - about different aspects concerning sexual life and

[3] "Knowledge, attitudes and practices about nuptiality, sexual activity, HIV/Aids and STD"

HIV/Aids. Results related to the execution of HIV diagnosis show that almost ¾ of the people who participated in the survey had never had the tests done (Ministry of Health and Social Welfare of Malabo, 2006). The fact that an important percentage of the population is not aware of their serological status aggravates the magnitude of the epidemic due to the existing risk of exponential growth, as a consequence of HIV transmission through people unaware of their seropositive status. Likewise, this study also stresses the vulnerability of this society towards the epidemic, since evidence shows that being aware of one's serological status is the first step to be taken in order to prevent and treat the disease.

Regarding the use of male condoms among the Guinean population, the CAP survey produced alarming results. Sexual intercourse is the main HIV transmission route in Equatorial Guinea. That is why, in this country, different social agents competent in HIV prevention have made tremendous efforts to extend and promote the use of male condoms when having sex in order to control this transmission route. In spite of the efforts made, the results of the CAP survey show that the use of the male condom has not been one of the prevention methods used by a vast majority of the Guinean population. Although 73% of those polled point out that they do know how to use male condoms as an HIV preventive measure, almost seven out of ten declared that they had not used them in the last twelve months when having occasional sex with different partners. The male condom was not used by 73% of those men who had sex with prostitutes either.

Generally, CAP results reveal that the Guinean population has taken few measures regarding HIV prevention.

4.2 Justification for the study

No sociological investigation considering HIV as a social phenomenon had been previously carried out in Equatorial Guinea. That is why there was no holistic or hermeneutic knowledge about the epidemic phenomenon in the country.

Until the completion of the ESEVIGUE study, there was no qualitative data about the epidemic. In this sense, the qualitative aspects of the epidemic constitute key elements to take into account when designing HIV prevention policies. For instance, there was no information about the meaning or possible meanings that the epidemic had acquired in society. Moreover, there was no information about the elements -whatever their nature: cultural, social, political, economic…-that could be interfering with the results of the implemented prevention strategies, acting like barriers and/or facilitators. In general, explanatory information about people's practices and behaviours related to the implemented prevention strategies was non-existent.

Given the absence of these data, the possibility to carry out an investigation in order to announce this situation arises. In the last analysis, the reasons why the preventive measures developed in the country got such results will be evaluated and explained. In this context, the ESEVIGUE comes into being with the general aim of: "understanding and generating knowledge about the epidemic phenomenon in Equatorial Guinea".

This study targeted the use of generated knowledge as support in order to direct the decision taking process, regarding the different strategies and measures to be implemented in the area of HIV prevention.

This research started in Bata in August 2009 and has been led jointly by MINSABBS, in Malabo, and the National Centre for Tropical Medicine of the Carlos III Health Institute, (Referential Centre for the Control of Endemic Diseases [CRCE], 2009) in Spain. This investigation has been carried out by a research team made up of professionals belonging to both institutions.

4.3 The basis of the methodological design

Although epidemiological methods have been traditionally regarded as the standard reference for the study of public health, these methodologies are based on a reductionist view of the world in which simple causality standards are established through statistical processes (Baum, 1997). Health and disease are the result of a complex interrelation of social, economical, political and environmental factors. Interpretative methods based on qualitative techniques are generally well prepared for the analysis of complex situations and contribute to a large extent to the study of public health (Baum, 1997).

The aim of the research was to observe the epidemic as a social phenomenon so that, considering biological investigative or medical approaches, a social perspective of the HIV study was adopted. The design of the investigation has been a qualitative one. The decision of carrying out a qualitative methological design was backed up by the adaptation that qualitative strategies have shown in order to generate holistic, deep and comprehensive knowledge of the real situation under study. Nowadays, in the area of public health, the effective use of qualitative techniques for the understanding and comprehension of factors and processes affecting health and disease is also sufficiently verified. To be more specific, many examples of qualitative methodology applied to the study of the HIV and its context can be found in scientific literature (Medicus Mundi, 2007). In this respect, it is worth mentioning that, confronting epidemiological and quantitative HIV medical study, this type of investigations have proliferated over the last decades.

The sample used in the investigation was a structural one. As in quantitative investigations, the sample design consitutes one of the first methodological aspects to be defined. However, its theoretical basis differs from the sample design in quantitative research. Whereas sample design in quantitative research is based on the concept of statistic representation, in qualitative research it is based on the social signification criteria of the individuals (Valles, 1997). In this sense, sample validity is not given by the number of individuals that make up the sample but by the pertinence of selected individuals in connection with the aims of the study.

Regarding the object of the study, a first general criterion of sample inclusion was established: Individuals aged between 13 and 60. Defining this section of age span became relevant due to the fact that the main HIV route of transmission is sexual intercourse. Therefore, in view of prevention, getting to know the meaning of the HIV epidemic phenomenon and other related aspects within the sexually active population in Guinea was considered to be pertinent.

In the second place, the sample was segmented according to certain variables of interest: being infected by HIV or not, sex, age, education level and place of residence. This segmentation was aimed at identifying and gathering different perceptions and experiences of the HIV. For instance, the initial hypothesis was that, in general terms, there would be differences between PLWHIV and those who do not, as regards perceptions, meanings and practices. Likewise, it was also considered to be pertinent to pay attention to the thoughts of different social groups so as to know the various conceptions of HIV that there may be throughout the whole variety of social groups that form the Guinean society. The objective was to adequate prevention strategies to the specific needs of each social group. For the purpose of this research, the sex and the gender of the individuals, their education level, etc. was taken into account.

Information gathering techniques applied in order to produce and collect information were: semi-structured individual interview and discussion group. These techniques are generically named qualitative techniques. In order to develop both techniques, the script item was outlined. The script item is a gathering information tool that contains qualitative techniques. This script item was drawn up through open questions that explored analytical dimensions related to the object of study. Now, in table 2, some of the analytical dimensions are shown:

ANALYTICAL DIMENSION	CATEGORIES AND QUESTIONS
Health meaning and value	What are the important things in your life? What does health mean to you?
Social Perception of the HIV	What do you think about the HIV? What do people say about the HIV?
Knowledge about the HIV	What is the HIV? Are the HIV and Aids the same disease? How can a person become infected by the HIV?

Table 2. Analytical Dimensions of the ESEVIGUE research

Before the fieldwork was performed, the script item was tested following preliminary interviews. The aim of testing this instrument was to check the validity of its technical design as regards the content of the questions, the format and the language.

4.3.1 The reasons why semi-structured interviews are applied

Semi-structured interviews were done to people living with the HIV. The application of this technique, in opposition to other group qualitative techniques like discussion groups, has the advantage of preserving anonymity and confidentiality about the serological status of the interviewee.

Semi-structured interview is performed on the basis of a face-to-face conversation between the interviewer and the interviewee. That involves immediate and personal norms of verbal interaction generating, therefore, a subjective knowledge of the observed reality (Alonso, 1994). The interview is a communicative tool that sets out to grasp meanings that are influenced by the constructions made by the individuals themselves according to their experience:

> *"Personal interview results very productive to the study of extreme or typical cases in which the attitudes of certain people embody, in every sense, the ideal model of a certain attitude much less crystallized in the average of the group of reference (Ortí, 1986)".*

So that this technique was carried out with the aim of getting to know the experiences and meanings felt by people living with the HIV. Therefore, its application in the ESEVIGUE resulted in the knowledge of the subjective aspect of suffering HIV. Also, this technique provided information about the phenomenon of the epidemic from the point of view of the people living with the HIV.

4.3.2 The reason why the discussion group is applied to the study

The discussion group was performed among the population segment of participants who did not know if they were seropositive and/or those whose blood tests results were negative. Since it is a group technique, it has the advantage of confronting and gathering discourse from the different social groups in one session. At the same time, in economical terms, this technique becomes more profitable

The different points of view of the studied reality regarding the position occupied by the individual in the social framework can be known through the application of discussion groups (ref.). This used to be a key aspect of the technical selection since it allowed the gathering of different HIV related discourses in order to produce and adapt prevention strategies to the specificities of each social group. Therefore, the application of such technique created diverse knowledge about the different social aspects regarding the HIV.

4.3.3 Fieldwork

Finally, fieldwork based on qualitative methodological strategies was done with the aim of generating knowledge about the HIV phenomenon. Prior to the phase of gathering information, the research team applied the non-participant observation technique. It was aimed at validating different aspects of the study protocol such as sample design or instruments to collect information. It was also aimed at later development of fieldwork.

Geographically, this research took place in Bata between January and April 2010 and it was carried out by a multidisciplinary working group made up of sociologists, doctors, nurses and lab assistants.

5. Conclusions

In terms of results achieved, the application of qualitative methodology has turned out to be very adequate and valid in order to generate holistic and comprehensive information of the HIV epidemic phenomenon in Equatorial Guiena. So that data has been generated in order to allow both evaluating some of the prevention strategies in the country and showing some of the key aspects to take into account in decision-making processes in the strategy to be implemented.

For instance, results show the inadequacy of massive HIV/Aids information and prevention campaigns carried out in Equatorial Guinea. The association established between the HIV, Aids and death has caused much alarm and fear among the population. Nowadays, it constitutes one of the main barriers for the population to have diagnostic tests done of their own free will. The conducted campaigns played a decisive role in the HIV social construction, which does not favour the integration of people living with Aids into society. Such social construction about people living with the HIV having abandoned the services of the HIV treatment and diagnosis, influenced the reasons given in order to explain why they decided to give up their treatment.

Results have also revealed the importance and necessity of implementing and carrying out prevention strategies considering already existing specificities and needs among different social groups. In this sense, interviewed women's and men's different ways of understanding health and facing the disease are shown. These aspects must be taken into account when designing prevention strategies in order to achieve maximal efficiency and effectiveness in results.

Nevertheless, the development of the methodology has not been exempt from difficulties and inconveniences. The first drawback was brought about by the application of this type of methodology in a context of low involvement of the population in social movements and slender culture of social discussion forums. In spite of counting on the collaboration and participation of MINSABS, occasionally people did not want to participate in group sessions for fear of attending politically oriented meetings. Likewise, this fear was also revealed through some of the participants' concerns regarding the confidentiality of the provided information related to personal assessment and opinions about the country.

Difficulties were also revealed due to the lack of tradition in qualitative research in the country. That is why human resources educated and/or qualified in this methodology can scarcely be found. As a consequence, identifying and integrating Guinean personnel into the research team was quite difficult.

To sum up, the HIV epidemic is a complex social phenomenon in the Guinean society. In this sense, the HIV epidemic phenomenon has acquired particular connotations that require specific interventions in this field. Moreover, it also reveals that working frameworks and multidisciplinary action is required in order to prevent and treat the epidemic.

6. Acknowledgment

To the people who took part in interviews and discussion groups, for sharing their time and HIV experiences with the research team. To Jesús Nzang for the generosity that he showed during the development of fieldwork. His dedication and collaboration made it possible to overcome the problems found during the data collection. To Catalina Mangue, Gaspar Nkoni and Luis Mbonio from the CRCE in Equatorial Guinea, for the support they gave me during the recruitment of participants. To Doctor Nemesio Abeso, Director of the MINSABS National Plan of Fight against Aids in Malabo, and Pilar Aparicio, for his support and confidence in the study for his support and confidence in the study. To Jose Luís Cenal, Leticia Díaz and Alberto Hedo from the Foundation for International Health and Cooperation of the National Health System of Spain, for his assistance in the logistic management of the project. And To the Spanish Agency for International Development Cooperation, for financing the study. The study was co-funded by the Instituto de Salud Carlos III, Spanish Research Network of Tropical Diseases (RICET;RD06/0021/0000), Ministry of Science and Innovation of Spain.

It has been possible to write these pages thanks to the contributions made by all these people and institutions.

7. References

Alonso, LE. (1994). Subject and Discourse: The place of the open interview in the practices of qualitative sociology. In: *The Qualitative look on sociology,* Síntesís, pp. 144-53, Madrid

Arachu & Pau. (2003). Aids and structural violence: The blaming of the victim. *Notebooks on Social Anthropology,* Vol.14, pp.29-47

Baum, F. (1997). Public health research: The debate about qualitative and quantitative methodologies. *Public health reviews,* Vol.5, pp.175-193

Bryman, A. (1984). The debate about quantitative and qualitative research: a question of method or epistemology?. *Br J Sociol,* Vol 35, pp. 33- 77

Caitlin, E.; Amy, K.; Medly, M.; Sweat, M. & Reilly, K. (2010). Behavioural Interventions for the prevention of HIV in developed countries: systematic revision and meta-analysis. *WHO bulletin,* Vol. 88, pp. 561-640

Campbell, M. ; Fitzpatrick, R. ; Haines, A.; Kinmonth, A. ; Sandecork, P. ; Spiegelhalter, D.; & Tyrer, P. (2000). Framework for the design and evaluation of complex interventions to improve health. *BMJ,* Vol.321, pp. 694–96

Centre of Reference for the Endemic disease Control. (2009) Presentation of the ESEVIGUE study in the MINSABS. Date of access, 1/4/2010. Available from: http://www.crceguinea.org/index.php?option=com_content&task=view&id=118 &Itemid=86

Conde, F. (1997). HIV/Aids future scenarios: from the disease «event» to the diffuse chronicity. From the moral stigma to the central areas of social vulnerability. *Public health magazine,* Vol.71, No.1, pp.1-7

Creese, A.; Floyd, K.; Alban, A.; & Guinness, L. (2002). Cost-effectiveness of HIV/Aids interventions in Africa: a systematic review of the evidence. *Lancet,* Vol.359, pp. 1635–42

Dodd, P.; Garnett, G. & Hallett, T. (2010). Examining the promise of HIV elimination by 'test and treat' in hyper-endemic settings. *AIDS,* Vol.24, pp. 729–35

Frame & Carlson. (1975). A critical review of periodic health screening using specific screening criteria. Part 4: selected miscellaneous diseases. *J Fam Pract.* Vol.2, No.4, pp.283-9

Granich, M.; Gilks, F.; Dye, C.; De Cock, M. & Williams, G. (2009). Universal voluntary HIV testing with immediate antiretroviral therapy as a strategy for elimination of HIV transmission: a mathematical model. *Lancet, Vol.* 373, pp. 48–57

Grulich & Kaldor. (2002). Evidence of success in HIV prevention in Africa. *The Lancet,* Vol. 360, pp.41-6

Quinn, C.; Wawer, J.; Sewankambo, N.; Serwadda, D.; Li, C.; Wabwire, F. & Meehan, M. (2000). Viral load and heterosexual transmission of human immunodeficiency virus type 1. *N Engl J Med,* Vol. 342, pp.921–29

Idasa. (2004).HIV/Aids and Democratic Governance in South Africa http://www.aceproject.org/ace-es/focus/fo_aids/onePage Consulted: 23/3/2011

Medicus Mundi. (2007). *Women, Aids and access to health in Sub-saharan Africa: Approach from Social Sciences,* (Medicus Mundi Barcelona), B-9865-2007, Spain

Salinero, J., García-Inés, M., Sánchez, I., Sidro, I. (2006). *Survey on knowledge, attitudes and practices about nuptiality, sexual activity, HIV/Aids and STD among the sexually active population in Equatorial Guinea.* (MINSABS). Malabo, Guinea Ecuatorial

Paltiel, A.; Weinstein, M.; Kimmel, A.; Seage, G.; Losina, E. & Zhang, H. (2005). Expanded screening for HIV in the United States. An analysis of cost-effectiveness. *N Engl J Med.* Vol.352, pp.586-95

Piot, P.; Bartos, M. & Larson, H. (2008). Coming to terms with complexity: a call to action for HIV prevention. *Lancet,* Vol.372, pp.845-59

Skinner & Mfecane.(2004). Stigma, discrimination and the implications for people living with HIV/Aids in South Africa. *Sahara J,* Vol.1.N3, pp.157-64

Unaids. (2010 a). Report on the global Aids epidemia. Available in: http://www.unaids.org/documents/20101123_GlobalReport_em.pdf Consulted: 29/11/2010

Unaids. (2010 b). National report on progresses made in the performance of UNGAS. Available in: http://www.unaids.org/en/dataanalysis/monitoringcountryprogress/2010progressreportssubmittedbycountries/equatorialguinea_2010_country_progress_report_es.pdf Consulted: 29/11/2010

Unpd. (2011). Human Devolopment Report 2010. Avaible in: http://hdr.undp.org/en/reports/global/hdr2011/ Consulted: 4/2/2011

Unpd. (2002). HIV/Aids and strategies for poverty reduction. Diponible en: http://www.pnud.cl/areas/4.asp Consulted: 4/3/2011

UN. (2000). Millenium Goals Declaration. Resolution 58/291. General Assembly. Available in: http://www.un.org/es/comun/docs/?symbol=A/RES/55/2. Consulted 29/11/2010 Consulted: 8/3/2011

Unesco.(2003). A cultural approach to HIV/Aids prevention and attention. Collection of methodological manuals N° 1

Ortí, A. (1986). The opening and the qualitative or structural approach: The semi-managerial open interview and the discussion group, In: *The analysis of social reality: methods and techniques of social investigation,* M. García, J. Ibañez & F. Alvira (comps.), pp. 171-203, Madrid

Valles, M. (1997). Qualitative techniques of social investigation: methodological reflexion and professional practice. Síntesis, Madrid

Who.(2010). Towards universal access: scaling up priority HIV/Aids interventions in the health sector. Progress report 2010. Available in: http://www.who.int/hiv/pub/2010progressreport/report/en/index.html Consulted: 23/3/2011

Who. (2009). Prioritary HIV/Aids interventions, prevention, treatment and care in the health sector. Available in: http://www.aidslex.org/site_documents/HP-0062F.pdf Consulted: 15/3/2011

Who. (2008). Epidemiological Country Profile on HIV and Aids. Available in: http://www.unaids.org/es/resources/unaidspublications/2008/ Consulted:12/02/2011

Who. (2007). Mortality country fact sheet 2006. Available in: http://www.unaids.org/es/resources/unaidspublications/2007/ Consulted:15/3/2011

Who. (2000). Guidelines for Second Generation Surveillance of HIV Infection. Geneva: Who and Joint United Nations Programme on HIV/Aids Available in:

http://www.unaids.org/es/resources/unaidspublications/2000/ Consulted:14/2/2011
Who.(1998). Public health approach for STD control. Available in: http://www.who.int/hiv/pub/sti/en/stdcontrol_sp.pdf Consulted: 15/2/2011